Oral Health Handbook

Oral Health Handbook

Edited by Philip Chiders

hayle medical
New York

Hayle Medical,
750 Third Avenue, 9th Floor,
New York, NY 10017, USA

Visit us on the World Wide Web at:
www.haylemedical.com

ISBN: 978-1-63241-473-1

Printed in China.

Cataloging-in-Publication Data

Oral health handbook / edited by Philip Chiders.
p. cm.
Includes bibliographical references and index.
ISBN 978-1-63241-473-1
1. Mouth--Care and hygiene. 2. Oral medicine. 3. Dentistry.
I. Chiders, Philip.
RC815 .O73 2018
617.522--dc23

Table of Contents

Preface IX

Chapter 1 **Influence of obesity on the outcome of non-surgical periodontal therapy** 1
Fabienne A. Gerber, Philipp Sahrmann, Oliver A. Schmidlin, Christian Heumann, Jürg Hans Beer and Patrick R. Schmidlin

Chapter 2 **Oral health and coronary heart disease** 21
Marc J. Mathews, Edward H. Mathews and George E. Mathews

Chapter 3 **Inequalities in the frequency of free sugars intake among Syrian 1-year-old infants** 31
Easter Joury, May Khairallah, Wael Sabbah, Kanaan Elias and Raman Bedi

Chapter 4 **The impact of a formal complaint on Dutch dentists' professional practice** 38
Josef J. M. Bruers, Brigitte A. F. M. van Dam, Ronald C. Gorter and Michiel A. J. Eijkman

Chapter 5 **PDGFRβ^+/c-kit$^+$ pulp cells are odontoblastic progenitors capable of producing dentin-like structure in vitro and in vivo** 47
Shiwei Cai, Wenjian Zhang and Wei Chen

Chapter 6 **Association between maximum occlusal force and 3-year all-cause mortality in community-dwelling elderly people** 58
Toshimitsu Iinuma, Yasumichi Arai, Michiyo Takayama, Yukiko Abe, Tomoka Ito, Yugaku Kondo, Nobuyoshi Hirose and Nobuhito Gionhaku

Chapter 7 **Oral-health-related background factors and dental service utilisation among Sudanese children with and without a congenital heart defects** 66
H. M. Ali, M. Mustafa, E. F. Nasir, S. A. Lie, S. Hasabalrasol, O. H. Elshazali, R. W. Ali and M. S. Skeie

Chapter 8 **Effect of the plant-based hemostatic agent Ankaferd Blood Stopper® on the biocompatibility of mineral trioxide aggregate** 78
Muzaffer Emir Dinçol, Hakan Ozbas, Bulent Yılmaz, Handan Ersev, Selcuk Gokyay and Vakur Olgac

Chapter 9 **A comparison of the shaping ability of three nickel-titanium rotary instruments: A micro-computed tomography study via a contrast radiopaque technique in vitro** 87
Zhao Wei, Zhi Cui, Ping Yan and Han Jiang

Chapter 10 **Comparison of occlusal caries detection using the ICDAS criteria on extracted teeth or their photographs** 94
P. Bottenberg , W. Jacquet, C. Behrens, V. Stachniss and A. Jablonski-Momeni

Chapter 11 **Utilization of dental care among patients with severe mental illness: A study of a National Health Insurance database** 102
Po-Ren Teng, Miao-Jean Lin and Ling-Ling Yeh

Chapter 12 **Relationship between risk assessment and payment models in Swedish Public Dental Service** ... 109
Gunnel Hänsel Petersson and Svante Twetman

Chapter 13 **Human cathelicidin LL-37 enhance the antibiofilm effect of EGCG on *Streptococcus mutans*** ... 115
Yi-jie Guo, Bo Zhang, Xue-song Feng, Hui-xun Ren and Ji-ru Xu

Chapter 14 **Current stress and poor oral health** ... 123
A. Vasiliou, K. Shankardass, R. Nisenbaum and C. Quiñonez

Chapter 15 **Dental anxiety in patients with borderline intellectual functioning and patients with intellectual disabilities** ... 131
Antonio Fallea, Rosa Zuccarello and Francesco Calì

Chapter 16 **Utilising daily diaries to examine oral health experiences associated with dentine hypersensitivity** ... 137
Jenny M. Porritt, Farzana Sufi and Sarah R. Baker

Chapter 17 **Patterns of use of oral health care services and barriers to dental care among ambulatory older Chilean** ... 148
Rodrigo Mariño and Rodrigo A. Giacaman

Chapter 18 **Reliability and diagnostic validity of a joint vibration analysis device** ... 155
Sonia Sharma, Heidi C. Crow, Krishnan Kartha, W. D. McCall Jr. and Yoly M. Gonzalez

Chapter 19 **Waist circumference and waist-to-height ratio are associated with periodontal pocketing—results of the Health 2000 Survey** ... 162
Sanna Kangas, Petra Timonen, Matti Knuuttila, Antti Jula, Pekka Ylöstalo and Anna-Maija Hannele Syrjälä

Chapter 20 **Less extrusion debris during the retreatment of curved canals using twisted files with higher rotational speeds: An *ex vivo* study** ... 169
Mengdong Liu, Shijiang Xiong, Fei Tan and Yi Liu

Chapter 21 **Temporal relationship between dysthymia and temporomandibular disorder: A population-based matched case-control study in Taiwan** ... 175
Shang-Lun Lin, Shang-Liang Wu, Shun-Yao Ko, Ching-Yu Yen, Wei-Fan Chiang and Jung-Wu Yang

Chapter 22 **The influence of adding modified zirconium oxide-titanium dioxide nano-particles on mechanical properties of orthodontic adhesive: An in vitro study** ... 181
Nayef H. Felemban and Mohamed I. Ebrahim

Chapter 23 **Response of human dental pulp cells to a silver-containing PLGA/TCP-nanofabric as a potential antibacterial regenerative pulp-capping material** ... 189
Barbara Cvikl, Samuel C. Hess, Richard J. Miron, Hermann Agis, Dieter Bosshardt, Thomas Attin, Patrick R. Schmidlin and Adrian Lussi

Chapter 24 **Prevalence of *Candida albicans* and non-*albicans* on the tongue dorsa of elderly people living in a post-disaster area** ... 199
Toshiro Sato, Mitsuo Kishi, Miki Suda, Kiyomi Sakata, Haruki Shimoda, Hiroyuki Miura and Akira Ogawaand Seiichiro Kobayashi

Chapter 25 **Effects of various debonding and adhesive clearance methods on enamel surface: An in vitro study** 209
Xiao-Chuan Fan, Li Chen and Xiao-Feng Huang

Chapter 26 **Assessing the progression of chronic periodontitis using subgingival pathogen levels: A 24-month prospective multicentre cohort study** 219
E. Kakuta, Y. Nomura, T. Morozumi, T. Nakagawa, T. Nakamura, K. Noguchi, A. Yoshimura, Y. Hara, O. Fujise, F. Nishimura, T. Kono, M. Umeda, M. Fukuda, T. Noguchi, N. Yoshinari, C. Fukaya, S. Sekino, Y. Numabe, N. Sugano, K. Ito, H. Kobayashi, Y. Izumi, H. Takai, Y. Ogata, S. Takano, M. Minabe, A. Makino-Oi, A. Saito, Y. Abe, S. Sato, F. Suzuki, K. Takahashi, T. Sugaya, M. Kawanami, N. Hanada, S. Takashiba and H. Yoshie

Chapter 27 **Prevalence of oral manifestations in children and adolescents with cancer submitted to chemotherapy** 227
Deise Berger Velten, Eliana Zandonade and Maria Helena Monteiro de Barros Miotto

Permissions

List of Contributors

Index

Preface

Oral health deals with the prevention, diagnosis, treatment and study of the diseases affecting the oral cavity, oral mucosa, maxillofacial area and the temperomandibular structure. Oral health is a vast area of study that includes sub-branches like geriatric dentistry, endodontics, oral medicine, periodontology, orthodontics, etc. This book is a valuable compilation of topics, ranging from the basic to the most complex advancements in the field of dentistry. From theories to research to practical applications, case studies related to all contemporary topics of relevance to this field have been included in the book. It presents this complex subject in the most comprehensible and easy to understand language. For all those who are interested in oral health, the text can prove to be an essential guide.

The information contained in this book is the result of intensive hard work done by researchers in this field. All due efforts have been made to make this book serve as a complete guiding source for students and researchers. The topics in this book have been comprehensively explained to help readers understand the growing trends in the field.

I would like to thank the entire group of writers who made sincere efforts in this book and my family who supported me in my efforts of working on this book. I take this opportunity to thank all those who have been a guiding force throughout my life.

Editor

1

Influence of obesity on the outcome of non-surgical periodontal therapy

Fabienne A. Gerber[1], Philipp Sahrmann[1], Oliver A. Schmidlin[2], Christian Heumann[3], Jürg Hans Beer[2] and Patrick R. Schmidlin[1*]

Abstract

Background: Obesity and periodontitis are important chronic health problems. Obesity is associated with an increased prevalence of periodontitis. Whether obesity also affects the outcome of non-surgical periodontal therapy is to date still unclear.

Methods: A systematic review of studies referenced in SCOPUS, MEDLINE, PubMed, Cochrane, CINAHL, Biosis and Web of Science was performed. Titles, abstracts and finally full texts were scrutinized for possible inclusion by two independent investigators. Quality and heterogeneity of the studies were assessed and the study designs were examined. Probing pocket depth reduction was analyzed as primary surrogate parameter for therapeutic success after non-surgical periodontal therapy.

Results: One-hundred-and-fifty-nine potentially qualifying studies were screened. Eight studies fulfilled the inclusion criteria and were analyzed. Three of eight studies failed to show an influence of obesity on pocket depth reduction after non-surgical therapy. The remaining five studies documented a clear negative effect on the outcome of non-surgical periodontal therapy. The finally included studies did not correspond to the highest level of quality (RCTs). Due to the heterogeneity of the data a meta-analysis was not possible.

Conclusion: The literature on the effect of obesity on the treatment outcome of non-surgical periodontal therapy remains controversial. The data, however, support that obesity is not only a factor associated with poorer periodontal health but might also result in inferior response to non-surgical treatment of periodontitis.

Keywords: Obesity, Chronic periodontitis, Non-surgical periodontal therapy, Outcome

Background

The prevalence of obesity is increasing worldwide and is becoming one of the most important health hazards [1], as obesity is highly associated with increased overall morbidity and mortality [2].

Obesity is defined with a body mass index (BMI; body weight in kilogram divided by the square of the height in meters (kg/m^2)) of at least 30.0 kg/m^2 [3], whereas overweight is defined with a BMI of 25–29.9 kg/m^2. Normal weight is characterized by a BMI ranging between 19 to 24.9 kg/m^2 [4]. In this context, BMI seems a valuable parameter to predict obesity-related disease risks in a wide range of populations [2]. There are, however, some limitations: Firstly, risk assessment by BMI is less applicable in persons over 65 years of age because they generally have a higher body fat content for the same BMI. Secondly, the abdominal (central, visceral, android) type of obesity, which is more often seen in men, is associated with higher morbidity than the rather female type of gluteofemoral (peripheral, gynoid) obesity and, thirdly, the BMI cut-off points for overweight and obesity are too high for Asian people [2]. In addition, current large studies have indicated that measurement of waist circumference (WC) or waist-to-hip-ratio (WHR) may be a better disease risk predictor than BMI [5, 6]. There is,

* Correspondence: patrick.schmidlin@zzm.uzh.ch
[1]Clinic of Preventive Dentistry, Periodontology and Cariology, Center of Dental Medicine, University of Zurich, Plattenstrasse 11, CH-8032 Zurich, Switzerland
Full list of author information is available at the end of the article

however, currently intensive research and debate as to whether BMI, WC, WHR, or all of them should be used to assess disease risk [2].

For the purpose of this systematic review, however, only BMI is the most frequently reported data of obesity in a large number of studies.

Adipose tissue contains usually 5-10 % macrophages, but the adipose tissue of obese patients shows up to 60 % macrophage infiltration [4]. Adipocytes secrete bioactive molecules called adipokines, that can modify or trigger inflammation and fat metabolism locally or systemically as signaling molecules to liver, muscle and endothelium [4]. Therefore, the adipose tissue can be considered as an important metabolically active endocrine organ [4].

This explains how obesity acts as a risk factor for several chronic diseases: Hypertension, type 2 diabetes, dyslipidemia, and coronary heart disease are so closely related to obesity that obesity itself is often considered to be a systemic disease. This disease also affects dental health [7]. Accordingly obese persons require attention of physicians and dentists [2].

Among dental pathologies, periodontitis is a very common, primarily bacterial inflammatory disease, which destroys teeth surrounding soft tissues and bone. It leads to pocket formation and ultimately to loss of teeth if no effective treatment is applied [8]. Periodontitis is no longer considered only an oral health issue but also a public health problem, as it constitutes a risk factor for cardiovascular conditions, poor glycemic control in diabetics and adverse outcome of pregnancy [4, 8]. These correlations coincide with obesity and general health.

Recently, it has been suggested that obesity is a possible risk factor for periodontitis [8]. One study identified obesity even as the second strongest risk factor for periodontitis preceded only by smoking [9]. The first report on the relationship between obesity and periodontal disease appeared in 1977. Perlstein and co-workers [10] found greater alveolar bone resorption in obese than in non-obese rats. Under healthy oral conditions, obesity itself did not promote periodontal damage, but in the presence of bacterial plaque accumulation periodontal inflammation was more severe in obese than in non-obese animals. With concomitant arterial hypertension, plaque accumulation caused even more pronounced periodontal destruction than with obesity alone. These results suggest that a combination of risk factors, such as the one defined by the metabolic syndrome, elicit a more severe periodontal effect [10, 11]. Chaffee et al. [12] found in their meta-analysis an increased prevalence odds ratio for obesity among subjects with periodontal disease of approximately one-third, a greater mean clinical attachment loss (CAL) among obese individuals, a higher BMI among subjects with periodontal disease, and a trend for linear increase in the odds of periodontal disease with increasing BMI [4, 12]. Finally the association reported between obesity and periodontitis was less strong than that reported between periodontal disease and adverse pregnancy outcomes [12, 13] or cardiovascular events [12, 14]. There seems, however, to be a stronger obesity-periodontitis association in women, non-smokers and younger individuals than in the general adult populations [12]. In addition, smoking remains another well-studied predisposing factor for periodontitis [12, 15, 16]. Thus, BMI and smoking share a complex relationship [17]. This relationship can be inverse in certain populations [12, 18, 19].

The biological mechanism by which obesity predisposes to periodontitis is not fully understood [8]. Compared to individuals with normal weight individuals with obesity have higher levels of circulating tumor necrosis factor-α (TNF-α) and interleukin-6 (IL-6), which are also secreted from adipose tissue and are involved in the pathophysiology of both obesity and periodontitis. Not surprisingly, serum levels of these cytokines decrease with loss of weight [20].

The objective of this systematic review was to study the hypothesis whether the clinical outcome, in terms of pocket depth reduction, after non-surgical periodontal therapy in non-obese is better than in obese individuals. To verify this hypothesis, we systematically reviewed all retrievable, qualitatively adequate clinical investigations, which focused on this topic.

Methods

The review was conducted according to the PRISMA criteria [21]. The research question was explored using the *PICO* method [22]. The focused question addressed was:

Does non-surgical periodontal therapy (I) have a different outcome in obese chronic periodontitis patients (P), than in non-obese chronic periodontitis patients (C), regarding periodontal pocket depth reduction as the main clinical periodontal parameter (O).

Search strategy and review process

An electronic search of SCOPUS, MEDLINE, PubMed, Cochrane, CINAHL, Biosis and Web of Science was carried out considering articles published up to January 2016 in English or German language. The search was performed in two steps. The first electronic search started at 20.11.14 and an update has been done at 5.1.16.

This is shown in Table 1. For the database search, a combination of subject headings (MeSH terms and CINAHL headings) and free text search was used. An example of a detailed strategy (Medline/OvidSP) is shown in Table 2.

The same search protocol was applied to all databases.

Table 1 Search protocols with the respective number of references dated from November 11 2014 (1) and January 1 2016 (2)

	References 1 & 2	References after deduplication 1 & 2
Scopus	40 + 14	9 + 5
Medline	42 + 8	39 + 7
PubMed	6 + 11	2 + 11
Cochrane	12 + 2	2 + 1
CINAHL	48 + 15	42 + 13
Biosis	25 + 7	10 + 1
Web of Science	38 + 13	16 + 1
Pool	211 + 70	120 + 39

After deduplication 159 references

Two of the authors (FAG, PRS) screened the titles for potential eligibility according to the inclusion criteria. Based on the abstract screening, 18 studies were selected for full text review. Scores were independently allocated by both authors to each publication according to their suitability for the present review (see inclusion criteria). Any discrepancies were resolved by consensus.

Table 2 Medline search strategy

Step	Query	Hits
1	Exp Periodontitis/AND (adult OR chronic*).ti,ab.	5703
2	Chronic periodontitis/OR periodontal pocket/	7004
3	2 OR 3	10454
4	((adult OR chronic*) adj3 periodontiti*).ti,ab.	5352
5	(attachment adj3 loss).ti,ab. AND ((clinical OR periodontal) adj3 attachment).ti,ab.	1305
6	(periodontal adj3 pocket).ti,ab.	1066
7	OR/3-7	12910
8	Dental scaling/ OR "root planing"/	3479
9	((subgingival OR root OR supragingival) adj3 (scaling* OR planing*)).ti,ab.	2288
10	(deep adj3 (scaling* OR cleaning)).ti,ab.	62
11	((conventional OR inital OR "non surgical" OR non-surgical OR nonsurgical) adj3 (treatment OR therapy)).ti,ab.	33417
12	OR/8-11	37131
13	7 AND 12	2184
14	Exp Obesity/	154540
15	Exp Body Weight/	369850
16	(overweight OR obese OR obesity OR adiposit* OR BMI OR "body mass index").ti,ab.	300847
17	(cardiolipin OR lipid* OR leptin).ti,ab.	395517
18	"waist to hip".ti,ab.	9048
19	(body adj3 weight).ti,ab.	163760
20	OR/14-19	954233
21	13 AND 20	42

The asterisk represents a wildcard and can be used in all search fields that allow words and phrases

Inclusion criteria

To be included studies had to be clinical interventional studies regarding the outcome of non-surgical periodontal therapy in obese or non-obese patients. The studies had to display the diagnosis of chronic periodontitis. Key parameters to be reported were data for pocket probing depth (PPD) and BMI.

Exclusion criteria

Studies were excluded for the following reasons: animal studies, case reports, commentaries, unsuitable exposure or outcome measures, confounding medical diagnoses (e.g. pregnancy or any systemic disease, such as diabetes, in addition to metabolic syndrome), confounding *systemic* medical treatments such as immunosuppressive treatments, cortisone or antibiotic treatment as well as confounding *local* treatments such as treatment of peri-mucositis, gingival overgrowth or surgical periodontal treatment. Studies including either the diagnosis of aggressive periodontitis or of peri-implantitis were excluded as well.

Outcome measures

The primary outcome measure is PPD after non-surgical periodontal treatment.

Data extraction

A list with exclusion reasons for each paper was generated. Total number of patients, demographic data, origin of study, outcome measurements 2, 3, 6 and 12 months after therapy and the impact of obesity on the treatment-outcome were extracted. In addition, the exact definition of chronic periodontitis, the assessment of the periodontal disease and the number of smokers included in the studies were summarized. Data on the individual definition of obesity and the systemic examinations were also collected. Non-surgical periodontal treatment measures, treatment time, periodontal maintenance and adverse events were also recorded for each study separately (Tables 3, 4, 5, 6 and 7).

The quality of the included studies was assessed through the Newcastle-Ottawa Quality Assessment Scale (Table 8).

Results

Selection of studies

Initially, 159 studies were identified by electronic search by the two reviewers (FAG, PRS). Full text analysis of the 18 potentially qualified reports led to exclusion of 10 other studies. Additional five titles [23–27] were identified by hand search but after full text analysis, all these articles had to be excluded based on the inclusion and exclusion

Table 3 Excluded studies

Excluded studies	Reason for exclusion
Europerio 4 2003 [37]	Not addressing research question
Abstracts for the Royal Australian and New Zealand College of Psychiatrists 2005 [38]	Not addressing research question
5th Joint Meeting of the European Tissue Repair Society and the Wound Healing Society 2009 [39]	Not addressing research question
Recently published abstracts [40]	Not addressing research question
DENTSPLY Posters 2012 [41]	Not addressing research question
HealthBeat 2007 [42]	Not addressing research question
Abstracts for Poster Presentations 2011 [43]	Not addressing research question
Abstracts for the International Symposium on Dental Hygiene 2013 [44]	Not addressing research question
Abou Sulaiman et al. 2010 [45]	Not addressing research question
Acharya et al. 2010 [46]	No PPD reduction data
Akpinar et al. 2013 [47]	Not addressing research question
Altay et al. 2013 [20]	No PPD reduction data
Armstrong et al. 2010 [48]	Not addressing research question
Arora et al. 2013 [49]	Not addressing research question
Basegmez et al. 2011 [50]	Not addressing research question
Bresolin et al. 2013 [51]	Not addressing research question
Bresolin et al. 2014 [52]	Not addressing research question
Caspersen et al. 2012 [53]	Not addressing research question
Caula et al. 2014 [54]	No comparison
Caula et al. 2014 [54]	Duplicate
Chapple et a. 2006 [55]	Not addressing research question
Chapple et al. 2007 [56]	Not addressing research question
Chandni et al. 2015 [57]	Not addressing research question
Chaston et al. 2014 [58]	Not addressing research question
Chee et al. 2008 [59]	Inclusion of diabetes
Chee et al. 2013 [60]	Missed intervention, inclusion of diabetes
Chen et al. 2012 [61]	Inclusion of diabetes
D'Aiuto et al. 2004 [62]	Not addressing research question

Table 3 Excluded studies *(Continued)*

D'Aiuto et al. 2004 [63]	Not addressing research question
D'Aiuto et al. 2005 [23]	No comparison
D'Aiuto et al. 2006 [64]	Not addressing research question
Deppe et al. 2010 [65]	Not addressing research question
Dodington et al. 2015 [66]	No obesity data
Draper et al. 2010 [67]	Not addressing research question
Duan et al. 2009 [24]	Written in Chinese
Edwards et al. 2006 [68]	Not addressing research question
Efurd et al. 2012 [69]	Not addressing research question
Elliott-Smith et al. 2011 [70]	Not addressing research question
Engebretson et al. 2014 [71]	Not addressing research question
Fairfield et al. 2010 [72]	Not addressing research question
Fang et al. 2015 [73]	Inclusion of end-stage renal disease patients
Fentoglu et al. 2010 [74]	Statin intake
Fine et al. 2007 [75]	Not addressing research question
Fokkema et al. 2012 [76]	Not addressing research question
Fu et al. 2015 [77]	No comparison
Garcia et al. 2010 [78]	Not addressing research question
Giblin et al. 2014 [79]	Inclusion of prediabetes
Giblin et al. 2014 [79]	Duplicate
Gluch et al. 2007 [80]	Inclusion of diabetes
Goldie et al. 2002 [81]	Not addressing research question
Goldie et al. 2004 [82]	Not addressing research question
Goldie et al. 2005 [83]	Not addressing research question
Griffin et al. 2012 [84]	Not addressing research question
Gurenlian et al. 2006 [85]	Not addressing research question
Gurenlian et al. 2009 [86]	Not addressing research question
Hammaker et al. 2010 [87]	Not addressing research question
Horwitz et al. 2007 [88]	Not addressing research question
Hovliaras-Delozier et al. 2008 [89]	Not addressing research question
Ide et al. 2004 [90]	No obesity data

Table 3 Excluded studies *(Continued)*

Ide et al. 2007 [91]	Not addressing research question
Iwamoto et al. 2003 [25]	Application of antibiotics
Jahn et al. 2004 [92]	Not addressing research question
Jahn et al. 2015 [93]	Not addressing research question
Jaiswal et al. 2015 [94]	No treatment (SRP)
Janket et al. 2014 [95]	Meta-analysis
Janket et al. 2014 [95]	Duplicate
Jared et al. 2008 [96]	Not addressing research question
Jared et al. 2008 [96]	Duplicate
Jiang et al. 2013 [97]	Not addressing research question
Kamil et al. 2011 [98]	No obesity data
Kamilov et al. 1998 [99]	Not addressing research question
Kapellas et al. 2013 [100]	No obesity data
Kardeşler et al. 2010 [26]	Inclusion of diabetes
Keller et al. 2015 [101]	Systematic review
Kiany et al. 2014 [102]	No obesity data
Kiany et al. 2015 [103]	Duplicate
Kipp et al. 2003 [104]	Not addressing research question
Kudva et al. 2010 [105]	Inclusion of diabetes
Kumar et al. 2015 [106]	Inclusion of diabetes
Kurti et al. 2007 [107]	Not addressing research question
Kurtis et al. 2007 [108]	Duplicate
Lee et al. 2014 [109]	Not addressing research question
Li et al. 2013 [110]	No obesity data
Ling et al. 2012 [111]	Inclusion of diabetes
Lo et al. 2011 [112]	Not addressing research question
Malhotra et al. 2012 [113]	No obesity data
Mancl et al. 2013 [114]	Not addressing research question
Martinez et al. 2014 [115]	Supplementation of ω-3 eicosapetaenoic acid
Martinez et al. 2014 [116]	One year of omega-3 supplementation
Matlock et al. 2012 [117]	No treatment (SRP)
McDaniel et al. 2013 [118]	Not addressing research question
Meharwade et al. 2014 [119]	Local drug delivery
Merchant et al. 2014 [120]	Inclusion of diabetes
Michalowicz et al. 2014 [121]	Inclusion of diabetes

Table 3 Excluded studies *(Continued)*

Mizrak et al. 2006 [122]	Not addressing research question
Moeintaghavi et al. 2012 [123]	Inclusion of diabetes
Moravec et al. 2011 [124]	No treatment (SRP)
Muthu et al. 2015 [125]	No obesity data
Nassar et al. 2012 [126]	Inclusion of diabetes
Newton et al. 2011 [127]	Not addressing research question
Nichols et al. 2001 [128]	Not addressing research question
Nielsen et al. 2000 [129]	Not addressing research question
Novakovic et al. 2013 [130]	Not addressing research question
Novakovic et al. 2014 [131]	Not addressing research question
Oliveira et al. 2011 [132]	Not addressing research question
Olsen et al. 2006 [133]	Not addressing research question
Paquette et al. 2008 [134]	Not addressing research question
Perayil et al. 2014 [135]	No obesity data
Perayil et al. 2014 [136]	Duplicate
Phillips et al. 2013 [137]	Not addressing research question
Pradeep et al. 2007 [138]	Not addressing research question
Price et al. 2010 [139]	Not addressing research question
Qiqiang et al. 2012 [140]	No obesity data
Radafshar et al. 2012 [141]	Not addressing research question
Radnai et al. 2009 [142]	Not addressing research question
Raghavendra et al. 2012 [143]	Not addressing research question
Ramirez et al. 2011 [144]	No obesity data
Rasch et al. 1995 [145]	Not addressing research question
Sadatmansouri et al. 2006 [146]	Not addressing research question
Saffi et al. 2013 [147]	Inclusion of patients with coronary disease
Saffi et al. 2013 [147]	Duplicate
Saffi et al. 2014 [148]	Inclusion of patients with coronary artery disease
Shruti et al. 2010 [27]	No obesity data
Sembene et al. 2000 [149]	Not addressing research question
Sengupta et al. 1990 [150]	Not addressing research question

Table 3 Excluded studies *(Continued)*

Sgolastra et al. 2013 [36]	Meta-Analysis
Shimada et al. 2010 [151]	No comparison
Shimoe et al. 2011 [152]	Case report
Singh et al. 2014 [153]	Not addressing research question
Siqueira et al. 2013 [154]	Not addressing research question
Stewart et al. 2001 [155]	Inclusion of diabetes
Talbert et al. 2006 [156]	Inclusion of diabetes
Tamaki et al. 2009 [157]	No obesity data
Tamaki et al. 2011 [158]	No obesity data
Tawfig et al. 2015 [159]	No comparison
Teles et al. 2012 [160]	No comparison
Toker et al. 2012 [161]	Not addressing research question
Tuter et al. 2007 [162]	Inclusion of patients with systemic disease
Vardar et al. 2003 [163]	Not addressing research question
Van Dyke et al. 2015 [164]	Not addressing research question
Vyas et al. 2000 [165]	Not addressing research question
Wahid et al. 2013 [166]	Not addressing research question
Wang et al. 2013 [167]	Inclusion of aggressive periodontitis
Wehmeyer et al. 2013 [168]	Not addressing research question
Wei et al. 2010 [169]	No obesity data
Williams et al. 2007 [148]	No obesity data
Williams et al. 2009 [170]	Not addressing research question
Williams et al. 2009 (171]	Not addressing research question
Wood et al. 2006 [172)	Not addressing research question
Wu et al. 2015 [173)	Not addressing research question
Zare et al. 2014 [174)	Not addressing research question
Zhou et al. 2013 [175]	Inclusion of patients with systemic disease
Zuza et al. 2011 [176)	No PPD reduction data

criteria (Table 3). Therefore, eight publications [8, 28–34] from the electronic and hand search fulfilled the criteria. However, it was not possible to compare the raw data so that we had to reduce our analysis to a qualitative analysis. This process is summarized in a flow-chart (Fig. 1).

Summary of studies: characteristics (PICO)

Total number of patients, demographic data, origin of study, outcome measurements 2, 3, 6 and 12 months after therapy and the impact of obesity on the treatment-outcome are summarized in Table 4.

Definition of chronic periodontitis, periodontal assessment and the amount of smokers included are depicted in Table 5.

The definition of obesity and systemic examination were summarized in Table 6. Non-surgical periodontal treatment, treatment time, periodontal maintenance and limitations are shown in Table 7.

Population

Of the eight finally analyzed studies, clinical trials comprised 516 participants. One study [8] enrolled only women. The prevalence of smoking among male patients affected with periodontitis was so high that Al-Zahrani and co-workers [8] were unable to correct for smoking in the male population. Accordingly, only women were included in their study. Overall the studies comprised between 26 up to 260 subjects (Table 4).

The inclusion criteria "age" was defined in all but one study [30]. Three investigations [28, 33, 34] defined the age ≥18 years. The other studies defined a minimum age of 30 years [31, 32] or 35 years [8]. Duzagac et al. defined an age range from 25 to 55 years (Table 4).

Suvan et al. [34] included smokers into their study. Lakkis et al. [33] and Eldin et al.(30] did not mention the smoking status of the patients. All other studies [8, 28, 29, 31, 32] excluded smokers (Table 5).

Patients with diabetes, another important modifier of periodontal health or disease [35] were excluded in seven studies [8, 28–32, 34]. Lakkis et al. [33] did not report the presence or absence of diabetes.

Intervention/Comparison

Each paper described the periodontal intervention as a non–surgical therapy. All studies [8, 28–34] applied scaling and root planing. Ultrasonic instruments and/or hand instruments were used in all studies (Table 7).

Two papers (8,34] reassessed the PPD 2 months after therapy. Two studies [29, 30] reassessed their patients after 3 months. Another two papers [28, 31] re-evaluated the patients after 3 and 6 months and one study [32] reassessed the PPD three, six and 12 months after therapy. Only Lakkis et al. [33] measured the periodontal pocket depths already 4 to 6 weeks after non-surgical therapy (Table 3). Oral hygiene was instructed additionally to the non–surgical periodontal therapy in all studies (Table 7).

Due to the heterogeneity of the study designs with respect to outcome measures and treatment protocol, as well as variation in study population, sample size, and/or

Table 4 Probing pocket depth (PPD [mm]) as primary outcome variable

Author & year	Total number of patients Age (mean ± SD) Country	Outcome after 2 months mean (± SD) at baseline – mean (± SD) at reassessment	Outcome after 3 months mean (± SD) at baseline – mean (± SD) at reassessment	Outcome after 6 months mean (± SD)at baseline – mean (± SD) at reassessment	Outcome after 12 months mean (± SD)at baseline – mean (± SD) at reassessment	Impact of obesity on the treatment - outcome mean – reduction of PPD (± SD)	
Al – Zahrani et al. 2012 [8]	Total number of patients: 40 (only women) Normal-weight: 20 Obese: 20 Age: Normal-weight: 43.4 (±7.8) Obese: 44 (±8.4) Country: Saudi Arabia	Total sample: 2.65 (±0.47) – 2.44 (±0.41) *p*-value = 0.001	n.r.	n.r.	n.r.	Normal-weight: 0.19 (±0.27) Obese: 0.23 (±0.33) *p*-value = 0.663 (n. sig.)	
Bouaziz et al. 2015 [28]	Total number of patients: 36 Normal-weight: 18 Obese: 18 Age: Range from 22 to 78 Normal-weight: 51.00 (±13.1) Obese: 51.3 (±16.7) p-value: n. sig. Country: France	n.r.	Normal-weight: 3.33 (±0.92) – 2.71 (±0.40) *p*-value: n. sig. Obese: 3.22 (±0.76) – 2.78 (±0.55) *p*-value: n. sig.	Normal-weight: 3.33 (±0.92) 2.45 (±0.53) *p*-value < 0.05 Obese: 3.22 (±0.76) – 2.43 (±0.49) *p*-value < 0.05	n.r.	Summary of Multivariable Analysis Results (Coefficient, 95 % CI): ▵ %PD > 5mm after 3 months to obese (Model 2): *p*-value = 0.02 ▵ %PD > 5mm after 6 months to obese (Model 2): *p*-value = 0.005 Nb ▵PD > 2mm after 3 months to Obese (Model 2); *p*-value = 0.02 Nb ▵PD > 2mm after 6 months to Obese (Model 2); *p*-value = 0.06 (n.sig.)	
Duzagac et al. 2015 [29]	Total number of patients: 45 Normal weight patients with periodontitis (CPNW): 15 Obese patients with periodontitis (CPO): 15 Normal weight periodontally healthy control subjects (PHNW): 15 Age: Range from 28 to 52 CPNW: 41.06 (±7.10) CPO: 40.66 (±7.98) PHNW: 39.66 (±6.53) *p*-value: n. sig. Country: Turkey	n.r.	CPNW: 3.19 (±0.38) – 2.51 – (±0.06) *p*-value = 0.001 CPO: 4.10 (±0.50) – 2.55 (±0.45) *p*-value = 0.001	n.r.	n.r.	Number of sites with PD < 4 mm: Baseline: CPO: 1706 CPNW: 1766 3 months: CPO: 2214 CPNW: 2206 % of sites with PD < 4 mm: Baseline: CPO: 75.4 CPNW: 77.9 3 months: CPO: 97.9 CPNW: 97.3 Similar clinical healing; (n. sig.)	Number of sites with PD ≥ 4 mm: Baseline: CPO: 556 CPNW: 502 3 months: CPO: 48 CPNW: 32 % of sites with PD ≥ 4 mm: Baseline: CPO: 48 CPNW: 22.1 3 months: CPO: 2.1 CPNW: 2.7 Similar clinical healing; (n. sig.)

Table 4 Probing pocket depth (PPD [mm]) as primary outcome variable *(Continued)*

Eldin et al. 2013 [30]	Total number of patients: 26 Overweight: 12 Obese: 14 Age: Range from 35 to 48 Country: Egypt	n.r.	Overweight: 0.6 (±1.29) – 0.75 (±2.12) *p*-value: n.r. Obese: 3.15 (±2.43) – 1.59 (±2.34) *p*-value: n.r.	n.r.	n.r.	Overweight: 0.784 Obese: 0.209 *p*-value = 0.326 (n. sig.)		
Gonçalves et al. 2015 [31]	Total number of patients: 39 Without obesity: 21 With obesity: 18 Age: Without obesity: 48.4(±9.5) With obesity: 48.8 (±5.9) p-value= 0.85 (n. sig.) Country: Brazil	n.r.	Without obesity: 3.4 (±0.6) – 3.0 (±0.5) *p*-value: sig. With obesity: 3.6 (±0.6) – 3.3 (±0.6) *p*-value: sig.	Without obesity: 3.4 (±0.6)- 2.7 (±0.6) *p*-value: sig. With obesity: 3.6 (±0.6) – 3.0 (±0.5) *p*-value: sig.	n.r.	Without obesity Full-mouth sites: 0-3 months: 0.44 (±0.06) 0-6 months: 0.73 (±0.07) Initially moderate sites (PD 4-6mm): 0-3 months: 0.87 (±0.12) 0-6 months: 1.38 (±0.14) Initially deep sites (PD ≥ 7mm): 0-3 months: 1.86 (±0.25) 0-6 months: 3.00 (±0.23)	With obesity Full-mouth sites: 0-3 months: 0.30 (±0.06) 0-6 months: 0.54 (±0.07) Initially moderate sites (PD 4-6mm): 0-3 months: 0.70 (±0.13) 0-6 months: 1.10 (±0.15) Initially deep sites (PD ≥ 7mm): 0-3 months: 1.22 (±0.26) 0-6 months: 2.30 (±0.24)	*p*-value (<0.05) 0.08 0.04 0.31 0.16 0.07 0.04
Gonçalves et al. 2015 [32]	Total number of patients: 40 Non-obese: 20 Obese: 20 Age: Non-obese: 48.5 (±9.3) Obese: 50.0 (±4.5) p-value = 0.52 (n. sig.) Country: Brazil	n.r.	Non-obese: 3.4 (±0.6) – 2.9 (±0.6) *p*-value: sig. Obese: 3.6 (±0.6) – 3.3 (±0.5) *p*-value: sig.	Non-obese: 3.4 (±0.6) – 2.7 (±0.6) *p*-value: sig. Obese: 3.6 (±0.6) – 3.0 (±0.5) *p*-value: sig.	Non-obese: 3.4 (±0.6) – 2.6 (±0.6) *p*-value: sig. Obese: 3.6 (±0.6) – 2.9 (±0.4) *p*-value: sig.	Mean PPD values (± SD): After 3 months: Non-obese: 2.9 (±0.6) Obese: 3.3 (±0.5) *p* = 0.25 (n. sig.) After 6 months: Non-obese: 2.7 (±0.6) Obese: 3.0 (±0.5) *p* = 0.04 After 12 months: Non-obese: 2.6 (±0.6) Obese: 2.9 (±0.4) *p* = 0.03		

Table 4 Probing pocket depth (PPD [mm]) as primary outcome variable *(Continued)*

Lakkis et al. 2011 [33]	Total number of patients: 30 Surgery: 15 Control: 15 Age: Surgery: 45.6 (±11.1) Control: 48.5 (±12.0) p-value = 0.778 (n. sig.) Country: USA (Cleveland, Ohio)	4-6 weeks after therapy! Surgery: 2.6 (±0.6) – 2.2 (±0.5) *p*-value < 0.001 Control: 3.1 (±0.8) – 2.8 (±0.7) *p*-value < 0.001	n.r.	n.r.	n.r.	Surgery: 0.45 Control: 0.28 *p*-value = 0.007
Suvan et al. 2014 [34]	Total number of patients: 260 Normal: 112 Overweight: 93 Obese: 55 Age: Normal: 46.30 (±8.38) Overweight: 47.27 (±8.93) Obese: 46.55 (±6.87) *p*-value = 0.701 (n. sig.) Country: Great Britain (London)	Summary of univariable GEE Analysis Results (Coefficient, 95 % CI): BMI [kg/m^2] to PPD at 2 months *p*-value = 0.055 Overweight to PPD at 2 months *p*-value = 0.372 (n. sig.) Obese to PPD at 2 months *p*-value = 0.064 (n. sig.) Summary of Multivariable GEE Analysis Results (Coefficient, 95 % CI): BMI [kg/m^2] to PPD at 2 months *p*-value = 0.013 Overweight to PPD at 2 months *p*-value = 0.63 (n. sig.) Obese to PPD at 2 months *p*-value = 0.031	n.r.	n.r.	n.r.	BMI and obesity were sig. associated with mean PPD after 2 months. ($p = 0.055$) Overweight was not sig. associated with PPD after 2 months ($p = 0.372$) BMI had a stat. sig. linear relationship with mean PPD after 2 months ($p = 0.013$). Overweight compared with normal BMI status did not demonstrate a stat. sig. association with mean PPD after 2 months (p = 0.63). Obesity compared with normal BMI status remained a stat. sig. predictor of mean PPD ($p = 0.031$) at 2 months in the same multivariable model.

CI confidence interval, *CPNW* normal weight patients with periodontitis, *CPO* obese patients with periodontitis, *kg* kilogram, *m* meter, *mm* millimeter, *Nb Δ PD* number of improving PD, *n.r.* not reported, *PD* probing depth, *PHNW* normal weight periodontally healthy control subjects, *PPD* periodontal pocket depth, *p* probability, *SD* standard deviation, *(n.) sig.* (not) significant, *stat.* statistically, *WHO* world health organisation

Table 5 Definition of periodontitis, periodontal assessment and definition of smoking

Author & year	Definition of chronic periodontitis	Periodontal assessment	Smokers
Al – Zahrani et al. 2012 [8]	≥ 20 teeth, CAL ≥ 3 mm at ≥ 30 of the sites (generalized moderate/severe chronic periodontits)	Full-mouth periodontal examination on all teeth excluding 3rd molars and partially erupted teeth	Smokers excluded
Bouaziz et al. 2015 [28]	≥ 12 teeth, ≥ 30 % of sites with CAL ≥ 3 mm (moderate-to-severe generalized chronic periodontitis)	Full-mouth clinical measurements included the following: 1) PI, 2) BOP, 3) PD (mm), 4) CAL (mm), PI, BOP, PD, and CAL measurements were performed using a manual periodontal probe at 6 sites per tooth, PD was defined as the distance from the free gingival margin to the bottom of the pocket/sulcus, and CAL was defined as the distance from the cemento-enamel junction to the bottom of the pocket/sulcus	Non-smoker or former smoker since ≥ 5 years
Duzagac et al. 2015 [29]	≥ 20 teeth, PD ≥ 4 mm in ≥ 30 % of periodontal sites, BOP in ≥ 50 % of periodontal sites, interproximal CAL > 2 mm in ≥ 20 % of periodontal sites, radiographic evidence of bone loss, as described by Armitage [177]	A Williams-type periodontal probe (UNC15, Hu-Friedy, Chicago, IL, USA) was used for the measurements of periodontal parameters, including PI (Silness–Löe) [178], GI (Löe–Silness) [179], BOP, PD and CAL, all clinical periodontal measurements were performed at 6 sites per tooth (mesiobuccal, mid-buccal, distobuccal, mesiolingual, mid-lingual and distolingual), excluding third molars	Smokers excluded
Eldin et al. 2013 [30]	n.r. (chronic periodontitis)	Full-mouth, 4 sites per tooth (mesio-buccal, mid-buccal, disto-buccal, mid-lingual) around each tooth	n.r.
Gonçalves et al. 2015 [31]	≥ 15 teeth excluding 3rd molars and teeth with advanced decay indicated for exodontia, >30 % of the sites with concomitant PD and CAL ≥4 mm and a minimum of 6 teeth distributed in the different quadrants presenting at least one site with PD and CAL ≥ 5 mm and BOP at baseline (generalized chronic periodontitis)	6 sites per tooth on all teeth excluding 3rd molars (distance between the gingival margin and the bottom of the sulcus/pocket [mm])	Smokers excluded
Gonçalves et al. 2015 [32]	≥ 15 teeth excluding 3rd molars and teeth with advanced decay indicated for exodontia, >30 % of the sites with concomitant PD and CAL ≥ 4 mm and a minimum of 6 teeth distributed in the different quadrants presenting at least one site with PD and CAL ≥ 5 mm and BOP at baseline (generalized chronic periodontitis)	6 sites per tooth (mesio-buccal, mid-buccal, disto-buccal, mesio-lingual, mid-lingual, disto-lingual) excluding third molars, with a manual periodontal probe (UNC15, Hu-Friedy, Chicago, IL, USA)	Current smokers excluded, smoking within the past 10 years excluded
Lakkis et al. 2011 [33]	≥ 20 teeth, mean CAL ≥ 2 mm (chronic periodontitis)	6 sites per tooth	n.r.
Suvan et al. 2014 [34]	PD > 5 mm and marginal alveolar bone loss > 30 % with > 50 % of the teeth affected (generalized severe periodontitis)	6 sites per tooth on all teeth present	Normal-group = 47 % smokers Overweight-group = 25 % smokers Obese-group = 15 % smokers p - value = 0.045 (sig. on $p \leq 0.05$)

BoP bleeding on probing, *CAL* clinical attachment level, *GI* gingival index, *mm* millimeter, *n.r.* not reported, *p* probability, *PD* probing depth, *PI* plaque index, *sig.* significant

statistical methods, a statistical synthesis of the results of the included studies was not possible. So the authors decided to analyze the papers on a qualitative way [22]. A meta-analysis was not possible.

Outcome

Generally obese patients were found to have deeper periodontal pockets at baseline in all studies.

Three [8, 29, 30] of the eight papers [8, 28–34] reported no major negative impact of obesity on response to periodontal therapy in terms of PPD reduction (mm). Al-Zahrani et al. [8] assessed the reduction of PPD (mm) comparing obese with normal–weighted women. There was no statistically significant effect of obesity on treatment outcome. Duzagac et al. [29] assessed the clinical response to non-surgical periodontal treatment,

Table 6 Definition of obesity and systemic examination

Author & year	Definition of obesity	Systemic examination
Al – Zahrani et al. 2012 [8]	Normal-weight: BMI: 18.5 to < 25 kg/m^2 Obese: BMI ≥ 30 kg/m^2	Weight in kilograms and height in meters were measured; BMI: (weight/height^2 [kg/m^2])
Bouaziz et al. 2015 [28]	Normal-weight: BMI ≥ 18.5 kg/m^2 and ≤ 25 kg/m^2 Obese: BMI ≥ 30 kg/m^2	Weight (kg), height (m), waist/hip circumferences (cm) weight was obtained using a calibrated scale,, height was measured using a measuring board, BMI: (weight/height^2 [kg/m^2]), waist measurements were taken at the level of the umbilicus (cm) hip measurements were taken at the greatest circumference with a measuring tape, WHR: ratio of waist to hip circumference
Duzagac et al. 2015 [29]	Normal-weight (CPNW): n.r. Obese (CPO): BMI ≥ 30 % and WHR > 0.95 for males and 0,80 for females	One trained examiner performed all anthropometric measurements: weight (kg), height (m), waist (cm), hip (cm), BMI: (weight/height^2 [kg/m^2]), WHR: ratio of waist to hip circumference, anthropometric measurements were repeated before the final follow-up visit to assess whether there was any change in BMI or WHR
Eldin et al. 2013 [30]	Overweight: BMI: 25-29.9 kg/m^2 Obese: BMI ≥ 30 kg/m^2 According to the WHO (3)	n.r.
Gonçalves et al. 2015 [31]	Without obesity: BMI 20-29.9 kg/m^2 and WHR < 0.85 for females and < 0.9 for males With obesity: BMI ≥ 30 kg/m^2 and < 40 kg/m^2 and WHR ≥ 0.85 for females and WHR ≥ 0.9 for males	BMI: (weight/height^2 [kg/m^2]) WHR: ratio of waist to hip circumference
	Non-obese: BMI: 20-24.9 kg/m2 and WHR below that determined for obesity (i.e. WHR < 0.85 for women and WHR < 0.90 for men) (World Health Organization 2008) Obese: BMI ≥ 30 and < 40 kg/m2 and concomitant WHR ≥0.85 for women and WHR ≥ 0.90 for men.	One trained examiner performed all anthropometric measurements: weight (kg), height (m), waist (cm) and hip circumferences (cm) BMI: (weight/height^2 [kg/m^2]), WHR: ratio of waist to hip circumference, anthropometric measurements were reassessed at all follow-up visits to verify that the patients did not change their obese or non-obese status during the course of the study
Lakkis et al. 2011 [33]	Control: obese (BMI ≥ 30 kg/m^2) Did not have the bariatric surgery nor did they lose weight to serve as a control group Surgery: obese (BMI ≥ 30 kg/m^2) and ≥ 40 % loss of their excess weight at ≥ 6 months after bariatric surgery	BMI: (weight/height^2 [kg/m^2]) Percentage of weight loss after BS
Suvan et al. 2014 [34]	Normal: BMI: 18.5-24.99 kg/m^2 Overweight: BMI: 25-29.99 kg/m^2 Obese: BMI ≥ 30 kg/m^2	BMI: (weight/height^2 [kg/m^2]) Based upon height and weight of the individual measured with a wall-mounted height measure and mechanical scales

BF body fat, *BMI* body mass index, *BS* bariatric surgery, *cm* centimeter, *CPNW* normal weight patients with periodontitis, *CPO* obese patients with periodontitis, *HDL* high-density lipoprotein, *kg* kilogram, *m* meter, *n. r.* not reported, *WC* waist circumference, *WHO* world health organization, *WHR* waist-hip-ratio

according to the severity of periodontitis based on probing depth < 4 mm vs. ≥ 4 mm. Patients with and without obesity showed similar clinical healing in terms of percentage and number of sites with probing depth < 4 mm and ≥ 4 mm. So they failed to show an effect of obesity on the treatment outcome dependent on the severity of the disease. Eldin et al. [30] also found no effect when comparing an overweight group with an obese group. The difference between the groups in reduction of PPD was not significant (Table 4).

Five [28, 31–34] of the eight papers showed a negative effect of obesity on the healing after non-surgical periodontal therapy. Bouaziz et al. [28] revealed that normal-weight patients had a better response to periodontal treatment than obese patients. This effect was specially observed for moderate-to-deep pockets. This fact suggests that the more severe the periodontitis the more pronounced is the negative effect of obesity on periodontal treatment outcome. They showed in the multivariate analysis that obesity was significantly associated with percentage changes of PD > 5 mm and numbers of improving sites ($p \leq 0.05$). In the univariate analysis all periodontal parameters improve more in patients suffering from more severe periodontitis at baseline. Other patient characteristics, like age, sex, obesity, and WHR, were not associated with periodontal parameter changes. Gonçalves et al. [31] showed that patients with obesity and chronic periodontitis had a lower PDD reduction than patients without obesity. The measurement of the

Table 7 Non-surgical periodontal treatment, treatment time and limitations

Author & Year	Non-surgical periodontal treatment	Treatment time; periodontal maintenance	Limitations
Al – Zahrani et al. 2012 [8]	Oral hygiene instructions, SRP performed by one operator	n.r.; n.r.	n.r.
Bouaziz et al. 2015 [28]	Oral hygiene instructions (brushing technique: Bass technique, use of interproximal hygiene devices, CHX mouthwash (0.12 %) twice a day for 7 days), SRP under local anesthesia using an ultrasonic device and manual curets, aim of each session was to remove biofilms and calculus of scaled roots, treatment protocol did not include antibiotic treatment, all treatments procedures were performed by the same periodontist (WB)	2-3 sessions for probing depth (PD) > 5 mm lasting 1 h each within 7 days; Oral hygiene was controlled at each appointment, hygiene instructions were repeated if needed at the 3-month examination, reinstruction of oral hygiene methods was performed if needed, and residual pockets ≥ 4 mm were systematically scaled and planed	During the study, two patients dropped out in each group for the following reasons: 1) two patients migrated; 2) one missed the 3-month examination; 3) one missed the final examination
Duzagac et al. 2015 [29]	Oral hygiene instructions, all kinds of dental treatments, such as fillings and adjustment of overhanging restorations, were completed immediately after patient enrollment, SRP using a reduced Gracey curette set (Gracey, SAS 5-6, SAS 7-8, SAS 11-12, SAS13- 14, Hu-Friedy) with an ultrasonic device (Dentsply/Cavitron, SPS, 30 K, TFI 1000, Dentsply, York, PA, USA) under local anesthesia, endpoint of treatment: a smooth tooth surface, patients received no adjunctive therapy (local or systemic antibiotics, NSAI, laser, ozonotherapy and mouth rinses), an experienced periodontist (EC) performed all treatment procedures (SRP, providing oral hygiene instructions and organizing patient recalls)	SRP in 4 sequential visits with 2 or 3 days intervals completed within 12 days, each appointment lasted 45 min; all patients received monthly periodontal maintenance, including oral hygiene reinforcement, scaling and polishing as necessary	8 were excluded for several reasons did not return for 3 months follow-up, pregnancy, weight loss
Eldin et al. 2013 [30]	Oral hygiene instructions, SRP	n.r.; periodontal maintenance (re-examination) performed weekly for 3 months after therapy	n.r.
Gonçalves et al. 2015 [31]	Oral hygiene instructions, Supragingival plaque and calculus removal, exodontia, filling overhang removal and provisional restoration as necessary, trained periodontist performed SRP with manual curets and ultrasonic device under local anesthesia, endpoint for each SRP appointment was "smoothness of the scaled roots."	4 to 6 appointments lasting ≈ 1 h each, periodontal therapy was completed in 14 days; periodontal maintenance at 3 and 6 months after therapy	3 patients from the group without obesity and 6 from the group with obesity did not return for the 3-months follow-up visit and were excluded.
Author & Year	Non-surgical periodontal treatment	Treatment time; periodontal maintenance	Adverse events
Gonçalves et al. 2015 [32]	Oral hygiene instructions regarding brushing technique and use of dental floss, supragingival plaque and calculus removal, exodontia, provisional restoration and filling overhang removal, as necessary, trained periodontist performed SRP using manual curettes (Hu-Friedy, Chicago, IL, USA) and ultrasonic device (Cavitron Select SPC, Dentsply professional, York, PA, USA), under local anaesthesia, without use of local and/or systemic antimicrobials.	4 to 6 appointments lasting approximately 1 h each, Periodontal therapy completed within 2 weeks; All patients received periodontal maintenance every 3 months post-therapy	There were no patient and sampled site dropouts during the course of the study.

Table 7 Non-surgical periodontal treatment, treatment time and limitations *(Continued)*

Lakkis et al. 2011 [33]	Oral hygiene instructions, SRP	n.r.; n.r.	n.r.
Suvan et al. 2014 [34]	Oral hygiene instructions, full-mouth mechanical periodontal debridement with hand and ultrasonic instruments performed with local anesthesia by the same clinician	Within a 24-h period of time; n.r.	No individuals in the sample had missing data for any of the covariates listed in this study.

CHX chlorhexidine, *min* minute, *mm* millimeter, *n.r.* not reported, *PD* pocket depth, *SRP* scaling and root planing

reduction in PPD (mm) at full-mouth sites showed after 3 months a not statistically significant difference ($p = 0.08$) between the obese group compared to the group without obesity. However after 6 months there was a statistically significant difference ($p = 0.04$). At this time point, especially deep sites (PPD ≥ 7 mm) showed a significantly better result in the group without obesity ($p = 0.04$). Another study of Gonçalves et al. [32] reported that patients with obesity had a significantly greater mean PD (6 months p-value = 0.04, 12 months p value = 0.03) than patients without obesity at six and 12 months post-therapy. The data of a study by Suvan et al. [34] corroborated these findings and showed that obesity was an independent impact value of poorer periodontal treatment outcome 2 months after therapy. The extent of the association between poorer periodontal treatment and obesity was similar to that of smoking ($p = 0.02$). They worked with 260 patients. This secondary analysis consisted of individuals participating in five clinical studies of non-surgical periodontal therapy over a 7-year period. Lakkis et al. [33] selected 30 patients who were obese; 15 of them had previously undergone bariatric surgery, whereas the other half ($n = 15$) did not loose any weight and served as a control group. The bariatric surgery group reached a statistically significant greater mean PPD reduction (0.45 mm versus 0.28 mm) compared with the control (no surgery) group ($p = 0.007$; Table 4).

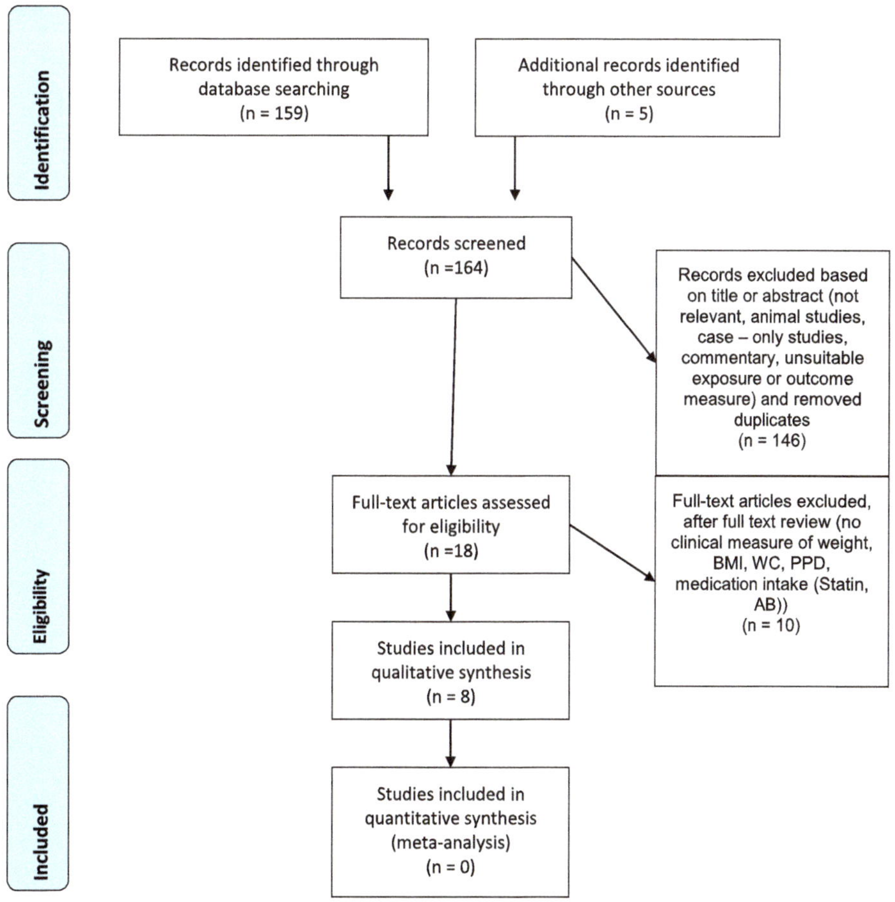

Fig. 1 PRISMA 2009 flow diagram

Table 8 Newcastle – Ottawa Quality Assessment Scale

	Al – Zahrani et al. 2012 [8]	Bouaziz et al. 2015 [28]	Duzagac et al. 2015 [29]	Eldin et al. 2013 [30]	Gonçalves et al. 2015 [31]	Gonçalves et al. 2015 [32]	Lakkis et al. 2011 [33]	Suvan et al. 2014 [34]
Selection								
1.) Is the case definition adequate?								
a) yes, with independent validation * b) yes, eg record linkage or based on self reports c) no description	*	*	*	*	*	*	*	
2) Representativeness of the cases								
a) consecutive or obviously representative series of cases * b) potential for selection biases or not stated	*	*	*	*	*	*	*	*
3) Selection of Controls								
a) community controls* b) hospital controls c) no description								
4) Definition of Controls								
a) no history of disease (endpoint) * b) no description of source								
Comparability								
1) Comparability of cases and controls on the basis of the design or analysis								
a) study controls for "smoking" * b) study controls for "diabetes mellitus"*	**	**	**	*	**	**		*
Exposure								
1) Ascertainment of exposure								
a) secure record * b) structured interview where blind to case/control status * c) interview not blinded to case/control status d) written self report or medical record only e) no description								
2) Same method of ascertainment for cases and controls								
a) yes * b) no	*	*	*	*	*	*		
3) Non-Response rate								
a) same rate for both groups * b) non respondents described c) rate different and no designation	*	*	*	*	*	*	*	*
Total	6x *	6x *	6x *	5x *	6x *	6x *	3x *	3x *

Stars represent "awards" for each quality item and serve as a quick visual assessment. A maximum of one 'star' for each item within the 'Selection'/'Exposure' categories and a maximum of two 'stars' for 'Comparability' can be awarded

Limitations

Some patients could not be reviewed or discontinued the study for personal reasons [28, 29, 31]. Weight loss and pregnancy were additional reasons to be excluded in the study of Duzagac et al. [29] (Table 7).

The quality of the included studies was evaluated through the Newcastle-Ottawa Quality Assessment Scale (Table 8).

Discussion

This review focused on obesity and the outcome after non-surgical periodontal therapy and has shown that currently there is no really robust scientific evidence to reach solid conclusions and recommendations.

Three papers [8, 29, 30] were found, which did not find any statistically significant negative impact of obesity on the response to non-surgical periodontal therapy, whereas five papers [28, 31–34] showed the opposite, i.e. a clearly negative influence of obesity on the treatment outcomes.

With regard to the quality of evidence, seven included papers [8, 28, 29, 31–34] reported some limitations.

Al-Zahrani et al. [8] included only women. Gonçalves and co-workers [31] did not consistently apply the accepted definitions of overweight and obesity, but rather included the waist-to-hip-ratio (WHR) for their definitions, probably leading to inclusion of patients with a BMI inferior to 30 kg/m^2 into the obesity group. Thus the results are difficult to interpret and compare with the other studies and are therefore not applicable for patients with a BMI ≥40 kg/m^2 [31]. Nonetheless, these studies still show a clearly better tendency with regard to the treatment response for patients without obesity as defined in their study. Lakkis et al. [33] chose another interesting way to find an impact of obesity on the outcome of non-surgical periodontal treatment. They compared obese people who had undergone bariatric surgery (BS) with obese who did not. After weight loss in the BS group, a reduction in total adipocytes might have resulted in a decrease in adipokines and pro-inflammatory mediators released by those adipose cells. This systemic inflammatory reduction might have played a role in reducing the insulin resistance resulting in a better outcome after periodontal therapy as suggested by the authors [33]. Some limitations in the specific profile of the obese patients (nondiabetic, non-smoker) in the paper of Bouaziz et al. (28) may restrict the extrapolation of the results to the whole obese population. Furthermore, the small sample size may also limit the power of this study. Duzagac et al. [29] failed to include a control group of periodontally healthy controls with obesity. Additionally the mean periodontitis parameters were within the limits of "moderate" periodontitis, and the WHR and BMI values of these obese patients were predominantly below those characterizing morbid obesity. So, the results of this study may not be extrapolated to those with severe periodontitis or morbid obesity. The second included study of Gonçalves and co-workers [32] assumes that the high inter-patient variance in adipokine levels may reduce the statistical power to detect treatment effects, as previously reported. The results presented by Suvan et al. [34] may have been influenced by study limitations linked with unequal numbers in BMI categories and sample size. In addition, there may have been limitations with regard to the interpretation associated with the *post hoc* secondary analysis experimental design, although variation in clinical assessment and treatment was minimized by examiner and treatment clinician stability. This study did not constitute a higher level of evidence in the context of evidence-based health care levels of scientific evidence [34].

Overall, obesity is an obvious, visible stigma so that the studies cannot be considered blinded. This may be another possible bias in each of the studies.

Five studies [8, 28, 29, 31, 32] excluded smokers. Since smoking influences periodontal health these studies are biased [9] and may not be fully representative for the typical overall population. Overall it appears, however, that a positive effect of normal weight is present in non-smokers [28, 31, 32] and in smokers [34].

As mentioned before, the included studies differed in statistical methods, populations, sample sizes, definition of chronic periodontitis, definition of obesity, time of outcome measurement, smoking status, periodontal assessment and non-surgical periodontal therapy. Therefore, it was not only impossible to perform a meta-analysis but also draw clear conclusions.

Nonetheless there is a consensus in the studies that obesity is associated with different baseline PPD levels. The large cohort in the study of Suvan et al. [34] and the long term results of Gonçalves et al. [31, 32] may lead to the conclusion that obesity is an important negative factor which influences non-surgical periodontal therapy.

In summary, all studies [8, 28, 29, 31–34] included in this review validated the efficacy of non-surgical periodontal therapy, except the study of Eldin and co-workers [30] who did not report any efficacy of the therapy (Table 3). Clinically, it appears obvious that a therapy is necessary to reach periodontal health independent of the patient's body mass index.

Because this systematic review provided only moderate evidence that obesity is an important factor for non-surgical periodontal therapy, future prospective cohort studies are needed to confirm these findings [36]. Such trials should be of high methodological quality. They should control important confounding factors such as smoking status, severity of chronic periodontitis, severity of obesity. Every patient should get the same periodontal treatment and periodontal maintenance. Overall, there is a possibility to solve the research question even though blinding of the examiners to obesity or non-obesity status is not practically possible.

Clinicians should know that obesity may have some influence on periodontal status and are likely to have a negative impact on the clinical outcome of conservative treatment, even if this systematic review found only five [28, 31–34] out of eight papers [8, 28–34] corroborating the influence of obesity on the clinical periodontal outcome focusing on PPD as surrogate parameter for periodontal healing.

Clinicians might consider a weight reduction diet as an additional treatment for periodontal health with a positive effect expected after 6 and 12 months [31, 32]. Also it should not be neglected that weight control has substantial other beneficial health effects which on their own justify such a recommendation.

Conclusion

This systematic review indicates a possible negative relationship between obesity and poorer treatment outcome in obese patients after non-surgical therapy based on the results of five out of eight studies. Three of these studies denied an impact of obesity on the treatment. The potentially inferior healing response could be based on pathophysiological inflammatory models.

Baseline levels showed also a poorer periodontal health in patients with obesity compared with non-obese patients.

No study found any better dental health parameters in obese than in non-obese individuals, and although dental health may not be the most important target for arriving at a near normal body weight, a person who can keep his or her body weight near normal might, in addition to all other established health benefits, count on having better periodontal health than if they are obese.

Acknowledgment
The authors would like to thank Mrs. Dr. Martina Gosteli, librarian of the main library of the University of Zurich who performed the electrical literature search. This study was supported by the Clinic of Preventive Dentistry, Periodontology and Cariology (Center of Dental Medicine) of the University of Zurich.

Authors' contributions
FAG and PRS conceived the study, participated in its design, did the literature search and drafted the manuscript. PS helped to supervise the methodological correctness of the performed study and the coordination. OAS and JHB provided the required medical theoretical background for this study and participated in the study design. CH helped with the statistical evaluation of the papers and the tables. All authors carefully read and approved the final text.

Competing interest
The authors declare that they have no competing interests.

Author details
[1]Clinic of Preventive Dentistry, Periodontology and Cariology, Center of Dental Medicine, University of Zurich, Plattenstrasse 11, CH-8032 Zurich, Switzerland. [2]Department of Internal Medicine, Cantonal Hospital Baden, Baden, Switzerland. [3]Department of Statistics, Ludwig-Maximilians-University of Munich, Munich, Germany.

References
1. Saito T, Shimazaki Y, Koga T, Tsuzuki M, Ohshima A. Relationship between upper body obesity and periodontitis. J Dent Res. 2001;80:1631–6.
2. Pischon N, Heng N, Bernimoulin JP, Kleber BM, Willich SN, Pischon T. Obesity, inflammation, and periodontal disease. J Dent Res. 2007;86:400–9.
3. Francesco Branca HNuTL. Die Herausforderung Adipositas und Strategien zu ihrer Bekämpfung in der Europäischen Region der WHO. 2007.
4. Suresh S, Mahendra J. Multifactorial relationship of obesity and periodontal disease. J Clin Diagn Res. 2014;8:ZE01–03.
5. Wang Y, Rimm EB, Stampfer MJ, Willett WC, Hu FB. Comparison of abdominal adiposity and overall obesity in predicting risk of type 2 diabetes among men. Am J Clin Nutr. 2005;81:555–63.
6. Yusuf S, Hawken S, Ounpuu S, Bautista L, Franzosi MG, Commerford P, et al. Obesity and the risk of myocardial infarction in 27,000 participants from 52 countries: a case-control study. Lancet. 2005;366:1640–9.
7. Słotwińska S. Host response, obesity, and oral health. Cent Eur J Immunol. 2015;40:201–5.
8. Al-Zahrani MS, Alghamdi HS. Effect of periodontal treatment on serum C- reactive protein level in obese and normal-weight women affected with chronic periodontitis. Saudi Med J. 2012;33:309–14.
9. Nishida NTM, Hayashi N, Nagata H, Takeshita T, Nakayama K, et al. Determination of smoking and obesity as periodontitis risks using the classification and regression tree method. J Periodontol. 2005;76:923–8.
10. Perlstein MI, Bissada NF. Influence of obesity and hypertension on the severity of periodontitis in rats. Oral Surg Oral Med Oral Pathol. 1977;43:707–19.
11. Koletsky S. Obese Spontaneously Hypertensive Rats-A Model for Study of Atherosclerosis. Exp Mol Pathol. 1973;19:53–60.
12. Chaffee BW, Weston SJ. Association between chronic periodontal disease and obesity: a systematic review and meta-analysis. J Periodontol. 2010;81:1708–24.
13. Wimmer GPB. A critical assessment of adverse pregnancy outcome and periodontal disease. J Clin Periodontol. 2008;35:380–97.
14. Blaizot A, Vergnes JN, Nuwwareh S, Amar J, Sixou M. Periodontal diseases and cardiovascular events: metaanalysis of observational studies. Int Dent J. 2009;59:197–209.
15. Tomar SL, Asma S. Smoking-attributable periodontitis in the United States: findings from NHANES III. National Health and Nutrition Examination Survey. 2000;71:743–51.
16. Tonetti MS. Cigarette smoking and periodontal diseases: etiology and management of disease. Ann Periodontol. 1998;1:88–101.
17. Arnaud Chiolero DF, Fred P, Jacques C. Consequences of smoking for body weight, body fat distribution, and insulin resistance. Am J Clin Nutr. 2008;87:801–9.
18. Fei Xu, BEcon, Xiao-Mei Yin BM, Youfa Wang. The association between amount of cigarettes smoked and overweight, central obesity among Chinese adults in Nanjing, China. Asia Pac J Clin Nutr. 2007;16:240-247.
19. Hou X, Jia W, Bao Y, Lu H, Jiang S, Gu H, Xiang K. Risk factors for overweight and obesity, and changes in body mass index of Chinese adults in Shanghai. BMC Public Health. 2008;8:389.
20. Altay U, Gurgan CA, Agbaht K. Changes in inflammatory and metabolic parameters after periodontal treatment in patients with and without obesity. J Periodontol. 2013;84:13–23.
21. David Moher AL, Tetzlaff J, Altman DG. Preferred Reporting Items for Systematic Reviews and Meta-Analyses: The PRISMA Statement. J Clin Epidemiol. 2009;62:1006–12.
22. Buset SL, Zitzmann NU, Weiger R, Walter C. Non-surgical periodontal therapy supplemented with systemically administered azithromycin: a systematic review of RCTs. Clin Oral Investig. 2015;19(8):1763–75.
23. D'Aiuto F, Nibali L, Parkar M, Suvan J, Tonetti MS. Short-term effects of intensive periodontal therapy on serum inflammatory markers and cholesterol. J Dent Res. 2005;84:269–73.
24. Duan JY, O-YX, Zhou YX. Effect of periodontal initial therapy on the serum level of lipid in the patients with both periodontitis and hyperlipidemia. Bejing Da Xue Xue Bao. 2009;41:36-39.
25. Iwamoto Y, Nishimura F, Soga Y, Takeuchi K, Kurihara M, Takashiba S, et al. Antimicrobial periodontal treatment decreases serum C-reactive protein, tumor necrosis factor-alpha, but not adiponectin levels in patients with chronic periodontitis. J Periodontol. 2003;74:1231–6.
26. Kardeşler BN, Cetinkalp S, Kinane DF. Adipokines and inflammatory mediators after initial periodontal treatment in patients with type 2 diabetes and chronic periodontitis. J Periodontol. 2010;81:24–33.
27. Tandon S, Lamba AK, Verma M, Munjal A, Faraz F. Effect of Periodontal Therapy on Serum Lipid Levels. Indian J Med. 2010;1:19–25.
28. Bouaziz W, Davideau JL, Tenenbaum H, Huck O. Adiposity Measurements and Non-Surgical Periodontal Therapy Outcomes. J Periodontol. 2015;86:1030–7.
29. Duzagac E, Cifcibasi E, Erdem MG, Karabey V, Kasali K, Badur S, et al. Is obesity associated with healing after non-surgical periodontal therapy? A local vs. systemic evaluation. J Periodontal Res. 2015. [Epub ahead of print]
30. Eldin AM, Nasr SA, Hassan NE. Effect of non-surgical periodontal therapy on interleukin-8(il-8) level in gingival crevicular fluid in overweight and obese subjects with chronic periodontitis. World J Med Sci. 2013;9:173–9.
31. Goncalves TE, Feres M, Zimmermann GS, Faveri M, Figueiredo LC, Braga PG, et al. Effects of scaling and root planing on clinical response and serum levels of adipocytokines in patients with obesity and chronic periodontitis. J Periodontol. 2015;86:53–61.
32. Goncalves TE, Zimmermann GS, Figueiredo LC, Souza Mde C, da Cruz DF, Bastos MF, et al. Local and serum levels of adipokines in patients with obesity after periodontal therapy: one-year follow-up. J Clin Periodontol. 2015;42:431–9.
33. Lakkis D, Bissada NF, Saber A, Khaitan L, Palomo L, Narendran S, et al. Response to periodontal therapy in patients who had weight loss after bariatric surgery and obese counterparts: a pilot study. J Periodontol. 2012;83:684–9.
34. Suvan J, Petrie A, Moles DR, Nibali L, Patel K, Darbar U, et al. Body mass index as a predictive factor of periodontal therapy outcomes. J Dent Res. 2014;93:49–54.
35. Genco RJ, Ho A, Nishimura F, Murayama Y. A proposed model linking inflammation to obesity, diabetes, and periodontal infections. J Periodontol. 2005;76:2075–84.

36. Sgolastra F, Severino M, Pietropaoli D, Gatto R, Monaco A. Effectiveness of Periodontal Treatment to Improve Metabolic Control in Patients With Chronic Periodontitis and Type 2 Diabetes: A Meta-Analysis of Randomized Clinical Trials. J Periodontol. 2013;84:958–73.
37. Europerio 4, Berlin, Germany, 19-21 June 2003. J Clin Periodontol. 2003;30:5-100.
38. Abstracts for the Royal Australian and New Zealand College of Psychiatrists 40th Congress. Psychiatry in a Changing World, Sydney, Australia, Sunday 22-Thursday 26 May, 2005. Aust N Z J Psychiatry. 2005;39:A97–186.
39. 5th Joint Meeting of the European Tissue Repair Society and the Wound Healing Society. Wound Repair Regen. 2009;17:A54–87.
40. Recently published abstracts. Altern Med Rev. 2010;15:369–80.
41. DENTSPLY. Posters. J Dent Hyg. 2012;86:322–6.
42. HealthBeat. Dent Assist. 2007;76:59–63. 55p.
43. Abstracts for Poster Presentations. 2nd North American/ Global Dental Hygiene Research Conference Bethesda, MD, October 20-22, 2011. J Dent Hyg. 2012;86:39–53. 15p.
44. Abstracts for the International Symposium on Dental Hygiene, Cape Town, South Africa, August 14-17, 2013. Int J Dent Hyg. 2013;11:156–73.
45. Abou Sulaiman AE, Shehadeh RMH. Assessment of Total Antioxidant Capacity and the Use of Vitamin C in the Treatment of Non-Smokers With Chronic Periodontitis. J Periodontol. 2010;81:1547–54.
46. Acharya A, Bhavsar N, Jadav B, Parikh H. Cardioprotective effect of periodontal therapy in metabolic syndrome: a pilot study in Indian subjects. Metab. 2010;8:335–41.
47. Akpinar A, Toker H, Ozdemir H, Bostanci V, Aydin H. The effects of non-surgical periodontal therapy on oxidant and anti-oxidant status in smokers with chronic periodontitis. Arch Oral Biol. 2013;58:717–23.
48. Armstrong BL, Sensat ML, Stoltenberg JL. Halitosis: a review of current literature. J Dent Hyg. 2010;84:65–74.
49. Arora N, Avula H, Avula JK. The adjunctive use of systemic antioxidant therapy (lycopene) in nonsurgical treatment of chronic periodontitis: A short-term evaluation. Quintessence Int. 2013;44:399–409.
50. Basegmez C, Berber L, Yalcin F. Clinical and Biochemical Efficacy of Minocycline in Nonsurgical Periodontal Therapy: A Randomized Controlled Pilot Study. J Clin Pharmacol. 2011;51:915–22.
51. Bresolin AC, Pronsatti MM, Pasqualotto LN, Nassar PO, Jorge AS, da Silva EAA, et al. Lipid profiles and inflammatory markers after periodontal treatment in children with congenital heart disease and at risk for atherosclerosis. Vasc Health Risk Manage. 2013;9:703–9.
52. Bresolin AC, Pronsatti MM, Pasqualotto LN, Nassar PO, Jorge AS, Da Silva EAA, et al. Effectiveness of periodontal treatment on the improvement of inflammatory markers in children. Arch Oral Biol. 2014;59:639–44.
53. Caspersen CJ, Thomas GD, Boseman LA, Beckles GLA, Albright AL. Aging, Diabetes, and the Public Health System in the United States. Am J Public Health. 2012;102:1482–97.
54. Caula AL, Lira-Junior R, Tinoco EM, Fischer RG. The effect of periodontal therapy on cardiovascular risk markers: a 6-month randomized clinical trial. J Clin Periodontol. 2014;41:875–82.
55. Chapple ILC. Oxidative stress, nutrition and neutrogenomics in periodontal health and disease. Int J Dent Hyg. 2006;4:15–21.
56. Chapple ILC, Brock GR, Milward MR, Ling N, Matthews JB. Compromised GCF total antioxidant capacity in periodontitis: cause or effect? J Clin Periodontol. 2007;34:103–10.
57. Chandni R, Mammen J, Joseraj MG, Joseph R. Effect of Nonsurgical Periodontal Therapy on Insulin Resistance in Patients with Type 2 Diabetes Mellitus and Chronic Periodontitis. Diabetes. 2015;64:A692.
58. Chaston R, Sabatini R, Koertge TE, Brooks CN, Schenkein HA. Serum anticardiolipin concentrations in patients with chronic periodontitis following scaling and root planing. J Periodontol. 2014;85:683–7.
59. Chee HK, Lim LP, Tay F, Thai AC, Sum CF. Non-surgical periodontal treatment and lipid levels in diabetic patients. Ann R Australas Coll Dent Surg. 2008;19:183.
60. Chee B, Park B, Bartold P. Periodontitis and type II diabetes: a two-way relationship. Int J Evid-Based Healthcare. 2013;11:317–29. 313p.
61. Chen L, Luo G, Xuan D, Wei B, Liu F, Li J, et al. Effects of non-surgical periodontal treatment on clinical response, serum inflammatory parameters, and metabolic control in patients with type 2 diabetes: a randomized study. J Periodontol. 2012;83:435–43.
62. D'Aiuto F, Parkar M, Andreou G, Brett PM, Ready D, Tonetti MS. Periodontitis and atherogenesis: causal association or simple coincidence? A pilot intervention study. J Clin Periodontol. 2004;31:402–11.
63. D'Aiuto F, Ready D, Tonetti MS. Periodontal disease and C-reactive protein-associated cardiovascular risk. J Periodontal Res. 2004;39:236–41.
64. D'Aiuto F, Parkar M, Nibali L, Suvan J, Lessem J, Tonetti MS. Periodontal infections cause changes in traditional and novel cardiovascular risk factors: results from a randomized controlled clinical trial. Am Heart J. 2006;151:977–84.
65. Deppe H, Hohlweg-Majert B, Holzle F, Schneider KT, Wagenpfeil S. Pilot study for periodontal treatment and pregnancy outcome: a clinical prospective study. Quintessence Int. 2010;41:e101–110.
66. Dodington DW, Fritz PC, Sullivan PJ, Ward WE. Higher Intakes of Fruits and Vegetables, beta-Carotene, Vitamin C, alpha-Tocopherol, EPA, and DHA Are Positively Associated with Periodontal Healing after Nonsurgical Periodontal Therapy in Nonsmokers but Not in Smokers. J Nutr. 2015;145:2512–9.
67. Draper C. Advances in technology and periodontal therapy. J Calif Dent Hyg Assoc. 2010;25:12–4.
68. Edwards J. Exploring the link between oral health & systemic disease. Access. 2006;20:15–20.
69. Efurd MG, Bray KK, Mitchell TV, Williams K. Comparing the Risk Identification and Management Behaviors between Oral Health Providers for Patients with Diabetes. J Dent Hyg. 2012;86:130–40.
70. Elliott-Smith S. Periodontal Disease: A Patient-by-Patient Approach. Access. 2011;25:28–32.
71. Engebretson SP, Hyman LG, Michalowicz BS. Hemoglobin a1c levels among patients with diabetes receiving nonsurgical periodontal treatment - Reply. JAMA. 2014;311:1921–2.
72. Fairfield C. Photodisinfection – innovative adjuntive therapy. J Calif Dent Hyg Assoc. 2010;25:20–2.
73. Fang F, Wu B, Qu Q, Gao J, Yan W, Huang X, et al. The clinical response and systemic effects of non-surgical periodontal therapy in end-stage renal disease patients: a 6-month randomized controlled clinical trial. J Clin Periodontol. 2015;42:537–46.
74. Fentoglu O, Sozen T, Oz SG, Kale B, Sonmez Y, Tonguc MO, et al. Short-term effects of periodontal therapy as an adjunct to anti-lipemic treatment. Oral Dis. 2010;16:648–54.
75. Fine JB. The influence of periodontal inflammation on systemic diseases and medical conditions. Access. 2007;21:14–9.
76. Fokkema SJ. Peripheral blood monocyte responses in periodontitis. Int J Dent Hyg. 2012;10:229–35.
77. Fu YW, Li XX, Xu HZ, Gong YQ, Yang Y. Effects of periodontal therapy on serum lipid profile and proinflammatory cytokines in patients with hyperlipidemia: a randomized controlled trial. Clin Oral Investig. 2015;20: 1263–9.
78. Garcia VG, Takano RY, Fernandes LA, de Almeida JM, Theodoro LH. Treatment of experimental periodontal disease by a selective inhibitor of cyclooxygenase-2 with scaling and root planing (SRP). Inflammopharmacology. 2010;18:293–301.
79. Giblin LJ, Boyd LD, Rainchuso L, Chadbourne D. Short-term effects of non-surgical periodontal therapy on clinical measures of impaired glucose tolerance in people with prediabetes and chronic periodontitis. J Dent Hyg. 2014;88 Suppl 1:23–30.
80. Gluch JI. Commentary on "The effect of periodontal therapy on TNF-alpha IL-6 and metabolic control in type 2 diabetics". Access. 2007;21:26–8.
81. Goldie MP. Perio trends. Dispelling myths about periodontal disease. Access. 2002;16:40.
82. Goldie MP. C-reactive protein, cardiovascular disease, and periodontal disease. Int J Dent Hyg. 2004;2:139–41.
83. Goldie MP. What is new in research? Antioxidants in oral health care: making the connection. Int J Dent Hyg. 2005;3:93–5.
84. Griffin SO, Jones JA, Brunson D, Griffin PM, Bailey WD. Burden of Oral Disease Among Older Adults and Implications for Public Health Priorities. Am J Public Health. 2012;102:411–8.
85. Gurenlian JR. Inflammation: the relationship between oral health and systemic disease. Access. 2006;20:1–9. 9p.
86. Gurenlian JR. Inflammation: the relationship between oral health and systemic disease. Dent Assist. 2009;78:8.
87. Hammaker BG. Pharmacologic interventions for controlling the inflammatory cascade in periodontal disease. Access. 2010;24:19.
88. Horwitz J, Hirsh I, Machtei EE. Oral aspects of Gaucher's disease: a literature review and case report. J Periodontol. 2007;78:783–8.

89. Hovliaras-Delozier CA. A common voice. Access. 2008;22:22–9.
90. Ide M, Jagdev D, Coward PY, Crook M, Barclay GR, Wilson RF. The short-term effects of treatment of chronic periodontitis on circulating levels of endotoxin, C-reactive protein, tumor necrosis factor-alpha, and interleukin-6. J Periodontol. 2004;75:420–8.
91. Ide M. Intensive periodontal treatment including extractions is associated with more immediate systemic inflammation but improved longer-term endothelial function compared to simple scaling. J Evid Based Dent Pract. 2007;7:162–4. 163p.
92. Jahn C. Diabetes and periodontal health. Dent Assist. 2004;73:24–9.
93. Jahn C. STANDARDS. Standard 1: Assessment: III. Risk Assessment. Access. 2015;29:19–23. 15p.
94. Jaiswal GR, Jain VK, Dhodapkar SV, Kumathalli KI, Kumar R, Nemawat A, et al. Impact of bariatric surgery and diet modification on periodontal status: A six month cohort study. J Clin Diagn Res. 2015;9:ZC43–5.
95. Janket SJ. Scaling and root-planing (SRP) may improve glycemic control and lipid profile in patients with chronic periodontitis (CP) and type 2 diabetes (DM2) in a specific subgroup: a meta-analysis of randomized clinical trials. J Evid Based Dent Pract. 2014;14:31–3.
96. Jared H, Boggess KA. Periodontal diseases and adverse pregnancy outcomes: a review of the evidence and implications for clinical practice. J Dent Hyg. 2008; 82:24–41.
97. Jiang H, Xiong X, Su Y, Zhang Y, Wu H, Jiang Z, et al. A randomized controlled trial of pre-conception treatment for periodontal disease to improve periodontal status during pregnancy and birth outcomes. BMC Pregnancy Childbirth. 2013;13:228.
98. Kamil W, Al Habashneh R, Khader Y, Al Bayati L, Taani D. Effects of nonsurgical periodontal therapy on C-reactive protein and serum lipids in Jordanian adults with advanced periodontitis. J Periodontal Res. 2011;46:616–21.
99. Kamilov KP. Relationship between chronic periodontitis clinical manifestation and lipid peroxidation in saliva. Uzbekiston Tibbiet Zhurnali. 1998;0:37–9.
100. Kapellas K, Do LG, Mark Bartold P, Skilton MR, Maple-Brown LJ, O'Dea K, et al. Effects of full-mouth scaling on the periodontal health of Indigenous Australians: a randomized controlled trial. J Clin Periodontol. 2013;40:1016–24.
101. Keller A, Rohde JF, Raymond K, Heitmann BL. Association between periodontal disease and overweight and obesity: a systematic review. J Periodontol. 2015;86:766–76.
102. Kiany F, Hedayati A. Evaluation of serum anti-cardiolipin antibodies after non-surgical periodontal treatment in chronic periodontitis patients. Odontology. 2014;103:203–9.
103. Kiany F, Hedayati A. Evaluation of serum anti-cardiolipin antibodies after non-surgical periodontal treatment in chronic periodontitis patients. Odontology. 2015;103:203–9.
104. Kipp A, Majeski J. New trends in perio. Access. 2003;17:10–5.
105. Kudva P, Tabasum ST, Garg N. Evaluation of clinical and metabolic changes after non surgical periodontal treatment of type 2 diabetes mellitus patients: A clinico biochemical study. J Indian Soc Periodontol. 2010;14:257–62.
106. Kumar M, Bandyopadhyay P, Mishra L, Das S, Kundu PK, Mistry S. Effect of periodontal therapy on glycemic control and circulating TNF-α in type 2 diabetic patients. Int J Diabetes Dev Ctries. 2015;35:96–102.
107. Kurti B, Tüter G, Serdar M, Pinar S, Demirel I, Toyman U. Gingival crevicular fluid prostaglandin E(2) and thiobarbituric acid reactive substance levels in smokers and non-smokers with chronic periodontitis following phase I periodontal therapy and adjunctive use of flurbiprofen. J Periodontol. 2007; 78:104–111.
108. Kurtis B, Tuter G, Serdar M, Pinar S, Demirel I, Toyman U. Gingival crevicular fluid prostaglandin E-2 and thiobarbituric acid reactive substance levels in smokers and non-smokers with chronic periodontitis following phase I periodontal therapy and adjunctive use of flurbiprofen. J Periodontol. 2007;78:104–11.
109. Lee HJ, Jun JK, Lee SM, Ha JE, Paik DI, Bae KH. Association between obesity and periodontitis in pregnant females. J Periodontol. 2014;85:e224–231.
110. Li X, Tse HF, Yiu KH, Zhang C, Jin LJ. Periodontal therapy decreases serum levels of adipocyte fatty acid-binding protein in systemically healthy subjects: a pilot clinical trial. J Periodontal Res. 2013;48:308–14.
111. Ling A, Wang P-W, Lin R-T, Hsieh C-J, Lee P-Y, Zhuang R-Y, et al. Evaluation of Periodontal Status and Effectiveness of Non-Surgical Treatment in Patients With Type 2 Diabetes Mellitus in Taiwan for a 1-Year Period. J Periodontol. 2012;83:621–8.
112. Lo JC, O'Ryan F, Yang J, Hararah MK, Gonzalez JR, Gordon N, et al. Oral Health Considerations in Older Women Receiving Oral Bisphosphonate Therapy. J Am Geriatr Soc. 2011;59:916–22. 917p.
113. Malhotra R, Kapoor A, Grover V, Grover D, Kaur A. Effect of Scaling and Root Planing on Erythrocyte Count, Hemoglobin and Hematocrit in Patients with Chronic Periodontal Disease. J Dent Hyg. 2012;86:195–203.
114. Mancl KA, Kirsner RS, Ajdic D. Wound biofilms: Lessons learned from oral biofilms. Wound Repair Regen. 2013;21:352–62.
115. Martinez GL, Koury JC, Brito F, Fischer RG, Gustafsson A, Figueredo CM. The impact of non-surgical periodontal treatment on serum levels of long chain-polyunsaturated fatty acids: a pilot randomized clinical trial. J Periodontal Res. 2014;49:268–74.
116. Martinez GL, Koury JC, Martins MA, Nogueira F, Fischer RG, Gustafsson A, et al. Serum level changes of long chain-polyunsaturated fatty acids in patients undergoing periodontal therapy combined with one year of omega-3 supplementation: a pilot randomized clinical trial. J Periodontal Implant Sci. 2014;44:169–77.
117. Matlock J, Ferguson K, Calef J, Abbott S. Obesity and Bariatric Surgery: Effects on the Oral Cavity. Access. 2012;26:8–11.
118. McDaniel JC, Roy S, Wilgus TA. Neutrophil activity in chronic venous leg ulcers-A target for therapy? Wound Repair Regen. 2013;21:339–51. 313p.
119. Meharwade VV, Gayathri GV, Mehta DS. Effects of scaling and root planing with or without a local drug delivery system on the gingival crevicular fluid leptin level in chronic periodontitis patients: a clinico-biochemical study. J Periodontal Implant Sci. 2014;44:118–25.
120. Merchant AT. Hemoglobin A1c levels among patients with diabetes receiving nonsurgical periodontal treatment [1]. JAMA. 2014;311:1919.
121. Michalowicz BS, Hyman L, Wei H, Oates Jr TW, Reddy M, Paquette DW, et al. Factors associated with the clinical response to nonsurgical periodontal therapy in people with type 2 diabetes mellitus. JADA. 2014;145:1227–39. 1213p.
122. Mizrak T, Guncu GN, Caglayan F, Balci TA, Aktar GS, Ipek F. Effect of a controlled-release chlorhexidine chip on clinical and microbiological parameters and prostaglandin E-2 levels in gingival crevicular fluid. J Periodontol. 2006;77:437–43.
123. Moeintaghavi A, Arab HR, Bozorgnia Y, Kianoush K, Alizadeh M. Non-surgical periodontal therapy affects metabolic control in diabetics: a randomized controlled clinical trial. Aust Dent J. 2012;57:31–37.
124. Moravec LJ, Boyd LD. Bariatric Surgery and Implications for Oral Health: A Case Report. J Dent Hyg. 2011;85:166–76.
125. Muthu J, Muthanandam S, Mahendra J, Namasivayam A, John L, Logaranjini A. Effect of Nonsurgical Periodontal Therapy on the Glycaemic Control of Nondiabetic Periodontitis Patients: A Clinical Biochemical Study. Oral Health Prev Dent. 2015;13:261–6.
126. Nassar PO, Walker CS, Salvador CS, Felipetti FA, Orrico SRP, Nassar CA. Lipid profile of people with Diabetes mellitus type 2 and periodontal disease. Diabetes Res Clin Pract. 2012;96:35–9.
127. Newton KM, Chaudhari M, Barlow WE, Inge RE, Theis MK, Spangler LA, et al. A population-based study of periodontal care among those with and without diabetes. J Periodontol. 2011;82:1650–6.
128. Nichols FC, Levinbook H, Shnaydman M, Goldschmidt J. Prostaglandin E2 secretion from gingival fibroblasts treated with interleukin-1beta: effects of lipid extracts from Porphyromonas gingivalis or calculus. J Periodontal Res. 2001;36:142–52.
129. Nielsen D, Walser C, Kodan G, Chaney RD, Yonkers T, VerSteeg JD, et al. Effects of treatment with clindamycin hydrochloride on progression of canine periodontal disease after ultrasonic scaling. Vet Ther. 2000;1:150–8.
130. Novakovic N, Cakic S, Todorovic T, Raicevic BA, Dozic I, Petrovic V, et al. Antioxidative Status of Saliva before and after Non-Surgical Periodontal Treatment. Srp Ark Celok Lek. 2013;141:163–8.
131. Novakovic N, Todorovic T, Rakic M, Milinkovic I, Dozic I, Jankovic S, et al. Salivary antioxidants as periodontal biomarkers in evaluation of tissue status and treatment outcome. J Periodontal Res. 2014;49:129–36.

132. Oliveira AM, de Oliveira PA, Cota LO, Magalhaes CS, Moreira AN, Costa FO. Periodontal therapy and risk for adverse pregnancy outcomes. Clin Oral Investig. 2011;15:609–15.
133. Olsen NC. Health Access. 2006;20:56–7. 52p.
134. Paquette DW, Ryan ME, Wilder RS. Locally delivered antimicrobials: clinical evidence and relevance. J Dent Hyg. 2008;82:10–5.
135. Perayil J, Suresh N, Fenol A, Vyloppillil R, Bhaskar A, Menon S. Comparison of Hba1c Levels in Non-Diabetic Healthy Subjects and Subjects With Periodontitis Before and After Non-Surgical Periodontal Therapy. J Periodontol. 2014:85:1658–66.
136. Perayil J, Suresh N, Fenol A, Vyloppillil R, Bhaskar A, Menon S. Comparison of glycated hemoglobin levels in individuals without diabetes and with and without periodontitis before and after non-surgical periodontal therapy. J Periodontol. 2014;85:1658–66.
137. Phillips A. Oral complications of diabetes: an under-recognized condition. Pract Nurs. 2013;24:562–6.
138. Pradeep AR, Manjunath SG, Swati PP, Shikha C, Sujatha PB. Gingival crevicular fluid levels of leukotriene B4 in periodontal health and disease. J Periodontol. 2007;78:2325–30.
139. Price T. Periodontal disease and adverse pregnancy outcomes: treatment recommendations for the pregnant woman. Access. 2010;24:20–3.
140. Qiqiang L, Huanxin M, Xuejun G. Longitudinal study of volatile fatty acids in the gingival crevicular fluid of patients with periodontitis before and after nonsurgical therapy. J Periodontal Res. 2012;47:740–9.
141. Radafshar G, Torabi F, Mirfarhadi N. Short-term effects of intensive non-surgical periodontal therapy and low-dose doxycycline on serum levels of IL-6, TNF-alpha and lipid profile in advanced periodontitis. Afr J Microbiol Res. 2012;6:355–60.
142. Radnai M, Pal A, Novak T, Urban E, Eller J, Gorzo I. Benefits of periodontal therapy when preterm birth threatens. J Dent Res. 2009;88:280–4.
143. Raghavendra NM, Pradeep AR, Kathariya R, Sharma A, Rao NS, Naik SB. Effect of non surgical periodontal therapy on gingival crevicular fluid and serum visfatin concentration in periodontal health and disease. Dis Markers. 2012;32:383–8.
144. Ramirez JH, Arce RM, Contreras A. Periodontal treatment effects on endothelial function and cardiovascular disease biomarkers in subjects with chronic periodontitis: protocol for a randomized clinical trial. Trials. 2011;12:46.
145. Rasch MS, Mealey BL, Prihoda TJ, Woodard DS, McManus LM. The effect of initial periodontal therapy on salivary platelet-activating factor levels in chronic adult periodontitis. J Periodontol. 1995;66:613–23.
146. Sadatmansouri S, Sedighpoor N, Aghaloo M. Effects of periodontal treatment phase I on birth term and birth weight. J Indian Soc Pedod Prev Dent. 2006;24:23–6.
147. Saffi MA, Furtado MV, Montenegro MM, Ribeiro IW, Kampits C, Rabelo-Silva ER, et al. The effect of periodontal therapy on C-reactive protein, endothelial function, lipids and proinflammatory biomarkers in patients with stable coronary artery disease: study protocol for a randomized controlled trial. Trials. 2013;14:283.
148. Williams KB. Effect of treating periodontal disease on cardiovascular markers. J Dent Hyg. 2007;81:49.
149. Sembene M, Moreau JC, Mbaye MM, Diallo A, Diallo PD, Ngom M, et al. Periodontal infection in pregnant women and low birth weight babies. Odontostomatol Trop. 2000;23:19–22.
150. Sengupta S, Fine J, Wu-Wang CY, Gordon J, Murty VLN, Slomiany A, et al. The relationship of prostaglandins to cAMP, IgG, IgM and alpha-2-macroglobulin in gingival crevicular fluid in chronic adult periodontitis. Arch Oral Biol. 1990;35:593–6.
151. Shimada Y, Komatsu Y, Ikezawa-Suzuki I, Tai H, Sugita N, Yoshie H. The effect of periodontal treatment on serum leptin, interleukin-6, and C-reactive protein. J Periodontol. 2010;81:1118–23.
152. Shimoe M, Yamamoto T, Iwamoto Y, Shiomi N, Maeda H, Nishimura F, et al. Chronic periodontitis with multiple risk factor syndrome: a case report. [Erratum appears in J Int Acad Periodontol. 2011 Oct;13(3):93]. J Int Acad Periodontol. 2011;13:40–7.
153. Singh N, Narula SC, Sharma RK, Tewari S, Sehgal PK. Vitamin E Supplementation, Superoxide Dismutase Status, and Outcome of Scaling and Root Planing in Patients With Chronic Periodontitis: A Randomized Clinical Trial. J Periodontol. 2014;85:242–9.
154. Siqueira MAD, Fischer RG, Pereira NR, Martins MA, Moss MB, Mendes-Ribeiro AC, et al. Effects of non-surgical periodontal treatment on the L-arginine-nitric oxide pathway and oxidative status in platelets. Exp Biol Med. 2013;238:713–22.
155. Stewart JE, Wager KA, Friedlander AH, Zadeh HH. The effect of periodontal treatment on glycemic control in patients with type 2 diabetes mellitus. J Clin Periodontol. 2001;28:306–10.
156. Talbert J, Elter J, Jared HL, Offenbacher S, Southerland J, Wilder RS. The effect of periodontal therapy on TNF-alpha, IL-6 and metabolic control in type 2 diabetics. J Dent Hyg. 2006;80:7–7.
157. Tamaki N, Tomofuji T, Ekuni D, Yamanaka R, Yamamoto T, Morita M. Short-Term Effects of Non-Surgical Periodontal Treatment on Plasma Level of Reactive Oxygen Metabolites in Patients With Chronic Periodontitis. J Periodontol. 2009;80:901–6.
158. Tamaki N, Tomofuji T, Ekuni D, Yamanaka R, Morita M. Periodontal treatment decreases plasma oxidized LDL level and oxidative stress. Clin Oral Investig. 2011;15:953–8.
159. Tawfig A. Effects of non-surgical periodontal therapy on serum lipids and C-reactive protein among hyperlipidemic patients with chronic periodontitis. J Int Soc Prev Community Dent. 2015;5:S49–56.
160. Teles FR, Teles RP, Martin L, Socransky SS, Haffajee AD. Relationships among interleukin-6, tumor necrosis factor-alpha, adipokines, vitamin D, and chronic periodontitis. J Periodontol. 2012;83:1183–91.
161. Toker H, Akpinar A, Aydin H, Poyraz O. Influence of smoking on interleukin-1beta level, oxidant status and antioxidant status in gingival crevicular fluid from chronic periodontitis patients before and after periodontal treatment. J Periodontal Res. 2012;47:572–7.
162. Tuter G, Kurtis B, Serdar M, Aykan T, Okyay K, Yucel A, et al. Effects of scaling and root planing and sub-antimicrobial dose doxycycline on oral and systemic biomarkers of disease in patients with both chronic periodontitis and coronary artery disease. J Clin Periodontol. 2007;34:673–81.
163. Vardar S, Baylas H, Huseyinov A. Effects of selective cyclooxygenase-2 inhibition on gingival tissue levels of prostaglandin E2 and prostaglandin F2alpha and clinical parameters of chronic periodontitis. J Periodontol. 2003;74:57–63.
164. Van Dyke TE, Hasturk H, Kantarci A, Freire MO, Nguyen D, Dalli J, et al. Proresolving nanomedicines activate bone regeneration in periodontitis. J Dent Res. 2015;94:148–56.
165. Vyas SP, Sihorkar V, Mishra V. Controlled and targeted drug delivery strategies towards intraperiodontal pocket diseases. J Clin Pharm Ther. 2000;25:21–42.
166. Wahid A, Chaudhry S, Ehsan A, Butt S, Khan AA. Bidirectional relationship between chronic kidney disease & periodontal disease. Pak J Med Sci. 2013;29:211–5.
167. Wang XE, Xu L, Meng HX, Lü D, Chen ZB, Lu RF. Long-term clinical and hematologic effects of non-surgical treatment on aggressive periodontitis. Zhonghua Kou Qiang Yi Xue Za Zhi. 2013;48:467–71.
168. Wehmeyer MM, Kshirsagar AV, Barros SP, Beck JD, Moss KL, Preisser JS, et al. A randomized controlled trial of intensive periodontal therapy on metabolic and inflammatory markers in patients With ESRD: results of an exploratory study. Am J Kidney Dis. 2013;61:450–8.
169. Wei D, Zhang XL, Wang YZ, Yang CX, Chen G. Lipid peroxidation levels, total oxidant status and superoxide dismutase in serum, saliva and gingival crevicular fluid in chronic periodontitis patients before and after periodontal therapy. Aust Dent J. 2010;55:70–8.
170. Williams KB. Periodontal disease and type 2 diabetes. J Dent Hyg. 2009;83:8–44.
171. Williams KB, Bray KK. Increasing patient engagement in care: motivational i nterviewing. Access. 2009;23:36–9.
172. Wood N. Oral health – how to reduce risks of periodontitis. Posit Health. 2006:30-35.
173. Wu Y, Chen L, Wei B, Luo K, Yan FH. Effect of Non-Surgical Periodontal Treatment on Visfatin Concentrations in Serum and Gingival Crevicular Fluid of Patients With Chronic Periodontitis and Type 2 Diabetes Mellitus. J Periodontol. 2015;86:795–800.
174. Zare Javid A, Seal CJ, Heasman P, Moynihan PJ. Impact of a customised dietary intervention on antioxidant status, dietary intakes and periodontal indices in patients with adult periodontitis. J Hum Nutr Diet. 2014;27:523–32. 510p.
175. Zhou SY, Duan XQ, Hu R, Ouyang XY. Effect of non-surgical periodontal therapy on serum levels of TNF-a, IL-6 and C-reactive protein in periodontitis subjects with stable coronary heart disease. Chin J Dent Res. 2013;16:145–51.

176. Zuza EP, Barroso EM, Carrareto AL, Pires JR, Carlos IZ, Theodoro LH, et al. The role of obesity as a modifying factor in patients undergoing non-surgical periodontal therapy. J Periodontol. 2011;82:676–82.
177. Armitage GC. Periodontal diagnoses and classification of periodontal diseases. Periodontology 2000. 2004;34:9–21.
178. Silness J, Löe H. Periodontal Disease in Pregnancy II. Correlation between oral hygiene and periodontal condition. Acta Odontol Scand. 1964;22:121–35.
179. Löe HSJ. Periodontal disease in pregnancy. I. Prevalance and severity. Acta Odontol Scand. 1963;21:533–51.

2

Oral health and coronary heart disease

Marc J. Mathews, Edward H. Mathews and George E. Mathews*

Abstract

Background: It is well documented that there is some correlation between poor oral health in the form of periodontal disease and coronary heart disease (CHD). It is unclear whether this correlation is due to a causal relationship or shared underlying disorder such as inflammation. A suitable integrated model of the CHD pathogenetic pathways relevant to periodontal disease may help to elucidate the association. Such a model is currently not available in literature.

Methods: A previously developed integrated model of CHD was used to investigate potential pathogenetic pathways linking periodontal disease to CHD biomarkers.

Results: The integrated model was created to provide insight into possible higher-order biological interactions underlying CHD and periodontal disease. In order to simplify these interactions a novel 'connection graph' was developed. It quantitatively illustrates the relationship between periodontal disease and various serological biomarkers of CHD. The pathogenesis of periodontitis shows various possible pathways which could link periodontitis to CHD pathogenesis.

Conclusion: An integrated model of CHD was developed which provides a summary of the potential CHD effects of periodontal disease. Further research must refine and validate the model.

Key words: Coronary heart disease, Periodontal disease, Biomarkers, Integrated model

Background

The largest cause of death globally is Coronary heart disease (CHD) [1]. It is also well documented that poor oral health in the form of periodontal disease is associated with an increased risk for CHD [2–6]. Whether this prevalence is directly linked to a causal effect of periodontitis or the effect of a shared underlying disorder such as inflammation has not been determined [7]. It is however clear that although there is a correlation between periodontal disease and CHD, the extent of this correlation and the usefulness thereof are not yet evident [2–7].

It may thus prove beneficial to quantify and elucidate the underlying pathogenetic effect of periodontal disease on the pathogenesis of CHD. Using a previously described integrated model of CHD [8] we therefore investigated the possible interconnectivity of periodontal disease and the pathogenesis and pathophysiological traits attributed to CHD.

The existing model graphically describes all the hypothetical pathogenetic pathways of CHD [8]. Some of these pathways can then be measured by serum biomarkers to give an indication of the degree of risk such a pathway represents. The model was used in this study to holistically review the interconnections between oral health pathogenesis and the pathogenesis of CHD. The theory is that where these conditions overlap there is the possibility for causal interaction which should be investigated in detail.

The vision behind the model is that it could be validated over time by calibrating it on a patient specific basis. Patients can be compared with themselves over time. Once the sample size of patient specific calibrated models is large enough the model could give new insight on the underlying workings of CHD. However, in the absence of existing studies of our model, using patient specific data, this paper attempts to gain some knowledge by looking at population based data. The data are in terms of risk ratios, the incidence of health factors and typical pathogenesis of CHD. Some interesting insights are revealed about possible interconnections of pathogenesis underlying both CHD and periodontal disease.

* Correspondence: 20270046@nwu.ac.za
CRCED, North-West University, P.O. Box 11207, Silver Lakes 0054, South Africa

Methods

An integrated model was developed as part of a larger research project [9]. This project was partially described in previous articles dealing with certain subsets of the research [8, 10, 11]. Briefly, an integrated model of CHD and health factors was developed from existing literature. The model was then used to describe the actions of some non-traditional health factors on CHD. This was achieved by using a connection graph which visually shows the relationship between CHD pathogenesis, measurable biomarkers and the health factors.

Integrated model development

The integrated model of CHD was developed using a systematic review of the literature for CHD pathogenesis, health factors, biomarkers and pharmacotherapeutics. Unless a publication was cited more than 50 times, the resulting dataset included results from 1998 until 2014 as these were deemed to contain the most relevant data. The studies were also selected based on how well they accounted for confounders such as age, sex, socio-economic status and others.

During the systematic literature review PubMed, Science Direct, Ebsco Host, and Google Scholar were searched for publications with "coronary heart disease" or "coronary artery disease" or "cardiovascular disease" or "CHD" as a keyword and combinations with "lifestyle effects", "relative risk prediction", "network analysis", "pathway analysis", "interconnections", "systems biology", "pathogenesis", "biomarkers", "conventional biomarkers", "drugs", "therapeutics", pharmacotherapeutics", "hypercoagulability", "hypercholesterolaemia", "hyperglycaemia", "hyperinsulinaemia", "inflammation", and "hypertension" in the title of the study.

Also searched were all major relevant specialty journals in the areas of cardiology, alcohol consumption, nutrition, cigarette smoking, physical exercise, oral health, psychological stress, depression, sleep disorders, endocrinology, psychoneuroendocrinology, systems biology, physiology, periodontology, CHD, the metabolic syndrome and diabetes.

This literature was consulted in detail and the research on the pathogenetic pathways of CHD was extracted therefrom. A total of 118 articles, books and studies were identified as important to the explanation of the pathogenesis of CHD. The information from these studies was thus combined in a graphical manner in order to develop the integrated model of CHD.

The integrated model was populated by considering health factors which were considered as either lifestyle effects or comorbid health disorders. Only health factors which have been associated with statistically significant increases or decreases in CHD risk were included in the model. The health factors considered were only those which are measurable through biomarkers and could conceivably be influenced by medication, prevention or other treatment. Thus, other factors such as socio-economic status were not considered. However, if future models are created for risk prediction more factors such as socio-economic status will have to be considered.

This resulted in nine health factors being considered in the model, namely Alcohol, Food, Exercise, Smoking, Oral health, Stress, Depression, Insomnia and Sleep Apnoea [8, 9].

In brief, the systematic review of literature revealed the pathological effects of various health factors on the pathogenesis of CHD. This information was combined to form a visual representation of the pathogenesis of CHD as it is affected by these health factors. In this study the integrated model was used to describe the possible integrated effects of periodontal disease on the pathogenesis of CHD.

The integrated model of CHD schematically illustrates the complexity of CHD and shows all theoretical pathogenetic pathways between the health factors and CHD. The model has been previously used to describe the effects of high carbohydrate diets on CHD [8], as well as the possible mechanisms through which antidepressants [11] and moderate alcohol consumption [10] may reduce CHD risk.

Furthermore, as the model is already complex, confounders were treated as follows: they were compensated for in the initial data but not included in the model. Therefore, when selecting the data used for the model, only the studies that best accounted for confounders such as age, sex, socio-economic status and others were used.

This encourages focus on a purely measurable biomarker driven model. Such a model, is not yet useful as a practical model for population based risk. It does however give a good indication of the way in which the interconnections between certain measurable factors (biomarkers) and the CHD risk correlate. Potential refining of the model is described in the Discussion section.

Biomarker identification

In order to allow the model to quantify the functionally measurable aspects of CHD pathogenesis, biomarkers were included in the integrated model [8, 9]. The biomarkers were only those whose measurement has been associated with statistically significant increases or decreases in CHD risk. This resulted in 23 biomarkers being considered in the model, namely triglycerides, low-density lipoprotein (LDL), high-density lipoprotein (HDL), apolipoprotein-B (Apo B), leptin, C-reactive protein (hsCRP), interleukin-6 (IL-6), tumour necrosis factor- α (TNF-α), growth-differentiation factor-15 (GDF-15), osteoprotegerin (OPG), myeloperoxidase

(MPO), B-type natriuretic peptide (BNP), homocysteine, fibrinogen, troponins, urinary albumin-to-creatinine ratio (ACR), glycosylated haemoglobin (HbA1c), insulin-like growth factor-1 (IGF-1), adiponectin, cortisol, brain-derived neurotrophic factor (BDNF) and insulin resistance.

Data selection

When selecting the data for the integrated model, only articles using the following risk measures: relative risk (RR), odds ratio (OR), or hazard ratio (HR) were considered. This study's intention was to create an overarching model rather than to conduct individual meta-analyses of the individual biomarkers or lifestyle effects. Thus, the risk data used in the model was taken from the most recent and relevant meta-analyses of each biomarker. A single high quality representative study was used where no meta-analysis for CHD risk was available for a specific biomarker or lifestyle effect.

The risk data used in the model was also further selected based on which meta-analysis adjusted for the most confounding variables such as age, sex, socio-economic status and others. This was done in order to ensure that the effects of most of the potential confounders were adjusted for. However, since not all the studies adjusted for the same confounders, this may, have increased the heterogeneity between studies..

For the effects of changes in biomarkers the relative risk (RR) was, where possible, extracted from the most recent meta-analysis conducted on the specific biomarker. If no relevant meta-analysis was available, a suitable high quality study was selected instead. The RR data included in the model was standardised to include only RR data that was given per increase of 1-standard deviation (SD) in the biomarker level. This was done in order to limit errors in comparisons between biomarkers and to prohibit the misrepresentation of risk due to the selection of extreme exposure contrasts [7].

Pathway characterisation

In this study the integrated model was used to elucidate the potential interactions between periodontal disease and the pathogenesis of CHD. To achieve this, the pathogenesis of CHD in which periodontal disease could play a role is described. A brief summation of the literature reviewed to develop the integrated model is presented as the "pathogenetic effects of periodontal disease" in the results section.

To simplify the importance of these interactions a connection graph was established for the relationship between periodontal disease and CHD. The connection graph is a graphic representation showing how the pathways underlying between CHD and periodontal disease are related to the CHD biomarkers.

The connection graph displays the RR for a 1-SD increase in all the biomarkers. Furthermore, the biomarkers were divided into eight classes, namely vascular function and neurohormonal activity, renal function, necrosis, coagulation, oxidative stress, lipids, metabolic and inflammation markers.

The pathogenesis of periodontal disease, as described by the pathways in the integrated model, was used to determine which of the biomarkers might be affected by periodontal disease. This was indicated on the connection lines between "Oral health" and the biomarkers.

Activation of the pathways can be analysed through measurement of the relevant biomarkers. Thus, to validate the connection graph, data from previous studies investigating changes in serum biomarker levels in patients with periodontal disease was corroborated with the biomarkers indicated in the connection graph.

Statistical analysis

Statistical analysis of the results was limited to the risk ratios which were extracted from published studies for the various biomarkers of CHD. All risk ratios were extracted to ensure that they were representative of a 1-SD change in the serum biomarker. All risk ratios extracted were converted to RR if given in odds or hazard ratios.

The study makes use of a non-traditional method of graphically displaying the RR indicating a decrease in risk. RR indicating an increasing risk is displayed as per normal. Decreasing RR is transformed by using the inverse of the typically presented RR.

The non-traditional method was used due to the problems of explaining relative risk to an untrained person as a result of the visual scaling of the traditional RR [8]. In this article a conventional RR = 3 is presented as per normal, as a 3-fold increase in risk while a conventional RR = 0.33 is presented as a 3-fold decrease in risk (1/0.33 = 3). This method was used to convert between the RR data extracted from studies and the bar graphs presented in this study.

Results

Integrated model of coronary heart disease

The integrated model of CHD which was developed in the previous studies [8–11]. It is presented in Figure One of the article by Mathews et al. [8]. In the integrated model the pathways (pathogenesis of CHD) can be tracked from where a specific health factor influences the relevant tissue, to the end state of CHD. The pathways of the integrated model are thus a visual representation of previously published knowledge on CHD pathogenesis.

The focus of this paper is on using the integrated model to describe the interconnections of periodontal disease on the pathogenesis of CHD. Thus, a more

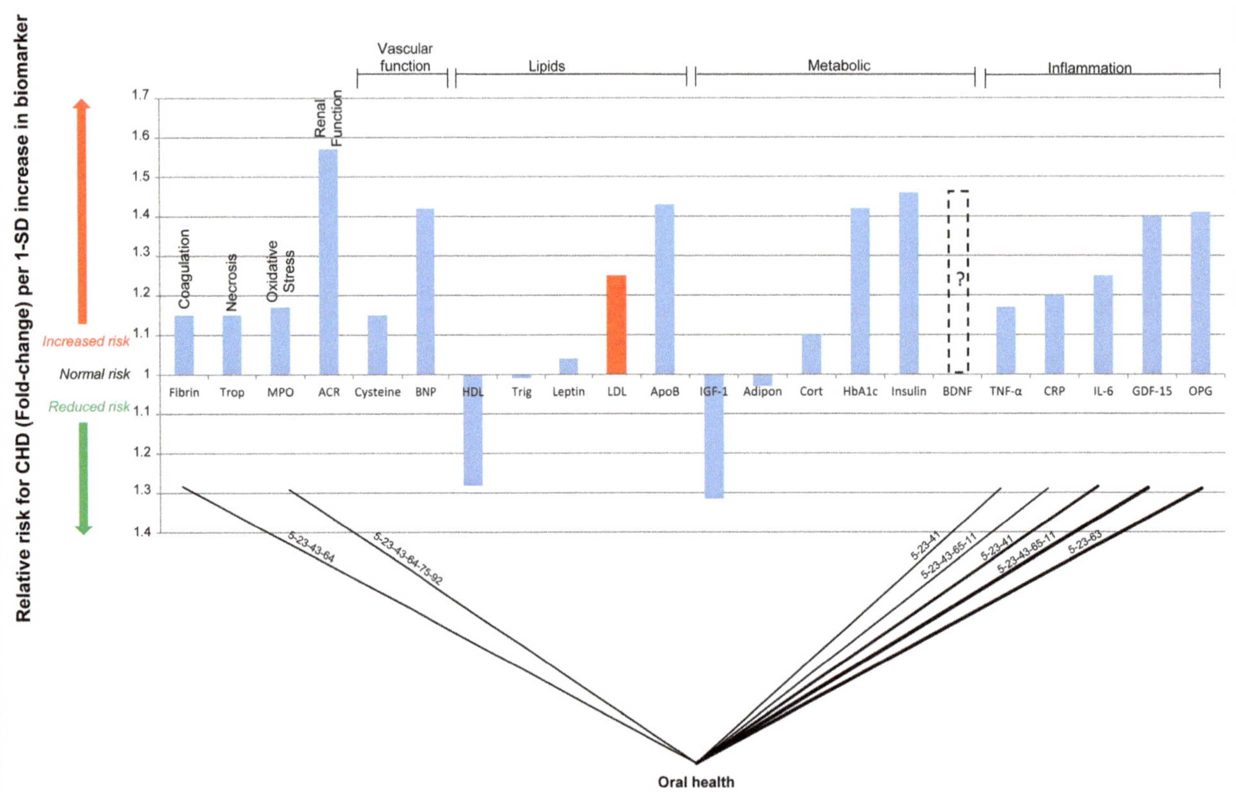

Fig. 1 Potential interconnection of relative risk effects of periodontal disease and serological biomarkers for CHD. "ACR" denotes, albumin-to-creatinine ratio; Trop, troponins; Fibrin, fibrinogen; MPO, myeloperoxidase; BNP, B-type natriuretic peptide; Cysteine, Homocysteine; HDL, high-density lipoprotein; LDL, low-density lipoprotein; Trigl, triglycerides; ApoB, Apolipoprotein-B; Adipon, adiponectin; HbA_{1c}, glycosylated haemoglobin A1c; Cort, cortisol; IGF-1, insulin-like growth factor-1; BDNF, brain-derived neurotrophic factor; GDF-15, growth-differentiation factor-15; CRP, C-reactive protein; IL-6, interleukin-6; TNF-α, tumour necrosis factor-α; RANKL or OPG, osteoprotegerin

detailed discussion of Figure One of Mathews et al. [8], relevant to periodontal disease, is given in following sections. This review therefore attempts to quantify the potential CHD effect of periodontal disease by the connection of these to an array of biomarkers which represent increasing or decreasing CHD risk.

Biomarkers of coronary heart disease

Biomarkers can be used as indicators of an underlying disorder and give an indication of the activation of pathogenetic pathways [12–14]. Furthermore, the prediction of the RR for CHD associated with a biomarker [12–14] is enabled by the measurement of said biomarker's levels. This can allow for an exploration of the possible effects of periodontal disease on the pathogenesis of CHD by considering the measurement of typically CHD biomarkers in patients with CHD.

The serological biomarkers which were used to simplify the integrated model are given in Table three of Mathews et al. [8]. Figure two of Mathews et al. [8] presents a comparison of the RR for CHD associated with these biomarkers per 1-standard deviation (SD) increase in the biomarker [8, 9].

Pathogenetic effects of periodontal disease

Figure One of Mathews et al. [8] indicates all possible pathogenetic pathways between the considered lifestyle effects and CHD. In the present paper we only appraise the possible CHD effects of periodontal disease. These are noted in Table 1 and will be described in detail.

Many of the potential pathogenetic effects of periodontal disease on CHD have been postulated to be due to the entry of bacteria or bacterial products into the blood stream [5]. A common periodontitis associated bacteria, *Porphyromonas gingivalis* (*P.gingivalis*), has been found to invade endothelial cells [15] as well as atheromatous tissues [16, 17]. This is one of the pathogenetic links between periodontal disease and CHD as shown by *pathway: 5-23- P.gingivalis* in the integrated model in Figure One of Mathews et al. [8]. In order to consider the overall effect of periodontal disease on CHD we will therefore consider all pathogenetic links between the two.

One of the possible links between *P.gingivalis* and CHD, supported by in vitro testing, is through increased platelet activity via a TLR2-dependent mechanism [18]. *Pathway 5-23-P. gingivalis-43-periodontitis-64-platelet*

Table 1 Putative effects of periodontal disease and salient CHD pathogenetic pathways

Pathways, and pathway numbers corresponding to those in Figure One of Mathews et al. [8]	Refs.
a. 5-23-↑P. gingivalis-43-↑periodontitis-64-↑platelet factors-73-↑hypercoagulability	a. [2, 4, 5, 64, 65]
b. 5-23-↑P. gingivalis-43-↑periodontitis-65-↑oxLDL-51-↑hypercholesterolaemia	b. [2, 4, 5, 64, 65]
c. 5-23-↑P. gingivalis-43-↑periodontitis-62-↑ROS-85-↑inflammatory state	c. [2, 4, 5, 64, 65]
d. 5-23-↑P. gingivalis-43-↑periodontitis-41-↑TNFα/IL6-↑inflammatory state	d. [4, 5, 64, 65]
e. 5-23-↑P. gingivalis-43-↑periodontitis-41-↑TNFα/IL6-↑inflammatory state-60-↑insulin resistance	e. [2, 64, 66, 67]
f. 5-23-↑P. gingivalis-43-↑periodontitis-41-↑TNFα/IL6-↑inflammatory state-60-↑insulin resistance-↑vasodilation	f. [68]

↑ denotes up regulation/increase, ↓ denotes down regulation/decrease, x-y-z indicates pathway connecting x to y to z. *FFA* free fatty acids, *IGF 1* insulin-like growth factor-1, *IL6* interleukin-6, *LDL* low-density lipoprotein, *MAPK* mitogen-activated protein (MAP) kinase, *MCP 1* monocyte chemoattractant protein-1, *NO* nitric oxide, *oxLDL* oxidised LDL, *P. gingivalis* Porphyromonas gingivalis, *PI3K* phosphatidylinositol 3-kinase, *PI3K:MAPK* ratio of PI3K to MAPK, *ROS* reactive oxygen species, *SMC* smooth muscle cell, *TNFα* tumour necrosis factor-α, *VCAM 1* vascular cell adhesion molecule-1

factors-73-hypercoagulability in Figure One of Mathews et al. [8] shows how increased platelet activity from periodontal disease can lead to an increased possibility for hypercoagulability, a hallmark of CHD.

Pathway *5-23-P. gingivalis-43-periodontitis-65-oxLDL-51-hypercholesterolaemia* in Figure One of Mathews et al. [8] shows how periodontal disease can have an effect on oxidised LDL cholesterol (oxLDL) due to the increased reactive oxygen species (ROS) associated with periodontal disease [19]. Increased ROS up regulates the oxidation of LDL cholesterol to form oxidised LDL [2].

Increased ROS may also play a crucial role in the link between periodontal disease and systemic inflammation. Pathway *5-23-P. gingivalis-43-periodontitis-62-ROS-85-inflammatory* in Figure One of Mathews et al. [8] shows how increased ROS can activate nuclear factor-κB (NF-κB) and consequent production of growth factors and pro-inflammatory cytokines [2] leading to systemic inflammation.

It is also possible that chronic systemic inflammation can further be up regulated by *P.gingivalis*, by causing increased elevations in C-reactive protein [20], fibrinogen [21], tumour necrosis factor-α (TNF- α) and intereukin-6 (IL-6) [4, 5] serum levels. These actions are shown in Figure One of Mathews et al. [8] by *5-23-P. gingivalis-periodontitis-41-TNFα/IL6-inflammatory state.*

Increased and systemic inflammation could link periodontal disease and a pro-atherogenetic state of insulin resistance. Pathway *5-23-P. gingivalis-43-periodontitis-41-TNFα/IL6-inflammatory state-60-insulin resistance* in Figure One of Mathews et al. [8] shows how the release of pro-inflammatory cytokines such as TNF-α, IL-6 and IL-1 from inflamed periodontal tissue could induce insulin resistance [22–24].

Pathway *5-23-P. gingivalis-43-periodontitis-41-TNFα/IL6-inflammatory state-60-insulin resistance-vasodilation* shows how periodontal disease could be linked to changes in vasodilation. Increased insulin resistance as a result of inflammation could affect vasodilation by impairing the vasodilation effect of insulin [25, 26].

It is thus evident from the integrated model that there are significant potential share underlying pathogenetic links between periodontal disease and CHD. These are largely in the form of increased inflammation and potential changes in hypercoagulability and insulin resistance. The rest of this paper will attempt to quantify the importance of the connections and links identified above by considering the changes in biological markers.

Effects of periodontal disease

In the previous section we elucidated the pathogenetic pathways underlying to CHD which are potentially activated by periodontal disease. Now we will link these pathways to measurable CHD biomarkers. It is possible that a pathogenetic pathway may be shared by both CHD and periodontal disease. However periodontal disease may not have a measured effect on CHD risk biomarkers for this pathway. This may indicate that the pathogenetic pathway is not influenced by periodontal disease in such a way which would increase CHD risk.

In an attempt to validate the theoretical pathways we considered existing literature which has shown measured differences in the serological biomarkers of CHD risk in patients with periodontal disease. Using this to describe the potential connection between periodontal disease and the serological biomarkers of CHD enables the simplification of the integrated model into a 'connection graph'. The connection graph in Fig. 1 shows all the potential connections between periodontal disease and the measurable serological biomarkers of CHD. The RR values linked with the relevant biomarkers were given in Table three of Mathews et al. [8].

The pathways from the integrated model (Figure One of Mathews et al. [8]) which are regulated by periodontal disease and described in Table 1 are thus shown on the connecting lines in Fig. 1. Each pathway suggests the manner in which the CHD biomarker is likely affected by periodontal disease. Previously published research on changes in serum biomarkers in patients with periodontal disease was used in an attempt to validate the connections between periodontal disease and the CHD biomarkers.

The explanation of the pathogenetic pathways in Table 1 would suggest that there should be a strong connection between periodontal disease and the markers of systemic inflammation. It is also evident from the connection graph of periodontal disease (Fig. 1), that there are a significant number of connections to the inflammatory biomarkers due to periodontal disease.

Numerous studies have noted increased serum levels of CRP in patients with periodontal disease compared to those without [20, 27–29]. One study [27] found elevations of CRP levels in the order of 30% when compared to patients without periodontal disease. Increased CRP levels are significantly associated with an increase in CHD risk (See Table three of Mathews et al. [8]).

Additionally, there is production of proinflammatory cytokines such as IL-6 and TNF-α in inflamed periodontal tissue [30, 31], which can further antagonise a systemic inflammatory response [32, 33]. Increased levels of IL-6 and TNF-α are both linked to increased risks for CHD (See Table three of Mathews et al. [8]).

In severe cases of inflammatory response, where inflammation has spread to the alveolar bone, proinflammatory cytokines can induce bone loss by increasing the expression of RANKL [34] and thus influence the levels of Osteoprotegerin (OPG) [35]. Decreased OPG levels, as a surrogate of RANKL levels, have been found to be significantly associated with increased CHD risk (see Table three of Mathews et al. [8]) [36]. It is thus possible that RANKL or OPG serum levels may serve as an indication of the severity of inflammation present due to periodontitis.

The connection graph in Fig. 1 shows that a strong connection between periodontal disease and inflammation is postulated and the abovementioned research confirms this. This indicates that it may be possible that a systemic inflammatory response to periodontal disease can antagonise CHD and CHD risk [12, 37].

Insulin resistance is postulated to be affected indirectly by periodontal disease through the actions of inflammatory cytokines [22–24]. Increased insulin resistance has indeed been found to be associated with the severity of periodontal infection [24]. Insulin resistance is however known to increase CHD risk [38] and Fig. 1 shows the connection between periodontal disease and insulin resistance with reference to the pathway from the integrated model of CHD (Figure One of Mathews et al. [8]).

It is known that chronic periodontal disease increases reactive oxygen species (ROS) generation which in turn depletes plasma antioxidants [2] and causes an oxidative stress situation [39]. This has been noted by increases in myeloperoxidase (MPO) in patients with chronic periodontal disease [40, 41] and is shown by the connection in Fig. 1. Oxidative stress induced by excess ROS could increases CHD risk due to the increased oxidation of LDL by ROS into oxidised LDL [42].

Oxidised LDL has been implicated in the pathogenesis of atherosclerotic plaques by facilitating cholesterol uptake by macrophages and the formation of foam cells in the endothelium [42, 43]. Therefore, MPO as an indicator of oxidative stress is attributed with a significant increased risk for CHD (See Table three of Mathews et al. [8]) [44].

Increases in serum fibrinogen levels have been found in patients with chronic periodontitis [45]. It is known that elevated serum levels of fibrinogen are implicated in poor CHD prognosis and increased CHD risk [46]. Increased fibrinogen caused by periodontal infection may cause an underlying increase in CHD risk by increasing the possibility for hypercoagulability as shown in Fig. 1.

Discussion

The use of an integrated systematic approach to better understand CHD elucidates the potential pathways which could lead to the hallmarks of CHD and a CHD event. It is evident that the pathological effects of periodontal disease are in some cases similar to or antagonise the pathogenesis of CHD.

It is apparent from Fig. 1 that there are several possible links between periodontal disease and CHD. Connections are evident between periodontal disease and CHD biomarkers through the hallmarks of hypercoagulability, and an inflammatory state.

From the connection graph (Fig. 1) it would appear that these connections may be relevant to CHD risk. However, what is not apparent is whether these connections are relevant to increased risk for CHD and if the relationship is causal. It is possible that these links may be mediated by direct pathological effects of periodontal bacteria or through the effects of underlying disorders such as inflammation.

These relationships should therefore be tested on a population basis in suitable trials. For instance, a study which determines the relationship between periodontal disease, CHD and serum biomarker levels would be needed to more clearly determine this relationship. Such a study would need to recruit a sample population having periodontal disease and note changes in the relevant biomarker levels with varying levels of periodontal disease. Furthermore, the study population must be large enough to limit confounding and the study period long enough for CHD incidents to occur. Unfortunately such studies are outside the scope of our research group.

Smaller studies could identify the effect of the successful treatment of periodontal disease on inflammatory markers, insulin sensitivity and markers of coagulation and oxidative stress (Fig. 1). While these will not substantiate a causal relationship between CHD and oral health they will show the relationship between the underlying pathogenetic pathways and periodontal disease with reference to known measurable CHD risk biomarkers.

Furthermore, the model presented may elucidate important CHD biomarkers which should be measured in patients with periodontal disease to more adequately screen for CHD risk, namely HOMA, TNF-α, CRP, IL-6, GDF-15, OPG, MPO and fibrinogen. This could lead to better treatment of patients at risk of CHD. In addition other risk confounders such as age, sex and socioeconomic status would need to be considered.

These other risk considerations are important for further development of the integrated model of CHD. For instance, it is known that some of the health factors we have included in the model are affected by confounders such as age, sex and socioeconomic status [47–49]. In particular, socioeconomic status is a substantial confounder to using the model on a population basis for risk prediction. It has the potential to present a significant confounding effect on all the health factors [49–53].

These further risk considerations should be included if the model is used for risk prediction on a population scale. It is important because these further considerations such as socioeconomic status are mediators of the health factors in the model and thus may present a top down approach to intervention.

Currently the integrated model is based purely on available measurable biomarker data and as such it is not meant as a practical model. Thus, the current model cannot be used for practical risk prediction of large populations until factors such as age, sex, socio-economic status and others are taken into account [54]. However, it is theorised that the model could be validated on a patient specific basis by comparing the patient specific biomarkers and health factors with themselves over time. Such an approach would circumvent the problem of confounders such as such as age, sex, socio-economic status by using the patient as their own 'control'.

A study could be conducted which attempts to validate the theoretical pathways by comparing a patient with themselves at different times where by different health factors or severity of health factors may be applicable. Such a study will require a smaller sample size but the results of the study would not likely be applicable to a greater population. However, it could validate the theoretical model to such a degree that large trials may prove worthwhile.

As such the current model is based entirely on a 'theoretical person' devoid of external factors. This theoretical model is built on data taken from external sources with an emphasis on having removed the most confounders in order to focus just on the underlying connections. The current integrated model is therefore more geared towards showing that these interconnections exist between health factors and CHD in a holistic sense. These should be studied further in preparation for the creation of a practical tool.

The intention of the model was to determine the likely method of action for a possible causal relationship between periodontal disease and CHD. In this regard the model itself shows why a causal relationship has not yet been demonstrated due to the interconnected nature of the disorders. The model shows how many variables mediate or confound the relationship. Each of these variables will have to be accounted for in studies of suitable size and design.

However, even with these shortcomings, numerous studies have alluded to the fact that periodontal disease is associated with a statistically significant increase in CHD risk [2–6]. The effect of periodontal disease on CHD biomarkers as shown in Fig. 1 indicates some of the effects which could serve to explain some of the risk for CHD. It is known that when increases in these biomarkers are considered in isolation they are associated with increased risk for CHD [36, 38, 46, 55, 56].

The importance of these relationships are however not immediately clear. An example may provide some context to their importance. An interesting comparison to make is between the relative risk for CHD associated with elevated LDL-cholesterol and the relative risk for CHD associated with periodontal disease. This in combination with the percentage of the population at risk of high cholesterol or periodontal disease should make the comparison interesting.

Previous studies have shown that the increased CHD risk attributed to periodontal disease is a relative risk of 1.34 (confidence interval 1.27 to 1.42) [6]. Other studies have shown that the risk for typical elevations (1-SD above the mean) in LDL-cholesterol is 1.25 (confidence interval 1.18 to 1.33) [57]. The study mean for LDL-cholesterol was 115.5 mg/dl and 1-SD was 35.0 mg/dl so this relative risk correlates to a LDL-cholesterol level of 150.5 mg/dl.

Considering that moderate periodontitis is present in 30.0% of the adult population of the United States [58] there is a significant 34% greater risk for them than those without periodontal disease. Knowing that LDL-cholesterol is widely regarded as the first indication of CHD risk [57, 59, 60] it would stand to reason that many more people are at risk due to high levels of LDL-cholesterol. If we look at the research 31.7% of the United States population is at risk of high LDL-cholesterol (above 130 mg/dl) [61]. This equates to an increased risk of less than 25% (1.25 for LDL greater than 150 mg/dl).

The CHD risk associated with LDL-cholesterol serum levels have resulted in substantial initiatives aimed at reducing LDL-cholesterol to reduce CHD risk [59, 62]. Considering that the potential CHD risk for periodontal disease may be even greater would it not be appropriate to engage in similar research undertakings to investigate if periodontal disease should be positioned as an important risk factor for CHD?

Various studies have investigated the effect of periodontal treatment on an array of CHD biomarkers. It was found that periodontal treatment significantly improved biomarkers of CHD [63]. However, causality between periodontal disease and CHD has not been suitably tested. If a causal relationship between periodontal disease and CHD could be substantiated it would elevate periodontal disease to an important CHD risk factor.

Conclusion

Although there is evidence that periodontal disease is associated with a higher risk of CHD, all the possible effects on CHD pathogenesis are not available in a detailed integrated model. Such a model should help provide further insight. A high level conceptual model was thus developed which shows possible links of periodontal disease with the pathogenesis, hallmarks and biomarkers of CHD.

It was shown that periodontal disease has significant physiological effects which are similar to or antagonise the pathogenesis of CHD. Important effects are increased inflammation, increased coagulation and insulin resistance. These pathological actions are backed up by the changes which have been noted through measured biomarkers.

These pathways and actions may explain why a significant risk for CHD has been observed in patients with periodontal disease. This is specifically important considering the large percentage of the United States population which have some form of periodontal disease. However, more research is needed to conclusively substantiate a causal link between periodontal disease and CHD.

Abbreviations

ACE: Angiotensin-converting-enzyme; ACR: Albumin-to-creatinine ratio; Apo B: Apolipoprotein-B; BDNF: Brain-derived neurotrophic factor; BNP: B-type natriuretic peptide; CHD: Coronary heart disease; COX: Cyclooxygenase; CRP: C-reactive protein; D-dimer: Fibrin degradation product D; FFA: Free fatty acids; GCF: Gingival crevicular fluid; GDF: Growth-differentiation factor; HbA_{1c}: Glycosylated haemoglobin A_{1c}; HDL: High-density lipoprotein; Hs: Homocysteine; ICAM: Intracellular adhesion molecule; IGF-1: Insulin-like growth factor-1; IL: Interleukin; LDL: Low-density lipoprotein; MAPK: Mitogen-activated protein kinase; MCP: Monocyte chemoattractant protein; MIF: Macrophage migration inhibitory factor; MMP: Matrix metalloproteinase; MPO: Myeloperoxidase; NF-κB: Nuclear factor-κB; NO: Nitric oxide; NO-NSAIDs: NO-non-steroidal anti-inflammatory drug; OPG: Osteoprotegerin; oxLDL: Oxidised LDL cholesterol; P. gingivalis: Porphyromonas gingivalis; PAI: Plasminogen activator inhibitor; PDGF: Platelet-derived growth factor; PI3K: Phosphatidylinositol 3-kinase; RANKL: Receptor activator of nuclear factor kappa-beta ligand; ROS: Reactive oxygen species; RR: Relative Risk; SCD-40: Recombinant human sCD40 ligand; SD: Standard deviation; SMC: Smooth muscle cell; SSRI: Serotonin reuptake inhibitors; TF: Tissue factor; TMAO: An oxidation product of trimethylamine; TNF- α: Tumour necrosis factor-α; VCAM: Vascular cell adhesion molecule; vWF: von Willebrand factor

Acknowledgements

The angel investor was Dr Arnold van Dyk. Prof Leon Liebenberg was involved in the initial research that led to the creation of the integrated model. We also acknowledge the fact that the integrated view is relevant to other lifestyle issues and for full comprehension will have to be replicated again in other articles describing these.

Funding

The research was funded by the authors.

Authors' contributions

All of the authors have been involved in the writing of this manuscript and have read and approved the final text.

Competing interests

The authors declare that they have no competing interests.

Consent for publication

Not applicable.

Ethics approval and consent to participate

Not applicable.

References

1. Mathers CD, Boerma T, Fat DM. Global and regional causes of death. Br Med Bull. 2009;92:7–32.
2. Granados-Principal S, El-Azem N, Quiles JL, Perez-Lopez P, Gonzalez A, Ramirez-Tortosa M. Relationship between cardiovascular risk factors and periodontal disease: current knowledge. In: Gasparyan AY, editor. Cardiovascular Risk Factors. 1st ed. Shanghai: InTech; 2012. p. 193–216.
3. Meurman JH, Sanz M, Janket S-J. Oral health, atherosclerosis, and cardiovascular disease. Crit Rev Oral Biol Med. 2004;15:403–13.
4. Persson GR, Persson RE. Cardiovascular disease and periodontitis: an update on the associations and risk. J Clin Periodontol. 2008;35:362–79.
5. Kebschull M, Demmer R, Papapanou P. "Gum bug, leave my heart alone!"-epidemiologic and mechanistic evidence linking periodontal infections and atherosclerosis. J Dent Res. 2010;89:879–902.
6. Blaizot A, Vergnes J-N, Nuwwareh S, Amar J, Sixou M. Periodontal diseases and cardiovascular events: meta-analysis of observational studies. Int Dent J. 2009;59:197–209.
7. Friedewald VE, Kornman KS, Beck JD, Genco R, Goldfine A, Libby P, Offenbacher S, Ridker PM, Van Dyke TE, Roberts WC. The American Journal of Cardiology and Journal of Periodontology Editors' consensus: periodontitis and atherosclerotic cardiovascular disease. J Periodontol. 2009;80:1021–32.
8. Mathews MJ, Liebenberg L, Mathews EH. How do high glycemic load diets influence coronary heart disease? Nutr Metab. 2015;12:6.
9. Mathews MJ. A systems engineering approach to coronary heart disease. PhD dissertation. Potchefstroom: North-West University; 2016.
10. Mathews MJ, Liebenberg L, Mathews EH. The mechanism by which moderate alcohol consumption influences coronary heart disease. Nutr J. 2015;14:33.
11. Mathews MJ, Mathews EH, Liebenberg L. The mechanisms by which antidepressants may reduce coronary heart disease risk. BMC Cardiovasc Disord. 2015;15:82.
12. Libby P. Inflammation in atherosclerosis. Nature. 2002;420:868–74.
13. Packard RR, Libby P. Inflammation in atherosclerosis: from vascular biology to biomarker discovery and risk prediction. Clin Chem. 2008;54:24–38.

14. Vasan RS. Biomarkers of cardiovascular disease molecular basis and practical considerations. Circulation. 2006;113:2335–62.
15. Deshpande RG, Khan MB, Genco CA. Invasion of aortic and heart endothelial cells byporphyromonas gingivalis. Infect Immun. 1998;66:5337–43.
16. Chiu B. Multiple infections in carotid atherosclerotic plaques. Am Heart J. 1999;138:S534–6.
17. Haraszthy V, Zambon J, Trevisan M, Zeid M, Genco R. Identification of periodontal pathogens in atheromatous plaques. J Periodontol. 2000;71:1554–60.
18. Blair P, Rex S, Vitseva O, Beaulieu L, Tanriverdi K, Chakrabarti S, Hayashi C, Genco CA, Iafrati M, Freedman JE. Stimulation of Toll-like receptor 2 in human platelets induces a thromboinflammatory response through activation of phosphoinositide 3-kinase. Circ Res. 2009;104:346–54.
19. Chapple IL, Matthews JB. The role of reactive oxygen and antioxidant species in periodontal tissue destruction. Periodontol 2000. 2007;43:160-–232.
20. Slade G, Offenbacher S, Beck J, Heiss G, Pankow J. Acute-phase inflammatory response to periodontal disease in the US population. J Dent Res. 2000;79:49–57.
21. Wu T, Trevisan M, Genco RJ, Falkner KL, Dorn JP, Sempos CT. Examination of the relation between periodontal health status and cardiovascular risk factors: serum total and high density lipoprotein cholesterol, C-reactive protein, and plasma fibrinogen. Am J Epidemiol. 2000;151:273–82.
22. Tilg H, Moschen AR. Inflammatory mechanisms in the regulation of insulin resistance. Mol Med. 2008;14:222–31.
23. Shoelson SE, Lee J, Goldfine AB. Inflammation and insulin resistance. J Clin Invest. 2006;116:1793–1801.
24. Demmer RT, Squillaro A, Papapanou PN, Rosenbaum M, Friedewald WT, Jacobs DR, Desvarieux M. Periodontal infection, systemic inflammation, and insulin resistance: results from the continuous National Health and Nutrition Examination Survey (NHANES) 1999–2004. Diabetes Care. 2012;35:2235–42.
25. Mather KJ, Steinberg HO, Baron AD. Insulin resistance in the vasculature. J Clin Invest. 2013;123:1003–4.
26. Anderson EA, Mark AL. The vasodilator action of insulin. Implications for the insulin hypothesis of hypertension. Hypertension. 1993;21:136–41.
27. Joshipura K, Wand H, Merchant A, Rimm E. Periodontal disease and biomarkers related to cardiovascular disease. J Dent Res. 2004;83:151–5.
28. D'Aiuto F, Ready D, Tonetti MS. Periodontal disease and C-reactive protein-associated cardiovascular risk. J Periodontal Res. 2004;39:236–41.
29. Slade GD, Ghezzi EM, Heiss G, Beck JD, Riche E, Offenbacher S. Relationship between periodontal disease and C-reactive protein among adults in the Atherosclerosis Risk in Communities study. Arch Intern Med. 2003;163:1172–9.
30. Lamster IB, Lalla E, Borgnakke WS, Taylor GW. The relationship between oral health and diabetes mellitus. J Am Dent Assoc. 2008;139:19S–24S.
31. Bretz WA, Weyant RJ, Corby PM, Ren D, Weissfeld L, Kritchevsky SB, Harris T, Kurella M, Satterfield S, Visser M, et al. Systemic inflammatory markers, periodontal diseases, and periodontal infections in an elderly population. J Am Geriatr Soc. 2005;53:1532–7.
32. Zhang J-M, An J. Cytokines, inflammation and pain. Int Anesthesiol Clin. 2007;45:27.
33. Watkins LR, Maier SF, Goehler LE. Immune activation: the role of pro-inflammatory cytokines in inflammation, illness responses and pathological pain states. Pain. 1995;63:289–302.
34. Nakashima T, Kobayashi Y, Yamasaki S, Kawakami A, Eguchi K, Sasaki H, Sakai H. Protein expression and functional difference of membrane-bound and soluble receptor activator of NF-κB ligand: modulation of the expression by osteotropic factors and cytokines. Biochem Biophys Res Commun. 2000;275:768–75.
35. Boyce BF, Xing L. Biology of RANK, RANKL, and osteoprotegerin. Arthritis Res Ther. 2007;9 Suppl 1:S1.
36. Mogelvang R, Pedersen SH, Flyvbjerg A, Bjerre M, Iversen AZ, Galatius S, Frystyk J, Jensen JS. Comparison of osteoprotegerin to traditional atherosclerotic risk factors and high-sensitivity C-reactive protein for diagnosis of atherosclerosis. Am J Cardiol. 2012;109:515–20.
37. Libby P. Inflammation in atherosclerosis. Arterioscler Thromb Vasc Biol. 2012;32:2045–51.
38. Gast KB, Tjeerdema N, Stijnen T, Smit JW, Dekkers OM. Insulin resistance and risk of incident cardiovascular events in adults without diabetes: meta-analysis. PLoS One. 2012;7:e52036.
39. Borges Jr I, Moreira EAM, De Oliveira TB, da Silva MBS, Fröde TS. Proinflammatory and oxidative stress markers in patients with periodontal disease. Mediators Inflamm. 2007;2007:ID 45794.
40. Hernández M, Gamonal J, Tervahartiala T, Mäntylä P, Rivera O, Dezerega A, Dutzan N, Sorsa T. Associations between matrix metalloproteinase-8 and −14 and myeloperoxidase in gingival crevicular fluid from subjects with progressive chronic periodontitis: a longitudinal study. J Periodontol. 2010;81:1644–52.
41. Över C, Yamalik N, Yavuzyilmaz E, Ersoy F, Eratalay K. Myeloperoxidase activity in peripheral blood, neutrophil crevicular fluid and whole saliva of patients with periodontal disease. J Nihon Univ Sch Dent. 1993;35:235–40.
42. Itabe H. Oxidative modification of LDL: its pathological role in atherosclerosis. Clin Rev Allergy Immunol. 2009;37:4–11.
43. Stoll G, Bendszus M. Inflammation and atherosclerosis novel insights into plaque formation and destabilization. Stroke. 2006;37:1923–32.
44. Rana JS, Arsenault BJ, Després J-P, Côté M, Talmud PJ, Ninio E, Jukema JW, Wareham NJ, Kastelein JJ, Khaw K-T. Inflammatory biomarkers, physical activity, waist circumference, and risk of future coronary heart disease in healthy men and women. Eur Heart J. 2009;32:336–44.
45. Loos BG. Systemic markers of inflammation in periodontitis. J Periodontol. 2005;76:2106–15.
46. Kaptoge S, Di Angelantonio E, Pennells L, Wood AM, White IR, Gao P, Walker M, Thompson A, Sarwar N, Caslake M, et al. C-reactive protein, fibrinogen, and cardiovascular disease prediction. N Engl J Med. 2012;367:1310–20.
47. Booth GL, Kapral MK, Fung K, Tu JV. Relation between age and cardiovascular disease in men and women with diabetes compared with non-diabetic people: a population-based retrospective cohort study. Lancet. 2006;368:29–36.
48. Barrett-Connor E. Sex differences in coronary heart disease Why are women so superior? The 1995 Ancel Keys Lecture. Circulation. 1997;95:252–64.
49. Schulman KA, Berlin JA, Harless W, Kerner JF, Sistrunk S, Gersh BJ, Dube R, Taleghani CK, Burke JE, Williams S. The effect of race and sex on physicians' recommendations for cardiac catheterization. N Engl J Med. 1999;340:618–26.
50. Hobdell M, Oliveira E, Bautista R, Myburgh N, Lalloo R, Narendran S, Johnson NW. Oral diseases and socio-economic status (SES). Br Dent J. 2003;194:91–6.
51. Adler NE, Ostrove JM. Socioeconomic status and health: what we know and what we don't. Ann N Y Acad Sci. 1999;896:3–15.
52. Baum A, Garofalo J, YALI A. Socioeconomic status and chronic stress: does stress account for SES effects on health? Ann N Y Acad Sci. 1999;896:131–44.
53. Sobal J, Stunkard AJ. Socioeconomic status and obesity: a review of the literature. Psychol Bull. 1989;105:260.
54. Baker SR, Gibson BG. Social oral epidemi (olog) 2y where next: one small step or one giant leap? Community Dent Oral Epidemiol. 2014;42:481–94.
55. Kaptoge S, Seshasai SRK, Gao P, Freitag DF, Butterworth AS, Borglykke A, Di Angelantonio E, Gudnason V, Rumley A, Lowe GDO, et al. Inflammatory cytokines and risk of coronary heart disease: new prospective study and updated meta-analysis. Eur Heart J. 2014;35:578–89.
56. Daniels LB, Clopton P, Laughlin GA, Maisel AS, Barrett-Connor E. Growth-Differentiation Factor-15 Is a Robust, Independent Predictor of 11-Year Mortality Risk in Community-Dwelling Older Adults The Rancho Bernardo Study. Circulation. 2011;123:2101–10.
57. Sniderman AD, Williams K, Contois JH, Monroe HM, McQueen MJ, de Graaf J, Furberg CD. A meta-analysis of low-density lipoprotein cholesterol, non-high-density lipoprotein cholesterol, and apolipoprotein B as markers of cardiovascular risk. Circ Cardiovasc Qual Outcomes. 2011;4:337–45.
58. Eke P, Dye B, Wei L, Thornton-Evans G, Genco R. Prevalence of periodontitis in adults in the United States: 2009 and 2010. J Dent Res. 2012;91:914–20.
59. Stone NJ, Robinson J, Lichtenstein AH, Merz CNB, Lloyd-Jones DM, Blum CB, McBride P, Eckel RH, Schwartz JS, Goldberg AC. 2013 ACC/AHA guideline on the treatment of blood cholesterol to reduce atherosclerotic cardiovascular risk in adults: a report of the American College of Cardiology/American Heart Association task force on practice guidelines. J Am Coll Cardiol. 2013; 63:2889-934.
60. Greenland P, Alpert JS, Beller GA, Benjamin EJ, Budoff MJ, Fayad ZA, Foster E, Hlatky MA, Hodgson JM, Kushner FG, et al. 2010 ACCF/AHA guideline for assessment of cardiovascular risk in asymptomatic adults: a report of the American College of Cardiology Foundation/American Heart Association Task Force on Practice Guidelines. J Am Coll Cardiol. 2010;56:e50–103.
61. Mozaffarian D, Benjamin EJ, Go AS, Arnett DK, Blaha MJ, Cushman M, de Ferranti S, Després J-P, Fullerton HJ, Howard VJ et al. Heart disease and stroke statistics—2015 update: a report from the American Heart Association. Circulation. 2014;3:e28-e292.
62. Perk J, De Backer G, Gohlke H, Graham I, Reiner Ž, Verschuren M, Albus C, Benlian P, Boysen G, Cifkova R. European Guidelines on cardiovascular

disease prevention in clinical practice (version 2012) The Fifth Joint Task Force of the European Society of Cardiology and Other Societies on Cardiovascular Disease Prevention in Clinical Practice (constituted by representatives of nine societies and by invited experts) Developed with the special contribution of the European Association for Cardiovascular Prevention & Rehabilitation (EACPR). Eur Heart J. 2012;33:ehs092.

63. Teeuw WJ, Slot DE, Susanto H, Gerdes VE, Abbas F, D'Aiuto F, Kastelein JJ, Loos BG. Treatment of periodontitis improves the atherosclerotic profile: a systematic review and meta-analysis. J Clin Periodontol. 2014;41:70–9.
64. Paquette DW, Brodala N, Nichols TC. Cardiovascular disease, inflammation, and periodontal infection. Periodontol 2000. 2007;44:113–26.
65. Machuca G, Segura-Egea JJ, Jiménez-Beato G, Lacalle JR, Bullón P. Clinical indicators of periodontal disease in patients with coronary heart disease: A 10 years longitudinal study. Med Oral Patol Oral Cir Bucal. 2012;17:e569.
66. Jackson SP. Arterial thrombosis-insidious, unpredictable and deadly. Nat Med. 2011;17:1423–36.
67. Rydén L, Standl E, Bartnik M, Van den Berghe G, Betteridge J, De Boer M-J, Cosentino F, Jönsson B, Laakso M, Malmberg K. Guidelines on diabetes, pre-diabetes, and cardiovascular diseases: executive summary. The Task Force on Diabetes and Cardiovascular Diseases of the European Society of Cardiology (ESC) and of the European Association for the Study of Diabetes (EASD). Eur Heart J. 2007;28:88–136.
68. Wang JC, Bennett M. Aging and atherosclerosis mechanisms, functional consequences, and potential therapeutics for cellular senescence. Circ Res. 2012;111:245–59.

3

Inequalities in the frequency of free sugars intake among Syrian 1-year-old infants

Easter Joury[1,2*], May Khairallah[2], Wael Sabbah[1], Kanaan Elias[3] and Raman Bedi[4]

Abstract

Background: High frequency of free sugars intake, during the first year of life is probably the greatest risk factor for early childhood caries. The latter is a global public health challenge. Very little is known about the social determinants of infant's frequency of free sugars intake, particularly in low-income countries. Thus, the present study aimed to assess the association between the frequency of free sugars intake among 1-year-old Syrian infants and each of parents' socioeconomic position (SEP), maternal frequency of free sugars intake and knowledge of infant's oral health behaviour.

Methods: Using a cross-sectional design, 323 1-year-old infants, attending vaccination clinics in 3 maternal and child health centres (MCHCs) in Damascus, Syria, were selected. A systematic random sampling was applied using the MCHCs' monthly vaccination registries. The 3 MCHCs were located in affluent, moderate and deprived areas. Infants' mothers completed a structured questionnaire on socio-demographics, infant's and mother's frequency of free sugars intake from cariogenic foods and beverages, and mother's knowledge about infant's oral health behaviour. Binary and multiple regression analyses were performed. The level of significance was set at 5 %.

Results: The response rate was 100 %. Overall, 42.7 % of infants had high frequency of free sugars intake (>4times a day). Infants whose fathers were not working were more likely to have high frequency of free sugars intake. Similarly, infants whose mothers had low level of knowledge about infant's oral health behaviour, or high frequency of free sugars intake were more likely to have high frequency of free sugars intake. The association between father's occupation and infant's frequency of free sugars intake attenuated after adjustment for mother's knowledge and frequency of free sugars intake (adjusted OR = 1.5, 1.8, 3.2; 95%CI = 0.5–4.8, 1.1–3, 1.4–7.4; respectively).

Conclusions: There are socioeconomic inequalities in the frequency of free sugars intake among Syrian 1-year-old infants. Integrated pre/post-natal interventions, targeting mothers from low SEP and aiming at reducing their free sugars intake and improving their knowledge about infant's oral health behaviour, will potentially reduce socioeconomic inequalities in infant's frequency of free sugars intake.

Keywords: Social determinants of health, Socioeconomic factors, Health literacy, Health behaviour, Dietary sugars, Infant, Syria

Abbreviations: SEP, Socioeconomic position; WHO, World Health Organization

* Correspondence: easter.joury@kcl.ac.uk
[1]Population and Patient Health, King's College London Dental Institute, Denmark Hill Campus, Bessemer Road, London SE5 9RS, UK
[2]Oral Medicine Department, Faculty of Dentistry, Damascus University, Damascus, Syria
Full list of author information is available at the end of the article

Background

Establishing oral health promoting behaviour at an early stage of life, especially during the first year, should be the foundation for maintaining lifelong health behaviour [1]. Low frequency of free sugars intake is an essential aspect of oral health promoting behaviour [2]. Free sugars are defined as monosaccharides and disaccharides added to foods by the manufacturer, cook or consumer, and sugars naturally present in honey, syrups, fruit juices and fruit concentrates [3]. High frequency of free sugars intake is well-recognised as a determinant of early childhood caries (ECC) [4–6]. The latter is a global public health challenge [7], particularly in low-income countries. For example, Syria, like other countries in the Middle East, had a high prevalence of the disease (86 % in 2013) and a dmft value of 7.7 in preschool children aged 3–5 years.

Children's frequency of free sugars intake is likely to be influenced by social factors such as parents' socioeconomic position (SEP), mother's knowledge of child's oral health behaviour as well as mother's own frequency of free sugars intake. Previous studies conducted on infants or pre-school children have demonstrated social inequalities in children's sugar intake [8, 9]. Children from low SEP were more likely to have sugar-containing beverages than their counterparts from high SEP [8]. In a cross-sectional survey, mother's perceived importance of controlling child's sugary snacking was positively associated with child's desirable sugary snaking behaviour [9].

Studies on infant's sugar intake have focused on dietary patterns or feeding practices [10–12]. For example, mothers whose own diet was characterised by high intakes of sweets, chips, white bread, crisps were more likely to have infants who have high intakes of biscuits, chips, savoury snacks and bread. Conversely, mothers who complied with dietary recommendations, and who had high intakes of fruit, vegetables, wholemeal bread, rice and pasta were more likely to have infants who have comparable diets (high intake of fruit, vegetables and home-prepared foods) [10]. When the presence of cariogenic feeding practices was investigated, infants whose mothers had low education were at 70 % higher risk to have such cariogenic feeding practices than their counterparts whose mothers had high education [12]. Despite the importance of such findings in relation to infant's dietary patterns, frequency of total free sugars intake holds paramount epidemiological and clinical relevance to dentistry [2, 3]. No previous study has investigated social inequalities in infant's frequency of total free sugars intake.

Acknowledging the broader social determinants of frequent free sugars intake among Syrian infants and identifying the groups more likely to engage in this behaviour will potentially enable developing and initiating health promotion policies and interventions to establish desirable low frequency of free sugars intake, early in the life course. Furthermore, information on the social patterning of frequent free sugars intake among infants will help identifying target groups that need tailored health promotion interventions [13]. Therefore, the aims of the present study were: (1) to assess the association of the frequency of free sugars intake among Syrian 1-year-old infants with parents' SEP, mother's knowledge of infant's oral health behaviour and her frequency of free sugars intake; and (2) to explore whether socioeconomic inequalities in infant's frequency of free sugars intake could be explained by differences in mother's knowledge of infant's oral health behaviour and her frequency of free sugars intake.

Methods

Definition of high frequency of free sugars intake

High frequency of free sugar intake was defined as more than 4 occasions per day of cariogenic foods or beverages intake. The latter is considered the point at which caries would most likely develop [14].

Study design, population and sampling

A cross-sectional study was conducted in 2012 on a sample of 1-year-old infants, attending vaccination clinics, at maternal and child health centres (MCHCs) in Damascus, Syria. Infants were selected from three MCHCs, by a systematic random sampling procedure using the MCHCs' monthly vaccination registries (for first birthday vaccinations). The current study's three MCHCs were located in three different areas: affluent, moderate and deprived areas, based on the average Real Estate value per square meter. The percentage of vaccination coverage in Damascus for infants aged 12–23 months was 89.4 % in 2011 [15]. This high percentage is explained by the fact that vaccination is mandatory in Syria and the child's vaccination card is required for school registration.

Sample size calculation

Determining the current study's sample size required an estimate of the prevalence of infant's high frequency of free sugars intake. There was no previous study conducted in Damascus city or Syria that investigated the frequency of free sugars intake in children under 3 years of age. Therefore, it was not feasible to determine *a priori* the aforementioned estimate. To address this, the present study conducted a pilot (on 60 infants; 20 from each MCHC) to draw an estimate of the prevalence of infant's high frequency of free sugars intake. Based on the pilot the prevalence was 40 %. The latter was used to calculate the sample size.

A minimum sample size of 323 was estimated to demonstrate 2-fold or greater odds ratio in explanatory variables between infants with high frequency of free sugars intake and their counterparts with low frequency of free sugars intake. The calculation assumed no less than 40 % of high frequency of free sugars intake's proportion. This calculation set the power of the test at 80 % and the level of significance at 5 %.

Data collection procedures

Mothers of the selected infants were approached by the researcher (MK), in the waiting room, before baby's vaccination. MCHCs usually run vaccination clinics once to twice a week in affluent/moderate and deprived areas, respectively. An informed letter explaining the study's nature and general purpose was distributed to the mothers of selected infants. Thereafter, mothers were asked to complete a questionnaire in the waiting room before baby's vaccination. Ten percent of the mothers were asked to complete the questionnaire again after baby's vaccination to assess the reliability of collected data. This 10 % of mothers were also asked to complete an infant's diet dairy to estimate the validity of infant's frequency of free sugars intake question. A pamphlet on promoting child's oral health was given to mothers after completing the questionnaire.

Questionnaire

Mothers completed a piloted pre-tested structured questionnaire including information on socio-demographic background, infant's frequency of free sugars intake and mother's knowledge about infant's oral health behaviour, as well as her frequency of free sugars intake.

Infant's and mother's frequency of free sugars intake measure

Infant's and mother's frequency of free sugars intake was measured using two questions (one was related to the infant and the other one was related to the mother) as follows: how many times your baby/you consume sugary foods or drinks, such as, biscuits, chocolate, candies/confectionary, soft drinks [including squashes, juices and fizzy drinks], ice-cream, cakes, cookies, crisps, honey, sugary syrups or table sugar [added to meals, milk or teas, or used as a dip for baby's pacifier], jam, halaweh [a tradition Syrian sweet food item], molasses, and other traditional sweets/desserts. The options were: (i) never, (ii) less than once a week. (iii) 1–6 times a week, (iv) 1–4 times a day, (v) more than 4 times a day. The cut off point, of 4 occasions or less per day of cariogenic foods or beverages, was used to dichotomise the frequency of free sugars intake into low [4 times or less a day] and high levels [more than 4 times a day].

Parents' socioeconomic position indicators

SEP information included parents' occupation, working status and educational level. The reason for adopting a number of indicators was due to the fact that socioeconomic position (SEP) is not directly measurable but rather operationalised indirectly by a number of indicators [16]. Parents' occupation included professional and manual occupations. Parents who do not work were grouped in one category. Education was measured by the highest qualification obtained [16] and dichotomised into two levels: high (post secondary school education) and low (secondary school or lower education).

Mother's knowledge about infant's oral health behaviour measure

Mother's knowledge about infant's oral health behaviour was measured by 17 items developed by the current study, based on the British evidence-based guidelines for prevention of caries in children aged 0–3 years [2]. The items covered mother's knowledge about: the importance of breastfeeding (1 item), appropriate time for bottle-feeding termination (around baby's first birthday; 1 items), the best means to provide baby's beverages (Sippy cup/ordinary cup; 1 item), baby's ready food is not the healthiest choice for baby (1 item), the high content of added sugars in baby's ready food (2 items), the potential harmful effect of adding sugars to baby's food and beverages or offering confectionary snacks between meals (3 items), the best time to start cleaning baby's teeth (since the first tooth erupted; 1 items), the best tool to clean baby's teeth (baby's toothbrush; 1 items), the best toothpaste to clean baby's teeth (fluoride toothpaste; 1 items), the correct amount of toothpaste (a smear; 1 item); the frequency of cleaning baby's teeth (at least twice a day; 1 item), the need for dentist consultation regarding professional preventive interventions (1 item), the importance of primary teeth (1 item), and the potential impact of dental caries on baby's general wellbeing (1 item). The correct answers of the aforementioned knowledge items were summed into a final score. Final scores were dichotomised into high and low levels of mother's knowledge about infant's oral health promoting behaviour. Subjects who achieved a score that was equal to or higher than the median were assigned to the high level group whereas subjects who achieved a score that was below the median were assigned to the low level group.

Data analysis

First, the presence of data entry errors was checked. Data were entered twice into separate files using the Statistical Package for Social Science software (SPSS version 20, IBM Corp., Armonk, NY, USA). When these two files were compared differences were highlighted. Any error identified was corrected by checking the infant's questionnaire.

Second, to assess the association between the current study explanatory variables (parents' SEP and mother's knowledge about infant's oral health behaviour and her frequency of free sugars intake) and infant's frequency of free sugars intake, binary logistic regression analyses were performed. Next, to assess the impact of mother's knowledge about infant's oral health behaviour and her frequency of free sugars intake on socioeconomic inequalities in infant's frequency of free sugars intake, a set of logistic regression models adjusted for mother's age, infant's gender and family size, was performed [17]. The most significant SEP indicator was selected for model 1. Socioeconomic position is considered the most distal factor in the causal chain. In model 2, mother's knowledge about infant's oral health behaviour was added. In model 3, mother's frequency of free sugars intake was added as the most proximal factor to infant's frequency of free sugars intake. Finally, model 4 was adjusted for the centre's level of deprivation to confirm the significance of identified social factors.

Results

The response rate was 100 %. Test-retest reliability of collected data on socio-demographic characteristics, infants' and mother's frequency of free sugars intake and mother's knowledge about infant's oral health behaviour was good (rho = 1), indicating perfect agreement. Agreement was also excellent (rho = 1) between the questionnaire and infant's diet diary regarding baby's frequency of free sugars intake (high versus low frequency).

The 323 infants included 151 (46.7 %) males and 172 (53.3 %) females; 83.3 % of infants had a birth weight ≥2500 g.

Overall, 42.7 % infants had high frequency of free sugars intake (more than 4 times a day).

The results of binary logistic regression between the current study social explanatory variables and infant's frequency of free sugars intake are summarised in Table 1.

Infants whose fathers were not working were almost three times more likely to have high frequency of free sugars intake than their counterparts whose fathers had professional occupation (Table 1). In contrast, infants whose mothers were housewives were less likely to have high frequency of free sugars intake than their counterparts whose mothers were working (Table 1). Infants whose mothers had low knowledge about infant's oral health behaviour or high frequency of free sugars intake were two and four times more likely to have high frequency of free sugars intake than their counterparts whose mothers had high knowledge about infant's oral health behaviour or low frequency of free sugars intake; respectively (Table 1).

Amongst SEP indicators, father's occupation was the most significant SEP indicator at the 0.2 level. Thus, it was selected to enter the regression models.

Table 1 Binary logistic regression to predict infant's high frequency of free sugars intake[a]

Variable	Base	Infant's high frequency of free sugars intake (%)	OR (95 % CI)[d]
Father's occupation			
Professional	224	96 (42.9)	1
Manual	74	26 (35.1)	0.7 (0.4–1.3)
Not working	19	13 (68.4)	2.9 (1.1–7.9)[b]
Missing	6		
Father's education[e]			
High	91	40 (44)	1
Low	232	98 (42.2)	0.9 (0.6–1.5)
Missing	0		
Mother's education[e]			
High	70	30(42.9)	1
Low	253	108 (42.7)	0.9 (0.6–1.7)
Missing	0		
Mother's working status			
Working	56	29 (51.8)	1
Housewife	267	109 (40.8)	0.6 (0.4–1.2)
Missing	0		
Mother's knowledge about infant's oral health behaviour[f]			
High	139	11 (8.2 %)	1
Low	181	88 (48.6 %)	1.9 (1.2–2.9)[b]
Missing	3		
Mother's frequency of free sugars intake[g]			
Low	287	112 (39 %)	1
High	36	26 (72.2 %)	4 (1.9–8.8)[c]
Missing	0		

[a] $n = 323$
[b] $P < 0.050$
[c] $P < 0.001$
[d] OR (95 % CI): odds ratios (95 % confidence intervals)
[e] High level refers to post secondary school education, whereas low level refers to secondary school or lower education
[f] Measured by 17 items developed by the current study, based on the British evidence-based guidelines for prevention of caries in children aged 0–3 years [2]. High level refers to scores equal to or higher than the median, whereas low level refers to scores below the median
[g] High level refers to > 4 times a day, whereas low level refers to 4 times or less a day

Regression models, adjusted for mother's age, infant's gender and family size, are presented in Table 2. When mother's knowledge about infant's oral health behaviour and her frequency of free sugars intake were added in model 2 and 3, respectively, the association between father's occupation and infant's frequency of free sugars intake had progressively attenuated and lost its significance (Table 2). The association between infant's frequency of free sugars intake, on the one hand, and mother's knowledge about infant's oral health behaviour

Table 2 A set of logistic regression models [c,d] to predict infant's high frequency of free sugars intake[a]

Variable	Adjusted OR (95 % CI)[e]			
	Model 1[c]	Model 2[c]	Model 3[c]	Model 4[d]
Father's occupation				
Professional	1	1	1	1
Manual	0.7 (0.4–1.3)	0.7 (0.4–1.2)	0.7 (0.4–1.3)	0.7 (0.4–1.3)
Not working	3.1 (1.1–8.5)[b]	2.6 (0.9–7.3)	1.5 (0.5–4.8)	1.4 (0.4–4.4)
Mother's knowledge about infant's oral health behaviour[f]				
High		1	1	1
Low		1.9 (1.2–3.1)[b]	1.8 (1.1–3)[b]	1.8 (1.1–3)[b]
Mother's frequency of free sugars intake[g]				
Low			1	1
High			3.2 (1.4–7.4)[b]	3.2 (1.4–7.4)[b]

[a] $n = 323$
[b] $P < 0.050$
[c] Model 1, 2 and 3 adjusted for mother's age, infant's gender and family size
[d] Model 4 additionally adjusted for centre's level of deprivation
[e] OR (95 % CI): odds ratios (95 % confidence intervals)
[f] Measured by 17 items developed by the current study, based on the British evidence-based guidelines for prevention of caries in children aged 0–3 years [2]. High level refers to scores equal to or higher than the median, whereas low level refers to scores below the median
[g] High level refers to >4 times a day, whereas low level refers to 4 times or less a day

and her frequency of free sugars intake, on the other hand, remained significant before and after adjustment.

Discussion

The current study demonstrated significant social inequalities in infant's frequency of free sugars intake. Socioeconomic inequalities in infant's frequency of free sugars intake were completey explained by mother's frequency of free sugars intake and knowledge of infant's oral health behaviour. To the best of our knowledge, this is the first study to investigate social inequalities in infant's frequency of total free sugars intake and explore whether socioeconomic inequalities in infant's frequency of free sugars intake would attenuate after adjusting for the effect of mother's knowledge about infant's oral health behaviour and her frequency of free sugars intake.

Inequalities in infant's frequency of free sugars intake, identified in the current study, are in line with previous studies on infant's dietary patterns and cariogenic feeding practices [10, 12]. It is worth mentioning that, amongst SEP indicators, mother's education showed inconsistent associations with infant's cariogenic feeding practices. For example, Feldens et al. reported that low maternal education was associated with higher risk of infant's cariogenic feeding practices [12]. In contrast, Contreras et al. found that high maternal education was associated with higher infant's consumption of highly processed snacks and sugar-sweetened beverages [11]. This variation in the relationship between maternal education and infant's sugar consumption is probably attributed to the studied populations. Contreras et al. study was conducted on a rural population where mothers with high education might have more economic capacity to purchase cariogenic foods and beverages, without having appropriate knowledge about the risk of these foods and drinks on baby's health [11]. Whereas Feldens et al. study was conducted on an urban population where mothers with high education might have better knowledge on the risk of cariogenic feeding practices and they might have more economic capacity to provide healthy alternatives to their babies [12].

In the current study, the association between father's occupation and infant's frequency of free sugars intake attenuated after adjustment for mother's knowledge about infant's oral health behaviour and her frequency of free sugars intake. This suggests a potential mediating role of mother's knowledge and frequency of free sugars intake in explaining socioeconomic inequalities in infant's frequency of free sugars intake.

The main limitation of the current study is its cross-sectional design. The significant associations found in this design do not imply causality. Furthermore, the direction of the association cannot be established. However, taking into account the context of the social determinants of health, it is unreasonable to assume that infant's frequency of free sugars intake impacts on social factors such as father's occupation. Despite efforts to minimise the possibility of recall bias by blinding the mothers to the current study's specific scope, this possibility, as in any other retrospective study, could not be completely ruled out in the present study. The current study used one question to estimate the frequency of free sugars intake. Although such question is widely used in oral health surveys and despite the current study's efforts to validate it against another dietary measure, more sophisticated instruments such as food frequency questionnaire might give a more precise estimate. Needless to say that such instruments are expensive to administer and time consuming. Another limitation pertains to the current study's estimates' precision. This is a common limitation of cross-sectional correlational studies that might not allow for a sufficient frequency distribution of different categories within a variable. In addition, correlational studies might not allow exploring all relevant associations. For example, the small numbers of working mothers did not allow exploring the impact of their type of occupation on their infant's frequency of free sugars intake. Yet, the current study serves as a starting point for more expensive prospective longitudinal studies with a larger sample size to confirm the presence of social inequalities and determine the pathways through which these social inequalities are translated into differences in Syrian infant's frequency of free sugars intake.

The current study's findings can only be generalised to the current study's Syrian infant's population. The fact that vaccination is mandatory in Syria supports the generalisability of the current study's findings to infants living in the catchment areas of selected MCHCs.

The importance of the present study's findings is linked to their implications for child's oral and general health in the short term and adult's oral and general health in the long term. Inequalities in infant's frequency of free sugars intake are likely to be translated into inequalities in early childhood caries and child's obesity. For example, infant's high frequency of sugary foods and beverages intake was independently associated with early childhood caries regardless of the frequency of sugars intake at later childhood age or oral hygiene practice [18, 19]. In addition, taste preference is established within the first 2 years of life [20]. Infants who develop a strong sweet taste preference such as that with free sugars might become more likely to have high frequency of free sugars intake in their later life stages [21, 22]. Therefore, it is very likely that such inequalities at an early stage of the life course might also lead to inequalities in adult's frequency of free sugars intake and its related adulthood diseases such as dental caries, obesity and type 2 diabetes.

The policy, research and health promotion programmes implications of the present study's findings could be summarised as follows: there is an urgent need for integrated oral health promotion interventions within the established Syrian national early childhood programmes, such as, breastfeeding and immunisation programmes. These whole population interventions should aim to reduce infant's frequency of free sugars intake. They should also work on improving mother's knowledge about infant's oral health behaviour. To reduce social inequalities in infant's frequency of free sugars intake, the aforementioned whole population programmes should be supported by other tailored oral health education and dietary interventions, targeting families from low SEP. Such interventions integrate the common risk factor approach into the social determinants framework [23], to promote infants' general and oral health. Interventions at the pre-natal stage seem to be of paramount importance [24]. The World Health Organization (WHO) is called to review its recommendation on adding little quantities of sugary items to baby's food [25].

Conclusions

There are significant social inequalities in Syrian infant's frequency of free sugars intake. Socioeconomic inequalities in infant's frequency of free sugars intake might be explained by differences in mother's knowledge about infant's oral health behaviour and her frequency of free sugars intake. Thus, reducing these socioeconomic inequalities might be achieved by designing integrated oral health education and dietary interventions, within Syrian national early childhood programmes, targeting families from low SEP, to improve mother's knowledge about infant's oral health behaviour and reduce her frequency of free sugars intake.

Acknowledgments
The authors wish to thank all Syrian mothers and infants who participated in the current survey, and the staff in the Maternal and Child Health Centres for their support. The authors also express their deep gratitude to Professor Wagner Marcenes and Professor Hyam Bashour for their valuable support and comments on an earlier version of this work.

Funding
The current study was funded by Damascus University. The fund covered the costs of printing the study's questionnaire and oral health education materials. The funding sponsor had no role in the design of the study and collection, analysis, and interpretation of data and in writing the manuscript.

Authors' contributions
EJ conceived the study, performed the statistical analyses, drafted the manuscript, and participated in the design of the study, planning data analyses and data interpretation. MK collected the data, and participated in the design of the study. WS participated in the planning of data analyses and interpreting the data. KE helped in the coordination of study. RB helped in interpreting the data. All authors read and approved the final manuscript and critically reviewed the manuscript.

Authors' information
EJ BDS, DOrth, MSc(Lond), PhD(Lond), MFDS RCPS(Glasg), FHEA, Assistant Professor of Dental Public health and Oral Epidemiology, Damascus University, and Teacher in Dental Public Health, Division of Population and Patient Health, King's College London Dental Institute; MK BDS, MSc, previous MSc candidate in Damascus University; WS BDS, DDPH, PhD, Senior Lecturer in Dental Public Health, Division of Population and Patient Health, King's College London Dental Institute; KE BDS, MSc(Lond), Honorary Lecturer in Restorative Dentistry, Eastman Dental Institute, University College London and Registered specialist with the GDC in Prosthodontics and Endodontics; RB BDS, MSc, DDS, hon DSc, DHL, FDSRCS (Edin), FDRCS (Eng), honFDSRCS (Glas), FGDP, FFPH; Head, Centre for International Child Oral Health, King's College London and Director, Global Child Dental Health taskforce.

Competing interests
The authors declare that they have no competing interests.

Consent for publication
Not applicable.

Ethics approval and consent to participate
Ethical approval was obtained from Damascus University Faculty of Dentistry Research Ethics Committee and the Syrian Ministry of Health (no. 196/2012). Informed written consent was obtained from all participants.

Author details
[1]Population and Patient Health, King's College London Dental Institute, Denmark Hill Campus, Bessemer Road, London SE5 9RS, UK. [2]Oral Medicine Department, Faculty of Dentistry, Damascus University, Damascus, Syria. [3]Eastman Dental Institute, University College London, London WC1X 8LD, UK. [4]Centre for International Child Oral Health, King's College London, 26-29 Drury Lane, Rooms 329-331, London WC2B 5RL, UK.

References

1. Australian Dental Association. Caring for teeth for life. Australian Dental Association. 2007. http://www.pbcexpo.com.au/baby/baby-development/caring-for-baby-teeth/. Accessed 23 July 2014.
2. Department of Health and British Association for the Study of Community Dentistry [BASCD]. Delivering Better Oral Health: an evidence-based toolkit for prevention. 2nd ed. London: Department of Health and British Association for the Study of Community Dentistry; 2009.
3. World Health Organization and Food and Agriculture Organization. Diet, nutrition and the prevention of chronic diseases; report of a joint WHO/FAO expert consultation. Geneva: WHO; 2002.
4. Harris R, Nicoll AD, Adair PM, Pine CM. Risk factors for dental caries in young children: a systematic review of the literature. Community Dent Health. 2004;21 Suppl 1:71–85.
5. McDonagh MS, Whiting PF, Wilson PM, Sutton AJ, Chestnutt I, Cooper J, et al. Systematic review of water fluoridation. BMJ. 2000;321:855–9.
6. Marinho VC. Cochrane reviews of randomized trials of fluoride therapies for preventing dental caries. Eur Arch Paediatr Dent. 2009;10:183–91.
7. Kassebaum NJ, Bernabé E, Dahiya M, Bhandari B, Murray CJ, Marcenes W. Global burden of untreated caries: a systematic review and metaregression. J Dent Res. 2015;94:650–8.
8. Wijtzes AI, Jansen W, Jansen PW, Jaddoe VW, Hofman A, Raat H. Maternal educational level and preschool children's consumption of high-calorie snacks and sugar-containing beverages: mediation by the family food environment. Prev Med. 2013;57:607–12.
9. Adair PM, Pine CM, Burnside G, Nicoll AD, Gillett A, Anwar S, et al. Familial and cultural perceptions and beliefs of oral hygiene and dietary practices among ethnically and socio-economically diverse groups. Community Dent Health. 2004;21(Suppl1):102–11.
10. Robinson S, Marriott L, Poole J, Crozier S, Borland S, Lawrence W, et al. Dietary patterns in infancy: the importance of maternal and family influences on feeding practice. Br J Nutr. 2007;98:1029–37.
11. Contreras M, Blandón EZ, Persson LÅ, Hjern A, Ekström EC. Socio-economic resources, young child feeding practices, consumption of highly processed snacks and sugar-sweetened beverages: a population-based survey in rural northwestern Nicaragua. BMC Public Health. 2015;15:25.
12. Feldens CA, Kramer PF, Sequeira MC, Rodrigues PH, Vitolo MR. Maternal education is an independent determinant of cariogenic feeding practices in the first year of life. Eur Arch Paediatr Dent. 2012;13:70–5.
13. Watt RG. Strategies and approaches in oral diseaseprevention and health promotion. Bull World Health Org. 2005;83:711–8.
14. Moynihan PJ, Kelly SA. Effect on caries of restricting sugars intake: systematic review to inform WHO guidelines. J Dent Res. 2014;93:8–18.
15. Central Bureau of Statistics. Family health survey in the Syrian Arab Republic, 2009-2010. 2011. http://www.cbssyr.sy/index-EN.htm. Accessed 2 Jan 2016.
16. Liberatos P, Link BG, Kelsey JL. The measurement of social class in epidemiology. Epidemiol Rev. 1988;10:87–121.
17. Altman DG. Practical statistics for medical research. London: Chapman and Hall; 1991.
18. Park S, Lin M, Onufrak S, Li R. Association of sugar-sweetened beverage intake during infancy with dental caries in 6-year-olds. ClinNutr Res. 2015;4:9–17.
19. Chaffee BW, Feldens CA, Rodrigues PH, Vítolo MR. Feeding practices in infancy associated with caries incidence in early childhood. Community Dent Oral Epidemiol. 2015;doi: 10.1111/cdoe.12158.
20. Ventura AK, Worobey J. Early influences on the development of food preferences. Curr Biol. 2013;23:R401–8.
21. Beauchamp GK, Moran M. Acceptance of sweet and salty tastes in 2-year-old children. Appetite. 1984;5:291–305.
22. Park S, Pan L, Sherry B, Li R. The association of sugar-sweetened beverage intake during infancy with sugar-sweetened beverage intake at 6 years of age. Pediatrics. 2014;134 Suppl 1:56–62.
23. Watt RG, Sheiham A. Integrating the common risk factor approach into asocial determinants framework. Community Dent Oral Epidemiol. 2012;40:289–96.
24. Plutzer K, Spencer AJ. Efficacy of an oral health promotion intervention in the prevention of early childhood caries. Community Dent Oral Epidemiol. 2008;36:335–46.
25. World Health Organization. Consultation on infants and young children feeding; a participant guide. 2006.http://applications.emro.who.int/dsaf/dsa719.pdf?ua=1. Accessed 12 May 2015.

4

The impact of a formal complaint on Dutch dentists' professional practice

Josef J. M. Bruers[1,2*], Brigitte A. F. M. van Dam[2], Ronald C. Gorter[1] and Michiel A. J. Eijkman[1]

Abstract

Background: A complaint from a patient can have a serious impact on the well-being of dentists. Little is known, however, about the nature and the extent of this impact.

Methods: Therefore in 2013 an anonymous survey was conducted among 955 dentists and dental specialists who were involved in a complaints procedure dealt with by the Complaints Committee of the Royal Dutch Dental Association (KNMT) in the period of mid-2008 to mid-2013.

Results: In total 413 (43 %) of these dentists participated in the study. As a result of a formal complaint 71 % of the respondents experienced a considerable impact in their professional practising, while 52 % stated that it had (also) seriously influenced their attitude towards colleagues and patients. Furthermore, 60 % (also) mentioned effects of a complaints procedure regarding their mental and/or physical well-being.

Conclusions: Being confronted with a formal complaint from a patient leads to a considerable impact on dentists' professional practice and personal well-being. It is remarkable this did not only pertain to a 'negative' impact, but also to a 'positive' impact. Despite unpleasant feelings, several dentists regarded the complaint as a 'wake-up call'. Furthermore, given the relatively high number of successful mediation attempts it can be concluded that this form of complaint handling appears to be a successful way of solving problems that have arisen between patients and dentists.

Keywords: Formal complaint, Patient dentist communication, General dental practice, Dentist

Background

This article is an edited translation of a previously published original article written in Dutch [1]. In 2012 nearly 8 out of 10 (77 %) Dutch citizens consulted a dentist, which they did on average 2.5 times [2]. By and large this amounts to well over 32.5 million contacts between patients and dentists per year. In general, these contacts go well and are satisfactory to the patient [3]. Nevertheless, it does happen that feelings of discomfort, annoyance, or anger about the care rendered arise in a patient. This may be the result of mistakes that may have been made, missed appointments, conduct experienced as a rebuff, too high expectations of the treatment, inadequate organisation of care, uncertainty about who performs the treatment, or a difference of opinion on the size of the bill [4]. Boers & Sanaan investigated 401 complaints dealt with by the Central Complaints Committee (CKC) within the complaints procedure of the Royal Dutch Dental Association (KNMT) in the period of 2005-2011 [5]. They categorised 826 complaint components, on which the CKC had given a verdict. It appeared that 49 % were related to dental technical and 50 % to organisational aspects or patient rights.

The complaints procedure of the KNMT meets the requirements such as laid down by the Dutch *Health Sector Client Complaints Act* and is meant for members of the KNMT, the largest professional organisation of dentists in the Netherlands with about 7,200 registered

* Correspondence: j.bruers@acta.nl
[1]Department of Social Dentistry and Behavioural Sciences, Academic Centre for Dentistry Amsterdam (ACTA), University of Amsterdam and VU University, Gustav Mahlerlaan 3004, 1081 LA Amsterdam, The Netherlands
[2]Department of Research and Information, Royal Dutch Dental Association (KNMT), Nieuwegein, The Netherlands

individual dentists and dental specialists [6, 7]. This amounts to 83 % of the total population of 9,258 dentists and dental specialists, aged 64 or younger with a home and/or work address in the Netherlands [8]. In addition, the second largest professional organisation, the Association of Dutch Dentists (ANT) also has a complaints procedure complying with the law. The ANT has a membership of approximately 2,300 registered individual dentists and dental specialists and their Dental Complaints Committee deals with patient complaints for 1,500 of their registered members [9].

An overview of the total number of complaints against Dutch dentists filed annually is not available. Besides the KNMT and ANT complaints procedures there is also the possibility to lodge a complaint with the regional health care disciplinary boards. Furthermore, an as yet unknown number of complaints are lodged against dentists in the civil courts and with the Public Health Care Inspectorate. In addition, when determining the number of complaints against dentists, the fact that more and more institutions have their own boards of complaint should be taken into consideration. However, in 2013 the KNMT complaints procedure dealt with 957 letters of complaint, 454 of which were in fact followed up in a procedure as a formal complaint [10]. In that year with the ANT this concerned 223 complaints, 111 of which were found viable with 50 resulting in a formal procedure [11]. In 2006 it was estimated that on average Dutch dentists are confronted with a complaint resulting in a procedure once in their professional career [12]. Based on the before mentioned figures it can be assumed that the average number of complaints has increased to several times in a dentists' career.

From some personal experiences it becomes clear that dentists are not often aware of the possibility that they could become involved in a complaint procedure and that, if this does happen, it may have a serious impact. Sleepless nights, thoughts going round in circles and health problems are mentioned, as well as the time a procedure takes and the stressful build-up to the hearing. Feelings of insecurity taking away the pleasure of work and the tendency to see every patient as a potential threat is also reported [13]. In this dentists are not unique: similar experiences of other Dutch care providers have been recorded [14]. Furthermore, several international studies also report that receiving a medical complaint has a significant negative impact on a doctor, ranging from stress, significant risks of moderate or severe depression and adjustment disorder to also drug and alcohol abuse, anxiety and other forms of physical illness [15–19].

While there is some data available on the nature and seriousness of the impact of a complaint on care providers, little is actually known when it concerns dentists. More knowledge is however desirable: it may contribute to raising awareness within the profession that one may be faced with a formal complaint and should be prepared how to best cope with this, both personally and professionally. In addition, more knowledge can be used to inform dentists - and dental students - about how complaints can best be prevented. Eventually this will contribute to a higher quality of patient care. Given the sparse knowledge on this topic, the aim of the present study was investigate the impact of a formal complaint (and the following procedure) on dentists' professional practising and personal well-being.

Methods

The study was built up in two phases. It started in the spring of 2012 with a pilot study, in which semi-structured oral interviews were held with 17 dentists and dental specialists who had been in a KNMT complaints procedure [13, 20]. The outcome of this pilot served as input for a quantitative investigation by a questionnaire among a larger group of dentists who faced a complaint which was dealt with via the KNMT complaints procedure. In view of the sensitivity of the topic it was decided to conduct this part of the study by means of an entirely anonymous survey in writing. The questionnaire was constructed based on the categories that emerged from the pilot study. The categories were on: (a) the nature of the complaint and the course of the procedure; (b) the consequences experienced in various aspects of the dentists' professional practising after the complaints (procedure); (c) the impact one's their mental and physical well-being; and (d) how the complaints procedure had been experienced. Because of the anonymous nature of the investigation, some general personal and practice characteristics were asked for. After the concept questionnaire was constructed, it was commented upon by an independent Research Committee of the KNMT, which led to some minor modifications.

The research group was defined by all Dutch dentists and dental specialists against whom a formal complaint had been lodged and dealt with via the KNMT complaints procedure in the period of 2008 up to and including the spring of 2013. For this occasion, exclusive permission from the KNMT Executive Board was granted to address this group. In this period 1 or more complaints against 1,013 dentists and dental specialists were dealt with via successful mediation by one of the Regional Mediation Boards (RBR) and/or via the Central Complaints Committee (CKC). The complaints procedure of the Royal Dutch Dental Association (KNMT) offers patients two options. The first option is mediation between the patient and the dentist by a Regional Mediation Board (RBR) or the Specialist Mediation Board (SBR). In case the mediation failed or the patient refuses to try mediation, the second option is for the patient to file a formal complaint with the Central Complaints Committee (CKC). The CKC can declare the complaint either entirely or partially legitimate or unfounded.

By the end of May 2013 this group was first contacted in writing. They received a letter in which the survey was announced and its background explained. Because the topic might trigger memories people were not overly keen to be questioned about, dentists who would rather not participate were offered the opportunity to report this: 58 prospective participants in the survey did so. The remaining 955 dentists and dental specialists received the questionnaire a few weeks later. Ultimately, after two reminders 413 (43 %) of them responded.

As for gender, age group and place of qualification the divisions within the group of respondents did not show significant differences from those in the intended research group. Comparison between respondents and non-respondents with regard to the way in which the complaint had been dealt with and, if applicable, the verdict from the Central Complaints Committee (CKC), also showed no significant differences.

It may safely be assumed that, as far as the aforementioned characteristics of the dentists and dental specialists in the survey are concerned, these constitute a reasonably representative reflection of the entire group of dentists and dental specialists against whom in the research period a complaint was dealt with via the KNMT complaints procedure. The data collected was analysed by means of SPSS [21].

Results

Nature and handling of the complaint

In the opinion of the dentists questioned, in 58 % of all cases the cause of the complaint had to do with dissatisfaction with treatment patient, while 29 % refers to patient behaviour ('an attempt by the patient to 'squeeze every last drop out of the situation'), 20 % to patient communication, 19 % to costs of treatment and 12 % to another aspect (Table 1).

More than half (51 %) of the dentists questioned said that the complaint against them had been dealt with via successful mediation by the Regional or Specialists Mediation Boards (RBR/SBR), whereas 17 % stated that the patient had withdrawn the complaint during the procedure. In all other cases (32 %) the complaint had been dealt with by the CKC, directly or after a failed attempt at mediation.

The complaints against 130 dentists who appeared before the CKC were declared entirely legitimate in 23 % of the cases, and partially legitimate in 18 %. 55 % of the cases were declared unfounded; in 3 % of the cases parties still agreed on a settlement and in 1 % the complaint was declared unsustainable. Looking at the total number of complaints that were mediated, withdrawn and dealt with this comes down to 13 % of (partially) legitimate complaints.

Table 1 Aspects related to the complaint lodged, according to dentists[a]

Regarding treatment		58 %
- No or insufficient result after treatment	24 %	
- Incorrect execution of (parts of) treatment	17 %	
- A complication after treatment, pain during treatment	15 %	
- Critical remarks from a another dentist about treatment rendered	14 %	
- No or insufficient aftercare	4 %	
- Wrong diagnosis	4 %	
- Discontentment about treatment delegated to the oral hygienist	2 %	
Regarding treatment		29 %
- An attempt by the patient to squeeze every last drop out of the situation	29 %	
Regarding treatment		20 %
- Incorrect attitude towards the patient	9 %	
- Insufficient or lacking information about treatment or treatment plan	8 %	
- Bad communication/rapport, incomprehension	5 %	
Regarding treatment		19 %
- Cost of treatment, bills, uncertainty about payments and/or reimbursements	19 %	
Regarding treatment		12 %

$n = 411$
[a]More than one response allowed

Table 2 shows that the perceived nature of a complaint was related to the handling of a complaint. Especially when a complaint was dealt with by the CKC relatively often (34 % versus 23 %) the complaint was related to multiple aspects (treatment, costs, communication and/or patient behaviour) and in relatively few cases to only costs. Furthermore, the perceived nature of a complaint showed no relation with gender and age of the dentists.

Experienced consequences of the complaint

Being confronted with a complaint had affected 29 % to a large extent or strongly in their personal professional practising, whereas 42 % reported they were affected somewhat. 29 % stated not to be affected (Table 3). Dentists who were involved in the CKC reported more frequently the effects on their professional practising than colleagues whose complaints had been dealt with via mediation (83 % against 65 %; $p < 0.05$).

Table 4 (A) offers an overview of the way in which the complaint had influenced their personal professional practising. With the exception of the experienced result 'the complaint was a blemish to my good reputation as a dentist' there proved to be little difference as to the nature in which the complaint was handled.

Table 2 Aspects related to the complaint lodged, according to dentists, in relation to the way in which the complaint was handled

Aspects related to the complaint lodged regarding:[a]	RBR/SBR or withdrawn	CKC	Total
Treatment	32 %	34 %	32 %
Treatment + costs, communication and/or patient behaviour	23 %	34 %	27 %
Costs	11 %	2 %	8 %
Costs + communication and/or patient behaviour	5 %	2 %	4 %
Communication	11 %	6 %	9 %
Communication + patient behaviour	2 %	3 %	2 %
Patient behaviour (+ some other aspect)	10 %	9 %	10 %
Some other aspect/unknown	6 %	10 %	8 %
n	278	130	408

[a]More than one response allowed
*Chi Square test: $p = 0.00$/Cramer's V = 0.22

As is shown in Table 3, more than half (52 %) of the respondents had experienced that the complaint had influenced the attitude and/or the feelings towards other colleagues at work. This was also more applicable to those who ended up with the CKC than to those whose complaint was dealt with through mediation (63 % against 47 %; $p < 0.05$).

From Table 4 (B) it appears that this mainly concerned the attitude and/or the feeling towards patients. Only the feeling of 'every (new) patient was seen as a possible risk', which occurred the most, was felt more frequently in dentists who were dealing with the CKC than in those whose complaint had been dealt with through mediation.

Furthermore, 60 % stated that the after effects of the complaint affected their mental and physical well-being (Table 2). Dentists who ended up with the CKC reported this more often than their colleagues whose complaints could be mediated (69 % against 57 %; $p < 0.05$). Table 4 (C) shows to what kind of mental and physical problems this pertained. Sleeping disorders and feelings of anxiety, stress and fatigue were experienced more by dentists who had been through the 'CKC trajectory' than by dentists who had undergone a 'mediation trajectory'.

All things considered it appears that 21 % of the dentists did not report any impact, 6 % only a positive impact, 42 % a mixed impact and 31 % only a negative impact (Table 5). Moreover dentists whose complaint was dealt with by the CKC reported more often only a negative or a mixed impact than dentists whose complaint had been dealt with through mediation (86 % versus 66 %; $p < 0.05$).

On the whole, 32 % of the respondents indicated that they were not burdened by unpleasant feelings as a result of the complaint. Others were troubled at the most for some weeks (26 %), some months up to a year (31 %), or longer than a year (11 %). It was noted that only one person was off sick as a result of the complaint, but just for a few days.

Table 3 Extent to which the complaint has affected dentists, in relation to the way in which the complaint was handled

	RBR/SBR or withdrawn	CKC	Total
Did the complaint affect your professional practising*			
- Not at all	35 %	17 %	29 %
- Somewhat	44 %	38 %	42 %
- Largely/strongly	21 %	45 %	29 %
Did the complaint affect your attitude/feelings towards patients, colleagues and/or co-workers*			
- Not at all	53 %	37 %	48 %
- Somewhat	37 %	45 %	39 %
- Largely/strongly	10 %	18 %	13 %
Did the complaint affect your mental and/or physical well-being*			
- Not at all	43 %	31 %	40 %
- Somewhat	42 %	43 %	42 %
- Largely/strongly	15 %	26 %	18 %
n	279	130	409

*Chi Square test: $p < 0.05$

Effects on rendering care

In most of the cases (75 %) the relationship between the dentist and the patient was permanently damaged as a result of the complaint and the complainant had left to go to another dentist; in practically all cases to another practice (Table 6). In 8 % this was not yet clear and also in another 8 % the complainant had left the practice some time ago, the complainant had been treated after referral, or elsewhere during a weekend, or the dentist himself had left and was already working somewhere else. In 9 % of the cases the complainant had remained with the dentist.

Nearly two thirds (64 %) of the dentists said that as a result of the complaint they had become more alert on certain aspects of care or had made changes. Table 7 shows that 53 % of these dentists have become more alert to signals of doubt from patients or too high expectations regarding the treatment. Besides, they are now documenting more accurately what has been discussed with patients about the results and risks of the treatment (49 %). It was also mentioned that they were going to document more treatment data in patient records (46 %), they would pay (even) more attention to patient communication (43 %) and/or better guard their own professional limits when following the patients' wishes (33 %).

Table 4 Extent to which being confronted with a complaint has affected somewhat, largely or strongly (A) the personal professional practising of dentists, (B) the attitude and/or feeling of dentists towards patients, colleagues and/or staff and (C) the mental and/or physical well-being of dentists, related to the way in which the complaint was handled

	RBR/SBR or with-drawn	CKC	Total
A personal professional practising[a]			
$_p$The complaint was a signal to improve/do things differently ('wake-up call')	41 %	37 %	39 %
$_n$The complaint was a blemish on my good reputation as a dentist*	29 %	44 %	35 %
$_n$I started frequent 'checking and double checking' during treatment	19 %	22 %	20 %
$_n$To me the complaint felt like a personal let down	17 %	17 %	17 %
$_n$I became unsure in my professional functioning	16 %	19 %	17 %
$_n$I became unsure when rendering certain (types of) treatment	9 %	15 %	12 %
$_n$I try to avoid/no longer do certain treatment	9 %	14 %	11 %
$_n$I felt indignation, anger, injustice[b]	11 %	8 %	10 %
$_n$I am more distrustful, cautious, insecure, selective towards patients[b]	5 %	6 %	5 %
-other	13 %	9 %	11 %
n	181	109	290
B attitude and/or feeling of dentists towards patients, colleagues and/or staff)[a]			
$_n$Started seeing every (new) patient as a possible risk*	38 %	55 %	44 %
$_p$The complaint has taught me to recognize dissatisfaction of patients earlier	34 %	22 %	29 %
$_n$Became more reserved when dealing with (certain similar) patients	26 %	32 %	28 %
$_n$Left dealing with certain patients if possible to colleagues or associates	9 %	9 %	9 %
$_p$Tried to recognize risky patients better (contact, treatment)[b]	5 %	5 %	5 %
$_n$Had less patience in contacts with patients	4 %	4 %	4 %
$_n$Felt insecure in my professional functioning towards colleagues or associates	8 %	8 %	8 %
$_n$Felt frustrated by disloyal behaviour from colleagues (who caused complaint)[b]	2 %	5 %	3 %
$_n$Felt towards my associates that my 'authority' as a dentist was undermined	2 %	5 %	3 %
$_n$Had less patience in contacts with colleagues or associates	1 %	2 %	1 %
-Other	17 %	16 %	16 %
n	131	82	213
C mental and/or physical well-being[a]			
$_n$I had feelings of anger and/or aggression	57 %	47 %	53 %
$_n$I felt powerless	44 %	52 %	47 %
$_n$I had sleep disorders*	22 %	34 %	26 %
$_n$I became suspicious of other people	22 %	18 %	20 %
$_n$I felt (continually) scared, tense or tired/stressed*	14 %	27 %	19 %
$_n$In the morning I (often) went to work reluctantly	14 %	17 %	15 %
$_n$I considered to quit work entirely	10 %	17 %	12 %
$_n$I had physical complaints, such as heart palpitations, headaches, sickness	8 %	11 %	9 %
$_n$I was afraid of getting a nervous breakdown	5 %	8 %	6 %
- Other	10 %	13 %	11 %
n	158	90	248

$_p$Considered as 'positive' impact

$_n$Considered as 'negative' impact

*Difference between dentists, according to the way in which the complaint was handled (RBR/SBR or withdrawn versus CKC), Chi Square test: $p < 0.05$

[a]More than one response allowed

[b]Spontaneous response (expressed in respondents own words)

Table 5 Impact of a formal complaint as reported by dentists, in relation to the way in which the complaint was handled

Reported impact	RBR/SBR or withdrawn	CKC	Total
Only positive impact	7 %	3 %	6 %
Both positive and negative impact	38 %	49 %	42 %
Only negative impact	28 %	37 %	31 %
No impact reported/impact unknown	26 %	11 %	21 %
n	279	130	409

Chi Square test: $p = 0.00$ / Cramer's $V = 0.21$

Table 7 Aspects of care dentists have changed or have become more aware of as a result of the complaint[a]

- More attentive to patients' signals of doubt or too high expectations of treatment	53 %
- More accurate documentation of what has been discussed with the patient about the results and risks of treatment	49 %
- More documentation of treatment data in patient records	46 %
- (Even) more attention for patient communication	43 %
- Better safeguarding one's own professional limits when following patients' wishes	33 %
- Documentation of patients' consent with regard to treatment	18 %
- Clearer procedures within the dental team about the recording of patient data	16 %
- Clearer procedures within the dental team about patient communication	15 %
- Earlier consultations with a colleague in case of problems with a patient	8 %
- Earlier consultations with a colleague about treatment or a treatment proposal	6 %
- More careful when expressing opinions to patients about the work of colleagues	3 %
- Other aspect	13 %

n = 265
[a]More than one response allowed

Discussion

In the present study the focus was on the consequences of a complaints procedure for dentists and dental specialists. The questions were not limited to information about the effects on the professional practising of these health care providers and their attitude towards patients, colleagues and/or staff, but also pertained to their mental and/or physical well-being. Eight out of 10 respondents indicated that they had experienced a considerable impact in at least one of these areas. It is remarkable this did not only pertain to a 'negative' impact, but also to a 'positive' impact. It is true that two thirds of the respondents mentioned unpleasant feelings as a result of the complaint, but at the same time 4 out of 10 dentists (also) regarded the complaint as a 'wake-up call'. So, the complaints procedure obviously also generates a 'spontaneous' effect on the profession with regard to the quality of care [7].

Several studies indicate that in relatively many cases complainants are not satisfied with the outcome of a formal complaint procedure [22]. This has to do with the circumstance that doctors often fail to respond in line with what complainants are looking for: in particular an explanation and/or an apology [23, 24]. The chances of getting an explanation and/or an apology are greater in a more informal handling of a complaint, which therefore seems beneficial to patients. Anyway, this study proves that the more informal 'mediation trajectory' leads to less dentists who experience a negative impact. Presumed that also more patients are positive about the outcome when the complaint was handled by mediation, the results of this survey suggest that a two-stage complaints procedure as described meets the needs of patients to some extent and enables them to hold dentists accountable when they are of the opinion that they have not been dealt with adequately [25]. Especially the relatively high number of successful mediation attempts indicates that this form of complaint handling appears to be a successful way of solving problems that have arisen between patients and dentists. In this way more burdensome procedures are being prevented, both for dentists and patients.

Table 6 Patient who lodged the complaint did or did not remain with the dentist for treatment, related to the way in which the complaint was handled

	RBR/SBR or withdrawn	CKC	Total
Yes, the patient remained with the dentist for treatment	11 %	3 %	9 %
No, the patient went to another dentist within the practice	1 %	2 %	1 %
No, the patient went to another dentist in another practice	71 %	80 %	74 %
This is not (yet) clear	8 %	9 %	8 %
Not applicable[a]	9 %	6 %	8 %
n	275	129	404

[a]Patient was just passing (weekend, transferred) or left to another dentist (long ago), or the dentist was already working in another practice

Thus from the many successful mediation results it can be derived that in dentist - patient communication there is room for improvement. About half of the respondents indicated they had learned to better improve at this point. This was also suggested by Boers and Sanaan and, for that matter, the respondents themselves also agreed [5]. Several respondents said that as a result of the complaint they are more alert to signals of doubt from patients or too high expectations of treatment, pay more attention to communication with patients, better safeguard their own professional limits when following patients' wishes and/or make procedures clearer within the dental team about patient communication. In a survey aimed at the way in which dentists deal with rules and regulations regarding patient communication it was noted earlier that there was room for improvement [26]. In connection to the above about half of the dentists questioned also said that in the future they will pay more attention to good documentation of what has been discussed and agreed upon with patients. Both careful communication and adequate documentation should be considered as major tools to help prevent a dentist from being confronted with a formal complaint procedure. It is strongly recommended to emphasize this in both graduate and postgraduate education.

Nobody looks forward to receiving a complaint and therefore it is not strange that unpleasant feelings arise when this happens. Many a dentist does not seem to be upset for too long and sees a complaint as a warning. But it also becomes clear that other dentists will still be seriously 'out of sorts' when they are confronted with a complaint. They feel their good reputation is blemished, experience the complaint as a personal let down, lose their self confidence in contacts with patients, colleagues and staff and/or become mentally unbalanced (stress, suspicious, insomnia). It is difficult to describe this in general, since personal characteristics naturally play a part. But that the impact is substantial in a number of cases has perhaps something to do with the fact that in oral health care it often concerns long treatment relationships in which trust has developed. This is in the interest of the patient, but also of the dentist. Silverman et al. point out that 'the development of a long term relationship with patients is experienced by most care providers as the most satisfying aspect of their work' [27]. A complaint is synonym to a violation to this. Therefore, it can lead to the strong impact dentists are mentioning, certainly when a complaint is lodged unexpectedly and when the patient goes to another dentist, which is often the case. This is also in accordance with the results of research on burnout among dentists which shows that a breach of trust with patients leads to more stress [28]. Here we must indicate that in this survey a relatively `dentist-friendly procedure' has been under investigation, without public hearings and serious measures. It may be assumed that the impact of a disciplinary hearing, which can have a considerably stronger and more formal character, will even be greater. All the more, since this survey already showed that the impact of a 'heavier' CKC trajectory had been greater than the impact of a 'lighter' mediation trajectory. All in all, the impact Dutch dentists experience when confronted with a formal complaint was in most cases unpleasant, but temporal and in any case less severe than the situation a physician gets after a serious adverse patient event. The impact of such an event is defined by the concept of 'second victim', e.g. a health care provider involved in an unanticipated adverse event, a medical error and/or a patient related injury who becomes victimized in the sense that he or she is seriously traumatized by the event [29]. The prevalence of second victims after an adverse event varies from 10 % up to 43 %. Common reactions can be emotional, cognitive, and behavioral [30]. None of the dentists in this survey has mentioned impact that could characterize him or her as a second victim. Generally, adverse events in oral health care are rare, not life-threatening or having serious consequences [31]. Besides, complaints about serious patient events in dentistry are brought to the Disciplinary board and seldom dealt with via the KNMT complaints procedure.

When it concerns patient complaints of course it always goes that prevention is better than the cure. Here, first and foremost, the responsibility lies with the dentist himself. The aspects of care in this survey that dentists have changed as a result of a complaint lodged against them can form a leitmotif for prevention. In short: consideration for and attentiveness towards patients, clear and thoughtful explanation of oral health and the pros and cons of treatment, 'informed consent' and adequate documentation can prevent complaints. The Institute of Medicine does not describe in vain good communications with patients as 1 in 6 criteria of good medical care [32]. In this way wishes and preferences of patients can be taken into account and decisions can be made by mutual agreement. In addition clear work procedures within the team and consultations with colleagues in case of troublesome and/or difficult treatment are also important points of attention in the prevention of complaints.

Here contributions can also be made at a more collective level. Of course this already starts in education. Van der Ven et al. advocate that dentists have to be imparted with sufficient knowledge on health care legislation and patient rights in their academic studies and later on via post academic education [7]. In addition, the professional oral health care organisations can also contribute, for example by providing their members with tools for good patient communications (information, training courses) and adequate documentation. All sorts of guidelines and other knowledge documents can help oral health care providers in rendering well-considered care to patients. Good patient information from the professional organisation, by means of a website or a telephone service, can also prevent complaints. That these initiatives emanate a preventive effect is already known from experiences with TIP, a telephone service in the Netherlands where patients can pose all kinds of questions about the treatment (plans) of their dentist. Thus, in 2012 the TIP answered calls from approximately 4,600 people. 58 % of these calls ended in the patient declaring that he/she intended to (re) open the discussion with the dentist, 17 % wanted consultations with a third party and 18 % refrained from further actions. The remaining 6 % (still) intended to lodge a complaint against their dentist [33].

In the perception of several dentists a complaint has to do with a patient who aims to squeeze every last drop out of a situation. From the data of this study it can't be determined whether this perception is correct. Probably this interpretation stems from the fact that in the Netherlands dental treatment is not or only partially reimbursed for adults. In case of a complaint regarding treatment it is conceivable that dentists experience that patients exploit the situation. Especially, because dentists tend to fail to fully explain the content and costs of a treatment.

This study has some weaknesses, which have to do with the type of data. First of all it concerns retrospective data, representing the recollection of dentists regarding thought, feelings and experiences they had in the past. For some the past could be a few years ago and for others some months ago. Respondents can under- or overestimate their earlier reactions. In any case, this forms a risk with regard to the reliability of the data.

Furthermore, because of the anonymous character of the data collection it is difficult to determine exactly to what extent these results are representative for all the dentists who were confronted with a complaint in the past few years. Besides, it must be kept in mind that patients can also lodge their complaints elsewhere, including e.g. with the regional health care disciplinary boards. In 2013 a total of 104 complaints against dentists were lodged with these disciplinary boards, 27 (26 %) of which were ultimately declared legitimate [34]. It is known, however, that these may include complaints that were also lodged with the KNMT or other complaints procedures. A straightforward comparison between these complaints procedures is therefore not possible. Finally the cross sectional design has its limitations. The study deals with the impact on dentists of a complaint. To fully understand this phenomenon a more comprehensive study in time is required.

Nevertheless, this study yields relevant and new information on the impact of complaints of patients on dentists. This information can be cons id ered acceptably representative since it covers the situation in the Netherlands nationwide over a period of several years. Moreover, from a comparison of a number of relevant characteristics it has been made plausible that the participants in this survey constitute a reasonable reflection of the total population of dentists and dental specialists who were confronted with a complaint through the KNMT complaints procedure.

Conclusions

Being confronted with a formal complaint from a patient has a serious impact on many dentists. This not only affects the different aspects of professional practise, but also mental and physical well-being. The handling of a complaint through mediation appears to be preferable to dealing with the complaint by means of a verdict from the CKC. Anyway, dentists for whom the complaint was successfully mediated reported fewer 'negative' consequences in certain respects. Moreover, it is not just a matter of 'negative' impact (stress, blemished reputations, anger etc.), a complaint is often also read as a signal to do things better. To a majority of dentists who are confronted with a complaint this is therefore the reason to change certain matters in the care they render. In doing so, a great deal of attention is paid to improve on communication with patients and on documentation of the care rendered. It is recommended to make this lesson learned also part of dental (post)graduate curricula.

Abbreviations

ACTA: Academic Centre for Dentistry Amsterdam; ANT: Association of Dutch Dentists; CKC: Central Complaints Committee; KNMT: Royal Dutch Dental Association; RBR: Regional mediation board; SBR: Specialists mediation board; TIP: Dental information point

Acknowledgements

Not applicable.

Funding

The study was funded by the KNMT (Royal Dutch Dental Association). A financial contribution was received from Legal Insurance Company ARAG (located in Leusden, the Netherlands), who financed half of the costs of the pilot study that was conducted in preparation of the main study.

Authors' contributions

All authors participated in the design of the pilot study. RG conducted the oral interviews and reported the results. JB and BD designed the quantitative investigation and ME and RG commented on the questionnaire. JB and BD took care of the acquisition of data and JB was responsible for the analysis and interpretation of data. JB drafted the manuscript and BD, RG and ME revisited it critically for important intellectual content. All authors read and approved the final manuscript.

Competing interests

The authors declare that they have no competing interests.

Consent for publication

Not applicable.

Ethics approval and consent to participate

The study protocol was approved by an independent review board of the KNMT (Royal Dutch Association of Dentists). Dentists eligible for participation received a written letter in which the survey was announced and its background explained. Those who would rather not participate were offered the opportunity to report this and were excluded from the research group. Those who didn't report any objections received a fully anonymous questionnaire. By completion and returning the written questionnaire (by freepost), dentists consented participation. Returned questionnaires could not be traced back to the dentist who answered the questions.

References

1. Bruers JJM, van Dam BAFM, Gorter R, Eijkman MAJ. Het welbevinden van tandartsen na een klachtenprocedure. Ned Tijdschr Tandheelkd. 2015;122: 41–8. doi:10.5177/ntvt.205.01.14152.
2. CBS Statistics Netherlands. Medische contacten, ziekenhuisopname, medicijnen; leeftijd, geslacht. Statline, [Internet] 2014 [updated 2014 Feb 1; cited 2014 Apr 3]. Available from: http://statline.cbs.nl/StatWeb/

publication/?DM=SLNL&PA=81178NED&D1=25-27&D2=1-2&D3=a&D4=0&D5=l&VW=T
3. 3 CBS Statistics Netherlands. Nederlanders tevreden over arts en fysiotherapeut. [Internet] 2012 [updated 2012 Sept 20; cited 2014 Apr 3]. Available from: http://www.cbs.nl/nl-NL/menu/themas/gezondheid-welzijn/publicaties/artikelen/archief/2012/2012-3693-wm.htm
4. Bismark MM, Spittal MJ, Gurrin LC, Ward M, Studdert DM. Identification of doctors at risk of recurrent complaints: a national study of healthcare complaints in Australia. BMJ Qual Saf. 2013;22(7):532–40.
5. Boers ME, Sanaan B. Klachten tegen tandartsen. Nederlands Tandartsenblad. 2013;69(01):26–9.
6. KNMT Royal Dutch Dental Association. National database of Dentists in the Netherlands. Nieuwegein: KNMT; 2014.
7. van der Ven JM, Eijkman MAJ, Brands WG. Dentistry and healthcare legislation 10. The law governing complaints: readily accessible filing procedures. Ned Tijdschr Tandheelkd. 2014;121:147–53. with summary in English.
8. KNMT Royal Dutch Dental Association. [Internet] 2014 [updated 2014 Feb 1; cited 2014 Apr 16]. Available from: http://www.staatvandemondzorg.nl
9. ANT Association Dutch Dentists. Klacht over uw tandarts? [Internet] 2014 [updated 2014 March 1; cited 2014 Apr 14]. Available from: https://www.ant-online.nl/patienten/klacht-over-uw-tandarts
10. KNMT Royal Dutch Dental Association. Annual report 2013. Nieuwegein: KNMT, 2014c
11. ANT Association Dutch Dentists. Annual report 2013 of the Complaints Committee Dentistry. Heemstede: ANT, 2014b
12. Doorakkers P. De impact van een klacht. Tuchtzaak vreet energie. Nederlands Tandartsenblad. 2005;61(05):17–8.
13. Doeleman A. Een klacht hakt er altijd in. Nederlands tandartsenblad. 2014;70(03):14–7.
14. Linthorst GE, Hoekstra JBL, Lauw FN, Hanekamp LA. Complaint to the disciplinary board about a resident. Ned Tijdschr Geneeskd. 2014;158:A6464. with summary in English.
15. Cunningham W. The immediate and long-term impact on New Zealand doctors who receive patient complaints. N ZMed J 2004 (117); 1198: URL: https://www.researchgate.net/publication/8384663_The_immediate_and_longterm_impact_on_New_Zealand_doctors_who_receive_patient_complaints. Accessed 25 Sept 2016.
16. Nash L, Tennant C, Walton M. The psychological impact of complaints and negligence suits on doctors. Australasian Psych. 2004;3:278–81.
17. Nash L, Curtis B, Walton M, Willcock S, Tennant C. The respons of doctors to a formal complaint. Australas Psychiatry. 2006;14:246–50.
18. Balch CM, Oreskovich MR, Dyrbye LN, Colaiano JM, Satele DV, Sloan JA, Shanafelt TD. Personal Consequences of Malpractice Lawsuits on American Surgeons. J Am Coll Surg. 2011;5:657–67.
19. Bourne T, Wynants L, Peters M, van Audenhove V, Timmerman D, van Caltser B, Jalmbrant M. The impact of complaints procedures on the welfare, health and clinical practise of 7926 doctors in the UK: a cross-sectional survey. BMJ Open. 2015;4:e006687. doi:10.1136/bmjopen-2014-006687.
20. van Dam B, Bruers J. De impact van een klacht. Nederlands Tandartsenblad. 2012;68(02):34–5.
21. IBM Corp. Released 2013. IBM SPSS Statistics for Windows. Version 22. Amonk, NY: IBM Corp.
22. Friele RD, Kruikemeier S, Rademakers JJ, Coppen R. Comparing the outcome of two different procedures to handle complaints from a patient's perspective. J Forensic Leg Med. 2013;20(4):290–5. doi:10.1016/j.jflm.2012.11.001. Epub 2012 Dec 13.
23. Friele RD, Sluijs EM. Patient expectations of fair complaint handling in hospitals: empirical data. BMC Health Serv Res. 2006;6:106.
24. Iedema R, Allen S, Britton K, Piper D, Baker A, Grbich C, Allan A, Jones L, Tuckett A, Williams A, et al. Patients' and family members' views on how clinicians enact and how they should enact incident disclosure: the '100 patient stories' qualitative study. BMJ. 2011;343:d4423.
25. Brands WG, van derVen JM, Eijkman MAJ. Dentistry and healthcare legislation 9. The dentist and the disciplinary court case. Ned Tijdschr Tandheelkd. 2014;121:115–20. with summary in English.
26. Schouten BC, Eijkman MA, Hoogstraten J, den Dekker J. Informed consent in Dutch dental practice: knowledge, attitudes and self-efficacy of dentists. Patient Educ Couns. 2001;42:185–92.
27. Silverman J, Kurtz S, Draper J. Skills for communicating with Patients. Oxon: Radcliffe Medical Press ltd; 2005.
28. Gorter RC, Albrecht G, Hoogstraten J, Eijkman MAJ. Measuring work stress among Dutch dentists. Intl Dent J. 1999;49:144–52.
29. Scott SD, Hirschinger LE, Cox KR. The natural history of recovery for the health care provider "second victim" after advers patients events. Qual Saf Health Care. 2009;18:325–30. doi:10.1136/qshc.2009.032870.
30. Seys D, Wu AW, Van Gerven W, Vleugels A, Euwema M, Panella M, Scott SD, Conway J, Sermeus W, Vanhaecht K. Health Care Professionals as Second Victims after Adverse Events: A Systematic Review. Eval Health Prof published online 12 September 2012. doi: 10.1177/0163278712458918.
31. Mettes T, Bruers J, van der Sanden W, Wensing M. Patient safety in dental care: A challenging quality issue? An exploratory cohort study. Acta Odontol Scand. 2013;71(6):1588–93. doi:10.3109/00016357.2013.777471. Epub 2013 Apr 29.
32. IOM Institute of Medicine. Crossing the quality Chasm: a new health system for the 21st century. Washington DC: Institute of Medicine (IOM); 2001.
33. van Dam B, Bruers J. Patiëntencontacten met het TIP. Nederlands Tandartsenblad. 2013;69(12):34–5.
34. Disciplinary Committee for Health Care and Committee Medical Oversight. Annual report 2013. Den Haag: Tuchtcolleges voor de Gezondheidszorg en het College Medisch Toezicht, 2014

PDGFRβ⁺/c-kit⁺ pulp cells are odontoblastic progenitors capable of producing dentin-like structure in vitro and in vivo

Shiwei Cai[1], Wenjian Zhang[2*] and Wei Chen[1]

Abstract

Background: Successful pulp regeneration depends on identification of pulp stem cells capable of differentiation under odontoblastic lineage and producing pulp-dentinal like structure. Recent studies demonstrate that platelet-derived growth factor (PDGF) plays an important role in damage repair and tissue regeneration. The aim of this study was to identify a subpopulation of dental pulp cells responsive to PDGF and with dentin regeneration potential.

Methods: Pulp tissues were isolated from 12 freshly extracted human impacted third molars. Pulp cells were sorted by their expression of PDGFRβ and stem cell marker genes via flow cytometry. For the selected cells, proliferation was analyzed by a colorimetric cell proliferation assay, differentiation was assessed by real time PCR detection the expression of odontoblast marker genes, and mineralization was evaluated by Alizarin Red S staining. GFP marked PDGFRβ$^+$/c-kit$^+$ pulp cells were transplanted into emptied root canals of nude rat lower left incisors. Pulp-dentinal regeneration was examined by immunohistochemistry.

Results: PDGFRβ$^+$/c-kit$^+$ pulp cells proliferated significantly faster than whole pulp cells. In mineralization media, PDGFRβ$^+$/c-kit$^+$ pulp cells were able to develop under odontoblastic linage as demonstrated by a progressively increased expression of DMP1, DSPP, and osteocalcin. BMP2 seemed to enhance whereas PDGF-BB seemed to inhibit odontoblastic differentiation and mineralization of PDGFRβ$^+$/c-kit$^+$ pulp cells. In vivo root canal transplantation study revealed globular dentin and pulp-like tissue formation by PDGFRβ$^+$/c-kit$^+$ cells.

Conclusions: PDGFRβ$^+$/c-kit$^+$ pulp cells appear to have pulp stem cell potential capable of producing dentinal like structure in vitro and in vivo.

Keywords: c-kit, Odontoblasts, Platelet-derived growth factor receptor, Pulp regeneration, Stem cell

Background

One of the ultimate goals of endodontic therapy is to retain natural dentition via predictably regenerating vital dental pulp which is lost as a consequence of pulp diseases or trauma [1]. The cellular and molecular mechanisms regulating the formation of pulp dentinal tissues during development as well as during pulp regeneration remain to be fully elucidated.

Dental pulp is a highly vascularized and metabolically active tissue with a large capacity for regeneration [2]. In vitro study finds that pulp tissue can be used to isolate post-natal stem cells, which presumably locate at perivascular area [3]. Pulpal injury stimulates the proliferation and differentiation of the progenitor/stem cells at this area with subsequent reparative dentin formation [4].

Dental pulpal stem cells (DPSCs) isolated by affinity purification using an antibody against STRO-1, an early marker of mesenchymal stem cells, are capable of generating dentin-like structures lined with human odontoblast-like cells surrounded by a pulp-like interstitial tissue [3, 5]. Majority of these DPSCs demonstrate a phenotype consistent with pericytes, and are found to be positive for α-smooth muscle actin, CD146, as well as a pericyte marker, 3G5 [3]. These findings indicate a possible common ontogeny between dental pulp tissue and pericytes,

* Correspondence: Wenjian.Zhang@uth.tmc.edu
[2]Department of Diagnostic and Biomedical Sciences, University of Texas School of Dentistry at Houston, 7500 Cambridge Street, Suite 5366, Houston, TX 77054, USA
Full list of author information is available at the end of the article

since both are believed to originate from migratory neural crest cells during embryogenesis [6].

DPSCs have been found to demonstrate many stem cell properties, such as clonogenic efficiency, self-renewal capability, high mitotic activity, and multi-lineage differentiation capacity [7]. Depending on the culture conditions, DPSCs are able to differentiate into osteoblasts, endotheliocytes, adipocytes, neural-like cells, as well as odontoblasts [5, 7–10]. Pag A fraction of dental pulp cells have been shown to express stem cell marker genes, including STRO-1 and c-kit [3, 10, 11], indicating that these markers could be used to identify stem/progenitor cells from dental pulp.

Various degrees of success have been achieved for pulp-dentin regeneration in pulpectomized dog teeth with transplantation of DPSCs supplemented with different growth factors [12–14]. In light of the heterogeneity of pulp cells and the complexity of microenvironment in dental pulp, identify the subpopulation of pulp cells and/or growth factors with the highest regenerative potential would help to achieve optimal pulp-dentin regeneration.

In damaged tissues, hemorrhage is followed by blood clot formation and platelet degranulation and release of growth factors including PDGF, TGF-β, and EGF [15–18]. PDGF induces fibroblast proliferation and differentiation and the formation of granulation tissue in soft-tissue wound-healing models [19]. PDGF is induced during bone fracture repair and stimulates cell replication and enhance matrix protein synthesis [20, 21]. PDGF appears to play important roles in wound repair and tissue regeneration.

PDGF is a disulfide-linked dimer of two related polypeptide chains, A and B, which are assembled as heterodimers (PDGF AB) or homodimers (PDGF AA and PDGF BB) [22]. PDGF exerts its biological activity by binding to alpha (−α) or beta (−β) PDGFRs resulting in their dimerization and the subsequent activation of intrinsic receptor tyrosine kinases required to initiate cytoplasmic signal transduction pathways. Activation of these pathways is necessary to stimulate the migration, proliferation, and differentiation of PDGF-responsive cells [23]. PDGF receptors have been found to be expressed by a variety of cells, including fibroblasts, smooth muscle cells, and dental pulp cells [24–26]. The α receptor binds both PDGF A and B chains, whereas the β receptor binds only PDGF B [27]. Studies have indicated that PDGF B subunit is more potent than the A unit, and PDGFRβ occupancy permits optimal PDGF-mediated biological effects [27–30].

Dental pulp cells exhibit increased proliferative activity in the presence of PDGF-BB [24]. PDGF BB/PDGFRβ pathway appears to play an important role during terminal odontoblast differentiation [30]. It is speculated that a subpopulation of dental pulp cells positive for PDGFRβ and stem cell marker expressions would be ideal candidate for pulp stem/progenitor cells with dentin regeneration potential. The aim of the present study is to isolate dental pulp cells expressing PDGFRβ and stem cell marker by fluorescence activated cell sorting (FACS), and evaluate their responses to different growth factors and ability to produce dentin/pulp like structure in vitro and in vivo. The knowledge gained from this study is expected to help optimize regenerative endodontics, a promising alternative to root canal or implant restoration in treating pulpal and periapical diseases, and to help achieve the ultimate goal of endodontic treatment in retaining natural dentition and improving overall oral health-related quality of life.

Methods

Human dental pulp samples

Pulp tissue from freshly extracted normal human impacted third molars (12 subjects, 18–25 years of age) was gently separated from the crown and root, and then digested in 3 mg/ml collagenase type I and 4 mg/ml dispase for one hour at 37 °C. Single-cell suspension was obtained by passing the cells through a 70-μm strainer several times. The cells were plated at 1×10^5/well into six-well gelatin coated plates in undifferentiation media, which contained 80 % Dulbecco's Modified Eagle's medium (DMEM) and 20 % knockout serum replacement (KSR) supplemented with 1 mM MEM nonessential amino acids, 0.1 mM β-mercaptoethanol, 2 ng/ml FGF, 2 ng/ml IGF, 1 mM L-glutamine, 100 units/ml penicillin, and 100 μg/ml streptomycin. The cells were cultured at 37 °C in 5 % CO_2 to maintain the undifferentiated status. Tooth extraction was performed with the understanding and written consent of each subject. The study was approved by the Institutional Review Board (IRB) of the University of Texas Health Sciences Center at Houston.

Flow cytometry

Dental pulp cells were labeled with and sorted by the reactivity to anti-PDGFRβ antibody. The PDGFRβ$^+$ dental pulp cells were further characterized by their expression of stem cell and other surface markers including CD34 and c-kit (markers of hematopoietic stem cells), STRO-1 (mesenchymal stem cell marker), vimentin (mesenchymal cell marker), NG_2 (mesenchymal cell marker), and CXCR4$^+$ (chemokine receptor). The sources of these antibodies were: phycoerythrin (PE)-conjugated anti-PDGFRβ (BD Pharmingen, Franklin Lakes, NJ, USA), APC conjugated anti-CD34 (BD Pharmingen, Franklin Lakes, NJ, USA), PE-Cy5 conjugated anti-c-kit (BD Pharmingen, Franklin Lakes, NJ, USA), fluorescerin isothiocyanate (FITC)-conjugated anti-STRO-1 (Santa Cruz Biotechnology, Inc., Santa Cruz, CA, USA), FITC-conjugated anti-vimentin (Santa Cruz Biotechnology, Inc., Santa Cruz, CA, USA), FITC-conjugated anit-NG_2 (Santa Cruz Biotechnology, Inc., Santa Cruz, CA, USA), and Allophycocyanin (APC)-conjugated anti-CXCR4$^+$ (BD Pharmingen, Franklin

Lakes, NJ, USA). Dental pulp cells were labelled with the antibodies for 30 min on ice followed by fluorescence sorting performed at 4 °C with a BD FACS Vantange Sorting Flow Cytometer using CELLQuest software (BD Biosciences, San Jose, CA, USA). Isotype IgG was used as control to assess background fluorescence. Isolated cells were expanded to passage 3 to ensure adequate quantity for further experiments. Figure 1 shows the flow chart for experimental setup.

Cell proliferation assays

Cell proliferation was measured by a colorimetric assay using CellTiter 96 Aqueous One Solution (Promega, Madison, WI, USA) according to the manufacturer's instruction. Briefly, whole pulp cells, PDGFRβ$^+$ pulp cells, PDGFRβ$^+$/c-kit$^+$ pulp cells, and PDGFRβ$^-$ cells were seeded at 2×10^3 cells per well in 48-well tissue culture plates in 0.2 mL of undifferentiation media. After overnight incubation to allow cellular attachment, the media were replaced with fresh media. On days 1 to 6, 20 μl of CellTiter 96 Aqueous One Solution was added to each well. The plates were incubated in darkness at 37 °C for 1 h. Then 200 μl of the mixed medium solution was transferred to 96-well plate, and the absorbance was read at 490 nm with a SPECTRAmax 190 multiplate reader with SOFTmax PRO version 3.0 (Molecular Devices, Sunnyvale, CA, USA). The mean absorbance from wells containing cell-free media was used as the baseline and was deducted from the absorbencies of other cell-containing wells. The readings from five individual wells were averaged for each cell type at assayed time point. The proliferation rate was calculated as the following for each cell type: (absorbance at assayed time point/absorbance on day 1) X100.

In vitro differentiation of pulp cells

To stimulate differentiation, PDGFRβ$^+$/c-kit$^+$ cells were cultured in mineralization media containing 90 % Minimum Essential Medium α (α – MEM) (Gibco/Thermo Fisher Scientific, Grand Island, NY, USA), 10 % fetal bovine serum (FBS), 1 mM L-glutamine, and supplemented with 50 μg/ml ascorbic acid, 10 mM β – glycerophosphate, and 10 nM dexamethasone. For concentration study, the cells were cultured in the presence and absence of 1, 10, 100, and 1000 ng/ml BMP2 or PDGF-BB for two days. The mRNA was extracted, and the expressions of odontoblast differentiation markers were detected by real-time PCR.

For the time-course study, PDGFRβ$^+$/c-kit$^+$ cells were cultured in mineralization media with the presence or absence of 10 ng/ml BMP2 or PDGF-BB for 2 weeks. The media were changed every other day. On days 3, 7, and 14, mRNA was extracted and real-time PCR was run to detect the expressions of odontoblast differentiation markers.

RNA isolation and real time PCR

Total RNA was isolated from PDGFRβ$^+$/c-kit$^+$ cell cultures by a Qiagen Rneasy Mini Kit (Qiagen Inc, Valencia, CA, USA) according to the manufacturer's instructions and purified via DNAse treatment. The extracted RNA had a A260/A280 ratio above 2.0. Reverse transcriptase treatment of RNA was performed at 42 °C for 80 min using 3 μg of RNA with oligo primers (Invitrogen, Carlsbad, CA, USA) and BD Sprint Powerscript (BD Biosciences, San Jose, CA, USA). The 10 μl PCR reaction mixture consisted of 4 μl cDNA dilution (40 ng cDNA), 1 μl primers (5 μM) and 5 μl 2X iQ SYBR Green Supermix (Bio-Rad Laboratories, Hercules, CA, USA). Each sample was amplificated for 40 cycles of 95 °C/10 s, 55 °C/15 s, and 72 °C/15 s with a Bio-Rad Real-Time PCR Detection System. Melting

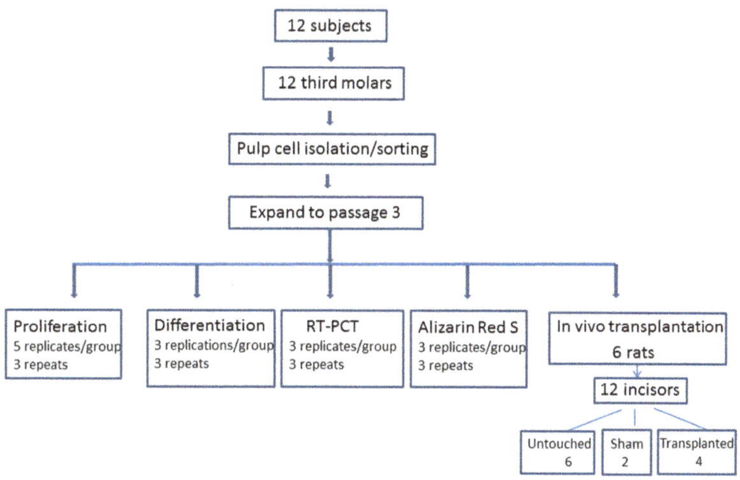

Fig. 1 Flow chart for experimental setup

curve analysis was performed on the products to ensure specificity of the reaction. After calibrator normalization and amplification efficiency correction, PCR products were quantified by comparing amplification of the gene of interest to that of glyceraldehyde 3-phosphate dehydrogenase (GAPDH) as a reference gene, using $2^{-\Delta\Delta Ct}$ method with the Relative Quantification Software version 1.0 (Bio-Rad Laboratories, Hercules, CA, USA). The genes detected were dentin matrix protein 1 (DMP1), dentin sialophosphoprotein (DSPP), osteocalcin (OCN), and alkaline phosphatase (ALP). The criteria for choosing primers included: 18–24 bases in length, GC content 50-60 %, avoid repeats of Gs or Cs longer than 3 bases, amplified region 60–150 bp, melting temperature 50-65 °C, avoid primer-dimer formation and secondary structure in the target sequence, and verifying specificity by blasting the primers' sequences. The primers were: DMP1, 5'- CAGG AGCACAGGAAAAGGAG and 5'- CTGGTGGTATCTT CCCCCAGGAG; DSPP, 5'- AGAAGGACCTGGCCAAA AAT and 5'- TCTCCTCGGCTACTGCTGTT; OCN, 5'- CATGAGAGCCCTCACA, and 5'- AGAGCGACACCC TAGAC; ALP, 5'- ACGTGGCTAAGAATGTCATC, and 5'- CTGGTAGGCGATGTCCTTA; and GAPDH, 5'- CG GAGTCAACGGATTTGGTCGTAT, and 5'- AGCCTTC TCCATGGTGGTGAAGAC.

Alizarin Red S staining (ARS)

PDGFRβ$^+$/c-kit$^+$ pulp cells were cultured in undifferentiation media or mineralization media with the presence or absence of 1, 10, 100, and 1000 ng/ml BMP2 or PDGF-BB. The media were changed every other day, and mineral formation of the cells was assessed with ARS on day 14. Briefly, the media were removed, and the cells were rinsed with distilled water twice and fixed with 50 % ethanol at 4 °C for 45 min. Following removal of the ethanol, the cells were rinsed with deionized water twice and stained with 1 % Alizarin Red S and 0.1 % ammonium hydroxide for 30 min at room temperature. The Alizarin Red S solution was then removed, and the cells were rinsed with water three times. The stained mineral nodules within each well were documented by photomicrography with Nikon E400 microscope (Nikon, Melville, NY, USA) at 100-200X magnification. To quantify the Alizarin Red S staining, the cells were rinsed with deionized water, washed in PBS while rocking for 15 min at room temperature, then destained for 30 min with 10 % (w/v) acetic acid and 20 % (v/v) methanol extraction solution. The absorbance of extracted Alizarin Red S solution was determined at 490 nm with a microplate spectrophotometer (Bio-Rad Laboratories, Hercules, CA, USA). The concentration of Alizarin Red S in each sample was quantified by comparing the absorbance of extraction solution with those from Alizarin Red S standards.

Plasmid constructs and transfection

The PDGFRβ clone was purchased from ATCC (Manassas, VA, USA). The cDNA of the PDGFRβ was isolated with Qiagen miniprep kit (Qiagen, Valencia, CA, USA). The cDNA of the PDGFRβ open reading frame was amplified, digested, and inserted into the pcDNA3.1/NT-GFP-ToPo plasmid vector (Invitrogen, Carlsbad, CA, USA). The recombinant PDGFRβ plasmid was transfected into PDGFRβ$^+$/c-kit$^+$ pulp cells using LipofectAMINE reagent and Opti-MEM (Invitrogen, Carlsbad, CA, USA) according to the manufacturer's instructions. Forty-eight hours after transfection, cells were harvested with 0.25 % trypsin/EDTA, resuspended in DMEM with 10 % FBS, washed with PBS, and filtered through a 35 μm nylon screen. The cells were then cultured in DMEM with 10 % FBS and 400 μg/ml G418 (Sigma-Aldrich, St. Louis, MO, USA) to select the ones with successful transfection. Two weeks later, transfection efficacy was examined with a fluorescent microscope, and the transfectants (GFP marked PDGFRβ$^+$/c-kit$^+$ cells) were used in in vivo root canal transplantation experiments.

In vivo root canal implantation

Six 8–10 week old NIH nude rats (NIH-Foxn 1/rnu), with body weight 150–225 g, were obtained from Charles River Laboratories (Wilmington, MA, USA). The rats were kept in isolated cages and provided with sterile housing, food, and drinking water under 12 h light/dark cycle. The animal surgery protocol was approved by the Animal Welfare Committee of the University of Texas Health Sciences Center at Houston. Animals were anesthetized with intraperitoneal injection of 135 mg/kg ketamine and 15 mg/kg xylazine. The apical region of the rat lower left incisor was surgically exposed by first making an incision through the skin and masseter using the corner of the mouth and the inferior border of the ear as landmarks, followed by removal of the external bony wall of the mandible using a high speed surgical hand piece and a #4 round long shank bur under sterile saline irrigation. The root apex and apical papillary tissues were removed by a #2 round bur and a small spoon excavator. Through the opened apex, a prebent #20 or #25 endodontic K file was advanced in an anterior direction into the presumed canal space, and a digital radiograph was taken to confirm the entrance of the endodontic file into the canal space. Pulpal tissue was removed with #30 or #35 barbed broaches and #20, #25, and #30 endodontic files, and the canal space was irrigated with sterile water to remove lose remnants. The procedure created an empty root canal space and adjacent bony crypt which was used as the recipient site for transplanted GFP marked PDGFRβ$^+$/c-kit$^+$ cells. 1×10^7 cells in 50 μl Chitosan Hydrogel (Sigma-Aldrich, St. Louis, MO, USA) were implanted in the root canal space and bony crypt. The crypt was then covered with an oval piece of Collatape

(Integra, Plainsboro, NJ, USA) to ensure the transplanted cells stay within the place prior to the surgical closing of the masseter and skin incision. Detailed surgical procedure is illustrated in Additional file 1: Figure S1, Additional file 2: Figure S2, Additional file 3: Figure S3, Additional file 4: Figure S4, Additional file 5: Figure S5, Additional file 6: Figure S6, Additional file 7: Figure S7, Additional file 8: Figure S8 and Additional file 9: Figure S9.

Immunohistochemistry

Ten weeks after transplantation, mandibles were harvested, fixed in 10 % neutral buffered formalin, and decalcified in 3.4 % Kristensen's sodium formate/15 % formic acid solution. Specimens were then dehydrated through increasing concentrations of alcohols, including 50, 70 , 95, and 100 % for 2 min each, followed by paraffin embedding. Sessions (6-micron thickness) cut through the middle of the rat incisor root canal space were mounted, deparaffinized with xylene, and rehydrated in descending concentrations of alcohols. Antigen retrieval was performed by incubation with 1 mg/ml proteinase K (Invitrogen, Carlsbad, CA, USA) for 10 min at RT. The slides were rinsed, and endogenous hydrogen peroxidase activity was blocked by incubation with PeroxyAbolish (Biocare Medical, Concord, CA, USA) for 10 min at RT. The slides were then treated with the primary antibodies overnight at 4 °C according to the manufacturers' instructions. The primary antibodies were 1:500 rabbit anti-GFP (Abcam, Cambridge, MA, USA), 1:200 rabbit anti-PDGFRβ$^+$, rabbit anti-DSP, and mouse anti-osteopontin (OPN) (Santa Cruz Biotechnology, Inc., Santa Cruz, CA, USA). Negative controls were the ones with exclusion of primary antibodies, and positive controls were the tissue samples with high level expressions for the detected proteins, such as human kidney for PDGFRβ, tooth for DSP, and bone for OPN. Sections were further incubated with 1:10,000 secondary antibodies diluted in blocking buffer. Finally, the sections were reacted with streptavidin peroxidase for 30 min at RT, stained with DAB substrate kit (Vector laboratories, Burlingame, CA, USA), and counterstained with hematoxylin (sigma-Aldrich, St. Louis, MO, USA) for 5 min.

Data analysis

All of the experiments were performed at a minimum of three times. Data was analyzed by Student's *t* test or ANOVA followed by a Tukey-Kramer multiple comparison test. Statistical significance was set at $p < 0.05$.

Results

Fractionation of pulp cells by surface markers

Twelve samples of adult human pulp cells were obtained from 12 individuals under 25 years of age. Cells from all 12 samples were reactive with PDGFRβ antibody, and this PDGFRβ$^+$ fraction represented approximately 0.8 % of the total pulp cell population. A stem/progenitor cell population was further selected by labeling these cells with specific antigens for stem cells. Not all of the PDGFRβ$^+$ cells from the 12 samples consistently reacted with STRO-1, NG_2, CD34, vimentin, or CXCR4. However, c-kit was found to be consistently expressed by PDGFRβ$^+$ cells of all 12 samples (0.15 % of the total pulp cell population) (Fig. 2). PDGFRβ$^+$/c-kit$^+$ cells were sorted and collected for further studies.

PDGFRβ$^+$/c-kit$^+$ cells proliferated faster than whole pulp cells

The proliferation of whole human dental pulp cells, PDGFRβ$^-$, PDGFRβ$^+$, PDGFRβ$^+$/c-kit$^+$ cells was analyzed by a colorimetric proliferation assay through a 6-day culture period. Approximately 3×10^3 cells were plated in 48-well plates instead of 96-well to prevent contact inhibition, which generated less than 90 % confluence for all the cell types at final time points. PDGFRβ$^+$/c-kit$^+$ and PDGFRβ$^+$ cells showed significantly faster proliferation

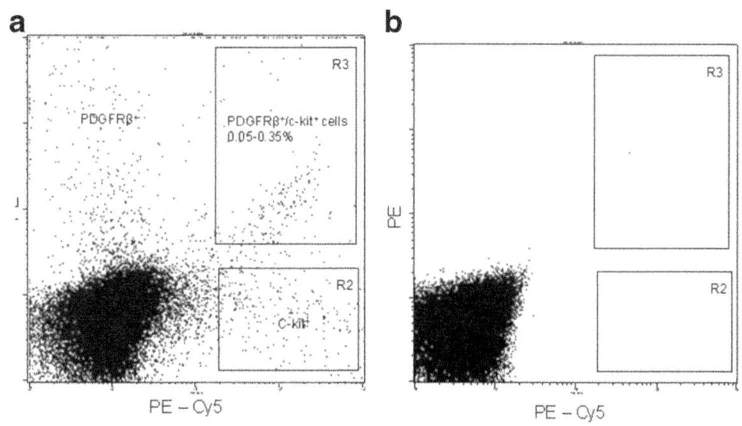

Fig. 2 Fractionation of human dental pulp cells by fluorescence activated cell sorting (FACS). **a** Fraction of PDGFRβ$^+$, c-kit$^+$, and PDGFRβ$^+$/c-kit$^+$ cells by cell surface fluorescence labeling. **b** Isotype IgG controls

from day 4 to day 6 compared with whole pulp cells and PDGFRβ⁻ cells ($p < 0.05$). There was no significant difference of cell growth between PDGFRβ$^+$/c-kit$^+$ and PDGFRβ$^+$ cells (Fig. 3).

PDGFRβ$^+$/c-kit$^+$ cells expressed odontoblast differentiation marker genes

For the concentration study, when PDGFRβ$^+$/c-kit$^+$ pulp cells were treated with 0, 1, 10, 100, and 1000 ng/ml BMP2, mRNA expressions of DMP1, OCN, and ALP were up-regulated by BMP2 in a concentration-dependent manner. DSPP was up-regulated by 1 ng/ml BMP2 (Fig. 4a).

When PDGFRβ$^+$/c-kit$^+$ pulp cells were treated with 0, 1, 10, 100, and 1000 ng/ml PDGF-BB, mRNA expressions of OCN was down-regulated by PDGF-BB in a concentration-dependent manner, the expressions of DMP1 and DSPP were inhibited in a non-concentration dependent manner, and the effects on ALP were varied (Fig. 4b).

For the time course study, when PDGFRβ$^+$/c-kit$^+$ pulp cells were cultured in mineralization media alone, the expression of DMP1, DSPP, and OCN reached the highest levels on day 14. BMP2 stimulated maximal DMP1 and OCN expressions on day 7, and DSPP expression increased continuously throughout the 14 day culture period. PDGF-BB showed a general inhibitory effect on the level of DMP1, DSPP, and OCN gene expressions compared with mineralization media alone in the time course study (Fig. 5a, b, and c).

PDGFRβ$^+$/c-kit$^+$ cells were able to produce mineralization in vitro

PDGFRβ$^+$/c-kit$^+$ pulp cells produced significantly more mineral nodules when cultured in mineralization media than that of the nondifferentiation media. Among the studied concentrations (1–1000 ng/ml), 1000 ng/ml BMP2 stimulated significantly more mineralization by PDGFRβ$^+$/c-kit$^+$ cells than in mineralization media alone. Interestingly, PDGF-BB suppressed the formation of mineral nodules in a concentration dependent manner than mineralization media alone (Fig. 6a, b).

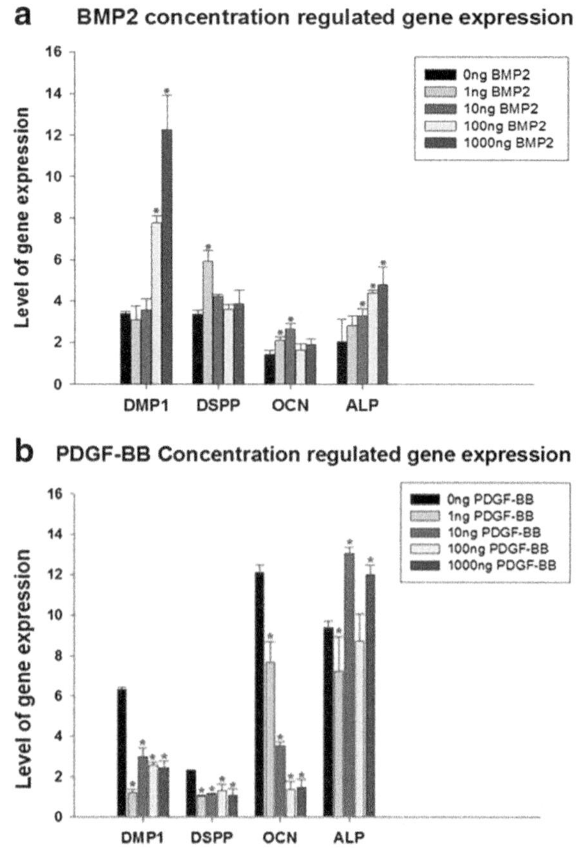

Fig. 4 Differentiation of PDGFRβ$^+$/c-kit$^+$ pulp cells under various concentrations of growth factors. **a** 0–1000 ng/ml of BMP2 treatment. Expressions of DMP1, OCN, and ALP were up-regulated by BMP2 in a concentration-dependent manner. DSPP was up-regulated by 1 ng/ml BMP2. * denotes $p < 0.05$ compared with 0 ng/ml BMP2. **b** 0–1000 ng/ml of PDGF-BB treatment. Expression of OCN was down-regulated by PDGF-BB in a concentration-dependent manner. DMP1 and DSPP were inhibited in a non-concentration dependent manner. The effects on ALP were varied. * denotes $p < 0.05$ compared with 0 ng/ml PDGF-BB

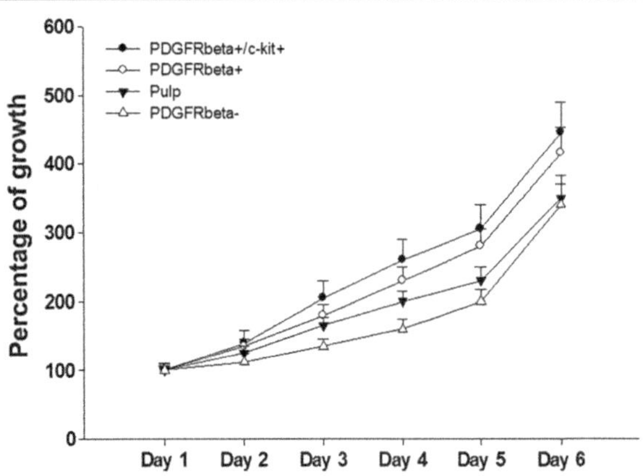

Fig. 3 Dental pulp cell proliferation assay. In a 6-day assay period, PDGFRβ$^+$/c-kit$^+$ and PDGFRβ$^+$ cells proliferated significantly faster than that of whole pulp cells and PDGFRβ$^-$ cells from day 4 to day 6

Transplanted PDGFRβ$^+$/c-kit$^+$ cells produced dentin-pulp like structure in vivo

Successful creation of recombinant PDGFRβ-GFP plasmid was confirmed by DNA sequencing. The recombinant plasmid was transfected into PDGFRβ$^+$/c-kit$^+$ cells, which were then transplanted into emptied rat incisor root canal. Unoperated rat lower incisors were included as negative controls (Fig. 7a). Ten weeks after transplantation, control animals that were sham-operated without transplantation of PDGFRβ$^+$/c-kit$^+$ pulp cells were not observed to undergo any dentinogenesis (Fig. 7b). For the animals received PDGFRβ$^+$/c-kit$^+$ pulp cells, some globular

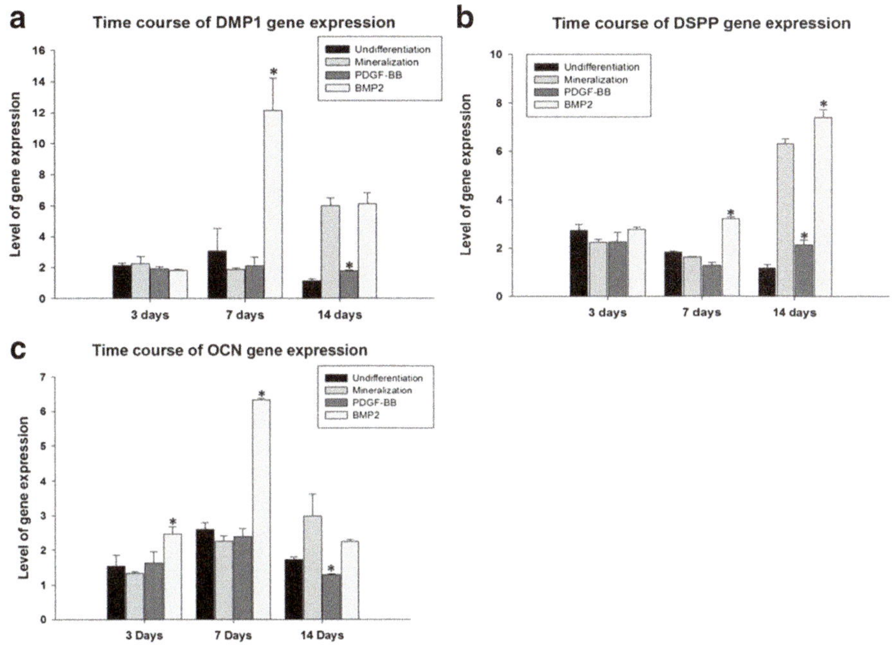

Fig. 5 Fourteen-day differentiation study of PDGFRβ$^+$/c-kit$^+$ pulp cells under 10 ng/ml growth factor treatments. **a** BMP2 stimulated maximal DMP1 expressions on day 7. PDGF-BB inhibited DMP1 on day 14 when compared with mineralization media alone. **b** Compared with mineralization media alone, BMP2 significantly enhanced DSPP expressions on day 7 and 14, and PDGF-BB greatly inhibited DSPP on day 14. **c.** Compared with mineralization media alone, BMP2 significantly increased OCN expressions on day 3 and 7, and PDGF-BB greatly inhibited OCN on day 14. * denotes $p < 0.05$ compared with mineralization media alone

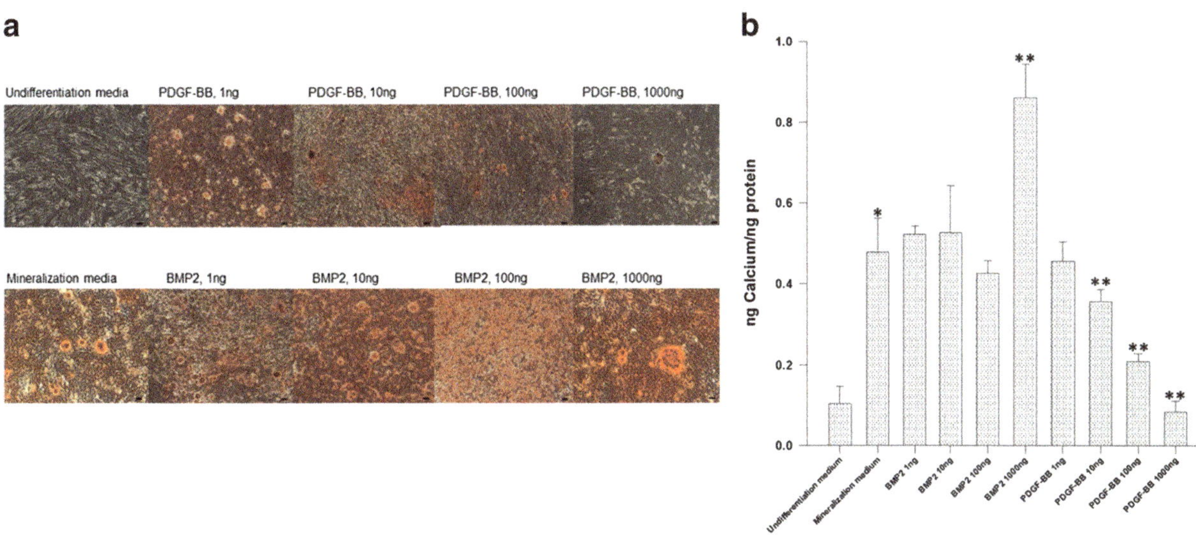

Fig. 6 BMP2 stimulated and PDGF-BB inhibited mineralization of PDGFRβ$^+$/c-kit$^+$ pulp cells. **a** Alizarin Red S staining. Dark red area indicates mineralization in the culture. Scale bar = 100 μm. **b** Quantitative Alizarin Red S analysis. PDGFRβ$^+$/c-kit$^+$ pulp cells produced significantly more mineralization when cultured in mineralization media than that of the nondifferentiation media. 1000 ng/ml BMP2 stimulated significantly more mineralization by PDGFRβ$^+$/c-kit$^+$ cells than in mineralization media alone. PDGF-BB suppressed mineralization in a concentration dependent manner when compared with mineralization media alone. * denotes $p < 0.05$ compared with undifferentiation media. ** denote $p < 0.05$ compared with mineralization media

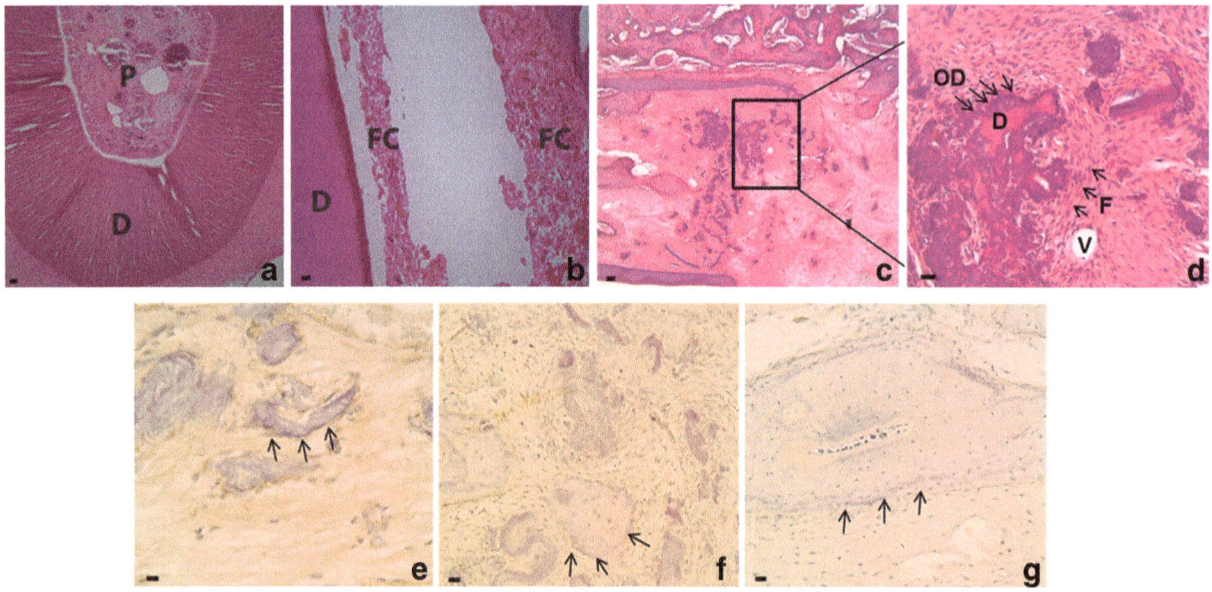

Fig. 7 Generation of dentin-pulp like structures by PDGFRβ$^+$/c-kit$^+$ cells transplanted in emptied rat incisor root canal. **a** An untouched rat lower incisor as negative control. **b** A sham operation control with transplantation of hydrogel alone in rat emptied incisor root canal. Notice largely void canal space with small amount residual fibrous tissue at the periphery. **c-g** Transplantation of PDGFRβ$^+$/c-kit$^+$ cells and hydrogel into emptied rat incisor root canal. The canal was filled with globular dentin like calcification lined by odontoblast-like cells surrounded by vascular and fibrous connective tissues. **c** Low magnification **d** High magnification of the boxed area in **c**. **e** Odontoblast-like cells (arrows pointed) were positive for GFP staining. **f** Odontoblast-like cells (arrows pointed) were positive for DSP staining. **g** Odontoblast-like cells (arrows pointed) were positive for OPN staining. D, dentin; F, fibroblasts; FC, fibrous connective tissue; OD, odontoblast-like cells; P, pulp; V, blood vessel. Scale bar = 100 μm

calcifications were developed in the emptied root canal space (Fig. 7c, d). The cells outlining the mineral surface had been shown to express moderate GFP (Fig. 7e), DSP (Fig. 7f), and weak OPN (Fig. 7g) by immunohistochemical staining. These globular dentin-like structures were surrounded by fibroblasts and vascular-like entities (Fig. 7d).

Discussion

Our study identified 0.15 % of the total pulp cells are positive for PDGFRβ/c-kit. C-kit, a stem cell marker, has previously been shown to be expressed in dental follicle and dental papilla in vivo and in human dental pulp cells in vitro [11, 31]. PDGF-PDGFR pathway is critical for tissue repair and regeneration [19, 20]. Our study is the first one to isolate and characterize pulps cells with co-expression of c-kit and PDGFRβ, and the results suggest a promising cellular source for endodontic regeneration. The PDGFRβ$^+$/c-kit$^+$ pulp cells are highly proliferative, and capable of generating dentin-like structure in vitro as well as in emptied root canal space. BMP2 and PDGF-BB counteract each other and are crucial in regulating the development of PDGFRβ$^+$/c-kit$^+$ pulp cells into dentin-forming cells.

During differentiation phase, odontoblasts express an array of differentiation markers. DMP1 and DSPP are generally considered to be specific markers of odontoblast differentiation [32–34]. Noncollagenous proteins such as alkaline phosphatase (ALP), osteocalcin (OCN), and osteopontin (OPN) are also found in odontoblasts during dentin matrix maturation and mineralization [35, 36]. In this study, PDGFRβ$^+$/c-kit$^+$ cells were able to develop under odontoblastic linage when cultured in mineralization media alone, as demonstrated by a general increased expression of DMP1, DSPP, and OCN during the 14-day culture period. BMP2 stimulated the expressions of DMP1, DSPP, ALP, and OCN, whereas PDGF-BB suppressed the expressions of DMP1, DSPP, and OCN, and had a variable effect on ALP depending on concentrations. These observations suggest that BMP2 enhances but PDGF-BB inhibits differentiation of PDGFRβ$^+$/c-kit$^+$ cells into odontoblastic like cells. Consistently, the quantitative mineralization assay demonstrated that PDGFRβ$^+$/c-kit$^+$ cells were able to produce mineralized nodules in mineralization media alone, and BMP2 enhanced but PDGF-BB inhibited the mineralization process.

Majority of our findings on the effects of BMP-2 and PDGF-BB on odontoblast differentiation and mineralization are consistent with what have been reported in the literature. BMP2 can stimulate the expressions of DSPP, ALP, and OCN of dental pulp cells, and induce dentin formation in pulp cultures and pulp cap therapy [37–40]. PDGF-BB has been found to stimulate pulp cell proliferation, suppress ALP and OCN expression, and decrease calcium content and the formation of dentin-like nodules in dental pulp cultures, although DSP expression has been enhanced [24, 26, 30, 41]. The discrepancy of the effect of PDGF-BB on DSP expression in our study could be due to differences in concentrations of the growth factor, culture method, or origin of the pulp cells. Our results seem to indicate that PDGF-BB is mainly to maintain primitive status and proliferative capacity of pulp progenitor cells.

In vivo transplantation of dental pulp progenitor cells for dentinogenesis has been established previously, such as subcutaneously [5, 7] or in renal capsules [42]. The root canal space of rat incisors has not been reported as a recipient site before. As rat incisor continuously erupts, the coronal access to its root canal is restricted. In addition, rat incisor has relatively large periapical tissue mass and apex opening, which limit it being used as a recipient site for pulp stem cell transplantation. However, some features of rats make them a good model to study pulpal regeneration, such as cost effectiveness, well-established genome and proteome, and readily availability for a variety of transgenic rat models [43, 44]. Nude rats are especially suitable for transplantation study, due to its immune tolerance. To cope with continuous eruption of rat incisors, a retrograde approach was used in this study to remove the apex and periapical growing apparatus. The existing dental pulp was removed and a large empty root canal space was prepared for transplantation of human dental pulp progenitor cells. It was discovered that transplantation of PDGFRβ$^+$/c-kit$^+$ pulp cells into nude rat emptied incisor root canal generated globular dentin like structure with surrounding odontoblastic cells and pulp-like tissues. Immunohistochemistry revealed expression of DSP and OPN in these "dentinogenic" cells. The interface between dentin wall of rat incisor root and the transplants was filled with fibrous connective tissue and scattered vascular-like structures, which, presumably, were derive from angiogenesis of PDGFRβ$^+$/c-kit$^+$ cells under stimulation of local growth factors. For sham operation with transplantation of hydrogel alone, the root canal space was largely void, with small amount of fibrous connective tissue seen at the periphery, which was likely to be residual tissue left off the operation. Together, these observations validate the feasibility of the emptied root canal as alternative recipient site for dentin regeneration, and revealed the stem/progenitor cell characteristic of PDGFRβ$^+$/c-kit$^+$ pulp cells with regenerative potential for dentin-pulpal complex.

One limitation of the current technique was lack of fully organized dentin-pulp formation in the emptied root canal space. PDGFRβ$^+$/c-kit$^+$ cells appeared to provide sufficient cellular resources to generate various components of dentin-pulp complex, supplementing with optimal scaffold system and/or morphogenic factors in the local environment might facilitate a more organized de novo dentin-pulp regeneration. A variety of scaffold materials have been tested in endodontic regeneration with variable results, including injectable hydrogels, platelet-rich plasma, bioceramic, and polymer scaffolds [45–48]. Future studies using PDGFRβ$^+$/c-kit$^+$ cells, functionalized scaffolds, and properly titrated morphogens are needed to optimize the technique to achieve a more successful de novo regeneration of dentin-pulp complex. This study, together with other investigations in the field, strives to fulfill the ultimate goal of endodontic therapy, to retain infected or traumatized nature dentition, and avoid the discomfort and complications resulting from tooth devitalization/extraction or prosthetic restorations.

Conclusions

In summary, the research described herein identified a subset of dental pulp cells (PDGFRβ$^+$/c-kit$^+$) with pulp stem cell properties such as highly proliferative and capable of producing dentin-like structures in vitro and in vivo. This knowledge will help us better understand the fundamentals of dentinogenesis and develop novel strategy for endodontic dentin/pulp regeneration.

Additional files

Additional file 1: Figure S1. General anesthesia. (JPG 22 kb)

Additional file 2: Figure S2 Incision. (JPG 17 kb)

Additional file 3: Figure S3. Locating of apical area of incisor. (JPG 18 kb)

Additional file 4: Figure S4. Removal of apex, access of root canal through apex, and removal of pulpal tissue. (JPG 21 kb)

Additional file 5: Figure S5. Radiograph shows removal of pulp and access to canal from apex. (JPG 13 kb)

Additional file 6: Figure S6. Mixture of pulpal stem cells and gel scaffold. (JPG 39 kb)

Additional file 7: Figure S7. Implantation of cells and scaffold into emptied root canal. (JPG 18 kb)

Additional file 8: Figure S8. Suture. (JPG 22 kb)

Additional file 9: Figure S9. Collecting specimen. (JPG 29 kb)

Abbreviations

ALP: Alkaline phosphatase; APC: Allophycocyanin; ARS: Alizarin red S staining; DMEM: Dulbecco's modified eagle's medium; DMP1: Dentin matrix protein 1; DPSCs: Dental pulpal stem cells; DSPP: Dentin sialophosphoprotein; FACS: Fluorescence activated cell sorting; FBS: Fetal bovine serum; FITC: Fluorescerin isothiocyanate; GAPDH: Glyceraldehyde 3-phosphate dehydrogenase; IRB: Institutional Review Board; KSR: Knockout serum replacement; OCN: Osteocalcin; OPN: Osteopontin; PDGF: Platelet-derived growth factor; PE: Phycoerythrin; α – MEM: Minimum essential medium α

Acknowledgements

Not applicable.

Funding

This research was supported in part by a Research Grant from the American Association of Endodontists Foundation awarded to SC and by an internal funding from University of Texas School of Dentistry at Houston designated to SC and WZ.

Authors' contributions

SC conceived of the study, participated in its design and data interpretation, and drafted the manuscript. WC carried out cell culture and animal studies, and collected the data. WZ helped with study design and data interpretation, and critically revised the manuscript.

Competing interests

The authors declare that they have no competing interest.

Consent for publication

Not applicable.

Ethics approval and consent to participate

The study was approved by the Institutional Review Board (IRB) and the Animal Welfare Committee of the University of Texas Health Sciences Center at Houston. Tooth extraction was performed with the understanding and written consent of each subject.

Author details

[1]Department of Endodontics, University of Texas School of Dentistry at Houston, 7500 Cambridge Street, Suite 5366, Houston, TX 77054, USA. [2]Department of Diagnostic and Biomedical Sciences, University of Texas School of Dentistry at Houston, 7500 Cambridge Street, Suite 5366, Houston, TX 77054, USA.

References

1. Baranwal KA. Regenerative Stem Cells for Endodontic Tissue Engineering: Past, Present and Future. Ann Prosthodont Restor Dent. 2015;1(1):20–5.
2. Pinzon RD, Toto PD, O'Malley JJ. Kinetics of rat molar pulp cells at various ages. J Dent Res. 1966;45(3):934–8.
3. Shi S, Gronthos S. Perivascular niche of postnatal mesenchymal stem cells in human bone marrow and dental pulp. J Bone Miner Res. 2003;18(4):696–704.
4. Tecles O, Laurent P, Zygouritsas S, Burger AS, Camps J, Dejou J, About I. Activation of human dental pulp progenitor/stem cells in response to odontoblast injury. Arch Oral Biol. 2005;50(2):103–8.
5. Gronthos S, Mankani M, Brahim J, Robey PG, Shi S. Postnatal human dental pulp stem cells (DPSCs) in vitro and in vivo. Proc Natl Acad Sci U S A. 2000;97(25):13625–30.
6. Canfield AE, Schor AM. Osteogenic potential of Vascular pericytes. Cambridge: Cambridge University Press; 1998.
7. Gronthos S, Brahim J, Li W, Fisher LW, Cherman N, Boyde A, DenBesten P, Robey PG, Shi S. Stem cell properties of human dental pulp stem cells. J Dent Res. 2002;81(8):531–5.
8. d'Aquino R, Graziano A, Sampaolesi M, Laino G, Pirozzi G, De Rosa A, Papaccio G. Human postnatal dental pulp cells co-differentiate into osteoblasts and endotheliocytes: a pivotal synergy leading to adult bone tissue formation. Cell Death Differ. 2007;14(6):1162–71.
9. Huang GT, Yamaza T, Shea LD, Djouad F, Kuhn NZ, Tuan RS, Shi S. Stem/progenitor cell-mediated de novo regeneration of dental pulp with newly deposited continuous layer of dentin in an in vivo model. Tissue Eng Part A. 2010;16(2):605–15.
10. Laino G, d'Aquino R, Graziano A, Lanza V, Carinci F, Naro F, Pirozzi G, Papaccio G. A new population of human adult dental pulp stem cells: a useful source of living autologous fibrous bone tissue (LAB). J Bone Miner Res. 2005;20(8):1394–402.
11. Gagari E, Rand MK, Tayari L, Vastardis H, Sharma P, Hauschka PV, Damoulis PD. Expression of stem cell factor and its receptor, c-kit, in human oral mesenchymal cells. Eur J Oral Sci. 2006;114(5):409–15.
12. Iohara K, Imabayashi K, Ishizaka R, Watanabe A, Nabekura J, Ito M, Matsushita K, Nakamura H, Nakashima M. Complete pulp regeneration after pulpectomy by transplantation of CD105+ stem cells with stromal cell-derived factor-1. Tissue Eng Part A. 2011;17(15–16):1911–20.
13. Zhu X, Wang Y, Liu Y, Huang GT, Zhang C. Immunohistochemical and histochemical analysis of newly formed tissues in root canal space transplanted with dental pulp stem cells plus platelet-rich plasma. J Endod. 2014;40(10):1573–8.
14. Zhu X, Zhang C, Huang GT, Cheung GS, Dissanayaka WL, Zhu W. Transplantation of dental pulp stem cells and platelet-rich plasma for pulp regeneration. J Endod. 2012;38(12):1604–9.
15. Antoniades HN, Scher CD, Stiles CD. Purification of human platelet-derived growth factor. Proc Natl Acad Sci U S A. 1979;76(4):1809–13.
16. Assoian RK, Grotendorst GR, Miller DM, Sporn MB. Cellular transformation by coordinated action of three peptide growth factors from human platelets. Nature. 1984;309(5971):804–6.
17. Childs CB, Proper JA, Tucker RF, Moses HL. Serum contains a platelet-derived transforming growth factor. Proc Natl Acad Sci U S A. 1982;79(17):5312–6.
18. Oka Y, Orth DN. Human plasma epidermal growth factor/beta-urogastrone is associated with blood platelets. J Clin Invest. 1983;72(1):249–59.
19. Pierce GF, Mustoe TA, Senior RM, Reed J, Griffin GL, Thomason A, Deuel TF. In vivo incisional wound healing augmented by platelet-derived growth factor and recombinant c-sis gene homodimeric proteins. J Exp Med. 1988;167(3):974–87.
20. Andrew JG, Hoyland JA, Freemont AJ, Marsh DR. Platelet-derived growth factor expression in normally healing human fractures. Bone. 1995;16(4):455–60.
21. Yu X, Hsieh SC, Bao W, Graves DT. Temporal expression of PDGF receptors and PDGF regulatory effects on osteoblastic cells in mineralizing cultures. Am J Physiol. 1997;272(5 Pt 1):C1709–16.
22. Hammacher A, Hellman U, Johnsson A, Ostman A, Gunnarsson K, Westermark B, Wasteson A, Heldin CH. A major part of platelet-derived growth factor purified from human platelets is a heterodimer of one A and one B chain. J Biol Chem. 1988;263(31):16493–8.
23. Williams LT. Signal transduction by the platelet-derived growth factor receptor. Science. 1989;243(4898):1564–70.
24. Denholm IA, Moule AJ, Bartold PM. The behaviour and proliferation of human dental pulp cell strains in vitro, and their response to the application of platelet-derived growth factor-BB and insulin-like growth factor-1. Int Endod J. 1998;31(4):251–8.
25. Heldin CH, Ostman A, Ronnstrand L. Signal transduction via platelet-derived growth factor receptors. Biochim Biophys Acta. 1998;1378(1):F79–113.
26. Rutherford RB, TrailSmith MD, Ryan ME, Charette MF. Synergistic effects of dexamethasone on platelet-derived growth factor mitogenesis in vitro. Arch Oral Biol. 1992;37(2):139–45.
27. Heldin CH, Backstrom G, Ostman A, Hammacher A, Ronnstrand L, Rubin K, Nister M, Westermark B. Binding of different dimeric forms of PDGF to human fibroblasts: evidence for two separate receptor types. EMBO J. 1988;7(5):1387–93.
28. Centrella M, McCarthy TL, Kusmik WF, Canalis E. Relative binding and biochemical effects of heterodimeric and homodimeric isoforms of platelet-derived growth factor in osteoblast-enriched cultures from fetal rat bone. J Cell Physiol. 1991;147(3):420–6.
29. Hart CE, Forstrom JW, Kelly JD, Seifert RA, Smith RA, Ross R, Murray MJ, Bowen-Pope DF. Two classes of PDGF receptor recognize different isoforms of PDGF. Science. 1988;240(4858):1529–31.
30. Yokose S, Kadokura H, Tajima N, Hasegawa A, Sakagami H, Fujieda K, Katayama T. Platelet-derived growth factor exerts disparate effects on odontoblast differentiation depending on the dimers in rat dental pulp cells. Cell Tissue Res. 2004;315(3):375–84.
31. Didilescu AC, Pop F, Rusu MC. c-kit positive cells and networks in tooth germs of human midterm fetuses. Ann Anat. 2013;195(6):581–5.
32. Andelin WE, Shabahang S, Wright K, Torabinejad M. Identification of hard tissue after experimental pulp capping using dentin sialoprotein (DSP) as a marker. J Endod. 2003;29(10):646–50.
33. Feng JQ, Luan X, Wallace J, Jing D, Ohshima T, Kulkarni AB, D'Souza RN, Kozak CA, MacDougall M. Genomic organization, chromosomal mapping, and promoter analysis of the mouse dentin sialophosphoprotein (Dspp) gene, which codes for both dentin sialoprotein and dentin phosphoprotein. J Biol Chem. 1998;273(16):9457–64.
34. Unterbrink A, O'Sullivan M, Chen S, MacDougall M. TGF beta-1 downregulates DMP-1 and DSPP in odontoblasts. Connect Tissue Res. 2002;43(2–3):354–8.
35. Butler WT. Dentin matrix proteins and dentinogenesis. Connect Tissue Res. 1995;33(1–3):59–65.
36. Yokose S, Kadokura H, Tajima Y, Fujieda K, Katayama I, Matsuoka T, Katayama T. Establishment and characterization of a culture system for enzymatically released rat dental pulp cells. Calcif Tissue Int. 2000;66(2):139–44.

37. Iohara K, Nakashima M, Ito M, Ishikawa M, Nakasima A, Akamine A. Dentin regeneration by dental pulp stem cell therapy with recombinant human bone morphogenetic protein 2. J Dent Res. 2004;83(8):590–5.
38. Nakashima M. Induction of dentin formation on canine amputated pulp by recombinant human bone morphogenetic proteins (BMP)-2 and –4. J Dent Res. 1994;73(9):1515–22.
39. Nakashima M, Nagasawa H, Yamada Y, Reddi AH. Regulatory role of transforming growth factor-beta, bone morphogenetic protein-2, and protein-4 on gene expression of extracellular matrix proteins and differentiation of dental pulp cells. Dev Biol. 1994;162(1):18–28.
40. Saito T, Ogawa M, Hata Y, Bessho K. Acceleration effect of human recombinant bone morphogenetic protein-2 on differentiation of human pulp cells into odontoblasts. J Endod. 2004;30(4):205–8.
41. Nakashima M. The effects of growth factors on DNA synthesis, proteoglycan synthesis and alkaline phosphatase activity in bovine dental pulp cells. Arch Oral Biol. 1992;37(3):231–6.
42. Yu J, Deng Z, Shi J, Zhai H, Nie X, Zhuang H, Li Y, Jin Y. Differentiation of dental pulp stem cells into regular-shaped dentin-pulp complex induced by tooth germ cell conditioned medium. Tissue Eng. 2006;12(11):3097–105.
43. Aitman TJ, Critser JK, Cuppen E, Dominiczak A, Fernandez-Suarez XM, Flint J, Gauguier D, Geurts AM, Gould M, Harris PC, et al. Progress and prospects in rat genetics: a community view. Nat Genet. 2008;40(5):516–22.
44. Baker H. The laboratory rat, vol. I. Academic Press; 1979.
45. Chandrahasa S, Murray PE, Namerow KN. Proliferation of mature ex vivo human dental pulp using tissue engineering scaffolds. J Endod. 2011;37(9):1236–9.
46. Erisken C, Kalyon DM, Zhou J, Kim SG, Mao JJ. Viscoelastic Properties of Dental Pulp Tissue and Ramifications on Biomaterial Development for Pulp Regeneration. J Endod. 2015;41(10):1711–7.
47. Piva E, Silva AF, Nor JE. Functionalized scaffolds to control dental pulp stem cell fate. J Endod. 2014;40(4 Suppl):S33–40.
48. Torabinejad M, Milan M, Shabahang S, Wright KR, Faras H. Histologic examination of teeth with necrotic pulps and periapical lesions treated with 2 scaffolds: an animal investigation. J Endod. 2015;41(6):846–52.

6

Association between maximum occlusal force and 3-year all-cause mortality in community-dwelling elderly people

Toshimitsu Iinuma[1*], Yasumichi Arai[2], Michiyo Takayama[3], Yukiko Abe[2], Tomoka Ito[1], Yugaku Kondo[1], Nobuyoshi Hirose[2] and Nobuhito Gionhaku[1]

Abstract

Background: Among the very elderly, poor oral health reduces life expectancy. In this study, differences in the magnitude of the maximum occlusal force (MOF) in the very elderly were examined in terms of effects on all-cause mortality in a 3-year follow-up.

Methods: We evaluated 489 community-living elderly individuals aged 85 years or older. MOF was measured using an occlusal force measuring device, and participants were classified into three groups according to gender- and dental status-sensitive tertiles. Demographic variables, cognitive, physical function, psychological status, oral health, comorbidity, and blood chemistry factors were assessed. One-way analyses of variance, χ^2 tests, and the Kruskal-Wallis test were used for statistical analyses. The relationship between MOF tertiles and 3-year all-cause mortality was examined using a multivariate Cox model analysis after adjusting for confounding factors.

Results: MOF tertiles were significantly associated with cognitive impairment, number of teeth, limitations on chewable foods, handgrip strength, timed up-and-go test, and diabetes mellitus. During the follow-up period, 74 subjects died. Subjects with the highest MOF had a significantly lower mortality rate than other groups (log rank $P = 0.031$). In the univariate Cox model, MOF tertiles were independently associated with a lower risk of death (HR = 0.69, 95 % CI = 0.51–0.91). Even after adjusting for various confounders in the multivariate Cox model (Model 1), MOF was independently associated with a lower risk of death (HR = 0.67, 95 % CI = 0.50–0.91). In model 2, we added handgrip strength as a confounder and found that the HR for MOF was attenuated (HR = 0.73, 95 % CI = 0.54–0.99), but still statistically significant.

Conclusions: In a cohort of the very elderly, MOF was independently associated with all-cause mortality after adjusting for various health issues. Moreover, this independent association remained after a further adjustment for handgrip strength; however, the HR was attenuated. This suggests that MOF and handgrip strength may share a common mechanism of a general decrease in muscle strength, possibly sarcopenia, which is a significant cause of mortality in the very old.

Keywords: Very elderly people, Bite force, All-cause mortality, Healthy life expectancy

Abbreviations: ADL, Activities of daily living; ALB, Albumin; BMI, Body mass index; CI, Confidence interval; CRP, C-reactive protein; HR, Hazard ratio; IL-6, Interleukin-6; IQR, Interquartile range; MMSE, Mini-Mental State Examination; MOF, Maximum occlusal force; SD, Standard deviation; TOOTH, The Tokyo Oldest Old Survey on Total Health; WHO-5, The World Health Organization-5 well-being index

* Correspondence: iinuma.toshimitsu@nihon-u.ac.jp
[1]Department of Complete Denture Prosthodontics, Nihon University School of Dentistry, Tokyo, Japan
Full list of author information is available at the end of the article

Background

Many studies of oral health status have examined factors such as number of teeth, oral hygiene, denture use status, saliva secretion, and masticatory function to clarify any relationship with mortality in the elderly [1–7]. In addition, masticatory function has been studied in terms of nutritional analysis from the diet, functional analysis by muscle activity involved in chewing, and analysis of the maximum occlusal force (MOF) [8–10].

There are several ways to measure masticatory function and chewing ability with objective indicators. These indicators include evaluation methods using questionnaires, a chewing efficiency determination method using samples (peanuts, chewing gum, and gummy jelly), and measuring MOF values [11–13]. Among them, MOF is a safe and easy way for subjects to be measured. Thus, it has been used in many studies. In addition, measurement of MOF is straightforward.

Though a significant relationship between MOF and physical function has been observed [10], few studies have investigated the relationship between MOF and mortality. Iwasaki et al. [14] investigated survival over 13 years in 70-year-old elderly people who participated in the Niigata study, where they divided subjects, first separated by gender, into tertiles according to maximum bite force to investigate its relationship with mortality. Male participants in the lower maximum bite force group showed increased risk of all-cause mortality compared with those in the upper maximum bite force group. The range of MOF is gender-sensitive and affected by the presence or absence of teeth [15–17]. Furthermore, as the average life span increases, further studies on very elderly people aged 85 years or older are required. Despite the increase in comorbidities and worsening of physical status, psychological status, and nutrition status [18–20] with increasing age, we hypothesized that MOF in the very elderly would be associated with their mortality independent of general health status.

In this study, we investigated the influence of the magnitude of MOF, classified by gender and number of teeth, based on survival at 3 years. Furthermore, we examined the relationships between MOF and physical and oral function. If our hypothesis is correct, MOF can be considered an indicator of the relationship between oral health and mortality in very elderly people.

Methods

Study population

The study analyzed data from participants in The Tokyo Oldest Old Survey on Total Health (TOOTH) study, which is an epidemiological survey involving very elderly people living in the Tokyo metropolitan area.

We recruited 542 subjects [236 men, 306 women; mean age ± SD, 87.8 + 2.2 (range 85–102) years] for a medical and dental survey. The participants were randomly selected from inhabitants between March 2008 and November 2009 [21].

Fifty-three participants without MOF measurements were excluded from the analyses for the following reasons: pain on biting, non-use of dentures, and current dental treatment. Consequently, data of 489 subjects were analyzed. The study protocol was reviewed and the survey was approved by the ethics committees at Nihon University School of Dentistry (No. 2003–20, 2008) and Keio University School of Medicine (No. 19–47, 2007). The TOOTH study has been registered in the UMIN-Clinical Trial Registry as UMIN-CTR ID UMIN000001842.

MOF

The MOF was measured using an occlusal force-measuring device (Occlusal Force-Meter GM10; Nagano Keiki, Tokyo, Japan, with a measuring range of 0 ~ 1000 N and accuracy of ±1 N) using a standard procedure. We calculated MOF as the average of three measurements of the first molar on the functional side. The subjects were seated in an unsupported natural position, and the users' dentures were inserted at that time. The intra-class correlation coefficients (ICC) for the reproducibility of the MOF measurements for intra- and inter-class reliability were 0.98 and 0.97, respectively [10].

MOF tertile classification

We classified the participants according to MOF tertile using the following three steps because MOF is sensitive to gender and dental status. First, we classified participants into four categories depending on gender and the presence or absence of teeth (edentulous male, dentulous male, edentulous female, and dentulous female). Then each category was classified into three groups based on MOF value (highest, middle, and lowest groups). Finally, to form three groups distinguished only by MOF, we merged the above four categories. (e.g., the MOF lowest tertile group included participants with MOFs in the lowest tertile within each group: edentulous male, dentulous male, edentulous female, and dentulous female). Accordingly, MOF could minimize the influence of gender, and presence or absence of teeth.

Oral health assessment

In face-to-face interviews and dental examinations, trained dentists assessed subjects' oral health status in terms of the number of remaining teeth, number of chewable foods, and degree of oral hygiene.

For the food intake questionnaire, 15 kinds of food were selected to evaluate chewing ability, and were categorized into three groups according to hardness and texture. Limitation of chewing ability was defined as being unable to eat one or more foods. In this study, we counted the total number of remaining teeth (range 0–32). Tongue surface plaque was examined to evaluate the degree of oral cleaning [22].

Demographics and general health assessment

At the same time as the dental examination, trained geriatricians assessed the subjects' demographic variables and general health, including medical conditions and physical functional status. Education was dichotomized according to whether participants had graduated from high school. Smoking and drinking were dichotomized in terms of whether participants had never or had ever smoked and whether they had ever or had never consumed alcohol, respectively. Ten indices of basic activities of daily living (ADL) were assessed using the Barthel index. A disability in ADL was defined as having a disability on one or more indices. Cognitive function was evaluated using the Mini-Mental State Examination (MMSE). Body mass index (BMI) was measured as an anthropometric parameter. The World Health Organization-5 (WHO-5) well-being index was used to assess psychological status [23]. To obtain the medical history, medical examinations conducted by geriatricians, personal interviews regarding available documentation including discharge summary and medication list, and personal interviews with the caregiver/proxy were used.

Self-reported medical conditions were classified according to the International Classification of Diseases, 10th Revision. Using non-fasting blood samples, we measured the plasma albumin (ALB) and C-reactive protein (CRP) concentrations using standard assay procedures. We used commercial ELISA kits (Quantikine HS, Human IL-6; R&D Systems, Minneapolis, MN) in duplicate to measure plasma interleukin-6 (IL-6) levels. The inter-assay CV for IL-6 was 9.43 %.

Physical function and activity

To assess lower extremity performance, the timed up-and-go test, which has been validated in older adults [24], was used. The test was performed by two examiners to prevent falls or injuries. A handheld dynamometer (Tanita 6103; Tanita, Tokyo, Japan) was used to measure handgrip strength of the dominant hand, and the average of twice measurements was calculated.

The physical activity was evaluated by asking whether participants walked more than 60 min per day.

Outcomes

The outcome of interest was death from any cause. All of the participants were followed by telephone contact or mail survey every 12 months to identify mortality. We also investigated the cause-specific mortality, including cancers, cardiovascular disease, pneumonia, and other causes. The survivors after 36 months were surveyed using the same protocol as at baseline.

Statistical analysis

Data are expressed as means [standard deviations (SDs)] or medians [interquartile ranges (IQRs)] for continuous variables or percentages for categorical variables, or were log-transformed for statistical analyses. The Kruskal–Wallis test was used to evaluate differences in continuous variables at baseline, and the chi-square test was used to assess categorical variables. Longitudinal analyses were performed using Kaplan–Meier survival curves according to MOF tertiles. The level of significance for prognostic results was defined as log-rank $P < 0.05$. Then, univariate and multivariate Cox proportional hazards regression models were used to identify the relative risk of mortality. First, biological and behavioral factors known to be associated with mortality (MOF, age, smoking and drinking status, cognitive impairment [MMSE < 24], ADL disability, low body mass index [<18.5], physical function [handgrip strength], physical activity [total walking time], oral hygiene [tongue plaque], nutrition [limited ability to chew foods], psychological status [WHO-5], and comorbidities [ischemic stroke, coronary heart disease, cancer], ALB, CRP, and IL-6) were assessed using the hazard ratio (HR) in univariate models. Those with significant associations ($P < 0.05$) were entered into the multivariate model. To eliminate multicollinearity between CRP and IL-6, these values were entered into the model separately. In all analyses, the level of statistical significance was set at $P < 0.05$. Analyses were performed using SPSS ver. 22.0 (SPSS, Chicago, IL, USA).

Results

The MOF tertiles are shown in Table 1. The median MOF was 14.0 kgf (IQR: 7.9–23.8 kgf) in males (219 participants) and 9.9 kgf (IQR: 5.4–16.7 kgf) in females (270 participants). There was a significant difference between the genders ($P < 0.001$). Regarding the presence or absence of teeth, the median MOF was 13.8 kgf (IQR: 8.0–22.3 kgf) in the dentulous (349 participants) and 7.7 kgf (IQR: 4.0–12.5 kgf) in the edentulous (140 participants); the difference was significant ($P < 0.001$). Baseline characteristics of subjects by MOF tertiles are shown in Table 2. MOF tertiles were significantly associated with cognitive impairment, number of teeth, limited ability to chew foods, handgrip strength, timed up-and-go test, and prevalence of diabetes mellitus ($P = 0.001$, $P < 0.001$, $P < 0.001$, $P = 0.006$, $P = 0.014$, and $P = 0.047$, respectively). During the 3-year follow-up period, 74 participants died (22 of cancer, 22 of cardiovascular disease, 16 of pneumonia, 11 of other causes, and three of unknown causes); four declined the follow-up survey. We

Table 1 Tertiles of MOF across age and dentulous status

	Maximum occlusal force groups (tertile)			
	All	1(lowest)	2	3(highest)
Characteristics	*n*=489	*n*=163	*n*=163	*n*=163
Maximum occlusal force, median [IQR], kgf				
Male dentulous (*n*=167)	15.7[8.9–26.1]	7.3[5.5–9.0]	15.7[13.1–18.8]	31.4[26.0–41.4]
Male edentulous (*n*=52)	11.2[4.7–16.3]	4.0[3.1–4.7]	11.2[8.4–12.4]	18.8[16.3–24.7]
Female dentulous (*n*=182)	11.9[7.2–18.6]	5.1[3.3–7.3]	11.9[10.1–14.2]	22.3[18.6–28.8]
Female edentulous (*n*=88)	6.6[3.6–10.9]	2.8[1.9–3.7]	6.6[5.4–8.1]	12.3[10.9–18.0]

plotted Kaplan–Meier survival curves for the cumulative incidence of all-cause mortality according to oral function (Fig. 1). The survival curve of MOF tertiles showed that subjects with the highest MOF had a significantly lower risk of all-cause mortality (log rank $P = 0.031$). Table 3 presents HRs and 95 % CI from Cox proportional hazards models for all-cause mortality. In the univariate Cox model, MOF tertiles (lowest as a reference) were associated with a lower HR of death (HR = 0.69, 95 % CI = 0.51–0.91). In addition, age, ADL disability, handgrip strength, total walking time, WHO-5 score, ALB, IL-6, and CRP were significantly associated with all-cause mortality. When we adjusted for age, ADL disability, total walking time, WHO-5, ALB, IL-6, and CRP in the multivariate Cox model (model 1), MOF was independently associated with a ~0.7-fold lower risk of 3-year survival (HR = 0.67, 95 % CI = 0.50–0.91). In model 2, we added handgrip strength as a confounder and found that the HR for MOF was attenuated (HR = 0.73, 95 % CI = 0.54–0.99), although the estimate was still statistically significant.

Discussion

This prospective study investigated community-dwelling very elderly people age ≥85 years, after minimizing the influence of effects of gender and the number of teeth present and adjusted for potential confounders. The results indicated that the risk of death in the subpopulation with the highest MOF conferred a 0.7-fold lower risk of death in three years versus the lowest MOF group (tertile). This suggests that the association between MOF and mortality is independent of gender, dental status, physical activity, psychological status, comorbidities, and serum levels of albumin and inflammatory biomarkers. Moreover, this independent association remained after a further adjustment for handgrip strength; however, the hazard ratio of MOF was attenuated. These results suggest that MOF and handgrip strength may at least partly share a common mechanism in the general decrease in muscle strength, possibly sarcopenia, a significant contributor to mortality in the very old. Moreover, we expect our results will be useful for the systematic evaluation of life expectancy in the very elderly.

Many studies of the elderly have investigated relationships between mortality and nutrition, lifestyle, comorbidities, physical status, and physical function [25–28]. Furthermore, factors concerning oral status, inflammation, and function have been investigated for the same purpose [29–31]. Recently, one study investigated the association between MOF and mortality in older Japanese adults, and reported that MOF was independently associated with all-cause mortality in males [14]. However, studies on the relationship between MOF and mortality are very limited, because it is generally considered that gender, age, remaining number of teeth, use of denture, and face morphology affect one's bite force [32, 33]. In fact, in the present study, significant differences were observed between men and women and between dentulous and edentulous subjects. This finding is partly consistent with the results of observational studies, which have demonstrated gender-sensitive effects on bite force and masticatory muscle thickness and their interactions [34, 35]. In this study, we took these factors into account by separating subjects into four categories. The participants were divided into three groups by MOF, gender, and dentulous versus edentulous. Even considering these factors, the 3-year all-cause mortality for the highest MOF group was significantly lower than the others. One reason why MOF affects mortality may be that a reduction of muscle activity from sarcopenia due to aging causes a decline in the skeletal muscle mass in the whole body [36]. In addition, a decrease in skeletal muscle function in the very elderly causes falls and leads to a reduction in ADL [37, 38]. Ling et al. [20] reported on 555 people who were followed for a period of 9.5 years in the Leiden 85-plus study. In their results, 80 % of the participants died, and handgrip strength was a predictor of all-cause mortality in the oldest old population. Raadsheer et al. [32] concluded that the size of the jaw muscles was significantly related to the size of the limb muscles; that is, a decrease in muscle mass of the whole body, due to sarcopenia, affected the muscle activity of the jaw muscles that express the bite force. In our study, MOF showed a significant association with handgrip strength and the timed up-and-go test, which are both physical functional

Table 2 Baseline characteristics of participants according to tertiles of MOF

	MOF groups (tertile)				
	All	1(lowest)	2	3(highest)	p^*
Characteristics	*n*=489	*n*=163	*n*=163	*n*=163	
Demographics					
Age, mean (SD)	87.3(2.2)	87.3(2.4)	87.5(2.3)	87.1(2.0)	0.264
Higher education, %[c]	26.5	26.1	27.2	26.1	0.968
Smoking, %[c]	40.6	35.8	44.3	41.6	0.294
Drinking, %[d]	48.8	45.0	49.4	52.2	0.431
Oral health status					
Number of teeth, median [IQR]	7.0[0.0–18.0]	5.0[0.0–11.0]	6.0[0.0–17.0]	15.0[0.0–24.0]	<0.001[a]
Limitation of chewable foods, %	46.9	60.7	50.0	30.1	<0.001
Tongue plaque, %	41.3	44.8	40.5	38.7	0.514
General health assessment					
MMSE, median [IQR][e]	27[25–29]	27[23–29]	27[25–29]	27[25–29]	0.072[a]
MMSE<24, %[e]	17.8	26.7	12.4	14.2	0.001
ADL disability, %[f]	22.8	24.4	24.1	20.0	0.581
BMI, mean (SD)	21.5(3.1)	21.1(3.0)	21.6(2.9)	21.9(3.4)	0.119
BMI<18.5, %	17.0	19.0	14.7	17.3	0.583
Psychological status					
WHO-5, median [IQR][d]	19.0[15.0–22.0]	19.0[15.0–22.0]	19.0[14.0–22.5]	20.0[17.0–22.0]	0.195[a]
Medical history, %					
Ischemic stroke	11.9	11.7	12.9	11.0	0.872
Coronary heart disease	11.2	11.0	10.4	12.3	0.866
Hypertension[g]	59.3	58.6	57.1	62.1	0.526
Diabetes mellitus	18.4	15.3	24.5	15.3	0.047
Cancer	18.6	19.0	19.0	17.8	0.947
Biochemical					
Albumin, g/dL (SD)[g]	4.1(0.3)	4.1(0.3)	4.1(0.3)	4.1(0.2)	0.372
IL-6, pg/ml, median [IQR][g]	1.69[1.29–2.46]	1.75[1.32–2.47]	1.72[1.33–2.54]	1.63[1.21–2.43]	0.568[b]
CRP, mg/dL, median [IQR][g]	0.09[0.04–0.18]	0.08[0.04–0.19]	0.10[0.04–0.21]	0.08[0.04–0.15]	0.594[b]
Physical functions					
Handgrip strength, median[IQR], kgf	19.3[15.5–24.0]	18.3[15.0–22.8]	19.0[15.5–23.3]	20.5[16.0–25.5]	0.006[a]
Time up & go test, median[IQR], second[h]	13.1[10.9–16.2]	13.8[11.3–18.7]	13.2[10.9–15.4]	12.7[11.0–15.2]	0.014[a]
Physical activity					
Total walking time>60 min/day, %[d]	37.2	36.3	40.0	35.2	0.649

[*]*P* values were calculated for categorical covariates using chi-square test, whereas P variables were calculated using one way analysis of variance (ANOVA) for continuous variables unless otherwise indicated. [a]Calculated using nonparametric Kruskal-Wallis test. [b]Calculated using ANOVA after logarithmic transformation [c-h]Data available for [c]472, [d]477, [e]484, [f]482, [g]486, and [h]432 people, respectively

measurement items. In addition, from the results obtained by adding handgrip strength as a confounding factor in the Cox hazard analysis, the correlation between MOF and death was affected. Based on these results, the pathogenesis of sarcopenia caused by aging could have the same impact on bite force, extremity muscle strength, and handgrip strength, and these might represent a significant mortality force among the very old. Hence, MOF is an important indicator of sarcopenia in the oral area in the very elderly. Thus, dental health professionals, there is a need for careful observation of very elderly concerning changes in the value of MOF in everyday clinical practice, because decreases in MOF may be associated with worsening physical health. Furthermore, the effects of aging on muscle activity may also be due to an attenuation of muscle strength

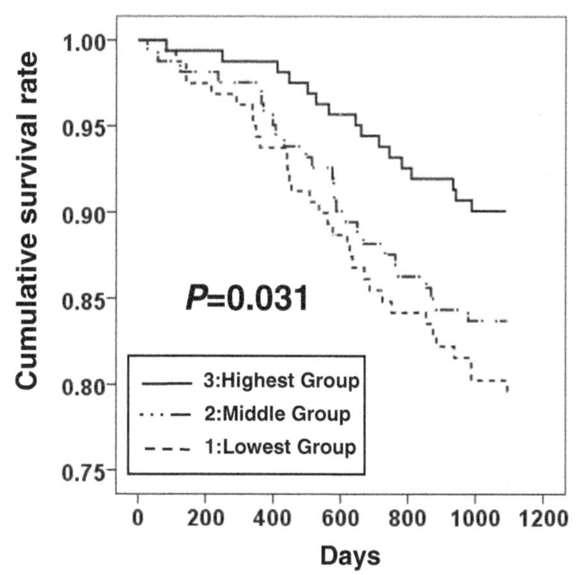

Fig. 1 MOF tertiles and 3-year all-cause mortality. Kaplan-Meier survival curves for the three maximum occlusal force groups ($P = 0.031$). Cumulative survival rate increased progressively in association with an increase in maximum occlusal force

(dynapenia) [39]. Further research is necessary to determine any such association.

MOF might affect meals and the nutritional value associated with food intake in the very elderly. In the present study, as an index of the variety of food intake in the diet of the very elderly, the proportion of those with no limit on food acceptance was significantly higher in the highest MOF group than in the other groups. However, MOF showed no significant correlation with serum levels of albumin or BMI <18.5, which are indices of malnutrition. From these results, we believe that a decline in MOF may limit the diversity of food acceptance rather than total calories from food. In this regard, there is substantial evidence that a decline in oral function is associated with a suboptimal diet that is low in fruits and vegetables, leading to micronutrient deficiencies [40]. Thus, there is a need to analyze any connection between MOF and nutrient intake.

This study had several limitations. First, the number of participants and areas of research were limited, as our study targeted very elderly people who lived in metropolitan Tokyo. Therefore, a larger-scale, separate cohort study that considers race, eating habits, and economic conditions should be conducted. Furthermore, to explore the underlying biological mechanism, it is important to study the relationship between MOF and cause-specific

Table 3 Hazard risk from univariate and multivariate cox models for mortality

	Univariate model			Multivariate model 1			Multivariate model 2		
Characteristics	HR	95 % CI	*p*-value	HR	95 % CI	*p*-value	HR	95 % CI	*p*-value
MOF (tertile)	0.69	[0.51–0.91]	0.010	0.67	[0.50–0.91]	0.010	0.73	[0.54–0.99]	0.040
Age	1.14	[1.06–1.23]	<0.001	1.11	[1.03–1.20]	0.006	1.08	[1.01–1.17]	0.038
Smoking	0.83	[0.51–1.35]	0.454						
Drinking	0.88	[0.55–1.41]	0.594						
Cognitive impairment (MMSE<24)	1.32	[0.76–2.30]	0.331						
ADL disability	1.70	[1.04–2.77]	0.035	1.11	[0.64–1.92]	0.714	1.05	[0.61–1.81]	0.866
BMI <18.5	1.15	[0.64–2.05]	0.645						
Handgrip strength (tertile)	0.72	[0.54–0.96]	0.026				0.58	[0.41–0.82]	0.002
Total walking time (>60min/day)	0.51	[0.30–0.88]	0.015	0.60	[0.34–1.06]	0.079	0.66	[0.37–1.16]	0.148
Limitation of chewable foods	1.46	[0.93–2.32]	0.103						
Tongue plaque	0.92	[0.58–1.46]	0.725						
WHO-5 (tertile)	0.72	[0.53–0.97]	0.032	0.77	[0.56–1.06]	0.114	0.79	[0.58–1.09]	0.152
Ischemic stroke	1.32	[0.70–2.51]	0.390						
Coronary heart disease	1.40	[0.74–2.66]	0.303						
Cancer	1.53	[0.91–2.58]	0.108						
ALB (tertile)	0.64	[0.47–0.87]	0.005	0.77	[0.55–1.08]	0.124	0.80	[0.57–1.11]	0.183
IL-6 (tertile)[a]	1.33	[1.00–1.76]	0.048	1.22	[0.90–1.66]	0.191	1.23	[0.90–1.66]	0.190
CRP (tertile)[a]	1.45	[1.09–1.94]	0.011	1.30	[0.96–1.76]	0.096	1.32	[0.97–1.80]	0.077

Model 1: Adjusted for age, ADL disability, MOF, Total walking time, WHO-5, ALB, IL-6, and CRP
Model 2: Adjusted for age, ADL disability, MOF, Total walking time, WHO-5, ALB, IL-6, CRP, and handgrip strength
[a]IL-6 and CRP were entered separately in the multivariate model. Tertile: lowest was a reference

mortality. However, this study did not include a sufficient number of individuals over a long enough period to analyze cause-specific mortality. Second, we classified the participants by the number of teeth as dentulous and edentulous. However, there is a need to subdivide by number of teeth and details. Third, we analyzed food variety. There is a need to examine the relevance of micronutrients. Finally, it is necessary to make a concrete plan to attempt to improve MOF in the very elderly, and also to advocate for their needs in an aging society.

Conclusions

In a cohort of the very elderly, MOF was independently associated with all-cause mortality after adjustment for various health elements, including ADL disability, physical activity, psychological status, and levels of albumin, interleukin-6, and C-reactive protein. These results suggest that MOF can be considered an important indicator of the relationship between oral health and mortality in very elderly people. Moreover, further adjustment for handgrip strength affected the HR of MOF, suggesting that age-related sarcopenia could at least partly mediate the association between MOF and mortality. The results of this study encourage dental health professionals to pay attention to MOF in the very elderly because decreases in MOF may reflect worsening physical health.

Acknowledgments

We wish to acknowledge the participant's cooperation and the support of Prof. Clive Langham, as well as the assistance of Ms. Miho Shimura. In addition to the authors, the following people contributed to data acquisition as TOOTH investigators: Yoshinori Ebihara, MD, PhD; Kenichiro Shimizu; MD, PhD; Ken Yamamura, MD, PhD; Susumu Nakazawa, MD; Midori Takayama, PhD; Kensuke Nishio, DDS, PhD; and Kentaro Urata, DDS, PhD.

Fundings

This study was funded by grants from the Grants-in-Aid for Scientific Research (C) (No. 22592347, 26463194, 20590706, 21590775, 23617024) from Japan Society for the Promotion of Science, by a grant from the Sato from Nihon University School of Dentistry, by a grant from Japan Health Foundation for the Prevention of Chronic Disease and the Improvement of QOL of Patients, by a grant from the Foundation for Total Health Promotion, by The Univers Foundation, and by the Chiyoda Mutual Life Foundation.

Authors' contributions

TI has full access to all the data in the study and takes responsibility for the integrity of the data and the accuracy of the data analysis. Study concept and design: TI, YA. Acquisition of data: TI, YA, MT, Y. Abe. Analysis and interpretation of data: TI, YA, MT, Y. Abe, NG. Drafting of the manuscript: TI, YA. Collection of biological specimen: YA. Data management: YA TI. Study oversee: NG, NH. All authors read and approved the final manuscript.

Competing interest

The authors declare that they have no competing interests.

Consent for publication

Not applicable.

Ethics approval and consent to participate

This study was approved by the ethics committees at Nihon University School of Dentistry (No. 2003–20, 2008) and Keio University School of Medicine (N0. 19–47, 2007). After we explained the purpose of the study, written informed consent was obtained from all participants.

Author details

[1]Department of Complete Denture Prosthodontics, Nihon University School of Dentistry, Tokyo, Japan. [2]Center for Supercentenarian Medical Research, Keio University School of Medicine, Tokyo, Japan. [3]Center for Preventive Medicine, Keio University School of Medicine, Tokyo, Japan.

References

1. Hayasaka K, Tomata Y, Aida J, Watanabe T, Kakizaki M, Tsuji I. Tooth loss and mortality in elderly Japanese adults: Effect of oral care. J Am Geriatr Soc. 2013;61:815–20.
2. Hirotomi T, Yoshihara A, Ogawa H, Miyazaki H. Number of teeth and 5-year mortality in an elderly population. Community Dent Oral Epidemiol. 2015; 43:226–31.
3. Liljestrand JM, Havulinna AS, Paju S, Männistö S, Salomaa V, Pussinen PJ. Missing teeth predict incident cardiovascular events, diabetes, and death. J Dent Res. 2015;94:1055–62.
4. Marín-Zuluaga DJ, Sandvik L, Gil-Montoya JA, Willumsen T. Oral health and mortality risk in the institutionalised elderly. Med Oral Patol Oral Cir Bucal. 2012;17:e618–23.
5. Iinuma T, Arai Y, Abe Y, Takayama M, Fukumoto M, Fukui Y, et al. Denture wearing during sleep doubles the risk of pneumonia in the very elderly. J Dent Res. 2015;94(3 Suppl):28S–36S.
6. Phillips AC, Carroll D, Drayson MT, Der G. Salivary immunoglobulin a secretion rate is negatively associated with cancer mortality: The West of Scotland Twenty-07 Study. PLoS One. 2015;10:e0145083.
7. Lee MS, Huang YC, Wahlqvist ML. Chewing ability in conjunction with food intake and energy status in later life affects survival in Taiwanese with the metabolic syndrome. J Am Geriatr Soc. 2010;58:1072–80.
8. Schimmel M, Katsoulis J, Genton L, Müller F. Masticatory function and nutrition in old age. Swiss Dent J. 2015;125:449–54.
9. Galo R, Vitti M, Santos CM, Hallak JE, Regalo SC. The effect of age on the function of the masticatory system – an electromyographical analysis. Gerodontology. 2006;23:177–82.
10. Iinuma T, Arai Y, Fukumoto M, Takayama M, Abe Y, Asakura K, et al. Maximum occlusal force and physical performance in the oldest old: The Tokyo oldest old survey on total health. J Am Geriatr Soc. 2012;60:68–76.
11. Takata Y, Ansai T, Awano S, Hamasaki T, Yoshitake Y, Kimura Y, et al. Relationship of physical fitness to chewing in an 80-year-old population. Oral Dis. 2004;10:44–9.
12. Nokubi T, Yoshimuta Y, Nokubi F, Yasui S, Kusunoki C, Ono T, et al. Validity and reliability of a visual scoring method for masticatory ability using test gummy jelly. Gerodontology. 2013;30:76–82.
13. Ikebe K, Matsuda K, Kagawa R, Enoki K, Yoshida M, Maeda Y, et al. Association of masticatory performance with age, gender, number of teeth, occlusal force and salivary flow in Japanese older adults: Is ageing a risk factor for masticatory dysfunction. Arch Oral Biol. 2011;56:991–6.
14. Iwasaki M, Yoshihara A, Sato N, Sato M, Taylor GW, Ansai T, et al. Maximum bite force at age 70 years predicts all-cause mortality during the following 13 years in Japanese men. J Oral Rehabil. 2016;43:565–74.
15. Kosaka T, Ono T, Kida M, Kikui M, Yamamoto M, Yasui S, et al. A multifactorial model of masticatory performance: The Suita study. J Oral Rehabil. 2016;43:340–7.
16. Varga S, Spalj S, Lapter Varga M, Anic Milosevic S, Mestrovic S, Slaj M. Maximum voluntary molar bite force in subjects with normal occlusion. Eur J Orthod. 2011;33:427–33.
17. Garner LD, Kotwal NS. Correlation study of incisive biting forces with age, sex, and anterior occlusion. J Dent Res. 1973;52:698–702.
18. Nilsson G, Ohrvik J, Lonnberg I, Hedberg P. Low Psychological General Well-Being (PGWB) is associated with deteriorated 10-year survival in men but not in women among the elderly. Arch Gerontol Geriatr. 2011;52:167–71.
19. McNaughton SA, Bates CJ, Mishra GD. Diet quality is associated with all-cause mortality in adults aged 65 years and older. J Nutr. 2012;142:320–5.

20. Ling CH, Taekema D, de Craen AJ, Gussekloo J, Westendorp RG, Maier AB. Handgrip strength and mortality in the oldest old population: The Leiden 85-plus study. CMAJ. 2010;182:429–35.
21. Arai Y, Iinuma T, Takayama M, Takayama M, Abe Y, Fukuda R, et al. The Tokyo Oldest Old Survey on Total Health (TOOTH): A longitudinal cohort study of multidimensional components of health and well-being. BMC Geriatr. 2010;10:35. doi:10.1186/1471-2318-10-35.
22. Abe S, Ishihara K, Adachi M, Okuda K. Oral hygiene evaluation for effective oral care in preventing pneumonia in dentate elderly. Arch Gerontol Geriatr. 2006;43:53–64.
23. Awata S, Bech P, Koizumi Y, Seki T, Kuriyama S, Hozawa A, et al. Validity and utility of the Japanese version of the WHO-Five Well-being Index in the context of detecting suicidal ideation in elderly community residents. Int Psychogeriatr. 2007;19:77–88.
24. Podsiadlo D, Richardson S. The timed "Up & Go:" a test of basic functional mobility for frail elderly persons. J Am Geriatr Soc. 1991;39:142–8.
25. Midlöv P, Calling S, Memon AA, Sundquist J, Sundquist K, Johansson SE. Women's health in the Lund area (WHILA) – Alcohol consumption and all-cause mortality among women: A 17-year follow-up study. BMC Public Health. 2016;16:22.
26. Odden MC, Peralta CA, Haan MN, Covinsky KE. Rethinking the association of high blood pressure with mortality in elderly adults: The impact of frailty. Arch Intern Med. 2012;172:1162–8.
27. Arnau A, Espaulella J, Méndez T, Serrarols M, Canudas J, Formiga F, Ferrer M. Lower limb function and 10-year survival in population aged 75 years and older. Fam Pract. 2016;33:10–6.
28. Legrand D, Vaes B, Matheï C, Adriaensen W, Van Pottelbergh G, Degryse JM. Muscle strength and physical performance as predictors of mortality, hospitalization, and disability in the oldest old. J Am Geriatr Soc. 2014;62: 1030–8.
29. Ansai T, Takata Y, Soh I, Awano S, Yoshida A, Sonoki K, et al. Relationship between tooth loss and mortality in 80-year-old Japanese community-dwelling subjects. BMC Public Health. 2010;10:386. doi:10.1186/1471-2458-10-386.
30. Avlund K, Schultz-Larsen K, Krustrup U, Christiansen N, Holm-Pedersen P. Effect of inflammation in the periodontium in early old age on mortality at 21-year follow-up. J Am Geriatr Soc. 2009;57:1206–12.
31. Ansai T, Takata Y, Soh I, Akifusa S, Sogame A, Shimada N, et al. Relationship between chewing ability and 4-year mortality in a cohort of 80-year-old Japanese people. Oral Dis. 2007;13:214–9.
32. Raadsheer MC, Van Eijden TM, Van Ginkel FC, Prahl-Andersen B. Human jaw muscle strength and size in relation to limb muscle strength and size. Eur J Oral Sci. 2004;112:398–405.
33. Bonakdarchian M, Askari N, Askari M. Effect of face form on maximal molar bite force with natural dentition. Arch Oral Biol. 2009;54:201–4.
34. Palinkas M, Nassar MS, Cecílio FA, Siéssere S, Semprini M, Machado-de-Sousa JP, et al. Age and gender influence on maximal bite force and masticatory muscles thickness. Arch Oral Biol. 2010;55:797–802.
35. Kiliaridis S, Georgiakaki I, Katsaros C. Masseter muscle thickness and maxillary dental arch width. Eur J Orthod. 2003;25:259–63.
36. Landi F, Liperoti R, Fusco D, Mastropaolo S, Quattrociocchi D, Proia A, et al. Sarcopenia and mortality among older nursing home residents. J Am Med Dir Assoc. 2012;13:121–6.
37. Janssen I, Heymsfield SB, Ross R. Low relative skeletal muscle mass (sarcopenia) in older persons is associated with functional impairment and physical disability. J Am Geriatr Soc. 2002;50:889–96.
38. Tanimoto Y, Watanabe M, Sun W, Sugiura Y, Hayashida I, Kusabiraki T, et al. Sarcopenia and falls in community-dwelling elderly subjects in Japan: Defining sarcopenia according to criteria of the European Working Group on Sarcopenia in Older People. Arch Gerontol Geriatr. 2014;59:295–9.
39. Clark BC, Manini TM. Sarcopenia =/= dynapenia. J Gerontol A Biol Sci Med Sci. 2008;63:829–34.
40. Bradbury J, Thomason JM, Jepson NJ, Walls AW, Mulvaney CE, Allen PF, et al. Perceived chewing ability and intake of fruit and vegetables. J Dent Res. 2008;87:720–5.

7

Oral-health-related background factors and dental service utilisation among Sudanese children with and without a congenital heart defects

H. M. Ali[1*], M. Mustafa[2], E. F. Nasir[3,2], S. A. Lie[1], S. Hasabalrasol[4], O. H. Elshazali[5], R. W. Ali[6] and M. S. Skeie[1]

Abstract

Background: Sudanese children with congenital heart defects (CHDs) were found to have poorer oral health than those without CHDs. The aims of this study were to: describe the patterns of oral-health-related background factors in children with and without CHD and explore any differences, and to evaluate the effects of background factors on caries and gingivitis prevalence and dental services utilisation.

Methods: In this analytical cross-sectional study, caregivers of children aged 3–12 years with (CHD cases $n = 111$) and without CHDs (Controls $n = 182$), underwent face-to-face interviews using a structured questionnaire. The questionnaire items covered several oral health background factors (independent variables) including: child's health status, oral hygiene practices, dental services utilization, mother's level of education, and caregiver's perception and awareness of their child's oral health. The relationship between these factors and occurrence of '*caries*' and '*gingivitis*' as well as '*child's dental services utilisation*' (dependent variables) were explored using multiple adjusted and hierarchal logistic regression analyses.

Results: Compared with controls, CHD cases had lower frequencies of brushing and use of fluoridated toothpaste, and their caregivers were less knowledgeable about caries. Among CHD cases, the variables (brushing and fluoridated toothpaste use) had significant impacts on caries prevalence (odd ratio (OR) =5.6, 95% confidence interval (CI): 1.4–22.8 and OR = 0.3, 95% CI: 0.1–0.8 for infrequent compared to frequent ones, respectively) as well as the mother's level of education (OR = 2.6, 95% CI: 1.0–6.4). When differences in background factors were controlled for, the adjusted ORs for caries and gingivitis prevalence in CHD cases compared with controls were 1.8, (95% CI: 1.1–3.2) and 5.3 (95% CI: 2.9–9.4), respectively. Among CHD cases, the child's age (8–12 years: OR = 11.9, 95% CI: 1.9–71.6), and the mother's level of education (lower education: OR = 0.2, 95% CI: 0.03–0.9) were significantly associated with the child's dental services utilisation.

Conclusions: Lower frequencies of brushing and use of fluoride tooth paste were reported among CHD cases, and brushing had the predominant significant impact on caries prevalence. The child's age and the mother's level of education were the main factors affecting the child's (CHD cases) dental services utilisation.

Keywords: Caries, Children, Congenital heart defects, Dental health services, Gingivitis, Oral health background factors

* Correspondence: Hiba.Mohammedali@student.uib.no
[1]Department of Clinical Dentistry, Faculty of Medicine and Dentistry, University of Bergen, Bergen, Norway
Full list of author information is available at the end of the article

Background

Congenital heart defects (CHDs) and structural abnormalities of the heart affect ~8 in 1000 live births worldwide [1]. Generally, caries and periodontal diseases have low mortality, however, both have high morbidity and are responsible for dental pain, teeth loss as well as being risk factors for other systemic complications especially among children [2]. Children with a CHD are at a disadvantage in that, because of their underlying medical condition, development of an oral disease can put their general health at risk [3]. The main risks and conditions caused by odontogenic bacteraemia are life-threatining conditions, including infective endocarditis and brain abcesses [4]. Recent changes in the recommendations for the prevention of infective endocarditis in children with a CHD have limited antibiotic prophylaxis to certain types of CHD and highlighted the importance of non-antibiotic prophylaxis [5, 6]. It has been emphasised that finding ways to prevent oral health problems in children with a CHD is more important than ever [5–7]. The role of the caregiver of a child with a CHD, in terms of practising daily oral health activities and possessing oral health knowledge, has been recognised to be more important than previously thought [6, 8–10].

Previous studies on the dental knowledge and attitudes of children with a CHD and their caregivers have yielded unsatisfactory results with regard to oral hygiene practices and the use of dental services [3, 11–13]. A study conducted in Brazil in 2002 found that 28.8% of children with a CHD had never visited a dentist [10]. The authors also reported that 47.1% of these children brushed their teeth more than once daily, which was below expectations despite the fact that brushing was performed with parental supervision [10]. A study undertaken in the UK in 1996 showed that caregivers of children with a CHD attended fewer regular dental check-ups for their children than caregivers of children with no medical problems [14]. In studies from several developing countries, caregivers of children with a CHD reported with less awareness about the link between CHDs and oral diseases and the increased risk of their children developing infective endocarditis [9, 10, 15]. However, in studies from other developed countries, caregivers had fairly better knowledge [16, 17].

Findings vary regarding the susceptibility to dental diseases of children with compared to children without a CHD resident in industrialised countries [14, 16, 18, 19]. In developing countries, few epidemiological studies have been conducted on children with a CHD and little information is available about their oral health status [9, 20, 21]. However, in a recent study in Khartoum state, Sudan, we found a significantly higher prevalence of caries and gingivitis among children aged 3–12 with a CHD years than among those without a CHD [22]. As a developing country, Sudan is markedly different from industrialised countries, not only in terms of cultural and socio-economic backgrounds, but also in terms of the dental care system [23, 24]. In Sudan, there is a lack of available and accessible regular dental care [25] and the provision of preventive dental care is not prioritised [25]. Thus, oral-health-related background factors may be distributed differently in Sudan compared with developed countries.

As in other countries, oral-health-related background factors can differ markedly among subgroups within the population [26, 27]. As stated earlier, our previous study in Khartoum state, Sudan, children with a CHD were found to exhibit poorer oral health than those without a CHD [22]. To gain a more in-depth understanding of this finding, detailed mapping of the underlying risks and oral health factors among that sample of children is required. Such mapping should consider oral hygiene practices, the caregiver's oral-health-related knowledge, and the availability and utilisation of dental services. Additional aspects of interest are the caregivers' perceptions of their children's oral health and how satisfied they are with it. Such a study will reveal inadequacies related to oral health background factors, and will enhance efforts towards provision of better oral health care for all children, especially among those with a CHD. Therefore, in this study, we aimed to: 1) describe the patterns of oral health background factors in children with and without a CHD and explore any differences; 2) evaluate the effects of background factors on the prevalence of caries and gingivitis among these children; and 3) evaluate the influence of background factors on their utilisation of dental services.

Methods

Ethical approval

For patients with a CHD, ethical approval was obtained from Ahmed Gasim Hospital (Sudan), Sudan Federal Ministry of Health, Research Ethical Committee at the University of Science and Technology (Sudan), and from the Regional Committee for Medical Research Ethics Western Norway (No. 2265). For the controls, ethical approval was obtained from the Sudan Ministry of Education (Khartoum), and Sudan Ministry of Primary and Pre-school Education in the three Khartoum localities (Khartoum city, Khartoum North and Omdurman). Ethical permission was obtained from the local offices of the Ministry of Education in each of the selected localities and permission letters were taken to each of the selected schools. Participants received verbal and written information about the study and confidentiality was ensured. They were also given the option of withdrawing from the study at any time without giving any reason. A translated consent form was then completed and signed by the participants' guardians upon agreement to participate (both CHD cases and controls).

Study design, setting and population

Study design

This was an analytical cross-sectional study among a group of children with CHDs (CHD cases), compared with children without CHDs (controls).

Sample size

The sample size was calculated initially to estimate the number of children needed to detect differences in caries between children with and without CHD. This was done using the sample size equation of two-sided Student's *t*-test (the test to be used for comparisons). The smallest difference to be detected in the mean (dmft/DMFT: decayed, missing and filled teeth) between the two groups was 1 and the variance was estimated to be 2.0 in the controls and 2.5 in the CHD cases. The level of significance was set at 0.05 and the power at 80%. The estimated sample size was 60 CHD cases and 60 controls in each age group: age group 1 (3–7 years) with deciduous teeth; and age group 2 (8–12 years) with permanent incisors and first molars. Altogether, the estimated sample consisted of 240 participants in the CHD case and control groups. Caregivers were invited to participate and answer the questionnaire while accompanying their children.

Sampling technique

One hundred and seventeen CHD cases and their caregivers from the Ahmed Gasim Cardiac Center in Khartoum, Sudan were invited to participate and 111 of them consented to participation (purposive sampling). Caregivers were included when they had a child with a confirmed diagnosis of CHD between the age of 3 and 12 years. The control group comprised children without CHD along with their caregivers; about 190 were invited and 182 consented to participate from schools and kindergartens in Khartoum State. A stratified random sampling technique was used to select controls through age and gender group matching to the CHD cases and the strata were rural–urban. Around 60 controls from each of the three localities of Khartoum State (Khartoum city, Khartoum North and Omdurman) were enrolled. All participants were approached once and since the response rates in both groups were sufficient no further attempts were undertaken.

Study population

Participants were the caregivers of children with a CHD (111 CHD cases, 62 girls) attending routine cardiac check-ups at the Ahmed Gasim Cardiac Centre, and the caregivers of 182 children (89 girls) without a CHD (controls) attending schools and kindergartens in the same state. The caregivers of children with and without a CHD were divided into age group 1 (caregivers of children aged 3–7 years [primary teeth]) and age group 2 (caregivers of children aged 8–12 years [permanent teeth]). The variable *'child's age'* was dichotomized to age 1 (0) if age was 3–7 years and age 2 (1) if age was 8–12 years. The variable *'child's gender'* was dichotomized to boy (0) or girl (1). More information on calibration and reliability tests for the clinical examinations is provided in our previous study, of which this study is a continuation [22].

Data collection tools

The data were collected through individual face-to-face interviews with the children's caregivers. Interviews were conducted by two trained research assistants, including the principle investigator, who initially approached and invited participants after they had been informed about the study by a cardiologist. Most of the items were adopted from a questionnaire used in 2009 to assess the oral health status of 12-year-old Sudanese children and was previously tested for validity, and reliability and recommended the use of face-to-face interviews [28]. However, the final structured and closed-ended questionnaire underwent some modifications and included some extra items to assess the caregivers' knowledge about dental caries. This resulted in a questionnaire consisting of 25 questions, which were directly translated from English into Arabic during the interview. Pilot testing of the questionnaire was not feasible because CHD cases were not easily available to complete the desired sample size within the study period. Therefore, CHD cases that met the inclusion criteria were included without having a pilot group. A similar questionnaire design was used earlier and the testing revealed no major flaws. Face-to-face interviews were preferred over a self-administered questionnaire because the presence of illiterate caregivers was anticipated, and this was recommended after the pilot testing of a similar questionnaire in the earlier mentioned study.

Independent variables

Status

The dichotomous variable *'status'* was categorised into the presence ('CHD case'; 1) or absence ('control'; 0) of a CHD.

Mother's education

The variable *'mother's education'* consisted of five items ranging from illiterate, primary schooling, secondary schooling to university or higher education. A significant difference in the number of illiterate mothers between CHD cases and controls (19.4 vs 3%) was identified in our previous study on the same sample [22]. The education variable was dichotomised into: low educational level (primary education or less) and high educational level (secondary education to university education) [29] and was included as a background variable in the present regression models.

Caregiver's perceptions

The two items that measured the caregiver's perceptions concerned the child's oral health and the appearance of the child's teeth. Two variables were constructed from the previous items; the variable *'perception of oral health'* was categorised into 'good oral health' (0) when the caregiver perceived that their child had 'good' or 'very good' oral health; 'moderate oral health' when the caregiver perceived their child to have 'neither bad nor good oral health' (1); and 'bad oral health' (2) when they perceived it as, 'bad' or 'very bad'. For the regression analyses, the variable was dichotomised into 'good oral health' (0) when the caregiver perceived their child to have 'good' or 'very good' oral health, and 'bad oral health' (1) when they perceived it as, 'neither bad nor good', 'bad' or 'very bad'. Similarly, *'perception of appearance'* was defined as the caregiver being 'satisfied' with the appearance of their child's teeth (0) when the caregiver responded 'agree' or 'strongly agree'; 'neutral' when the responses were 'neither agree nor disagree' (1); or as 'dissatisfied' (2) when the responses were, 'disagree' or 'strongly disagree'. For the regression analyses, the variable was dichotomised into 'satisfied' with the appearance of their child's teeth (0) when the caregiver responded 'agree' or 'strongly agree', or as 'dissatisfied' (1) when the responses were 'neither agree nor disagree', 'disagree' or 'strongly disagree'.

Caregiver's awareness

Four items were used to assess the caregiver's awareness of oral health, which consisted of statements that the respondents were asked to agree (yes) or disagree (no) with: 1) not cleaning teeth can cause tooth decay 2) using fluoridated toothpastes can prevent tooth decay 3) frequent intake of sugared foods and drinks can cause tooth decay and 4) Sugared milk/drinks in a bottle during the night can cause tooth decay.

The variable constructed based on the score for these four items was called *'caregiver's caries knowledge'* and was dichotomised into 'poor knowledge' (1) for respondents who did not answer any question correctly or who gave only one correct answer, and 'good knowledge' (0) for those who answered 2–4 of the questions correctly.

Oral hygiene practices (child and caregiver)

The items for oral hygiene practices concerned both the child and the caregiver. Three constructed variables defining the frequency of tooth brushing for the child *'brushing'* and the caregiver *'caregiver's brushing'* and the frequency of using fluoridated toothpaste for the child *'fluoride'* were categorised as 'frequent' (0) when the activities were performed 'several times a day' or 'daily' and 'not frequent' (1) when brushing and fluoridated toothpaste use was 'seldom or never'.

Dental services utilisation (child and caregiver)

The utilisation of dental services by both the child and the caregiver was covered by three constructed variables: *'child's dental services utilisation', 'caregiver's dental services utilisation'* and *'dentist availability'* nearby, which were categorised into 'yes' (0) and 'no' (1). The subjective need for dental care was based on items that assessed the caregiver's reports about their child's oral complaints during the 6 months preceding the interview (toothache, abscess related to a carious tooth, dry mouth, infected sore gums, bleeding gums, tooth decay or a broken tooth). The constructed variable *'complaint'* was constructed based on these complaints and dichotomised into 'yes' (1) when the caregiver reported that the child had a complaint regarding any of these issues, and 'no' (0) when they had no complaints. In addition, a set of items was used to clarify the child's medical history for the 3 months prior to the study, which covered: 1) antibiotic use; 2) history of hospitalisation; 3) current treatment; and 4) history of medication. The constructed variable *'child's medical history'* was dichotomised into 'yes' (1) when the caregiver responded affirmatively to any of the four items or 'no' (0) when the responses were no in the all medical history items.

Dependent variables (Outcomes variables)

Two dichotomous dependent variables were used in separate logistic regression analyses: 1) *'caries'* (DMFT/dmft > 0 or DMFT/dmft = 0); and 2) *'gingivitis'* (gingival index [GI] > 2 or ≤ 2 [median used as a cut-off]), which were categorised as high (1) or low (0) according to Rios et.al. [30]. Both *'caries'* and *'gingivitis'* were significantly more prevalent among CHD cases than controls in our previous study [22] (caries: 66.6 vs 46.7% and gingivitis: 57.3 vs 42.7%, respectively). Additional information on examination methods, diagnostic criteria and findings concerning caries and gingivitis can be found in the previous study [22]. The caries examination was based on the World Health Organization criteria and was recorded by using the dmft/DMFT indices [31]. A simplified form of GI [32] was used to measure gingivitis in the following teeth (55/16, 51/11, 65/26, 75/36, 71/31 and 85/46).

A third variable, *'child's dental services utilisation',* categorised as 'yes' (0) if the child had ever used dental services and 'no' (1) if they had not, was used as an independent variable to evaluate the relationship with the dependent variables *'caries',* and thereafter on *'gingivitis'*. The variable was also used as a dependent variable in a logistic regression analysis; this time to evaluate the influence of that the various background factors had on the child's dental services' utilisation.

Anderson's model

Anderson's model is a behavioural model which was developed to investigate factors influencing the utilisation of health services [33]. The model proposed that the use of health service is not only influenced by the individual's need for care (need-related factors), but it's also the function of several other factors including the sociodemographic (predisposing factors), socioeconomic and other individual-family factors (enabling factors), and the interplay of these factors [33].

The dichotomised independent background variables under examination for their association with the dependent variable *'child's dental services utilisation'* were arranged into categories according to the modified health service use model by Anderson (Fig. 1) [33], which was used in a previous study in adults in Sudan [34]. Variables were categorised into: predisposing factors *('mother's education,' 'child's age'* and *'child's sex')*; enabling factors (*'caregiver's caries knowledge,' 'perception of oral health,' 'perception of appearance,' 'brushing'* and *'fluoridated toothpaste use'*); and need-related factors (*'caries,' 'gingivitis,' 'complaint'* and *'child's medical history'*).

Statistical methods

Data were analysed using SPSS version 22 (IBM Corp., Armonk, NY, USA), followed by data cleaning and management. Frequency and percentage tables were created for descriptive statistics for categorical variables. The χ^2 test was performed to compare statistical differences between CHD cases and controls, except when the expected value in one of the categories occurred in fewer than five children; in which case, Fisher's exact test was applied. All background variables that differed significantly between CHD cases and controls were included in two separate multiple (adjusted) logistic regression analyses to investigate their effect on the dependent variables (*'caries'* and *'gingivitis'*) among CHD cases and then among controls. A further multiple (adjusted) logistic regression analysis was performed to determine the adjusted differences between CHD cases and controls *'status'* in the dependent variables (*'caries'* and *'gingivitis'*) while controlling for the effect of background factors. Also, a hierarchical logistic regression model was developed to examine the effect of predisposing, enabling and need-related factors on the third dependent variable *'child's dental services utilisation'* in a separate regression analysis. In the model, Step 1 controlled for predisposing factors and then enabling and need-related factors were entered in Steps 2 and 3, respectively. Odds ratios (ORs) with 95% confidence

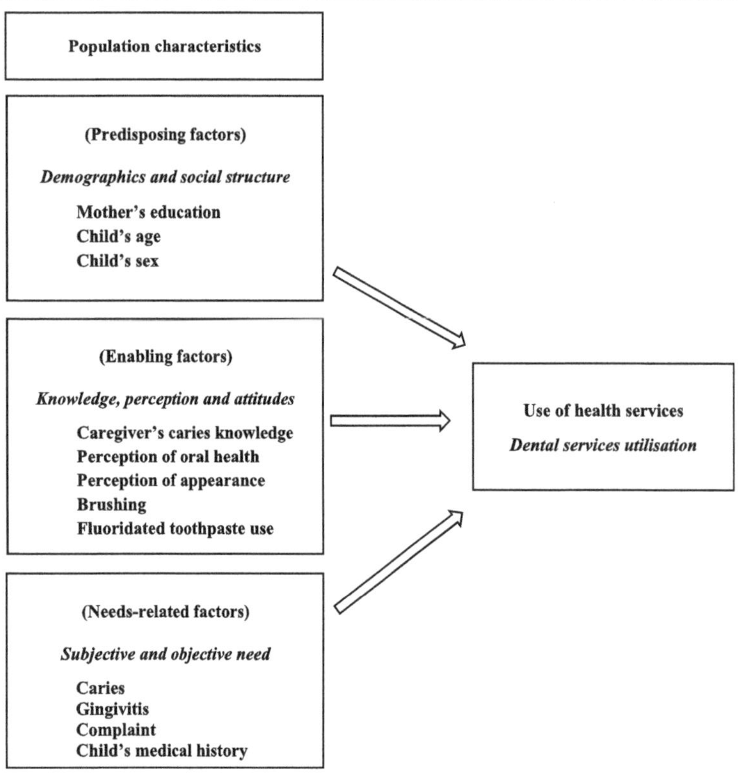

Fig. 1 Modified health service use according to Anderson's model

intervals (CIs) were used to estimate the association. $p < 0.05$ were considered statistically significant. Nagelkerke R^2 values were presented to indicate the amount of variation in the dependent variable explained by the model.

Results

The response rates for CHD cases and controls were 95.7 and 94.8%, respectively. The mean ages of CHD cases and controls were 7.1 years (standard deviation [SD 3]) and 7.2 years (2.8), respectively.

Frequency distribution of oral-health-related background variables among CHD cases and controls

Table 1 shows that the frequency distribution of oral-health-related background variables differed significantly between CHD cases and controls in both age groups. In age group 1, a significantly lower percentage of caregivers perceived that their child had good oral health among CHD cases than among controls. In both age groups, good knowledge of caries among caregivers and frequent brushing and use of fluoridated toothpaste by the child were significantly less common among CHD cases than among controls.

Regarding dental services utilisation, caregivers of CHD cases reported significantly less availability of a nearby dentist compared with the caregivers of controls in both age groups. In age group 2, a significantly higher percentage of the caregivers of controls reported attending the dentist compared with the caregivers of CHD cases. Regarding the *'complaint'* variable, a significantly higher percentage of CHD cases compared with controls in age group 1 reported having a dry mouth (25.8% CHD cases vs 4% controls) and infected gums (14.8% CHD cases vs 5% controls). Regarding the child's medical history, 19% of CHD cases versus 2.7% of controls reported a history of hospitalisation, whereas 46.8% of CHD cases versus 45.6% of controls reported antibiotic use during the 3 months preceding the study. Also,

Table 1 Frequency distribution of oral- health-related background variables in age groups 1 and 2

	Age group 1 (3–7 years)			Age group 2 (8–12 years)		
	CHD cases	Controls	*p*- value	CHD cases	Controls	*p*- value
Caregiver's perceptions about their child's dental conditions						
Perception of oral Health						
Good	35 (57.4%)	76 (76%)	0.027*	31 (63.3%)	47 (59.9%)	ns
Moderate	9 (14.8%)	5 (5%)		7 (14.3%)	7 (8.9%)	
Bad	17 (27.9%)	19 (19%)		11 (22.4%)	25 (31.6%)	
Perception of appearance						
Satisfied	46 (75.4%)	77 (77%)	ns	31 (63.3%)	51 (64.6%)	ns
Neutral	6 (9.8%)	3 (3%)		5 (10.2%)	6 (7.6%)	
Unsatisfied	9 (14.8%)	20 (20%)		13 (26.5%)	22 (27.8%)	
Caregiver's awareness (caregiver's caries knowledge)						
Good knowledge	52 (85.2%)	97 (97%)	0.010*	45 (93.8%)	75 (100%)	0.001**
Oral hygiene practices						
Brushing						
Frequent	46 (74.2%)	93 (93%)	0.002**	42 (85.7%)	78 (98.7%)	0.003**
Fluoride						
Frequent	27 (43.5%)	72 (72%)	0.001**	27 (55.1%)	61 (77.2%)	0.011*
Caregiver's brushing						
Frequent	62 (100%)	100 (100%)	ns	49 (100%)	76 (97.4%)	ns
Utilisation of dental services						
Child's dental services utilisation						
Yes	5 (8.1%)	11 (11%)	ns	19 (38.8%)	28 (34.6%)	ns
Dentist availability						
Yes	41 (66.1%)	89 (89%)	0.001**	32 (65.3%)	62 (81.6%)	0.040*
Caregiver's dental services utilisation						
Yes	20 (32.3%)	37 (37%)	ns	14 (28.6%)	46 (59.0%)	0.001**

Age group 1 (CHD cases: $n = 62$; controls: $n = 101$) and age group 2 (CHD cases: $n = 49$; controls: $n = 81$). The $\chi 2$test was used for the comparisons. (ns) denotes not significant, *denotes significance at $p < 0.05$ and **significance at $p < 0.01$

about 20.7% of CHD cases were chronic users of medication and 30.6% were currently receiving treatment; both of these items were related to their cardiac defects.

Impact of independent variables on dependent variables 'caries' and 'gingivitis' within CHD cases and controls and between CHD cases and controls

The effects of background factors (independent variables) on the dependent variables *'caries'* and *'gingivitis'* (within CHD cases and within controls) are shown in Tables 2 and 3, respectively. In CHD cases, the *'brushing'* and *'fluoride'* variables had a significant effect on the prevalence of caries, with ORs of 5.6 (95% CI: 1.4–22.8) and 0.3 (95% CI: 0.13–0.8), respectively, among infrequent brushers and fluoride toothpaste compared with frequent users, as well as the mother's level of education (OR = 2.6, 95% CI: 1.0–6.4). In controls, the variable *'mother's education'* had a significant effect on the dependent variable *'gingivitis'*, with an OR of 2.2 (95% CI: 1.1–4.6) for those with an uneducated mother compared with those with an educated mother.

No significant interaction effects between background factors and having a CHD were evident for the dependent variables *'caries'* and *'gingivitis'* (Additional file 1: Tables S1 and Additional file 2: Table S2). Tables 4 and 5 show the adjusted differences in the prevalence of caries and gingivitis between the CHD cases and controls while controlling for background factors (adjusted ORs). The adjusted ORs for *'caries'* and *'gingivitis'* in CHD cases compared with controls were 1.8 (95% CI: 1.1–3.2) and 5.3 (95% CI: 2.9–9.4), respectively, when all other background factors were controlled for.

Table 2 Multiple logistic regression analysis of oral- health-related background factors (independent variables) against caries (dependent variable) within cases and controls

Independent variables	CHD cases ($n = 111$) Multiple analysis Adjusted OR (95% CI)	Controls ($n = 182$) Multiple analysis Adjusted OR (95% CI)
Brushing		
Frequent (R)	1	1
Not frequent	5.60 (1.38–22.81)**	4.09 (0.72–23.32)
Fluoride		
Frequent (R)	1	1
Not frequent	0.32 (0.13–0.84)*	0.98 (0.46–2.09)
Caregiver's caries knowledge		
Good knowledge (R)	1	1
Low knowledge	3.082.05 (0.38–11.06)	2.78 (0.25–31.79)
Mother's education		
Higher education (R)	1	1
Lower education	2.59 (1.04–6.44)**	1.04 (0.51–2.10)
Child's dental services utilisation		
Yes (R)	1	1
No	1.82 (0.65–5.10)	0.66 (0.32–1.37)

Oral-health-related background factors (independent variables) were regressed against the dependent variable (Decayed, missed and filled teeth; DMFT/dmft > 0 and DMFT/dmft = 0). Multivariate analyses were performed using logistic regression, where R denotes the reference for analysis with odd ratio OR = 1. *denotes significance at $p < 0.05$ and **significance at $p < 0.01$

Table 3 Multiple logistic regression analysis of oral- health-related background factors (independent variables) against gingivitis (dependent variable) within cases and controls

Independent variables	CHD cases ($n = 111$) Multiple analysis Adjusted OR (95 % CI)	Controls ($n = 182$) Multiple analysis Adjusted OR (95 % CI)
Brushing		
Frequent (R)	1	1
Not frequent	1.90 (0.54–6.75)	1.08 (0.18–6.49)
Fluoride		
Frequent (R)	1	1
Not frequent	1.07 (0.42–2.72)	0.56 (0.24–1.32)
Caregiver's caries knowledge		
Good knowledge (R)	1	1
Low knowledge	1.16 (0.28–4.86)	0.87 (0.07–10.43)
Mother's education		
Higher education (R)	1	1
Lower education	1.22 (0.49–3.02)	2.21 (1.06–4.60)**
Child's dental services utilisation		
Yes (R)	1	1
No	0.28 (0.08–1.07)	0.86 (0.39–1.87)

Oral-health-related background factors (independent variables) were regressed against the dependent variable (gingivitis: gingival index GI > 2 and GI ≤ 2). Multivariate analyses were performed using logistic regression, where R denotes the reference for analysis with odd ratios OR = 1.
**donates significance at $p < 0.01$

Impact of independent variables on dependent variable 'child's dental services utilisations'

The effects of background factors on the child's use of dental services (*'child's dental services utilisation'*), based on hierarchical logistic regression analyses are presented in Table 6. This shows that the predisposing factors in Step 1 explained 19.4% (Nagelkerke's R^2, $p < 0.05$) of the variation in the child's dental services utilisation (in the total sample). This increased to 27.5% (Nagelkerke's R^2, $p < 0.01$) in Step 2, with the addition of enabling factors and to 33.4% (Nagelkerke's R^2, $p < 0.01$) when need-related factors were added in Step 3. The stratified analyses showed that the model explained 49.7% of the variation in the dental services utilisation among CHD cases, whereas it explained 34.6% of the variation among controls.

The factors that significantly affected the child's dental services utilisation among CHD cases were: 1) the child's age, with an OR of 11.9 (95% CI: 1.9–71.6) for children in age group 2 compared with children in age group 1; and 2)

Table 4 Adjustment for effect of oral-health-related background factors on difference in dependent variable 'caries' between cases and controls

	Crude analysis Unadjusted OR (95% CI)	Multiple analysis Adjusted OR (95% CI)
Status		
Controls (R)	1	1
CHD cases	2.28 (1.39–3.73) **	1.84 (1.07–3.16) **
Brushing		
Frequent (R)	1	1
Not frequent	5.08 (1.89–13.64)**	5.02 (1.71–14.74)**
Fluoride		
Frequent (R)	1	1
Not frequent	1.15 (0.71–1.86)	0.63 (0.35–1.22)
Caregiver's caries knowledge		
Good knowledge (R)	1	1
Low knowledge	3.68 (1.02–13.36)**	2.46 (0.64–9.47)
Mother's education		
Higher education (R)	1	1
Lower education	1.46 (0.69–3.11)	0.97 (0.88–2.61)
Child's dental services utilisation		
Yes (R)	1	1
No	1.01 (0.58–1.77)	0.91 (0.51–1.65)

Logistic regression analysis (bivariate and multivariate) was used to determine whether there was a difference in the prevalence of caries (Decayed, missed and filled teeth; DMFT/dmft > 0 and DMFT/dmft = 0) between CHD cases ($n = 111$) and controls ($n = 182$) while controlling for the different oral- health-related background variables (independent variables). Odds ratios (ORs) are presented with 95% confidence intervals (CIs).
**donates significance at $p < 0.01$

Table 5 Adjustment for effect of oral-health-related background factors on difference in dependent variable 'gingivitis' between cases and controls

	Crude analysis Unadjusted OR (95% CI)	Multiple analysis Adjusted OR (95% CI)
Status		
Controls (R)	1	1
CHD cases	5.61 (3.32–9.47)**	5.29 (2.98–9.39)**
Brushing		
Frequent (R)	1	1
Not frequent	2.39 (1.09–5.29)**	1.51 (0.58–3.97)
Fluoride		
Frequent (R)	1	1
Not frequent	1.39 (0.86–2.27)	0.72 (0.39–1.33)
Caregiver's caries knowledge		
Good knowledge (R)	1	1
Low knowledge	2.24 (0.74–6.72)	0.98 (0.29–3.38)
Mother's education		
Higher education (R)	1	1
Lower education	4.34 (1.81–10.38)**	1.74 (0.99–3.07)*
Child's dental services utilisation		
Yes (R)	1	1
No	0.77 (0.44–1.36)	1.58 (0.84–2.95)

Logistic regression analyses (bivariate and multivariate) were used to ascertain the exact difference in the prevalence of gingivitis (gingival index GI > 2 and GI ≤ 2) between CHD cases ($n = 111$) and controls ($n = 182$) while controlling for the different oral- health-related background variables (independent variables). Odds ratios (ORs) are presented with 95% confidence intervals (CIs). *denotes significance at $p < 0.05$ and **significance at $p < 0.01$

mother's level of education with an OR of 0.16 (95% 0.03–0.89) for children with lower educated mothers compared with children with higher education mothers.

Regarding the controls, the child's age (age group 2: OR = 5.2, 95% CI: 1.9–3.5) had a significant effect on the child's dental visits as well as the caregiver's perceptions of their child's dental appearance, with an OR of 2.9 (95% CI: 1.1–7.6) for caregivers who were unsatisfied with their child's dental appearance compared with caregivers who were satisfied with their child's oral health. The *'complaint'* variable also had a significant impact on the dental services utilisation among controls, with an OR of 6.4 (95% CI: 1.9–20.6) for children with complaints compared with those without complaints.

Discussion

This study investigated the oral-health-background factors and dental services utilisation among Sudanese children with CHDs. These children constitute a high-risk group with high susceptibility to oral diseases that may directly influence their general health, therefore they warrant investigation. The study was undertaken to provide the authorities with important information and highlight areas of insufficiency for future preventive oral health programmes that might reduce the injurious consequences of oral disease among this group. The current study revealed that children with a CHD exhibited a significantly higher percentage of dental risk predictors for both caries and gingivitis than their healthy peers did. More than 20% of the caregivers of CHD cases reported that their children did not brush their teeth frequently, which was significantly higher than the figure recorded for the controls. The constructed variable *'brushing'* in the logistic regression analyses showed a predominant significant association with the dependent variable *'caries'* among CHD cases, with an OR of >5 among CHD cases, in accordance with an earlier UK-based study [35]. This indicates that a child with CHD who is an infrequent brusher has a risk of caries five times higher than a child with CHD who is a frequent brusher. Also, two UK-based and one Indian study among children with a CHD have reported similar low brushing frequencies that were considered unsatisfactory [3, 13, 14]. Additionally, caregivers

Table 6 Child's dental services utilisation regressed on predisposing, enabling and need-related factors

	Total sample	CHD cases (111)	Controls (182)
Step 1: Predisposing factors	Adjusted OR (95% CI)	Adjusted OR (95% CI)	Adjusted OR (95% CI)
Mother's education			
Higher education (R)	1	1	1
Lower education	0.36 (0.16–0.80)*	0.16 (0.03–0.89)*	0.62 (0.211.85)
Child's age			
Age 1 (R)	1	1	1
Age 2	5.26 (2.40–11.52)**	11.89 (1.98– 71.56)**	5.17 (1.86– 14.38)**
Child's sex			
Boy (R)	1	1	1
Girl	1.46 (0.74–2.89)	1.78 (0.45–7.02)	1.46 (0.61– 3.46)
Nagelkerke's R^2	0.194	0.248	0.169
Step 2: Enabling factors			
Caregiver's caries knowledge			
Good knowledge (R)	1	1	1
Low knowledge	0.48 (0.06–4.27)	0.88 (0.07–10.51)	-
Perception of oral health			
Good (R)	1	1	1
Bad	1.32 (0.61–2.84)	3.82 (0.89–16.39)	0.69 (0.25–1.91)
Perception of appearance			
Satisfied	1	1	1
Unsatisfied	1.89 (0.92–3.92)	1.04 (0.28–3.88)	2.95 (1.14–7.59)*
Brushing			
Frequent (R)	1	1	1
Not frequent	0.88 (0.24–3.33)	1.05 (0.19–5.77)	0.76 (0.06–10.12)
Fluoride			
Frequent (R)	1	1	1
Not frequent	0.85 (0.39–1.88)	0.61 (0.15–2.48)	0.97 (0.32–2.95)
Nagelkerke's R^2	0.275	0.421	0.231
Step 3: Need-related factors			
Caries			
DMFT = 0 (R)	1	1	1
DMFT > 0	1.15 (0.53–2.49)	0.51 (0.12–2.37)	1.83 (0.68–4.91)
Gingivitis			
GI > 2 (R)	1	1	1
GI ≤ 2	0.86 (0.41–1.80)	8.23 (0.52–28.60)	0.39 (0.15–1.05)
Complaint			
No (R)	1	1	1
Yes	4.41 (1.78–10.87)**	6.71 (0.99–45.25)	6.36 (1.96–20.63)**
Child's past medical history			
No (R)	1	1	1
Yes	1.33 (0.68–2.61)	2.13 (0.54–8.45)	1.14 (0.48–2.70)
Nagelkerke's R^2	0.334	0.497	0.346

Hierarchical logistic regression analyses for effect of oral-health-related background variables categorised according to Anderson's model into predisposing, enabling and need-related factors. Analyses were performed on the total for CHD cases and controls. Odds ratios (ORs) are presented with 95% confidence intervals (Cis).
*denotes significance at $p < 0.05$ and **significance at $p < 0.01$

of CHD cases achieved significantly lower caries knowledge scores compared with the caregivers of the controls. Those findings indicated a clear lack of adequate oral hygiene measures among the CHD cases as well as lack of sufficient oral health knowledge among their caregivers.

The previously reported higher prevalence of caries and gingivitis among children with a CHD compared with those without a CHD in our previous study [22] has been strengthened by the results of the present logistic regression analyses. The CHD cases had a higher likelihood (ORs) of caries and gingivitis compared with the controls, even after controlling for the effects of differences in background factors. Notably, this could merit further investigation of other background factors not examined in the current study that might have an impact on those children's oral health. Hierarchical logistic regression analyses showed that the child's age and mother's level of education were significantly associated with the dental services utilisation among CHD cases. These findings also indicate that it is essential to encourage caregivers of children with a CHD to utilise dental services. Beyond doubt, these findings will be of use for any targeted future preventive oral health care programmes for children with a CHD in the studied population. There are reasons to believe that the findings are representative of the Khartoum State as a whole. Participation response rates were excellent; the controls were well adjusted to the CHD cases because they were selected from several schools and kindergartens in Khartoum State using stratified random sampling and were matched to CHD cases by group matching [22].

More than 40% of the caregivers of CHD cases were aware of the deterioration of their child's dental health (constructed variable *'perception of oral health'*), yet they had not taken their child to a dentist. Indeed, in our previous study [22], two children with a CHD exhibited swelling and sinus discharge related to carious teeth at the time of data collection and had never been taken to a dentist. In addition, the caregivers of CHD cases were less knowledgeable about caries, but this might indicate a lack of proper dental health information. In Sweden and the UK, as a comparison, the caregivers of children with a CHD who are registered with a dental practitioner have significantly better dental knowledge than the caregivers of children who are not registered [17]. Also, children with CHD and their caregivers are given comprehensive dental care and participate in a robust programme on the prevention of caries [16]. Nevertheless, most interventions for caries in the Swedish children took place after caries progression, because continuous hospital admissions delayed their ability to attend a dentist for treatment [16].

In terms of children's complaints, the percentages of those with dry mouth and infected sore gums were higher among CHD cases than controls. This may be explained by the use of medication related to underlying cardiac problems in the CHD cases; some of which are known to cause xerostomia [35, 36] and, consequently, sore gums.

The mother's level of education is known to be an important predictor of children's oral health [37, 38]. In this study, this variable was found to have a significant effect on the prevalence of caries among CHD cases and gingivitis among controls.

An unexpected finding was the effect that use of fluoridated toothpaste had on the prevalence of caries among CHD cases. Children with a CHD who frequently used fluoridated toothpaste had a significantly higher likelihood of caries than infrequent users. One explanation may be that the amount of fluoride in the toothpaste and frequency of brushing were insufficient to confer full protection. Also, the CHD cases represent a group in need of extra means of fluoride application. Another possible explanation may be that the contribution of other background factors to the deterioration of the oral health of children with a CHD might have reduced the effectiveness of fluoride against dental caries.

About 20% of the caregivers of CHD cases reported that they had visited a dentist to seek dental treatment for their child's complaint, but never for preventive check-ups, whereas the remaining 80% stated that they had never visited the dentist with their child for regular preventive check-ups or for dental treatment. Thus, the percentage of those who had never visited a dentist was much higher compared with that in three previous UK-based studies on dental visits among children with a CHD (18, 9 and 19% of had never visited a dentist, respectively) [3, 12, 14] and a recent Brazilian study (29% had never visited a dentist) [10].

A significantly higher percentage of caregivers of CHD cases in both age groups reported that they had no available nearby dental care, in significantly higher percentages compared with controls. CHD cases and controls were considered to live in similar surroundings; therefore, the higher proportion of caregivers reporting the unavailability of nearby dental care was challenging to interpret. One possible explanation is that the burden on the caregiver of the health condition of their child may have had a negative effect on their awareness of the availability of nearby dental care. Another possible explanation is that, in general, Sudanese people seldom seek dental services because of lack of public funding and insurance coverage for most dental treatment and the high cost of the treatment available [25, 34]. In addition, many children with a CHD are more fearful of medical staff, so the idea of dental treatment itself, together with a lack of dental staff knowledgeable in handling such CHD cases, may also have had an impact on attendance at dental clinics [35].

Regarding the dental services utilisation, Anderson's model is one of the extensively used models that investigated factors influencing families' and individuals' utilisation of the health services [39]. This model was developed by Anderson during the 60s and went through several developments since then [33]. The model had also been applied in the field of dentistry [40, 41] and had been recently used among Sudanese adults in Khartoum State, Sudan [34]. Therefore, the same model was chosen for the categorisation of the variables in the current hierarchical logistic analysis. Hierarchical logistic regression analysis showed that the mother's level of education, and the child's age were the most significant factors in explaining the child's dental services utilisation among both CHD cases and controls. This regression analysis also highlighted that, among CHD cases, a higher level of mother's education and older age of the child equated to a higher number of dental visits. The influence of age may be explained by a tendency to focus more on the child's permanent dentition than on primary teeth when seeking dental care.

Conclusions

The patterns of the oral-health-background factors differed significantly between CHD cases and controls with lower frequencies of brushing and fluoridated toothpaste use among CHD cases as well as their caregivers' lower scores regarding knowledge of caries. The effects of 'brushing' and 'mother's level of education' were significantly influencing caries prevalence among CHD cases and those children still had higher likelihood for both caries and gingivitis compared with controls even after controlling for their differences in the background factors. Finally, the influences of 'child's age' and 'mothers' level of education' in the child's utilisation of dental services were significant among CHD cases with higher reported dental visits among those aged 8–12 years and those having mothers with higher education.

The study findings indicate that there is a need in Sudan for preventive oral health programmes for children with a CHD, focusing on oral hygiene education as well as regular preventive dental visits.

Additional files

Additional file 1: Table S1. Interaction effects of oral-health-related background factors and having a CHD on prevalence of caries (DMFT/dmft > 0 and DMFT/dmft = 0). Interaction effects of oral-health-related background variables on prevalence of caries were ascertained using bivariate logistic regression analysis of the variables among CHD cases and controls. Odds ratios (ORs) are presented with 95% confidence intervals (CIs). (ns) denotes not significant, *denotes significance at $p < 0.05$ and **significance at $p < 0.01$. (DOCX 15 kb)

Additional file 2: Table S2. Interaction effects of oral-health-related background factors and having a CHD on the prevalence of gingivitis (gingival index GI >2 and ≤2). Interaction effects of oral- health-related background variables on prevalence of gingivitis were ascertained using bivariate logistic regression analysis of the variables among CHD cases and controls. Odds ratios (ORs) are presented with 95% confidence intervals (CIs). (ns) denotes not significant, *denotes significance at $p < 0.05$ and **significance at $p < 0.01$. (DOCX 15 kb)

Abbreviations

CHDs: Congenital heart defects; CI: Confidence interval; dmft/DMFT: Decayed missed and filled teeth; GI: Gingival index; OR: Odd ratio; SD: Standard deviation

Acknowledgements

This work was supported by the Faculty of Medicine and Dentistry, Department of Clinical Dentistry, University of Bergen, the University of Science and Technology, Omdurman, Sudan and the Ahmed Gasim Cardiac Centre, Khartoum, Sudan. The contributions of Dr Samih Salah and the study participants are gratefully acknowledged. The authors would also like to thank Associate. Professor Olav Bøe, University of Bergen for providing statistical advice before and during the study.

Funding

The work was supported by the Faculty of Medicine and Dentistry, Department of Clinical Dentistry, University of Bergen.

Authors' contributions

The study was designed by HMA, MM, EFN, RW and MSS. OHS and SH contribution was the recruitment of CHD participants in their referral clinic and confirmed their diagnosis, both contributed also to the discussion of the paper. HMA and MM collected the data from children with CHD and their caregivers, HMA collected the data from the controls and their caregivers. RWA and EFN were responsible for the project logistics (Ethical approvals, instruments and questionnaire materials) and also contributed to the discussion of the paper. HMA, SAL and EFN contributed to data analyses and SAL contributed with the statistical advices. HMA wrote and MSS edited and revised the manuscript. HMA, MM, RW, OHS, SH, SAL, EFN and MSS edited, revised and approved the final draft of the manuscript.

Competing interests

The authors declare that they have no competing interests.

Consent for publication

Not applicable.

Ethics approval and consent to participate

Ethical approvals for the CHD cases recruitment were obtained from the Ahmed Gasim Hospital, from the Sudanese Federal Ministry of Health, the Research Ethics Committee at the University of Science and Technology and from the Regional Committee for Medical Research Ethics, Western Norway (No. 2265). Ethical approvals were also obtained from the State Ministry of Education (Khartoum) and the State Ministry of Primary and Pre-school Education in the three Khartoum districts for the controls recruitment. Consent forms were completed and signed by the caregivers of the study participants after obtaining verbal agreement and the confidentiality was ensured for both CHD cases and controls.

Author details

[1]Department of Clinical Dentistry, Faculty of Medicine and Dentistry, University of Bergen, Bergen, Norway. [2]Oral Health Centre of Expertise in Western Norway, Hordaland, Bergen, Norway. [3]Department of Community Dentistry, University of Science and Technology, Khartoum, Sudan. [4]Ahmed Gasim hospital, Khartoum Teaching Hospital, Khartoum, Sudan. [5]Ahmed Gasim hospital, Faculty of Medicine University of Khartoum, Khartoum, Sudan. [6]Department of Periodontics, University of Science and Technology, Khartoum, Sudan.

References

1. van der Linde D, Konings EE, Slager MA, Witsenburg M, Helbing WA, Takkenberg JJ, Roos-Hesselink JW. Birth prevalence of congenital heart disease worldwide: a systematic review and meta-analysis. J Am Coll Cardiol. 2011;58(21):2241–7.

2. Slavkin HC, Baum BJ. Relationship of dental and oral pathology to systemic illness. JAMA. 2000;284(10):1215–7.
3. Saunders C, Roberts G. Dental attitudes, knowledge, and health practices of parents of children with congenital heart disease. Arch Dis Child. 1997;76(6):539–40.
4. Parahitiyawa NB, Jin LJ, Leung WK, Yam WC, Samaranayake LP. Microbiology of odontogenic bacteremia: beyond endocarditis. Clin Microbiol Rev. 2009; 22(1):46–64. Table of Contents.
5. Wilson W, Taubert KA, Gewitz M, Lockhart PB, Baddour LM, Levison M, Bolger A, Cabell CH, Takahashi M, Baltimore RS. Prevention of Infective Endocarditis Guidelines From the American Heart Association: A Guideline From the American Heart Association Rheumatic Fever, Endocarditis, and Kawasaki Disease Committee, Council on Cardiovascular Disease in the Young, and the Council on Clinical Cardiology, Council on Cardiovascular Surgery and Anesthesia, and the Quality of Care and Outcomes Research Interdisciplinary Working Group. Circulation. 2007;116(15):1736–54.
6. Baltimore RS, Gewitz M, Baddour LM, Beerman LB, Jackson MA, Lockhart PB, Pahl E, Schutze GE, Shulman ST, Willoughby R. Infective endocarditis in childhood: 2015 update a scientific statement from the American heart association. Circulation. 2015;132(15):1487–515.
7. Haag F, Casonato S, Varela F, Firpo C. Parents' knowledge of infective endocarditis in children with congenital heart disease. Rev Bras Cir Cardiovasc. 2011;26(3):413–8.
8. Poutanen R, Lahti S, Tolvanen M, Hausen H. Parental influence on children's oral health-related behavior. Acta Odontol Scand. 2006;64(5):286–92.
9. Rai K, Hegde AM. Oral health status of children with congenital heart disease and the awareness, attitude and knowledge of their parents. J Clin Pediatr Dent. 2009;33(4):315–8.
10. da Silva DB, Souza IP, Cunha MC. Knowledge, attitudes and status of oral health in children at risk for infective endocarditis. Int J Paediatr Dent. 2002; 12(2):124–31.
11. Berger EN. Attitudes and preventive dental health behaviour in children with congenital cardiac disease. Aust Dent J. 1978;23(1):87–90.
12. Lowry L, Evans D, Lowry R, Welbury R. Under-registration for dental care of children with heart defects in the north-east of England: a comparative study. Prim Dent Care. 1996;3(2):68–70.
13. Suvarna R, Rai K, Hegde AM. Knowledge and oral health attitudes among parents of children with congenital heart disease. Int J Clin Pediatr Dent. 2011;4(1):25–8.
14. Franco E, Saunders CP, Roberts GJ, Suwanprasit A. Dental disease, caries related microflora and salivary IgA of children with severe congenital cardiac disease: an epidemiological and oral microbial survey. Pediatr Dent. 1996;18(3):228–35.
15. Suma G, Usha MD, Ambika G, Jairanganath. Oral health status of normal children and those affiliated with cardiac diseases. J Clin Pediatr Dent. 2011; 35(3):315–8.
16. Grahn K, Wikstrom S, Nyman L, Rydberg A, Stecksen-Blicks C. Attitudes about dental care among parents whose children suffer from severe congenital heart disease: a case-control study. Int J Paediatr Dent. 2006;16(4):231–8.
17. Balmer R, Bu'Lock FA. The experiences with oral health and dental prevention of children with congenital heart disease. Cardiol Young. 2003; 13(05):439–43.
18. Tasioula V, Balmer R, Parsons J. Dental health and treatment in a group of children with congenital heart disease. Pediatr Dent. 2008;30(4):323–8.
19. Stecksen-Blicks C, Rydberg A, Nyman L, Asplund S, Svanberg C. Dental caries experience in children with congenital heart disease: a case-control study. Int J Paediatr Dent. 2004;14(2):94–100.
20. Pimentel EL, Azevedo VM, Castro Rde A, Reis LC, De Lorenzo A. Caries experience in young children with congenital heart disease in a developing country. Braz Oral Res. 2013;27(2):103–8.
21. Agbelusi G, Nwhator S, Okoromah C. Oral health status and treatment needs of children with congenital cardiac disease in Lagos, Nigeria. Tanzania Dental Journal. 2007;14(2):65.
22. Ali HM, Mustafa M, Hasabalrasol S, Elshazali OH, Nasir EF, Ali RW, Berggreen E, Skeie MS: Presence of plaque, gingivitis and caries in Sudanese children with congenital heart defects. Clinical oral investigations 2016 [Epub ahead of print].
23. Kandelman D, Arpin S, Baez RJ, Baehni PC, Petersen PE. Oral health care systems in developing and developed countries. Periodontol 2000. 2012;60(1):98–109.
24. Thorpe S. Oral health issues in the African region: current situation and future perspectives. J Dent Educ. 2006;70(11 suppl):8–15.
25. Khalifa N, Allen PF, Abu-Bakr NH, Abdel-Rahman ME, Abdelghafar KO. A survey of oral health in a Sudanese population. BMC Oral Health. 2012;12(1):5.
26. Steele J, Shen J, Tsakos G, Fuller E, Morris S, Watt R, Guarnizo-Herreño C, Wildman J: The Interplay between Socioeconomic Inequalities and Clinical Oral Health. Journal of dental research 2014:0022034514553978
27. Watt RG. Social determinants of oral health inequalities: implications for action. Community Dent Oral Epidemiol. 2012;40(s2):44–8.
28. Nurelhuda NM, Trovik TA, Ali RW, Ahmed MF. Oral health status of 12-year-old school children in Khartoum state, the Sudan; a school-based survey. BMC Oral Health. 2009;9:15.
29. Lasheras C, Patterson AM, Casado C, Fernandez S. Effects of education on the quality of life, diet, and cardiovascular risk factors in an elderly Spanish community population. Exp Aging Res. 2001;27(3):257–70.
30. Rios FS, Costa RS, Moura MS, Jardim JJ, Maltz M, Haas AN. Estimates and multivariable risk assessment of gingival recession in the population of adults from Porto Alegre, Brazil. J Clin Periodontol. 2014;41(11):1098–107.
31. World Health Organization. Oral health surveys, Basic Methods, Geneva. 1997.
32. Ainamo J, Bay I. Problems and proposals for recording gingivitis and plaque. Int Dent J. 1975;25(4):229.
33. Andersen RM. Revisiting the behavioral model and access to medical care: does it matter? J Health Soc Behav. 1995;36(1):1-10.
34. Nasir EF, Åstrøm AN, David J, Ali RW. Utilization of dental health care services in context of the HIV epidemic-a cross-sectional study of dental patients in the Sudan. BMC Oral Health. 2009;9(1):30.
35. Busuttil Naudi A, Mooney G, El-Bahannasawy E, Vincent C, Wadhwa E, Robinson D, Welbury RR, Fung DE. The dental health and preventative habits of cardiac patients attending the Royal Hospital for Sick Children Glasgow. Eur Arch Paediatr Dent. 2006;7(1):23–30.
36. da Fonseca MA, Evans M, Teske D, Thikkurissy S, Amini H. The impact of oral health on the quality of life of young patients with congenital cardiac disease. Cardiol Young. 2009;19(03):252–6.
37. Christensen LB, Twetman S, Sundby A. Oral health in children and adolescents with different socio-cultural and socio-economic backgrounds. Acta Odontol Scand. 2010;68(1):34–42.
38. Mattila M-L, Rautava P, Sillanpää M, Paunio P. Caries in five-year-old children and associations with family-related factors. J Dent Res. 2000;79(3):875–81.
39. Babitsch B, Gohl D, von Lengerke T. Re-revisiting Andersen's Behavioral Model of Health Services Use: a systematic review of studies from 1998–2011. GMS Psycho-Social-Medicine. 2012;9:Doc11.
40. Newman JF, Gift HC. Regular pattern of preventive dental services—a measure of access. Soc Sci Med. 1992;35(8):997–1001.
41. Tennstedt SL, Brambilla DL, Jette AM, McGuire SM. Understanding dental service use by older adults: sociobehavioral factors vs need. J Public Health Dent. 1994;54(4):211–9.

8

Effect of the plant-based hemostatic agent Ankaferd Blood Stopper® on the biocompatibility of mineral trioxide aggregate

Muzaffer Emir Dinçol[1*], Hakan Ozbas[1], Bulent Yılmaz[1], Handan Ersev[1], Selcuk Gokyay[1] and Vakur Olgac[2]

Abstract

Background: Due to the detrimental effect of blood contamination on the physico-chemical properties of mineral trioxide aggregate (MTA), obtaining an effective hemostasis in the surgical crypt during apical surgery is of paramount importance. The purpose of this in vivo study was to analyze the effect of Ankaferd Blood Stopper® (ABS) contamination on the biocompatibility of MTA.

Methods: Forty of 56 Wistar–Albino rats were divided randomly and equally into two groups (MTA and MTA-ABS) according to whether or not a hemostatic agent was used. The remaining 16 rats were designated as the control group. Rats in the experimental groups received freshly mixed MTA-Angelus in polyethylene tubes, which were inserted into monocortical bore holes created in their tibias. In the MTA-ABS group only, 0.5 mL of ABS solution was administered topically on the defect sites followed by implantation of MTA tubes. Inflammation, foreign-body reaction (FBR), necrosis, fibrosis, and new bone formation (NBF) were studied 7, 30, 60, and 90 days after implantation.

Results: On day7, statistically significant differences were found in tissue reactions with regard to NBF and necrosis ($p = 0.044$ and $p = 0.024$, respectively), the latter being observed in 40 % of the samples only in the MTA-ABS group. Slight inflammation in all groups was confined to day-7 only. Mild necrosis was present in the MTA-ABS group only on day-7. Severity of the foreign body reaction and fibrosis was limited. New bone formation increased gradually over time in all groups, reaching a maximum on day-90.

Conclusions: MTA and ABS-contaminated MTA are equally biocompatible. ABS does not impair the properties of MTA.

Keywords: Ankaferd blood stopper, Biocompatibility, Mineral trioxide aggregate

Background

Periapical surgery is commonly comprised of root-end resection, apical cavitation, and root-end filling to seal the communication between the periapical tissues and the root canal system [1]. An "ideal" root-end filling material should have properties like; easy handling, good biocompatibility and apical sealability at the root apex to prevent the egress of bacteria, and bacterial byproducts [2, 3]. It should also be insoluble in body fluids such as blood, saliva, and tissue fluid [4, 5]. Unfortunately, there is no ideal material that fulfills all of these requirements.

Various root-end filling materials have been suggested [6]. The calcium silicate-based compound mineral trioxide aggregate (MTA) has been compared with other root-end filling materials and hypothesized to be a "near-to-ideal substance" [7]. MTA is used widely in root-end filling, pulp capping, perforation repair, and in the treatment of immature apices. MTA is employed in these conditions because of its biocompatibility, antibacterial nature, ability to set in moist environments, and because it acts as a potential seal against bacterial penetration [8].

* Correspondence: muzafferemir@yandex.com
[1]Faculty of Dentistry, Department of Endodontics, Istanbul University, 34093, Fatih, Istanbul, Turkey
Full list of author information is available at the end of the article

In endodontic surgery, blood comes into contact with (and often becomes incorporated into) MTA during or after its placement. This contamination has detrimental effects on its surface microhardness, compressive strength, bond strength and marginal adaptation [9]. Blood contamination of unset MTA adversely affects the setting reaction and mechanical strength of the material [10]. When considering the clinical uses of MTA, its physical properties are important factors in achieving a good seal between the root canal and the external surface of the root [9]. Therefore, in using MTA, attempts should be made to control bleeding [9, 10].

Various local hemostatic agents have been used in oral and maxillofacial surgery [11]. Ankaferd Blood Stopper® (ABS) (Ankaferd Sağlık ürünleri A.Ş., Istanbul, Turkey) is an extract from medicinal plants that have been used for centuries in Turkish traditional medicine as a hemostatic agent. ABS consists of a standardized mixture of several plants: *Urtica dioica* (6.0 g/100 ml), *Vitis vinifera* (8.0 mg/100 ml), *Alpinia officinarum* (7.0 mg/100 ml), *Thymus vulgaris* (5.0 mg/100 ml) and *Glycyrrhiza glabra* (7.0 mg/100 ml) [12]. Each of these plants has an impact on cellular proliferation, vascular dynamics, angiogenesis, blood cells, cell mediators and endothelia [13]. Each constituent, if used separately, has interesting biologic effects. *U.diocia* can elicit vasorelaxation (mediated by the release of endothelial nitric oxide and the opening of potassium channels) as well as a negative inotropic action. *Vitis vinifera* exerts anticarcinogenic and antiatherosclerotic effects. *Alpina officinarum* inhibits nitric oxide production in macrophages. *Thymus vulgaris* has antioxidative actions such as prevention of peroxidation. *Glycyrrhiza glabra* has anti-inflammatory, antithrombin, antiplatelet, antioxidant, antiatherosclerotic, and anticarcinogenic effects [13, 14]. In addition, ABS has been found to be as effective as Surgicel® for achieving hemostasis in animal models [15, 16]. Moreover, ABS can be used to create a blood-free tooth surface during application of brackets on surgically exposed impacted teeth [13, 14]. ABS has also been used successfully for: dental extractions in patients undergoing antithrombotic treatment with acetylsalicylic acid and warfarin sodium without interrupting and/or altering the anticoagulant regimens [17]; in patients with hemorragic diathesis [18]; and in the treatment of acute and profuse bleeding of the gastrointestinal tract [19].

Reactions in tissues caused by hemostatic agents are important for the reliability of the materials used [20, 21]. Although ABS is widely used in endodontic surgery as a hemostatic agent [13], data regarding to its effects on root-end filling materials in animal experiments (devised for the investigation of their biocompatibility) are lacking. Thus, the aim of the present in vivo study was to evaluate and compare the effect of ABS on the early and long-term tissue reactions of MTA in a wound healing model at rat tibias. This is the first histopathologic study to ascertain whether ABS, when used as an hemostatic agent, affects the biocompatibility of MTA.

Methods

Animal care and sample grouping

The study was carried out in various departments within Istanbul University (Istanbul, Turkey). Care and use of laboratory animals was according to the criteria set by the Committee on Animal Research within Istanbul University (protocol number: 43/09). Rats were obtained from the Center of Experimental Medical Research of Istanbul University.

Fifty-six Wistar–Albino male rats (4–6 months, 250–300 g) were housed in groups of four per cage, fed standard pellets and water in a temperature-regulated room (22 °C, 55 % humidity, 12-h light–dark cycle), and allowed to mobilize freely. Forty rats were divided randomly and equally into two experimental groups according to whether or not a hemostatic agent was used. The remaining 16 rats were designated as the control group.

Intraosseous surgical procedure

Each animal underwent a general anesthetic procedure by the injection of ketamine hydrochloride (10 %; Alfamine®; 15 mg/kg body weight, i.m.) and xylazine hydrochloride (2 %; Alfazyne®; 60 mg/kg, i.m.). After shaving the left and right hind limbs, rats were positioned in the ventral decubitus position. Antisepsis (10 % povidone-iodine solution (Isosol®, Central Laboratory, Istanbul)) was carried out over shaved areas. An incision (≈15 mm) was made at the lateral aspect of the anterior border of the tibia until the tibia was reached. After reflection of the periosteum, a monocortical circular defect (diameter, 1.5 mm) was created at the anterior portion of the diaphysis of both tibias until the bone marrow was reached. These defects were drilled using a round carbide burr in a low-speed handpiece under constant irrigation with physiologic (0.9 %) sterile saline solution to prevent overheating and necrosis of bone tissue.

MTA-Angelus (Angelus Indústria de Produtos Odontológicos, Londrina, Brazil) was mixed according to the manufacturer's instructions. Then, the freshly mixed cement was introduced into sterile polyethylene (non-toxic, intravenous catheter, 18 G) tubes (external diameter, 1.2 mm; length, 10 mm; sealed at one end) with the aid of a syringe having a needle compatible with the inner diameter of the tubes. Empty tubes were used for rats in the control group. Tubes were introduced so that they projected into the bone-marrow compartment and their lateral walls were parallel to the long axis of the tibia with the closed ends pointing towards the knee joint [22].

In the MTA-ABS group, 0.5 mL of ABS solution was administered topically on the defect sites using an insulin syringe, after which the tubes containing MTA-Angelus were implanted into the right tibias. In the MTA group, local hemostasis was achieved with direct packing with gauze on the defect sites, and then the tubes containing MTA-Angelus were implanted into the left tibias. In the control group, local hemostasis was maintained in the same manner as that in the MTA group, and then empty tubes were inserted into both tibias. The muscle layer was sutured with absorbable 4/0 gut sutures, and the skin closed with 3/0 silk thread (M.E.D). No antibiotic was given and the rats were observed postoperatively. All animals survived the indicated time periods without complications.

Histological procedures

After each time period (7, 30, 60, and 90 days), 14 rats were sacrified with an overdose of ketamine hydrochloride (50 mg/kg). Entire tibias were isolated by gross dissection, fixed in 10 % formalin for 24 h, decalcified in 20 % formic acid, and processed for embedding in paraffin. Sections were cut parallel to the long axis of the tubes at 7 μm, mounted on slides, and stained with hematoxylin and eosin (H&E). Slides were analyzed and photographed at different magnifications in five areas with a light microscope (Eclipse E600; Nikon, Tokyo, Japan) coupled with a digital camera, by an oral pathologist (V.O) blinded to the study protocol.

Morphometric analysis

To estimate the level of inflammation and recovery in bone-marrow tissue adjacent to the open end of each tube, all sections were analyzed to evaluate inflammation, FBR, fibrosis, NBF, and necrosis. When evaluating

Table 1 Comparison of results belonging to the study groups at study intervals for the 5 events assessed

Histologic events	Experimental periods	Study groups			*p*
		MTA	MTA-ABS	Control	
Inflammatory response (Mean ± SD)	7 days	1 ± 0	1 ± 0	0,75 ± 0,46	**0,075**
	30 days	0 ± 0	0 ± 0	0 ± 0	**1,000**
	60 days	0 ± 0	0 ± 0	0 ± 0	**1,000**
	90 days	0 ± 0	0 ± 0	0 ± 0	**1,000**
	p	**0,001***	**0,001***	**0,001***	
Foreign body reaction (Mean ± SD)	7 days	0,2 ± 0,42	0,3 ± 0,48	0 ± 0	**0,262**
	30 days	0,1 ± 0,32	0,2 ± 0,42	0 ± 0	**0,407**
	60 days	0 ± 0	0,1 ± 0,32	0 ± 0	**0,407**
	90 days	0 ± 0	0 ± 0	0 ± 0	**1,000**
	p	**0,276**	**0,281**	**1,000**	
Fibrosis (Mean ± SD)	7 days	1 ± 0	1,4 ± 0,52	1,25 ± 0,46	**0,097**
	30 days	0,7 ± 0,48	0,4 ± 0,52	0,38 ± 0,52	**0,300**
	60 days	0,1 ± 0,32	0,1 ± 0,32	0,25 ± 0,46	**0,603**
	90 days	0,2 ± 0,42	0,5 ± 0,53	0,75 ± 0,46	**0,071**
	p	**0,001***	**0,001***	**0,004***	
New bone formation (Mean ± SD)	7 days	1,7 ± 0,48	1,6 ± 0,52	1,13 ± 0,35	**0,044*****
	30 days	2,3 ± 0,48	2,2 ± 0,42	2,38 ± 0,74	**0,681**
	60 days	2,7 ± 0,48	2,6 ± 0,52	2,25 ± 0,46	**0,154**
	90 days	3 ± 0	3 ± 0	3 ± 0	**1,000**
	p	**0,001***	**0,001***	**0,001***	
Necrosis [n(%)]	7 days	0(%0)	4(%40)	0(%0)	**0,024*****
	30 days	0(%0)	0(%0)	0(%0)	-
	60 days	0(%0)	0(%0)	0(%0)	-
	90 days	0(%0)	0(%0)	0(%0)	-
	p	-	**0,009****	-	

MTA Mineral trioxide aggregate, *ABS* Ankaferd blood stopper, *SD* Standart deviation; *Significant difference within the groups at $p < 0.05$; **Significant difference within the groups at $p < 0.01$; ***Significant difference among the groups at $p < 0.05$; Bold data confines only to *p* values both within or among the groups

FBR, the presence of foreign body giant cells and when evaluating inflammation, that of lymphocytes and plasmocytes were considered as basis. In the NBF, the trabecular, web-like woven bone or the thin lamellar bone tissue which tends to cover the area adjacent to the open end of the tube were considered as essentials. The bone trabecules without osteoblasts around, were considered as structures belonging to pristine bone and were neglected. While evaluating necrosis, at the open end of the tubes, the loss of the characteristic staining capability of cellular nuclei and disappearance of the details of cellular morphology, forming the classical appearance of cell death was considered as necrosis. Scores for these reactions (except for necrosis) were estimated by measuring the magnitude of the areas occupied by the tissue reactions in a standardized microscopic field at x40 magnification at the open end of the tubes by using an image analysis software (Olympus analySİS FIVE, Tokyo, Japan). A cell percentage of 0–25 % was scored semiquantitatively as "none" (0), 25–50 % as "mild" (1), 50–75 % as "moderate" (2), and 75–100 % as "severe" (3), [6, 13]. Scores for necrosis were determined according to its presence (1) or absence (0), [6].

Statistical analysis

Values for the severity of inflammation, FBR, fibrosis as well as the level of NBF were compared using the Kruskal–Wallis and the Mann–Whitney U non-parametric tests. Values for the presence or absence of necrosis were compared with the Fisher–Freeman–Halton test. Analyses were done using SPSS v22.0 (IBM, Armonk, NY, USA) with ($p < 0.05$) being considered significant.

Results

At the end of all time periods, wound healing was satisfactory for all rats and all implanted biomaterials remained in situ. Scores and percentages for inflammation, FBR, necrosis, fibrosis, and NBF in all groups are shown in Tables 1–2 and illustrated in Fig. 1 (see Additional file 1, for a detailed version of scores as raw data). Representative histologic images of specimens in all study groups at all times are illustrated in Figs. 2, 3 and 4.

Table 2 Distribution of new bone formation and fibrosis grades in the study groups at study intervals

Histologic events	Study groups	Intensity of reaction	Experimental periods			
			7 days	30 days	60 days	90 days
New Bone Formation	MTA (%)	Severe	0	30	70	100
		Moderate	70	70	30	0
		Mild	30	0	0	0
		None	0	0	0	0
	MTA-ABS (%)	Severe	0	20	60	100
		Moderate	60	80	40	0
		Mild	40	0	0	0
		None	0	0	0	0
	Control (%)	Severe	0	50	25	100
		Moderate	12.5	37.5	75	0
		Mild	87.5	12.5	0	0
		None	0	0	0	0
Fibrosis	MTA (%)	Severe	0	0	0	0
		Moderate	0	0	0	0
		Mild	100	70	10	20
		None	0	0	0	0
	MTA-ABS (%)	Severe	0	0	0	0
		Moderate	40	0	10	0
		Mild	60	40	0	50
		None	0	0	0	0
	Control (%)	Severe	0	0	0	0
		Moderate	25	0	0	0
		Mild	75	37.5	25	75
		None	0	0	0	0

MTA Mineral trioxide aggregate, *ABS* Ankaferd blood stopper

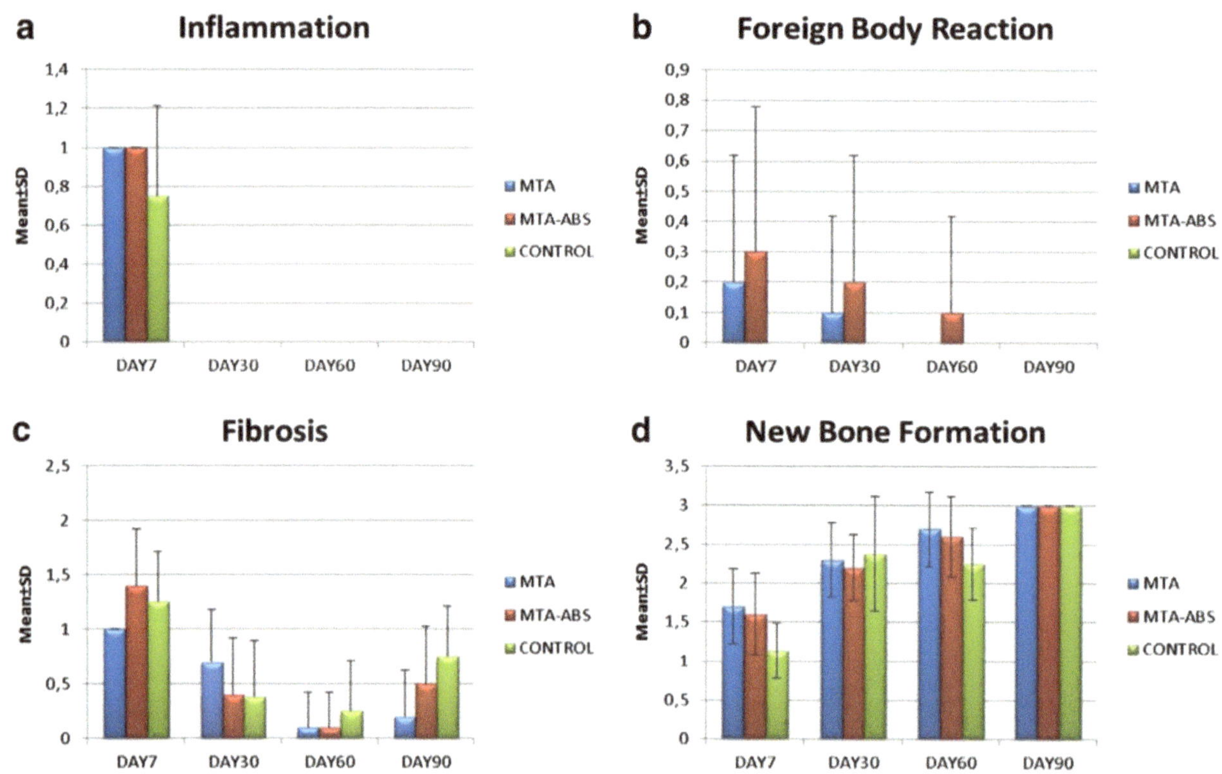

Fig. 1 The mean and standart deviation of reaction scores in all groups at time intervals. **a** Inflammation; **b** Foreign body reaction; **c** Fibrosis and **d** New bone formation

An inflammatory reaction was observed in the MTA, MTA-ABS and the control groups only at the first study interval on day 7, being absent in the remaining study intervals. No such reaction was present in any of the groups at 30, 60, or 90 days. There were no significant differences ($p > 0.05$) among the study groups on day-7, whereas significant differences ($p < 0.05$) were detected when day-7 was compared with the inflammation at 30, 60, or 90 days.

At the open ends of the inserted tubes, macrophages in the connective tissue were detected to phagocyte the implanted biomaterial at the junctional area, where the connective tissue came in touch with the biomaterial, forming foreign body giant cells which induced a foreign body reaction and which was observed in two samples in the MTA group and in three samples in the MTA-ABS group on day 7; in one sample in the MTA and in two samples in the MTA-ABS groups on day 30; and only in one sample in the MTA-ABS group on day 60. Extent of FBRs among groups was not significant ($p > 0.05$) at 7, 30, 60, or 90 days. At these intervals, a FBR was not present in the control group. There were no significant differences ($p > 0.05$) among time periods in any group.

There was no necrosis in the MTA group or the control group on day-7. Necrosis was present in the MTA-ABS group only on day-7 and differences between this group and the other two groups were significant ($p < 0.05$). A significant difference ($p < 0.01$) was present only in the MTA-ABS group on day-7 among the time intervals used.

With regard to the severity of fibrosis, no significant differences ($p > 0.05$) were present among MTA, MTA-ABS, and control groups at 7, 30, 60, or 90 days. However, significant differences ($p < 0.05$) were detected among time periods in all groups. Distribution of percentages of fibrosis in each study group at time intervals is shown in Table 2.

Intensity of NBF showed a significant difference ($p < 0.05$) among the study groups only on day-7. In the control group, the prevalence of NBF was significantly lower than either of the MTA and the MTA-ABS groups, but differences in NBF between these two groups were not significant at 30, 60, or 90 days. Comparison of the prevalence of NBF among groups showed significant differences ($p < 0.05$) during time periods, but the prevalence of NBF of specimens in each group varied with time (Table 2).

Discussion

Intraosseous models provide an appropriate environment for in vivo testing of the biomaterials used in endodontic surgery. The biomaterials to be tested for

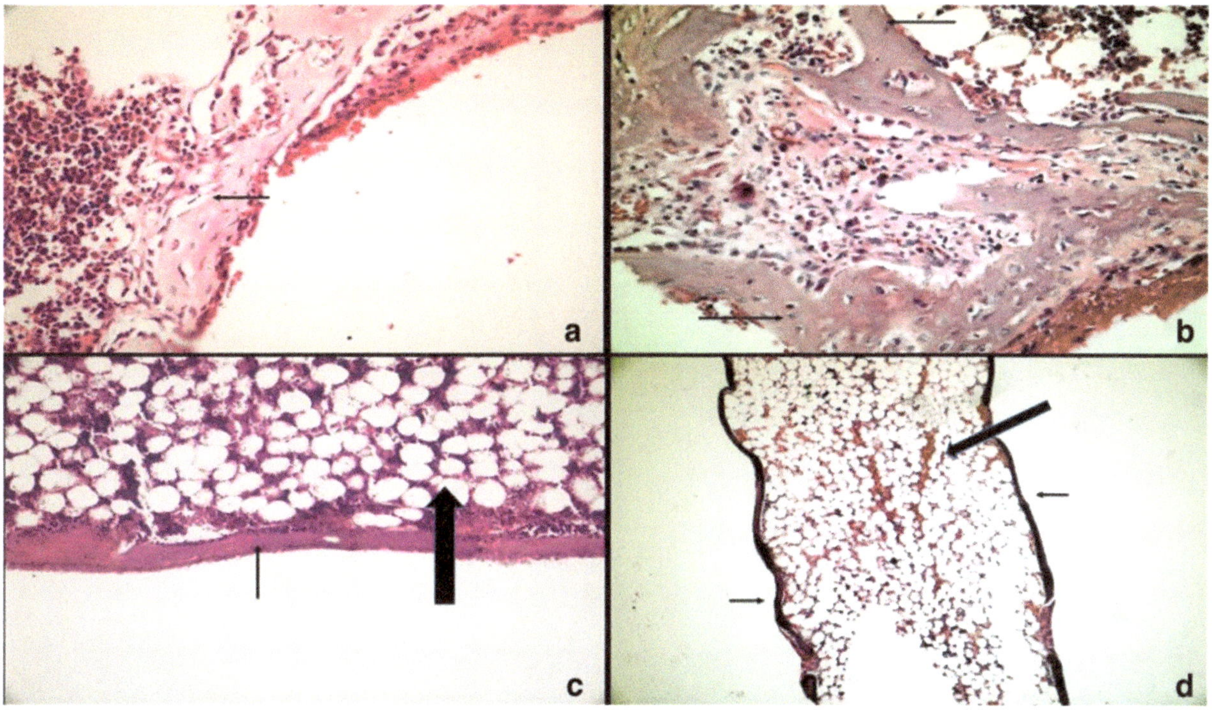

Fig. 2 Tissue reactions in the control group. 7 days: **a** Thin trabeculae of new bone (*arrow*) was observed at the open end of the tube (H&E,x400). 30 days: **b** New bone formation (*arrows*) adjacent to the tube end (H&E,x400). 60 days: **c** New bone became lamellar (*arrow*) at the open end of the tube. Normocellular bone marrow (*bold arrow*) is seen under the bone (H&E,x200). 90 days: **d** Lamellar bone (*arrows*) surrounding fatty bone marrow (*bold arrow*) getting into the tube (H&E,x40)

biocompatibility by intraosseous implantation are usually placed into the tibias and femurs of small laboratory animals like rats and guinea-pigs [13, 18, 22–24]. When a root end filling material is placed into the root end cavity, it comes into contact with periradicular tissues. Therefore, the reaction of bone to a biomaterial allows one to evaluate its biocompatibility. Thus, we have preferred to test the osseous reaction to our materials using the tibias of Wistar rats in a similar manner as reported in the endodontic literature [3, 7, 13, 22, 23]. Also in these studies, one can see that the study periods vary from author to author and there are no standart time points. If one desires immediate or early reactions, 7-day, 15-day and 30-day intervals are chosen. For long term reactions, the study intervals like 60 and 90-days can be added. Olsen et al. [22] have selected 7-14-21-56-100 days for time points.

A mild temporary inflammatory reaction was limited to 7 days in all groups. The inflammatory reaction in the control group was attributed only to the trauma produced during the tube placement [25]. However, in MTA and MTA-ABS groups, the high pH (owing to the release of calcium hydroxide when MTA was mixed with water), production of heat by an exothermic reaction during the setting of MTA, release of proinflammatory cytokines such as interleukin-1 and 6 during the process, and the aluminium content of the MTA, had additive effects on the inflammation caused by the surgical trauma [2, 3, 26].

Necrosis can be caused by almost any type of severe injury. In this study, tissue necrosis was only found, on day 7, in 4 samples of the MTA-ABS group where the possible cause may be the irritating effect of the material itself and the contamination with ABS. The disappearance of necrosis on day 30 may be related to the elimination of the acute irritating potential of the implanted material. Nevertheless, it has been shown that ABS is not toxic or allergenic, but has antibacterial and anti-inflammatory properties. ABS did not cause necrosis in bone tissue or defect areas according to histology. Moreover, ABS has been shown to reduce the prevalance of inflammation and necrosis in animal experiments [13, 18, 27]. Thus, ABS may not have caused this inflammation.

A FBR can occur if a foreign material is inserted into tissues. Fibroblasts proliferate and surround the foreign body. However, the latter is insoluble or indigestible by phagocytes, and is isolated by connective tissue [28]. FBRs were documented in the MTA and the MTA-ABS groups. In addition to all these, the FBR in the MTA-ABS group was found to be higher than that of the MTA group, the difference being statistically insignificant which may be

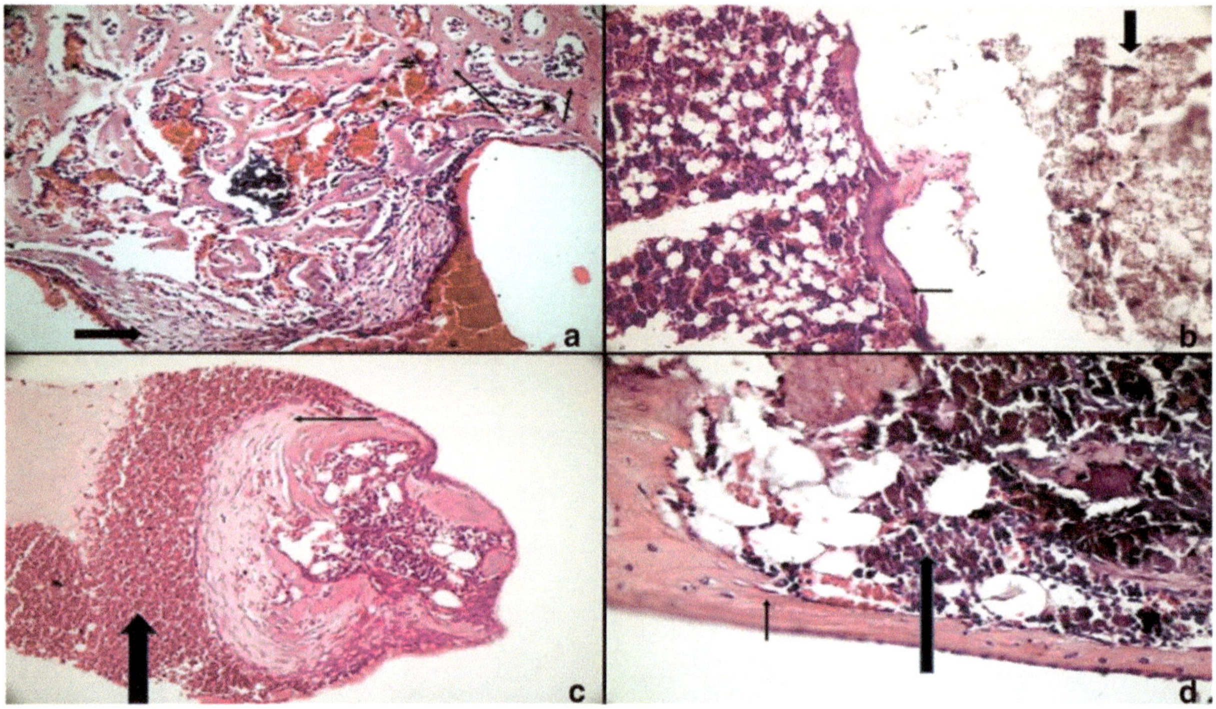

Fig. 3 Tissue reactions in the MTA group. 7 days: **a** Fibrous connective tissue (*bold arrow*) and new bone trabeculae (*arrows*) were seen at the open end of the tube (H&E,x200). 30 days: **b** Lamellar bone formation (*arrow*) and residual MTA (*bold arrow*) were observed (H&E,x100). 60 days: **c** New bone formation (*arrow*) and normocellular bone marrow (*bold arrow*) were seen at the open end (H&E,x200). 90 days: **d** Mature lamellar bone (*arrow*) and normocellular bone marrow (*bold arrow*) (H&E,x200)

attributed to the limited number of rats allowed due to ethical considerations. In the control group, a FBR was not detected at any time interval. In our opinion, the FBR in these two groups was owing to modified cells (epitheloid cells), remnants, constituents of mineral origin (waxy or oily remains), or complex polysaccharides and polymers [29].

Fundamentally, a connective-tissue reaction is a response of tissues to injury, and the damage tends to be repaired [29]. Severity of fibrosis among MTA, MTA-ABS, and control groups was very mild and was not significant at any time interval. Hence, the inflammation observed on day-7 was not persistent, and subsided in a short time. A stepwise increase in NBF was detected in all groups but a significant difference was not observed at any interval. In the control group, NBF increased but to a lesser extent. Distribution of NBF variations at time intervals is shown in Table 2.

All materials evoked an inflammatory reaction on day-7, this finding is in accordance with those of other studies [2, 3, 7]. Slight inflammation on day-7 and its absence at 30 days suggest that MTA and ABS-contaminated MTA had acceptable biocompatibility [8]. Absence of inflammation followed by NBF in surrounding areas owing to their osteoconductive properties, seems to be the best proof of biocompatibility for MTA and ABS-contaminated MTA [23].

An acceptable level of biocompatibility of a material ranges between no inflammatory response upon implantation, to an initial severe response that diminishes over time [30]. A biocompatibility scale has been devised by Moretton et al. [2] comprising of four levels, each associated with the severity of inflammation and its variation over time. This scale is used to assess the clinical relevance of findings of implantation experiments in animals whereby the first three levels denote an acceptable degree of biocompatibility. In the present study, the inflammatory response was mild and confined to the first week. According to the biocompatibility scale, MTA and ABS-contaminated MTA were biocompatible materials with almost identical effects on neighboring tissues. This mild response shows that both materials had better biocompatibility than those reported by Moretton et al. [2] and other scholars [3, 31–34]. The "gold standard" of biocompatibility is bone formation [24]. The absence of inflammation, together with a greater amount of hard-tissue formation against MTA and ABS-contaminated MTA, indicates their biocompatibility [8, 23].

MTA and ABS-contaminated MTA had similar effects throughout this 90-day study. Accordingly, ABS neither increased nor decreased the characteristic features of

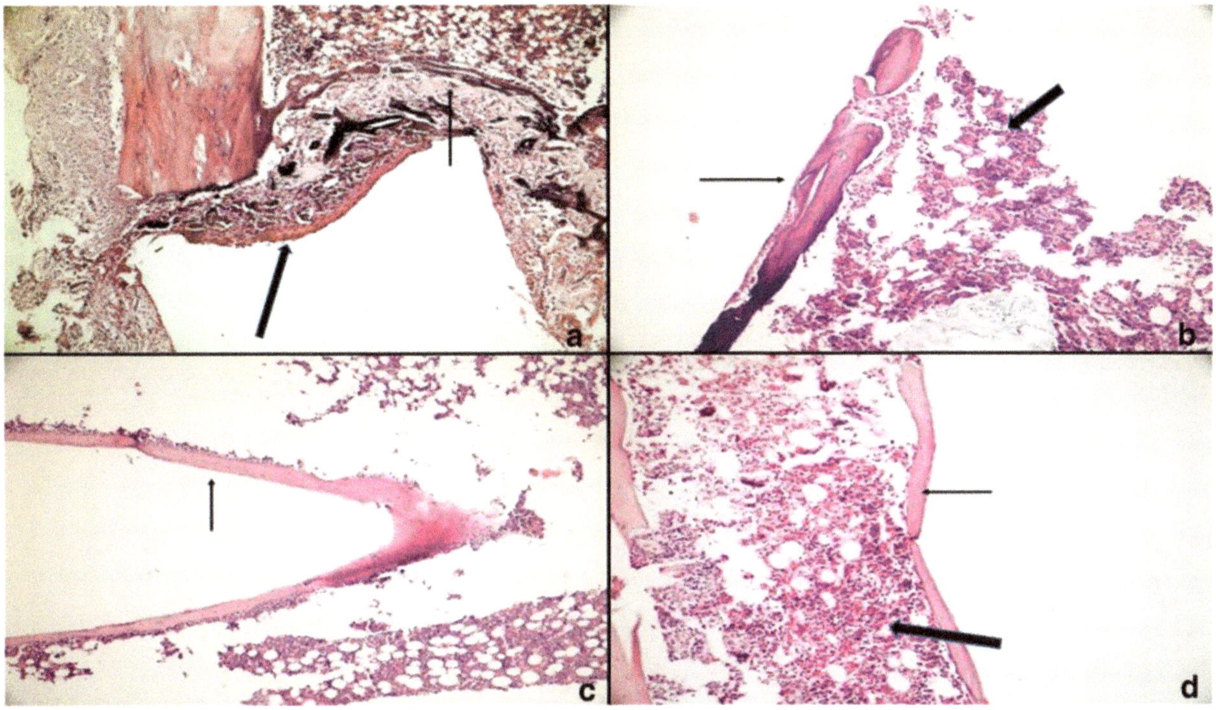

Fig. 4 Tissue reactions in the MTA-ABS group. 7 days: **a** Fibrous band of connective tissue (*bold arrow*) and tiny bone trabeculae (*arrow*) adjacent to the open end (H&E,x100). 30 days: **b** Lamellar bone (*arrow*) and bone marrow (*bold arrow*) at the open end of the tube (H&E,x200). 60 days: **c** Mature lamellar bone (*arrow*) surrounding the open end of the tube (H&E,x200). 90 days: **d** Mature lamellar bone (*arrow*) and bone marrow (*bold arrow*) (H&E,x100)

MTA but exerted a hemostatic effect. The "ideal" hemostatic agent is one that is safe, sterile, easy to apply, visible in the cavity, easy to remove, non-irritant, dissolves and degrades without interfering with periapical healing, and is an integral part of current surgical protocols [11, 17, 21].

Interestingly, ABS possesses features or functions not dissimilar to those mentioned above. Emes and colleagues, using an in vitro cell-culture model of rat fibroblasts, [35] stated that ABS, fibrin glue, and tranexamic acid may negatively affect tissue healing. However, other scholars have stated that ABS increases NBF in the early bone-healing period [13, 18]. Our findings show that ABS neither promoted nor inhibited the NBF of MTA. In our opinion, this potent hemostatic agent may be used in endodontic surgery owing to its biologic properties. However, further research is needed to clarify its beneficial effects and to detect potential unfavorable features.

Conclusions

Consequences of contamination of MTA with a new plant-based hemostatic agent, ABS, was investigated in an in vivo system to assess if it had an impact on MTA function. ABS had no deleterious effects on the mode of action of this root-end filling material.

Abbreviations

ABS: Ankaferd Blood Stopper; FBR: Foreign body reaction; MTA: Mineral trioxide aggregate; NBF: New bone formation

Acknowledgements

All authors declare that there is no funding in the current study.

Authors' contributions

MED performed animal experimentations and wrote the manuscript. HO and BY contributed to planning and designing the study, in the data analysis and submission of the mansucript. HE is supervisor of the study and assisted in drafting of the manuscript. SG participated in all stages of the research and helped to perform the animal experimentations. VO participated in the methodology by suggesting the implantation of the tubes into the medullary compartment and has microscopically examined the specimens without any knowledge of the kind, composition and function of the biomaterials. All authors have read and approved the final manuscript.

Competing interests

The authors declare that they have no competing interests.

Consent for publication

Not applicable.

Ethics approval and consent to participate

This in vivo, experimental study was conducted with the approval of the Local Ethics Committee on Animal Research Laboratory of Istanbul University (Vote number: 43/2009). Therefore, the informed concent was not applicable.

Author details

[1]Faculty of Dentistry, Department of Endodontics, Istanbul University, 34093, Fatih, Istanbul, Turkey. [2]Institute of Oncology, Department of Tumor Pathology and Cytology, Istanbul University, 34093, Fatih, Istanbul, Turkey.

References

1. Martínez Lalis R, Esaín ML, Kokubu GA, Willis J, Chaves C, Grana DR. Rat subcutaneous tissue response to modified Portland cement, a new mineral trioxide aggregate. Braz Dent J. 2009;20:112–7.
2. Moretton TR, Brown Jr CE, Legan JJ, Kafrawy AH. Tissue reactions after subcutaneous and intraosseous implantation of mineral trioxide aggregate and ethoxybenzoic acid cement. J Biomed Mater Res. 2000;52:528–33.
3. Zhang W, Peng B. Tissue reactions after subcutaneous and intraosseous implantation of iRoot SP, MTA and AH Plus. Dent Mater J. 2015;34:774–80.
4. Nekoofar MH, Oloomi K, Sheykhrezae MS, Tabor R, Stone DF, Dummer PM. An evaluation of the effect of blood and human serum on the surface microhardness and surface microstructure of mineral trioxide aggregate. Int Endod J. 2010;43:849–58.
5. Scarano A, Artese L, Piattelli A, Carinci F, Mancino C, Iezzi G. Hemostasis control in endodontic surgery: a comparative study of calcium sulfate versus gauzes and versus ferric sulfate. J Endod. 2012;38:20–3.
6. Cintra LT, Ribeiro TA, Gomes-Filho JE, Bernabé PF, Watanabe S, Facundo AC, et al. Biocompatibility and biomineralization assessment of a new root canal sealer and root-end filling material. Dent Traumatol. 2013;29:145–50.
7. Rahimi S, Mokhtari H, Shahi S, Kazemi A, Asgary S, Eghbal MJ, Mesgariabbasi M, et al. Osseous reaction to implantation of two endodontic cements: Mineral trioxide aggregate (MTA) and calcium enriched mixture (CEM). Med Oral Pathol Oral Cir Bucal. 2012;17:907–11.
8. Saidon J, He J, Zhu Q, Safavi K, Spångberg LS. Cell and tissue reactions to mineral trioxide aggregate and Portland cement. Oral Surg Oral Med Oral Pathol Oral Radiol Endod. 2003;95:483–9.
9. Rahimi S, Ghasemi N, Shahi S, Lotfi M, Froughreyhani M, Milani AS, et al. Effect of blood contamination on the retention characteristics of two endodontic biomaterials in simulated furcation perforations. J Endod. 2013; 39:697–700.
10. Oloomi K, Saberi E, Mokhtari H, Mokhtari Zonouzi HR, Nosrat A, Nekoofar MH, et al. Evaluation of the effect of blood contamination on the compressive strength of MTA modified with hydration accelerators. Restor Dent Endod. 2013;38:128–33.
11. Sauveur G, Roth F, Sobel M, Boucher Y. The control of haemorrhage at the operative site during periradicular surgery. Int Endod J. 1999;32:225–8.
12. Cinar C, Odabaş ME, Akca G, Işik B. Antibacterial effect of a new haemostatic agent on oral microorganisms. J Clin Exp Dent. 2012;4:151–5.
13. Işler SC, Demircan S, Cakarer S, Cebi Z, Keskin C, Soluk M, et al. Effects of folk medicinal plant extract Ankaferd Blood Stopper® on early bone healing. J Appl Oral Sci. 2010;18:409–14.
14. Trakyali G, Oztoprak MO. Plant extract Ankaferd Blood Stopper effect on bond strength. Angle Orthod. 2010;80:570–4.
15. Karakaya K, Ucan HB, Tascilar O, Emre AU, Cakmak GK, Irkorucu O, et al. Evaluation of a new hemostatic agent Ankaferd Blood Stopper in experimental liver laceration. J Invest Surg. 2009;22:201–6.
16. Okumus M, Yuksel KZ, Ozbag D, Cıralık H, Yılmaz Z, Gumusalan Y, et al. Medicinal plant extract (Ankaferd Blood Stopper) application in deep tissue injuries in rats: histopathological investigation of the effect on regional and systemic tissues. Turkish Eur J Trauma Emerg Surg. 2013;19:1–7.
17. Çakarer S, Eyüpoğlu E, Günes ÇÖ, Köseoğlu BG, Berberoğlu HK, Keskin C. Evaluation of the hemostatic effects of Ankaferd Blood Stopper during dental extractions in patients on antithrombotic therapy. Clin Appl Thromb Hemost. 2013;19:96–9.
18. Simşek HO, Tüzüm MŞ, Baykul T, Gürer IE, Başsorgun Cİ. Experimental investigation of the effects of a blood stopper agent (Ankaferd Blood Stopper) on bone surfaces. Turk J Haematol. 2013;30:177–83.
19. Kurt M, Oztas E, Kuran S, Onal IK, Kekilli M, Haznedaroglu IC. Tandem oral, rectal, and nasal administrations of Ankaferd Blood Stopper to control profuse bleeding leading to hemodynamic instability. Am J Emerg Med. 2009;27:631.
20. Jang Y, Kim H, Roh BD, Kim E. Biologic response of local hemostatic agents used in endodontic microsurgery. Restor Dent Endod. 2014;39:79–88.
21. Jensen SS, Yazdi PM, Hjørting-Hansen E, Bosshardt DD, von Arx T. Haemostatic effect and tissue reactions of methods and agents used for haemorrhage control in apical surgery. Int Endod J. 2010;43:57–63.
22. Olsen FK, Austin BP, Walia H. Osseous reaction to implanted ZOE retrograde filling materials in the tibia of rats. J Endod. 1994;20:389–94.
23. Torabinejad M, Ford TR, Abedi HR, Kariyawasam SP, Tang HM. Tissue reaction to implanted root-end filling materials in the tibia and mandible of guinea pigs. J Endod. 1998;24:468–71.
24. Tassery H, Pertot WJ, Camps J, Proust JP, Déjou J. Comparison of two implantation sites for testing intraosseous biocompatibility. J Endod. 1999; 25:615–8.
25. Yavari HR, Shahi S, Rahimi S, Shakouie S, Roshangar L, Abassi MM, et al. Connective tissue reaction to white and gray MTA mixed with distilled water or chlorhexidine in rats. Iran Endod J. 2009;4:25–30.
26. Saghiri MA, Tanideh N, Garcia-Godoy F, Lotfi M, Karamifar K, Amanat D. Subcutaneous connective tissue reactions to various endodontic biomaterials: an animal study. J Dent Res Dent Clin Dent Prospect. 2013;7:15–21.
27. Tasdelen Fisgin N, Tanriverdi Cayci Y, Coban AY, Ozatli D, Tanyel E, Durupinar B, et al. Antimicrobial activity of plant extract Ankaferd Blood Stopper. Fitoterapia. 2009;80:48–50.
28. Cunha SA, Rached Jr FJ, Alfredo E, León JE, Perez DE. Biocompatibility of sealers used in apical surgery: a histological study in rat subcutaneous tissue. Braz Dent J. 2011;22:299–305.
29. Cotran RS, Kumar V, Robbins SL. Robbins pathologic basis of disease. Volume chapter 2. UK: Harcourt Brace Jovanovich Inc; 1989.
30. Scarparo RK, Haddad D, Acasigua GA, Fossati AC, Fachin EV, Grecca FS. Mineral trioxide aggregate-based sealer: analysis of tissue reactions to a new endodontic material. J Endod. 2010;36:1174–8.
31. Lotfi M, Vosoughhosseini S, Saghiri MA, Mesgariabbasi M, Ranjkesh B. Effect of white mineral trioxide aggregate mixed with disodium hydrogen phosphate on inflammatory cells. J Endod. 2009;35:703–5.
32. Eghbal MJ, Asgary S, Baglue RA, Parirokh M, Ghoddusi J. MTA pulpotomy of human permanent molars with irreversible pulpitis. Aust Endod J. 2009;35:4–8.
33. Samiee M, Eghbal MJ, Parirokh M, Abbas FM, Asgary S. Repair of furcal perforation using a new endodontic cement. Clin Oral Investig. 2010;14:653–8.
34. Gomes-Filho JE, Watanabe S, Bernabe PF, de Moares Costa MT. A mineral trioxide aggregate sealer stimulated mineralization. J Endod. 2009;35:256–60.
35. Emes Y, Aybar B, Vural P, İşsever H, Yalçin S, Atalay B, et al. Effects of hemostatic agents on fibroblast cells. Implant Dent. 2014;23:641–7.

9

A comparison of the shaping ability of three nickel-titanium rotary instruments: a micro-computed tomography study via a contrast radiopaque technique in vitro

Zhao Wei[1], Zhi Cui[1], Ping Yan[1*] and Han Jiang[2*]

Abstract

Background: Micro-CT (μCT) studies that combine simulated canals with meglucamine diatrizoate to evaluate the shaping ability of nickel-titanium (NiTi) rotary instruments are lacking in the literature. The purpose of this study was to evaluate the shaping ability of three new different nickel-titanium rotary instruments in simulated root canals using μCT.

Methods: Thirty simulated root canals with a curvature of 60° were randomly allocated into the following 3 groups ($n = 10$): Group 1, ProTaper Universal (PTU) rotary system; Group 2, Reciproc single-file system; and Group 3, K3XF rotary system. Pre- and post-instrumented images of simulated canals were scanned with μCT via a radiopaque contrast technique to build a 3-dimensional (3D) model. Canal transportation, volumetric change and centring ability were evaluated in each group. Instrument failure and preparation time were also recorded. The Kruskal-Wallis test was used for statistical analysis and the significance level was set at $p = 0.05$.

Results: Reciproc produced greater volume change in the apical part of the canals compared with PTU and K3XF ($p < 0.05$). K3XF exhibited less transportation and better centring ability at the 2- and 3-mm levels from the apical foramen compared with PTU and Reciproc ($p < 0.05$). There were no significant differences in the centring ratio and transportation between PTU and Reciproc. Preparation time was significantly shorter in the Reciproc group ($p < 0.05$).

Conclusions: Under the conditions of our study, all of the canals were 3D reconstructed successfully via the radiopaque contrast technique. Reciproc showed enhanced apical volume changes and K3XF exhibited better centring ability when compared with other groups.

Keywords: Meglucamine diatrizoate, Micro-computed tomography, Nickel-titanium rotary instruments, Shaping ability, Simulated root canals

Background

Successful root canal therapy relies on the effective shaping and debridement of the root canal system without damaging the original configuration [1]. Preparation by using manual or rotary instrumentation techniques in a canal may lead to procedural errors, such as transportation, ledging, zipping and elbowing, however, various studies showed that NiTi rotary instruments maintained original canal shape better than stainless steel files [2, 3]. The elasticity and resistance to torsional fracture of NiTi rotary instruments make it possible to prepare curved canals in a relatively effective and safe manner [4, 5]. Over the decades, various NiTi rotary systems have been introduced to the market and each of them has a different design for its tip, taper, pitch, and rake and helical angles. In attempts to reduce the incidence of fracture and enhance the shaping ability, recent research has focused on new methods or techniques to

* Correspondence: WB000275@whu.edu.cn; jhqwe55@hotmail.com
[1]Department of Endodontics, School and Hospital of Stomatology, Wuhan University, 237 Luoyu Road, Wuhan 430079, China
[2]The State Key Laboratory Breeding Base of Basic Science of Stomatology (Hubei-MOST) and Key Laboratory of Oral Biomedicine Ministry of Education, School and Hospital of Stomatology, Wuhan University, Luoyu Road 237, Wuhan 430079, China

improve the mechanical properties of NiTi instruments, including the use of R-phase or M-wire alloys and modifications in the design of the cross-section, reciprocating or rotary working motion.

The ProTaper Universal (PTU) rotary system (Dentsply Maillefer Ballaigues, Switzerland) was launched several years ago. According to the manufacturer, the convex cross-sectional design with a shallow U-shaped groove in each convex triangular edge seeks to improve the flexibility of instruments and reduce apical transportation. The cross section of finishing files F3, F4, and F5 are designed as concave shape for increasing the flexibility. Reciproc (VDW, Munich, Germany) is made of M-wire alloy that presents a higher fatigue resistance with a reduced risk for instrument fracture. With an S-shaped cross-section design and non-cutting tip, this single file works in a reciprocating motion. It was suggested that the use of reciprocating techniques could reduce the incidence of fracture. The K3XF rotary system (SybronEndo, Orange, CA) has been available with an updated alloy design compared with the K3 system. The mechanical properties are modified by the special heat treatment (R-phase technology) on the alloy during the manufacturing process. This system was reported to have a higher fracture resistance than traditional NiTi rotary files [6]. The differences in the metallurgy and design of these modified NiTi instruments may produce different shaping abilities, and clinicians are often confused about which is better for an individual case to produce more centred preparations and minimize apical root canal transportation.

Various techniques involving simulated canals or extracted teeth have been used to evaluate the shaping ability of endodontic instruments. Traditionally, the evaluation of the shaping ability of endodontic instruments are usually performed using two-dimensional (2D) techniques, which rely on precisely fixed devices for taking radiographs/images and using software for calculation [7–9]. These 2D techniques are inexpensive and allow for the simultaneous comparison of the root canal morphology before and after preparation; however, the results of these studies are inaccurate and volumetric information was not disclosed.

Micro-computed tomography (μCT) is a non-invasive method for the three-dimensional evaluation of the shaping ability and the basic geometric parameters of the tooth's internal morphology [8, 10]. Data generated by μCT scanning can be analysed quantitatively and qualitatively with software, which can provide accurate information on volumetric changes, surface area, canal transportation, and canal diameter. Ounsi et al. reported that μCT is more sensitive to the changes in the canal space compared with 2D techniques [11]. μCT scanning is always used in extracted human teeth to evaluate the shaping ability of instruments. Notably, there is evidence to show the correlation between the complexity of root canal anatomy and the quality of root canal instrumentation [12]. Although it is often ignored characterizing, the heterogeneity of data drawn from extracted teeth with anatomic variations is very important for evaluating the shaping ability of endodontic instruments. This problem could be addressed by using standardized canals in resin blocks with the same length, taper, diameter and radius of curvature for data analysis. The reliability of the simulated canal as an ideal model for the analysis of instrumentation techniques has been validated [13]. However, due to the high radiolucency of resin blocks and the difficulty of 3D image reconstruction of simulated canals, few studies have been conducted to compare the shaping ability of endodontic instruments using μCT reconstruction techniques with standardized simulated canals.

Meglucamine diatrizoate is a water-soluble radiocontrast medium widely used for contrast-enhanced CT examination in patients for radiographic diagnosis and treatment [14]. It was verified that the combination of spiral CT and meglucamine diatrizoate could produce high-quality images for data analysis of 3D-reconstructed moulds [15].

Until now, μCT studies that combine simulated canals with meglucamine diatrizoate are lacking in the literature. In addition, no study to date has directly compared PTU, Reciproc and K3XF with regard to their shaping ability. The aim of our study was to comparatively analyse the canal shaping ability of PTU, Reciproc and K3XF by μCT in simulated canals via the meglucamine diatrizoate radiocontrast technique. The null hypothesis was that there would be no difference among the 3 rotary file systems regarding the analyzed parameters.

Methods

Simulated canals

Thirty simulated root canals with a single curvature in clear resin blocks (Endo Training Bloc; Dentsply Maillefer, Ballaigues, Switzerland) were used for this study. All canals were produced with a 0.15 mm apical foramen, 0.02 taper, 16.5 mm canal length, a 60°curvature (4.5 mm radius) and a 10-mm straight section before the curve [16]. Subsequently, the blocks were randomly assigned to 3 groups (n = 10): PTU, Reciproc and K3XF. We defined the direction of the apical foramen as distal.

Instrumentation of simulated canals

The instrumentation of all blocks was carried out by one experienced operator. Each instrument was only used to shape one canal. The patency of the root canals was confirmed with a stainless steel #10 K-file (Dentsply Maillefer). And a glide path was established in each canal using #13, #16 and #19 PathFiles (Dentsply Maillefer) at 300 rpm to the working length (WL), which was determined by inserting #10 K-file to the canal terminus and subtracting 0.5 mm from the measurement. The instrumentation sequences were then carried out as follows:

Group 1
Root canals were prepared with the PTU system. According to manufacturer's guidelines, all canals assigned to this group were shaped from S1 to F2 using the crown-down technique in full clockwise rotation by using X-Smart Plus endodontic motor (Dentsply Maillefer) with a 16:1 reduction handpiece. The torque and rotational speed were adjusted according to the manufacturer's recommendations. The F2 was used to standardize the diameter at the end-point of preparation to 0.25 mm, and the canal taper was 0.08.

Group 2
Reciproc files (R25, #25/0.08) were used in this group. Files were operated in a programmed slow in-and-out pecking, reciprocating motion according to the manufacturer's instructions. The flutes of the instrument were cleaned after 3 movements and then the canal was irrigated with sterile water. X-Smart Plus endodontic motor in the "RECIPROC" mode was used in this procedure.

Group 3
K3XF were used in this group. Ten blocks were prepared with a 16:1 reduction handpiece powered by the X-Smart Plus endodontic motor, set at 350 rpm and 3 Ncm torque. The following crown-down sequence was used: 25/10: 11 mm, 25/08: 14 mm, and 25/06: 16 mm (WL).

Following each file, patency was verified with #10 K-file and canal was irrigation with sterile water using a 27-gauge side-vented needle. The time for instrumentation was recorded which included only the time for active instrumentation. The number of permanently deformed instruments and fractured instruments during these procedures were also recorded.

Micro-CT (μCT) scanning and measurements
Pre- and post-instrumented images were scanned by μCT (μCT-50; Scanco Medical, Bassersdorf, Switzerland) with a resolution of 30 μm. Before scanning, all of the canals were brimming with 60% meglucamine diatrizoate injection. The parameters for the μCT scanner were 90 kVp and 88 μA. The cross-sectional images were segmented, visualized, registered, and quantified using analysis software (VGStudio Max version 2.2.0; Volume Graphics, Heidelberg, Germany). We selected the region extending from the constriction of the orifice to the apex as the area of interest. According to the number of cross-sectional slices, the artificial canals were equally divided into three parts, namely the coronal-, mid- and apical thirds of the canals.

Measurement of canal volume
The volume change between pre- and post- instrumentation of the three parts of each canal were computed separately using VGStudio Max 2. 2. 0.

Measurement of canal transportation
To evaluate the degree of canal transportation in the mesio-distal direction, these cross-sections were determined using perpendicular lines made by the canal axes at 1, 2, 3, 5, and 7 mm. Images of the cross-sections pre- and post- instrumentation were superimposed and recorded to determine the canal transportation and centring ability. The absolute value was calculated for each cross-section using the following formula [17]:

$$|(X1-X2)-(Y1-Y2)|$$

We designated the direction of the apical foramen as distal. X1 is the shortest distance from the distal edge of the blocks to the distal periphery of the pre-instrumented canal, and *X*2 represents the minimum distance between the distal of the block to the distal periphery of the instrumented canal. Y1 is the shortest distance from the mesial edge of the blocks to the corresponding periphery of the pre-instrumented canal, and Y2 represents the minimum distance between the mesial edges of the block to the mesial periphery of the instrumented canal (Fig. 1). A result of zero indicated no canal transportation, while other results indicated transportation towards the mesial or distal aspect of the canal.

Measurement of centring ability
The centring ratio was calculated using the following formula [17]:

$$(X1-X2)/(Y1-Y2) \text{ or } (Y1-Y2)/(X1-X2)$$

The denominator for the formula was the larger of the two numbers (X1–*X*2 or Y1–Y2). The closer the result was to one, the better the ability of the instrument to remain centred.

Statistical analysis
The statistical analysis was performed with SPSS (IBM SPSS Statistics 21; SPSS Inc., Chicago, IL). The mean difference and standard deviations for different parameters of the three parts of the canal were measured for each group. The Kruskal-Wallis test was performed to analyse the data due to non-normal distribution of the values. $P < 0.05$ was recognized as the level of statistical significance.

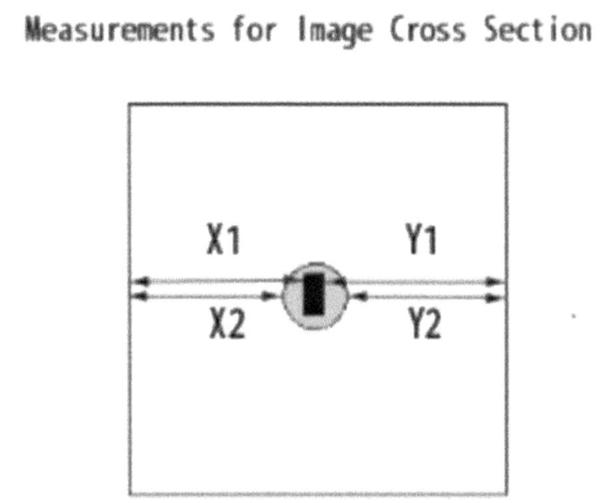

Fig. 1 Representation drawing of tooth section showing how transportation and centring ratio were derived. Dark shaded area represents original canal space, and grey shaded area represents canal's shape after instrumentation. X1 = shortest distance from the distal edge of the blocks to the distal periphery of the pre-instrumented canal; X2 = minimum distance between the distal of the blocks to the distal periphery of the instrumented canal; Y1 = shortest distance from the mesial edge of the blocks to the corresponding periphery of the pre-instrumented canal; and Y2 = the minimum distance between the mesial edge of the blocks to the mesial periphery of the instrumented canal

Results

No instrument showed macroscopic deformation or fracture in this study. Three-dimensional moulds were reconstructed for each simulated canal (Fig. 2).

Volume change

Table 1 shows the root volume change in the three parts of the canal before and after instrumentation. The Reciproc system produced greater volume change than the PTU and K3XF system in the apical third of the canals ($p < 0.05$). K3XF presented the smallest mean increase in apical volumetric change ($p < 0.05$).

Canal transportation

The difference of transportation in different parts of the canals between PTU and Reciproc was not statistically significant, which is shown in Table 2. Additionally, significantly less transportation was noted in the K3XF group.

Centring ratio

As shown in Table 3, the K3XF group showed significantly better centring ability than the PTU and Reciproc groups.

Instrumentation time

The Reciproc was significantly faster than PTU and K3XF, and the time spent by the PTU was the longest one ($p < 0.05$). The mean instrumentation time was 121.6 ± 11.9 s for PTU, 74.3 ± 4.2 s for K3XF and 73.8 ± 10.3 s for Reciproc.

Discussion

The present study describes a new method for precisely measuring canal contour before and after canal preparation in vitro. In this study, all of the simulated canals were reconstructed successfully via the radiopaque contrast technique. This method has a significant advantage over the existing methods because it allows for the non-invasive 3D evaluation of the samples with a standardization of canal length, radius and degree of curvature, taper and diameter of the apical foramen. The credibility of resin blocks for analysis of endodontic preparation and preparation techniques had been validated by previous study [9] and the materials were easily acquired, even though there were limitations with this model. A major drawback of using rotary instruments in resin blocks is the different hardness between resin and dentin. Another disadvantage is the heat generated, which might distort the canal, reduce the cutting efficiency and lead to separation of the instrument. In order to rectify this situation, syringe irrigation was applied continually during root canal preparation [18]. This method was thought to be the first attempt to compare the shaping ability of PTU, Reciproc, and K3XF by reconstructing simulated canals via the radiopaque contrast technique. This kind of model has wide application prospects in future researches. Firstly, the new method could be widely used in evaluation of root canal preparation techniques. In addition, simulated root canals included a wide range of items and C-shaped canals or lateral canals in clear resin blocks could be constructed based on the technique described by Dummer et al. [19]. Therefore, it should be possible to evaluate the quality of gutta-percha filling, the irrigating efficiency in standardized complex root canals. Moreover,it also has advantages in pre-clinical dental education because of easiness of sample obtainment.

The results of the present study revealed that the use of Reciproc instruments resulted in significantly greater volumetric change in the apical part of root canals. Reciproc R25 has the same tip taper and diameter as PTU F2 at 3 mm from their working tips. You et al. evaluated the shaping ability of continuous rotating motion in comparison to reciprocating motion in curved canals and the results showed that the type of motion had little effect on changes in root canal volume and curvature [20]. Thus, different modes of motion may not explain our study's results, but differences in instrument designs

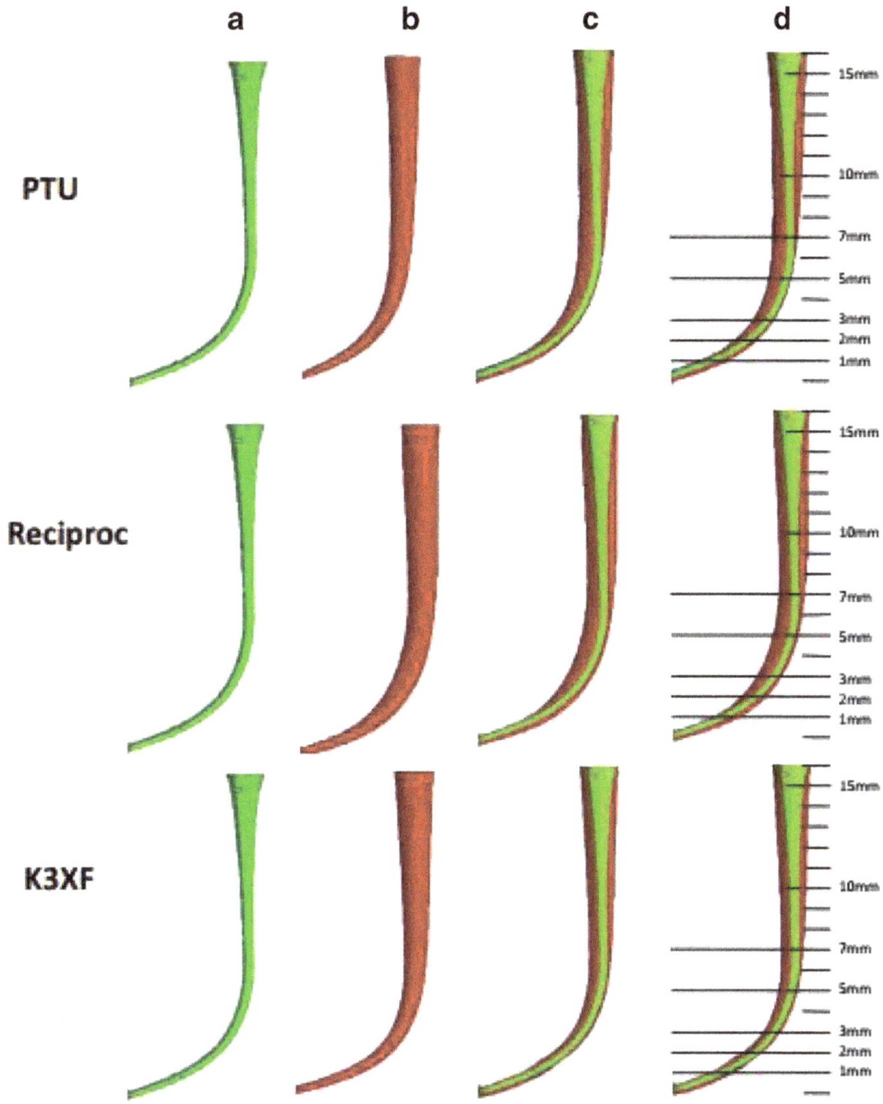

Fig. 2 Three-dimensional panels of the simulated canals in the PTU (ProTaper Universal, top), Reciproc (middle) and K3XF (bottom) groups. **a** Preoperative reconstruction of the simulated canal; **b** Postoperative reconstruction of the simulated canal; **c** Superimposed reconstructions of the simulated canal; **d** The points at which the canal width was measured after superimposition of pre- and post-operative images. The green colour indicates the canal before instrumentation, and the red colour represents the canal after instrumentation

Table 1 Volume (mm^3) change in three part of the canals (mean ± SD) with different files

Group ($n = 10$)	Apical third	Middle third	Coronal third
PTU†	0.15 ± 0.03	0.36 ± 0.03	0.40 ± 0.07
Reciproc	0.21 ± 0.05*	0.38 ± 0.04	0.42 ± 0.05
K3XF	0.09 ± 0.01*	0.24 ± 0.04	0.32 ± 0.09

†, ProTaper Universal
* Mean values represented by different superscript letters are significantly different according to the Kruskal-Wallis test ($P < .05$)

Table 2 Canal transportation (μm) of the canals after instrumentation at different measurement levels (mean ± SD)

Group ($n = 10$)	Canal transportation (mm from the apex)				
	1 mm	2 mm	3 mm	5 mm	7 mm
PTU†	0.03 ± 0.02	0.04 ± 0.02	0.06 ± 0.02	0.02 ± 0.02	0.03 ± 0.02
Reciproc	0.04 ± 0.02	0.06 ± 0.03	0.06 ± 0.03	0.03 ± 0.02	0.02 ± 0.02
K3XF	0.02 ± 0.01	0.01 ± 0.01*	0.02 ± 0.01*	0.01 ± 0.01	0.02 ± 0.01

†, ProTaper Universal
* Mean values represented with different superscript letters are significantly different according to the Kruskal-Wallis test ($P < .05$)

Table 3 Different measurement levels of centring ratio values for tested groups (mean ± SD)

Group ($n = 10$)	Centring ratio (mm from the apex)				
	1 mm	2 mm	3 mm	5 mm	7 mm
PTU[†]	0.76 ± 0.19	0.69 ± 0.17	0.52 ± 0.15	0.79 ± 0.17	0.72 ± 0.11
Reciproc	0.70 ± 0.12	0.54 ± 0.11	0.53 ± 0.15	0.80 ± 0.12	0.84 ± 0.11
K3XF	0.77 ± 0.15	0.82 ± 0.10*	0.81 ± 0.13*	0.86 ± 0.13	0.84 ± 0.13

[†], ProTaper Universal
* Mean values represented with different superscript letters are significantly different according to the Kruskal-Wallis test ($P < .05$)

on cross-section and cutting angles may lead to this result. Reciproc system has a double-cutting edge with S-shape geometry. Previous studies have confirmed that instruments with S-shape cross sections were associated with enhanced cutting efficiency [21, 22]. Another important attribute of instruments is debris removal to release the clogged cutting blades. S-shaped cross-sections allow for more space between the canal walls and the instrument [23]. The lowest volume change was recorded when K3XF instruments were used. This may be partially explained by the smallest apical taper of K3XF (size 25/0.06).

The enlargement of the apical area is conducive to reducing or eliminating the number of microorganisms in complex root canals. Gomes et al. concluded that the mechanical action of instruments eliminated more than 47% of oral bacterial endotoxins against the dentin wall [24]. On the one hand, with more volumetric changes, the irrigating needle can be placed into deeper apical sites, yielding a better irrigating effect [25, 26]. It is widely accepted that irrigation with the flow and backflow of the flushing fluid is directly related to the disinfection effect of root canals [27]. Nevertheless, previous studies noted that dentin thickness could affect the incidence of vertical root fracture, and it is safe for dentists when the canal width was controlled within 30% of the total root width [28].

Canal transportation and centring ability could be influenced by factors including different designs of instruments and the type of alloy [29, 30]. K3XF exhibited the least transportation and the best centring ability at 2 and 3 mm from the apical foramen in this study. This may be explained by smallest apical taper of K3XF (size 25/.06) compared with PTU F2 and Reciproc R25 (size 25/.08). Furthermore, R-phase (K3XF) technology makes the alloy more flexible than M-wire (Reciproc) and conventional alloy (PTU), which can minimize canal transportation in curved canals [29]. Wu et al. reported that apical transportation over 0.3 mm could compromise the outcome of the root canal filling [31]. In our study, all the transportation values obtained from different instruments were not over 0.3 mm. There were no significant differences in canal transportation and centring ability between the Reciproc and PTU groups, which were coincident with studies conducted by Capar et al. and Bürklein et al. [32, 33]. One of the reasons is that both of the instruments have non-cutting tips that only act as a guide to penetration [34]. However, Yoo et al. found that the Reciproc R25 maintained the original canal curvature better than the PTU system up to F2 in standardized plastic blocks [35]. This can be explained by the different study models used.

Instrumentation time relies on the numbers of used files, the technique and the experience of the operator. In our study, the numbers of the used files was the most influential factor. Obviously, Reciproc, which is a single-file system, required less time for instrumentation than PTU and K3XF that may because of the omission of the file change. This result was in agreement with previous studies [32, 33, 35].

Conclusions

The combination of μCT and simulated canals provided a method for the evaluation of the shaping properties of NiTi rotary instruments. Under the conditions of our study, the null hypothesis was rejected. PTU, Reciproc and K3XF instruments shaped simulated canals without any significant shaping error. Reciproc resulted in increased apical volume changes and significantly shorter instrumentation time compared with K3XF and PTU. K3XF exhibited less transportation and better centring ability at 2 and 3 mm from the apical foramen than PTU and Reciproc.

Abbreviations
NiTi: Nickel-titanium; PTU: ProTaper Universal; μCT: Micro-CT

Acknowledgements
The authors deny any conflicts of interest related to this study.

Funding
No funding was received.

Authors' contributions
Conceived and designed the experiment: HJ, PY. Performed the experiment: ZW, ZC. Analyzed the data: HJ ZC. Wrote the paper: PY, ZW. All authors read and approved the final manuscript.

Competing interests
The authors declare that they have no competing interests.

Consent to publish
Not applicable.

Ethics approval and consent to participate
Not applicable.

References

1. Sjögren U, Hagglund B, Sundqvist G, Wing K. Factors affecting the long-term results of endodontic treatment. J Endod. 1990;16:498–504.
2. Pereira AG, Santos RM F d, Mendes Azevedo KC, Raposo LH, Biffi JC. Asessment of influence of flexion angles of files in apical stop preparation by using manual and rotaryinstrumentation techniques. J Endod. 2012;38: 1383–86.
3. Alrahabi M. Comparative study of root-canal shaping with stainless steel and rotary NiTi files performed by preclinical dental students. Technol Health Care. 2015;23:257–65.
4. Kazemi RB, Stenman E, Spångberg LS. Machining efficiency and wear resistance of nickel-titanium endodontic files. Oral Surg Oral Med Oral Pathol Oral Radiol Endod. 1996;81:596–602.
5. Thompson SA. An overview of nickel-titanium alloys used in dentistry. Int Endod J. 2000;33:297–310.
6. Shen Y, Riyahi AM, Campbell L, Zhou H, Du T, Wang Z, et al. Effect of a combination of torsional and cyclic fatigue preloading on the fracture behavior of K3 and K3XF instruments. J Endod. 2015;41:526–30.
7. Southard DW, Oswald RJ, Natkin E. Instrumentation of curved molar root canals with the Roane technique. J Endod. 1987;13:479–89.
8. Gekelman D, Ramamurthy R, Mirfarsi S, Paqué F, Peters OA. Rotary nickel-titanium GT and ProTaper files for root canal shaping by novice operators: a radiographic and micro-computed tomography evaluation. J Endod. 2009; 35:1584–8.
9. Goldman M, Sakurai-Fuse E, Turco J, White RR. A silicone model method to compare three methods of preparing the root canal. Oral Surg Oral Med Oral Pathol. 1989;68:457–61.
10. Moinzadeh A, De Bruyne M. Re: A micro-computed tomographic evaluation of apical root canal preparation using three instrumentation techniques. Int Endod J. 2010;43:451–3.
11. Ounsi HF, Franciosi G, Paragliola R, Al-Hezaimi K, Salameh Z, Tay FR, et al. Comparison of two techniques for assessing the shaping efficacy of repeatedly used nickel-titanium rotary instruments. J Endod. 2011;37:847–50.
12. Peters OA, Peters CI, Schönenberger K, Barbakow F. ProTaper rotary root canal preparation: effects of canal anatomy on final shape analysed by micro CT. Int Endod J. 2003;36:86–92.
13. Lim KC, Webber J. The validity of simulated root canals for the investigation of the prepared root canal shape. Int Endod J. 1985;18:240–6.
14. Choi HK, Law WL, Ho JW, Chu KW. Value of gastrografin in adhesive small bowel obstruction after unsuccessful conservative treatment: a prospective evaluation. World J Gastroenterol. 2005;11:3742–5.
15. Choi AD, Joly JM, Chen MY, Weigold WG. Physiologic evaluation of ischemia using cardiac CT: current status of CT myocardial perfusion and CT fractional flow reserve. J Cardiovasc Comput Tomogr. 2014;8:272–81.
16. Silva EJ, Muniz BL, Pires F, Belladonna FG, Neves AA, Souza EM, et al. Comparison of canal transportation in simulated curved canals prepared with ProTaper Universal and ProTaper Gold systems. Restor Dent Endod. 2016;41:1–5.
17. Gambill JM, Alder M, Del RC. Comparison of nickel-titanium and stainless steel hand-file instrumentation using computed tomography. J Endod. 1996;22:369–75.
18. Kum KY, Spångberg L, Cha BY, Jung IY, Lee SJ, Lee CY. Shaping ability of three ProFile rotary instrumentation techniques in simulated resin root canals. J Endod. 2000;26:719–23.
19. Dummer PM, Alodeh MH, al-Omari MA. A method for the construction of simulated root canals in clear resin blocks. Int Endod J. 1991;24(2):63–6.
20. You SY, Kim HC, Bae KS, Baek SH, Kum KY, Lee W. Shaping ability of reciprocating motion in curved root canals: a comparative study with micro-computed tomography. J Endod. 2011;37:1296–300.
21. Cecchin D, de Sousa-Neto MD, Pecora JD, Gariba-Silva R. Cutting efficiency of four different rotary nickel: Titanium instruments. J Conserv Dent. 2011; 14:117–9.
22. Bürklein S, Benten S, Schäfer E. Shaping ability of different single-file systems in severely curved root canals of extracted teeth. Int Endod J. 2013;46:590–7.
23. Plotino G, Giansiracusa RA, Grande NM, Testarelli L, Gambarini G. Cutting efficiency of Reciproc and waveOne reciprocating instruments. J Endod. 2014;40:1228–30.
24. Gomes BP, Martinho FC, Vianna ME. Comparison of 2.5% sodium hypochlorite and 2% chlorhexidine gel on oral bacterial lipopolysaccharide reduction from primarily infected root canals. J Endod. 2009;35:1350–3.
25. Sedgley CM, Nagel AC, Hall D, Applegate B. Influence of irrigant needle depth in removing bioluminescent bacteria inoculated into instrumented root canals using real-time imaging in vitro. Int Endod J. 2005;38:97–104.
26. Shen Y, Gao Y, Qian W, Ruse ND, Zhou X, Wu H, et al. Three-dimensional numeric simulation of root canal irrigant flow with different irrigation needles. J Endod. 2010;36:884–9.
27. Martinho FC, Chiesa WM, Marinho AC, Zaia AA, Ferraz CC, Almeida JF, et al. Clinical investigation of the efficacy of chemomechanical preparation with rotary nickel-titanium files for removal of endotoxin from primarily infected root canals. J Endod. 2010;36:1766–9.
28. Wilcox LR, Roskelley C, Sutton T. The relationship of root canal enlargement to finger-spreader induced vertical root fracture. J Endod. 1997;23:533–4.
29. Peters OA, Paque F. Root canal preparation of maxillary molars with the self-adjusting file: a micro-computed tomography study. J Endod. 2011;37:53–7.
30. Olivieri JG, Stober E, Garcia FM, González JA, Bragado P, Roig M, et al. In vitro comparison in a manikin model: increasing apical enlargement with K3 and K3XF rotary instruments. J Endod. 2014;40:1463–7.
31. Wu MK, Fan B, Wesselink PR. Leakage along apical root fillings in curved root canals. Part I: effects of apical transportation on seal of root fillings. J Endod. 2000;26:210–6.
32. Capar ID, Ertas H, Ok E, Arslan H, Ertas ET. Comparative study of different novel nickel-titanium rotary systems for root canal preparation in severely curved root canals. J Endod. 2014;40:852–6.
33. Bürklein S, Hinschitza K, Dammaschke T, Schäfer E. Shaping ability and cleaning effectiveness of two single-file systems in severely curved root canals of extracted teeth: Reciproc and WaveOne versus Mtwo and ProTaper. Int Endod J. 2012;45:449–61.
34. Dummer PM, Hutchings R, Hartles FR. The effect of using files with altered tips in a sonic handpiece: an in vitro study. Int Endod J. 1993;26:209–17.
35. Yoo YS, Cho YB. A comparison of the shaping ability of reciprocating NiTi instruments in simulated curved canals. Restor Dent Endod. 2012;37:220–7.

10

Comparison of occlusal caries detection using the ICDAS criteria on extracted teeth or their photographs

P. Bottenberg[1*], W. Jacquet[1,2], C. Behrens[3], V. Stachniss[4] and A. Jablonski-Momeni[3]

Abstract

Background: Using photographs of occlusal surfaces instead of extracted teeth for the detection of caries can be useful in multicenter studies or education. Using a panel of observers, ICDAS scores on teeth or photographs were evaluated against the histological gold standard. The hypothesis was that both outcomes were equivalent.

Methods: Four examiners with different experience in ICDAS scored photographs of occlusal surfaces of 100 extracted teeth on a monitor using ICDAS criteria. Two of the examiners had previously scored extracted teeth prior to photography. Digital images of histological sections of the teeth were observed by all examiners and consensus scores were given for each investigation site (gold standard). Kappa statistics and Spearman correlation coefficients as well as repeated measure ANOVA were performed. ROC curves were constructed for each examiner and the areas under the ROC-curves (AUC) of both scoring techniques (extracted teeth, digital images) were compared ($\alpha = 0.05$).

Results: Intra- and inter-rater kappa for ICDAS on teeth were 0.81–0.94 and on photographs 0.54–0.88, respectively. Correlation with histology was 0.58– 0.61 for the teeth and 0.50–0.62 for the photographs. AUC of ICDAS scores of extracted teeth (mean 0.89) were slightly higher than those for photographs (mean 0.84). However, both AUC values were not statistically significant ($p = 0.38$).

Conclusion: Using photographs to assess occlusal surfaces with the ICDAS criteria was not statistically different from scoring the extracted teeth.

Keywords: Caries detection, Occlusal caries, ICDAS, Digital images, ROC curves

Abbreviations: ANOVA, Analysis of variance; AUC, Area under the curve; ICDAS, International Caries Detection and Assessment System; ROC, Receiver-operating characteristics

Background

Visual-tactile caries detection remains a process in which a human observer judges differences in color, texture, transparency or radiolucency to come to a conclusion about the presence and extent of pathological processes under the tooth surface. Until the advent of methods which automatically and directly detect demineralization in a reliable and affordable way, caries detection relies on the clinician as final signal processing tool. Each individual observer is liable to have a different interpretation of these signals based on visual acuity, neurological signal processing, experience or education.

The well-established ICDAS ("International Caries Detection and Assessment System") visual caries detection system enables lesions at various stages to be clinically detected [1]. ICDAS was introduced to standardize the interpretation of the visual signs of caries detection. Besides the score of "0" (caries free), six different stages of lesion severity are registered. This method exhibits good reproducibility and a clinically acceptable specificity and sensitivity to the detection of occlusal caries [2].

However, as with all methods, observers have to be trained in using ICDAS correctly. This is logistically demanding when ICDAS is to be used in other settings than small groups of intensively calibrated and trained

* Correspondence: pbottenb@vub.ac.be
[1]Department of Oral Health Sciences, Vrije Universiteit Brussel, Laarbeeklaan 103, 1090 Brussels, Belgium
Full list of author information is available at the end of the article

observers as was the practice in scientific reports hitherto. The logistical challenge is much greater in larger groups such as dentists with different backgrounds and experience participating in epidemiologic surveys or training of graduate students.

Moreover, organizing multi-center studies necessitates travels of trainers and examiners to perform the examinations. The logistics involved generally limited the number of observers.

However, it is preferable to use the same set of teeth in order to compare all participants. Physically sending teeth to different centers can lead to damage or bias due to desiccation of the samples. This also limits the repetitive use of extracted teeth in student education.

When calibration or evaluation of detection methods is performed, a reference standard is needed. Frequently, this is achieved by histological examination [3]. This leads to irreversible loss of the teeth.

In order to overcome this problem, teeth can be photographed before sectioning to keep them at least virtually available all by having a reference standard at hand. Development of digital photography has allowed producing photographs of high quality which can be reproduced, viewed and distributed nearly limitless and without loss of quality. This was demonstrated in a study for the histological reference standard but not yet for the occlusal surfaces of the teeth used in that study [4]. In several studies, photographs of teeth or tooth surfaces have been used for the purpose of epidemiology [5], detection of caries [6–8] or enamel disorders [9]. The comparison with a reference standard has shown that sensitivity and specificity obtained on photographs and extracted teeth were comparable [6]. Furthermore, in studies using clinical examinations [10], photographs allow the calibration of multiple observers or in repetition without putting undue stress on the volunteers, especially children [11], however without being able to use a histological reference standard. Comparing caries detection on teeth and photographs has been done before, however not using the full scale of ICDAS scores. Boye et al. [6] used a comparatively simple scoring system for caries for the purpose of epidemiological surveys. The score was the presence or absence of dentine caries. The study showed a good correlation. However, ICDAS, with a more elaborate scale of lesion severities could produce different results. Gomez et al. [12] showed no difference in detection of non-cavitated lesions between teeth or their photographs. In this study, a general agreement was studied using correlation and kappa analysis.

The aim of this study was to evaluate the performance of ICDAS scores obtained on extracted teeth compared to their photographs using histology as a reference standard. The working hypothesis was that there is no statistical difference between the diagnostic performances of both techniques. Furthermore, the effect of observer's different background and experience was evaluated by using photographs of teeth. The hypothesis was that the training of the examiner has an influence on detection ability. Therefore two other dentists with less experience in cariology research or ICDAS were added to the panel.

Methods

Sample selection and preparation

Teeth were selected from a collection extracted for periodontal or orthodontic reasons at University of Dundee and Marburg university dental schools in 2007. Oral consent of the patients was obtained according to the ethical rules of that time. In the meantime, Brussels University medical ethical committee allowed collection of teeth extracted in the framework of routine patient treatment for diagnostic research purposes (ref. B14320096266). 100 unrestored posterior teeth were selected from a batch of extracted and cleaned teeth stored in a thymol solution. Selection was performed based on visual criteria to obtain a number of sound teeth and a range of occlusal carious lesions in different states. Teeth with discoloration not due to carious changes were excluded since this was not a part of the hypothesis under study. Prior to examination or taking of photographs, the tooth surfaces were carefully dried with compressed air. Teeth were then immediately returned to containers with 100 % humidity. High resolution photographs were taken from the occlusal surfaces under standardized conditions with a digital camera and anti-dazzle macro lens (EOS 30 D, MP5; f = 65 mm, Canon Comp, Krefeld, Germany). The teeth were illuminated using an oblique incident light from a ring-shaped fluorescent tube which reproduced daylight. The resolution of the camera chip was 3.5 mega pixels [4]. After performing caries detection using the ICDAS criteria [13], serial sections of the teeth were provided for the establishment of a reference standard and digital images were obtained referring to a published protocol [4]. In brief, one to four histological sections and their images were assigned to each examination site. All images of the selected sections for each investigation site were analyzed by all four examiners using the following histological classification [14]: 0 = No enamel demineralization or narrow surface zone of opacity, 1 = Enamel demineralization limited to the outer 50 % of enamel, 2 = Demineralization involving the inner 50 % of enamel, up to the enamel–dentine junction (EDJ), 3 = Demineralization involving the outer 50 % of dentine, 4 = Demineralization involving the inner 50 % of dentine.

The histological score assigned to each investigation site represented the worst classification observed in the representative sections. Emphasis was placed on differentiating pulp–dentine complex reactions with dental tissues affected by caries. Consensus score between all examiners for each examination site served as reference standard [4].

The teeth were dried and examined by a panel of trained observers using the ICDAS criteria. The sites were recorded as: 0 = sound; 1 = first visible sign of non-cavitated lesion seen only when the tooth is dry; 2 = visible non-cavitated lesion seen when wet and dry; 3 = localized enamel breakdown without visual signs of dentine involvement; Code 4 = underlying dark shadow from dentine with or without localized enamel breakdown; Code 5 = distinct cavity with visible dentine; Code 6 = extensive cavitated lesion with visible dentine [13].

The digital photographs were saved on a CD-ROM and made accessible to 4 examiners. Two of them (AJM and VS) were identical to a panel of observers from a previous study [4], while two other examiners were newly recruited (PB and CB). Three of the observers had research experience in caries detection (AJM, VS and PB), one was last year student from dental school (CB). Of the examiners, 3 received extensive training in ICDAS (AJM, VS, CB) while one used the e-learning program for ICDAS [15] only (PB). Each examiner viewed the digital images on a LCD color monitor at a constant observation distance (60 cm).

Scoring according to the ICDAS criteria was performed on a computer screen without magnification or other image manipulations using a standard image viewing software (IrfanView). A printout at lower resolution indicating the sites to be scored per tooth and a form for the recording of the scores was presented to the examiner. Two consecutive scorings were performed with a four-week interval. The results of an earlier study of ICDAS scores [4] performed by visual inspection on the original extracted teeth (with 2 of the observers of the original 4-person panel, AJM and VS) served as comparison.

Statistical analysis

In total 169 sites were evaluated. Forty-three teeth had one site, 46 two, 10 teeth three and one tooth had four investigation sites. In order to exclude potential confounding factors by caries extending below the surface to neighboring sites, only one site per tooth was selected after scoring, using computer-generated random numbers. Analysis was performed via sensitivity and specificity (expressed as receiver-operating characteristic (ROC)-curves) and repeatability (expressed as intra-rater kappa). Variability between observers was estimated using Bland-Altman plots and repeated measures ANOVA. In all statistical hypothesis tests, a p-value of 0.05 or lower was chosen as a limit for significance.

Sensitivity and specificity were calculated (cutoff: dentine caries, histology D3 and ICDAS = 3) and ROC curves were established. Statistical comparison between correlated ROC-AUC values of both scoring techniques was performed using the tooth surface (and not the global result of one observer) as unit [16]. Further analysis was performed using kappa statistics between observers (inter-rater) and between both repeat scorings (intra-rater). Intra-rater kappa statistics was also calculated separately for histologically sound teeth and those with enamel or dentine caries. These calculations were performed with the R software (version 2.15.1, The R Foundation for Statistical Computing). Furthermore Bland-Altman-plots were established (Prism version 5.0, GraphPad, LaJolla, USA) between observers scoring photographs and histology as well as between the two observers having scored both teeth and photographs. A repeated measure ANOVA was performed to evaluate the effect of the observer with histological lesion category as covariate. A significant ($p < 0.001$) Mauchly test indicated that the compensation according to Greenhouse-Geiser was to be used for the calculation of within-subject effects. These statistical calculations were performed using SPSS (version 22.0, SPSS inc, Armonk, NY).

Results

Four teeth were lost during histological preparation, leaving 96 teeth for further evaluation. Of the 96 sites selected, 27 were histologically sound, 16 had shallow and 16 deep enamel caries, 26 had superficial and 11 deep dentine caries.

Correlation coefficients between histology and ICDAS scores varied between 0.55 and 0.71.

Scoring of the original teeth yielded Az values of the ROC curves of 0.9 and 0.89 respectively, scoring of the photographs resulted in Az values ranging from 0.8 to 0.88 (Table 1). There was no significant difference between both modalities ($p > 0.05$).

Specificity and sensitivity varied, especially in the case of the less experienced observers 3 and 4. The results of the Kappa statistics can be found in Table 2. Kappa values varied according to the histological reference standard of the tooth. Intra-rater kappa values were systematically higher than inter-rater. Values for sound and dentine caries also were higher than for enamel caries. Global Inter-rater (Fleiss) kappa values (all surfaces) were 0.261 for the first scoring and 0.221 for the second scoring ($p < 0.05$). Bland-Altman plots are shown in Fig. 1. The derived parameters (bias and limits of agreement) are given in Table 3.

The results of the repeated measure ANOVA showed that for the observers scoring both teeth and photographs, the variable "operator" (observer 1 or 2) had a F-value of 0.63, $p = 0.43$, "modality" (tooth or photograph) yielded a F-value of 1.57, $p = 0.21$. The two-way interaction effects yielded significant effect (modality*operator F = 40.57, $p < 0.001$) and (modality*histology F = 3.25, $p = 0.015$). In the case of the four observers scoring

Table 1 Sensitivity and specificity and ROC-AUC (Az) calculated for different cut-off values and modalities

Observer and modality	Cut-off histology = 1, ICDAS = 1		Cut-off histology = 3, ICDAS = 4,		
	Sensitivity	Specificity	A_z	Sensitivity	Specificity
Obs. 1, tooth	0.94	0.44	0,89	1.00	0.27
Obs. 2, tooth	0.72	0.48	0,9	0.97	0.52
Obs. 1, photo	0.86	0.56	0.88	0.97	0.41
Obs. 2, photo	0.94	0.41	0.84	0.97	0.24
Obs. 3, photo	0.77	0.63	0.80	0.84	0.45
Obs. 4, photo	1.00	0.19	0.84	1.00	0.08

photographs, observer was the most prominent variable (F = 10.56, $p < 0.001$).

In Fig. 2, representative samples of teeth and the corresponding histological sections are presented for different ICDAS scores.

Statistical power was calculated using a specific method for ROC analysis [16]. Based on Az values and their standard errors a power ranging from 0.14 to 0.29 for a difference of 5 % between raters and 0.39 to 0.80 for a difference of 10 % in Az value between raters could be calculated. For a difference between methods (tooth vs photograph) power was calculated to range between 0.28 and 0.40 for a 5 % difference between methods and 0.79 to 0.93 for a 10 % difference.

Discussion

In this in vitro study it could be shown that visual caries detection according to the ICDAS on extracted teeth and their photographs achieved a good agreement and had AUC values in the ROC curves exceeding 0.73 and acceptable to good intra- and inter-rater agreement. Direct observation scored somewhat better (ROC 0.84). The fact that in the direct observation higher (but not significantly so) AUC values were found could be attributed to the high scores they showed in the previous study from which the data were taken [4]. The training and discussion of the observers in the preparation of that study is certainly a major reason. Training and calibration of these two observers may also be the reason that no observer effect was found in the ANOVA for the direct observation of teeth. Nevertheless, in the previously performed study [4] the aim was to evaluate examiner reproducibility in the assessment of caries lesion depth when viewing images of histological sections on a computer monitor compared to direct microscopy.

In the present study in no case, a perfect detection was possible. Consistently, several histologically sound sites were scored as carious and vice versa (Fig. 2). In

Table 2 Kappa values, inter and intra-rater. O1 to O4: observers. Results are linearly weighted kappa

Modality		Histological state of the surface							
Inter-rater		Sound		Enamel		Dentine		Total	
		k ± S.E.	Sig.	k ± S.E.	Sig.	k ± S.E.	Sig.	k ± S.E.	Sig.
O1-O2	tooth	0.41 ± 0.16	*	0.33 ± 0.10	**	0.65 ± 0.07	***	0.64 ± 0.04	***
O1-O2	photo	0.55 ± 0.12	**	0.26 ± .14	*	0.46 ± 0.10	***	0.57 ± 0.05	***
O1-O3	photo	0.44 ± 0.12	*	0.02 ± 0.14	ns	0.17 ± 0.12	ns	0.39 ± 0.06	***
O1-O4	photo	0.30 ± 0.13	*	0.20 ± 0.13	ns	0.33 ± 0.11	**	0.44 ± 0.05	***
O2-O3	photo	0.53 ± 0.12	**	0.31 ± 0.11	*	0.32 ± 0.12	**	0.52 ± 0.05	***
O2-O4	photo	0.51 ± 0.12	**	0.25 ± 0.10	ns	0.52 ± 0.10	***	0.58 ± 0.05	***
O3-O4	photo	0.40 ± 0.14	**	0.15 ± 0.12	ns	0.26 ± 0.12	*	0.42 ± 0.06	***
Intra-rater		Sound		Enamel		Dentine		total	
O1	tooth	0.82 ± 0.07	***	0.54 ± 0.09	***	0.86 ± 0.06	***	0.85 ± 0.03	***
O2	tooth	0.54 ± 0.12	*	0.49 ± 0.09	**	0.75 ± 0.06	***	0.74 ± 0.04	***
O1	photo	0.62 ± 0.15	**	0.54 ± 0.11	***	0.67 ± 0.10	***	0.74 ± 0.04	***
O2	photo	0.50 ± 0.11	**	0.34 ± 0.14	*	0.53 ± 0.10	***	0.61 ± 0.05	***
O3	photo	0.44 ± 0.16	*	0.29 ± 0.12	*	0.81 ± 0.07	***	0.59 ± 0.05	***
O4	photo	0.82 ± 0.07	***	0.57 ± 0.15	***	0.73 ± 0.06	***	0.78 ± 0.04	***

Significance levels are given as follows: ns: not significant ($p > 0.05$), * $p < 0.05 > 0.01$, ** $p < 0.01.0.001$, *** $p < 0.001$

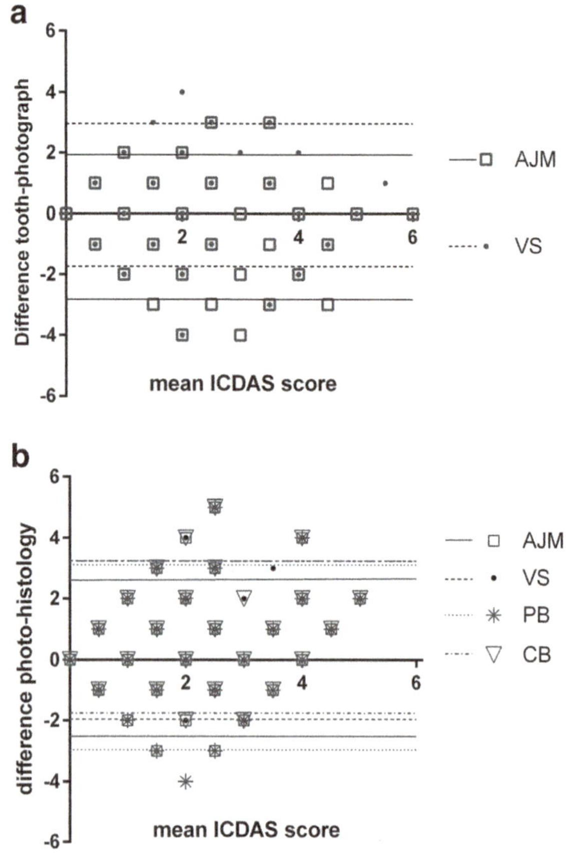

Fig. 1 Bland-Altman plot of ICDAS scores of extracted teeth versus their photographs (**a**) and ICDAS scores of photographs versus the histological reference standard (**b**) showing the variation between observers (initials as given in the text). The *lines* show the upper and lower limits of the 95 % CI per observer

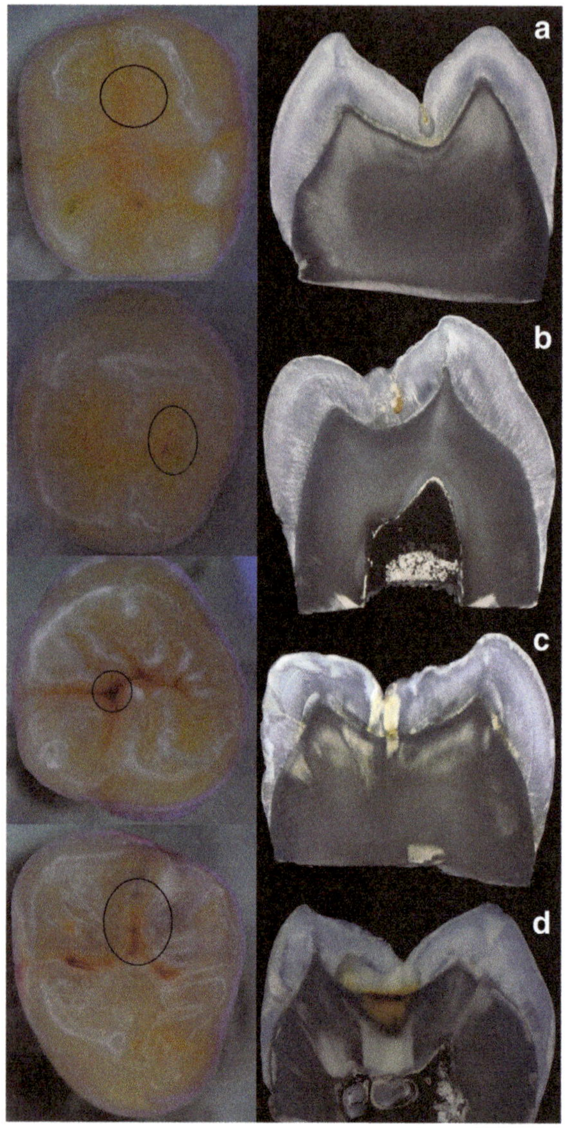

Fig. 2 a-d Examples of different teeth used in the study. The investigation sites are marked with a circle: **a** Example of a tooth being scored as sound while being histologically carious. **b** Tooth with ICDAS score 2 and corresponding histological images. **c** Tooth with ICDAS score 3 and corresponding histological images. **d** Tooth with ICDAS score 4 and corresponding histological images

Table 3 Results of the Bland-Altman test for different modalities and observers. Bias: asymmetric distribution of the discrepancies between the modalities. Limits of agreement: 95 % of the data fall between these limits

Modality	Bias (±SD)	95 % limits of agreement	
		Lower	Upper
Observer 1, tooth vs histo	−0.46 ± 1.30	−3.00	2.08
Obs. 2, tooth vs histo	0.0 ± 1.38	−2.70	2.70
Obs 1, tooth vs photo	0.43 ± 1.19	−1.90	2.75
Obs 2, tooth vs photo	−0.60 ± 1.21	−1.90	2.75
Obs 1, photo vs histo	0.03 ± 1.17	−2.25	2.31
Obs 2, photo vs. histo	0.59 ± 1.31	−1.98	3.16
Obs 3, photo vs histo	0.15 ± 1.54	−2.68	3.15
Obs 4, photo vs histo	0.67 ± 1.24	−1.74	3.10

the case of false-positive scores, discoloration and deep-narrow fissures with stain accumulation were involved. This phenomenon has been described as a "typical pitfall" for ICDAS by Altarakehma et al. [17].

Hintze et al. [18] proposed a minimum quantity of either surfaces/sites or observers in order to reach significant differences between radiographic detection methods. This calculation was based on an experimental design in which the individual observer's ROC curve is used as variable as unit of statistical calculation. In the present study, calculation and comparison of ROC curves was performed using the tooth as unit resulting in a larger data base for statistical comparisons.

A potential weakness of the experimental design was that the original research team was not more available and teeth were already sectioned. So we were not able to assess the scores of trained examiners on scoring photographs or less experienced observers of scoring the original teeth. With using the surface as unit, however, we believe that the statistical material would have been sufficient to demonstrate a difference with just these two remaining observers.

The power of the present study design was rather low. However, power calculations are intended to be applied for the demonstration of a possible difference, not for equivalence as was the aim of the present study.

The effect of photograph on observer's performance has already been examined and showed no significant difference in sound surfaces or those with ICDAS scores 1–4 [12]. With our data, we could show the same for the whole range of ICDAS scores. What seemed more important however, was the disparity between observers. Observer 4 had a very high sensitivity but a low specificity, notwithstanding the cut-off value used (Table 1).

Recently, Altarakehma et al. [17] and Qudeimat el al. [19] stressed the importance of the contribution of the individual observer to the result. Using photographs would allow to further explore this hypothesis as the material can be made accessible to larger groups of observers also by using digital media. Thus, studies would be less dependent on logistical aspects [8]. This is beneficial for multi-centre studies [4], teaching purposes and it also helps increasing the number of participants for such type of studies and hence to achieve valid power for interpreting the data.

Another interesting finding is that inter- and intra-rater kappa values varied according to the histological state of the tooth (Table 2). Intra-rater values were lowest for ICDAS 1–3 lesions. The same applied for inter-rater. The kappa values were close to nothing when the inexperienced observers (3 and 4) were matched against the experienced ones. The same was reflected in the Bland-Altman plots and analysis. This was in contrast to the findings of Diniz et al., [20] and may have been a result of a different balance between histological grades. The advantage of using photographs would be in this context that a balance can be made between histological grades before undertaking the experiment and letting the observers score the selected photographs. It would also allow studying the effect of different balances of histological gradation, for instance such as in a given population and compare this to a selection favoring a numerical balance.

Only very few teeth were scored differently to histology in only one modality. This is reflected in the small difference in ROC curve AUC for both methods. Photographs, although not (yet) being able to give a three-dimensional image, seem to be suitable for caries detection [6]. Also in other domains such as dental material evaluation, standardized photographs seem to be valuable tools of observation [21]. Standardization is important if texture and color (as used in the ICDAS definition) has to be judged. However the method used in this study did not use an elaborate color standardization protocol as the one described by Bengel [22] for the evaluation of bleaching techniques. It was deemed that strict color standardization was not needed because no consecutive evaluation of color change was intended.

One shortcoming of using photographs is the fact that the ICDAS scores should be determined after air drying the tooth surface. Hence in the present study proper differentiation of scores ICDAS1 and ICDAS 2 would not be possible. The question whether there is a benefit of using pictures of wet and dry tooth surfaces for detection of initial lesions on digital images was addressed by Jablonski-Momeni et al. [23, 24]. The authors showed that the diagnostic performance of the examinations (AUC) was consistent with a good to very good diagnostic performance irrespective of whether the surface was photographed wet or dry [23]. There was no considerable difference in the diagnostic accuracy of the ICDAS when the performance was evaluated either on images of wet or dried tooth surfaces [24]. In a recently published manual there are also suggestions to merge the ICDAS codes for the purpose of caries management [25]. Here the ICDAS codes 1 and 2 are categorized as initial stage of caries and are explained as "First or distinct visual changes in enamel seen as a carious opacity or visible discoloration (white spot lesion and/or brown carious discoloration) not consistent with clinical appearance of sound enamel (ICDAS code 1 or 2) and which show no evidence of surface breakdown or underlying dentine shadowing". Specifically for pits and fissures "the carious discoloration is apparent starting in the base of the fissure or pit and may extend up the wall of the pit/fissure but no distinct loss of enamel is apparent, i.e. the pit/fissure retains its original anatomical appearance. Appearance not consistent with stained pits/fissures (ICDAS code 0)". Hence the differentiation of initial and moderate lesions might still be possible when tooth images are used. The effect of grey value vision has been forwarded as possible source of bias in caries detection on radiographs [26] and it remains to be demonstrated if a similar phenomenon pertaining to color perception may have played a role in this study. Notwithstanding which method is used, caries detection methods rely upon the human eye and mind as tool for interpretation of mainly visual signs. In future studies a higher number of observers with a different background should be used for data generation in order to obtain a realistic appreciation of a method. Fortunately with the present data and also based on the study of Gomez et al. [12], photographs can be advantageously used to increase the number of observers. This hypothesis will be the object of future continuation of this research work.

Conclusions

The modality of scoring ICDAS (original teeth or their digital photographs) differs less than the observers among each other. Using photographs can facilitate the logistic aspect of multi-center studies and increase the number of observers next to being useful in clinical training and teaching.

Parts of this manuscript have been presented as a poster on the ORCA conference in Liverpool, 2013 (abstract nr. 92).

Acknowledgements

Funding

No funding was obtained for this study.

Authors' contributions

AJM conceived and supervised the study; CB conceived the study, supervised and coordinated the scoring procedure; VS performed the histology and supervised the gold standard scoring; WJ performed the statistical analysis; PB prepared the manuscript draft, participated in data analysis and prepared figures and tables. All authors participated in the final version of the manuscript and approved its form and content.

Competing interest

The authors declare that they have no competing interests.

Consent for publication

Not applicable

Ethical review

Our team has obtained the permission of the ethical committee of Vrije Universiteit Brussel (VUB) to use extracted human teeth for scientific studies in cariology (ref. B14320096266). The document (in Dutch) is to be found with the dataset: https://figshare.com/s/782b4fa6a2fa92a05e66

Author details

[1]Department of Oral Health Sciences, Vrije Universiteit Brussel, Laarbeeklaan 103, 1090 Brussels, Belgium. [2]Depatment of Educational Sciences EDWE-LOCI, Vrije Universiteit Brussel, Pleinlaan 2, 1050 Ixelles, Brussels, Belgium. [3]Dental School, Department of Pediatric and Community Dentistry, Philipps University of Marburg, Marburg, Germany. [4]Dental School, Department of Restorative Dentistry, Philipps University of Marburg, Georg-Voigt-Straße 3, D-35039 Marburg, Germany.

References

1. Pitts N. "ICDAS"- an international system for caries detection and assessment being developed to facilitate caries epidemiology, research and appropriate clinical management. Community Dent Health. 2004;21:193–8.
2. Jablonski-Momeni A, Stachniss V, Ricketts DN, Heinzel-Gutenbrunner M. Reproducibility and accuracy of the ICDAS-II for detection of occlusal caries. Caries Res. 2008;42:79–87.
3. Huysmans M, Longbottom C. The challenges of validating diagnostic methods and selecting appropriate gold standards. J Dent Res. 2004; 83(Spec Iss C):C48–52.
4. Jablonski-Momeni A, Ricketts DNJ, Stachniss V, Maschka R, Heinzel-Gutenbrunner M, Pieper K. Occlusal caries: evaluation of direct microscopy versus digital imaging used for two histological classification systems. J Dent. 2009;37:204–11.
5. Boye U, Willasey A, Walsh T, Tickle M, Pretty IA. Comparison of intra-oral photographic caries assessment with an established visual caries assessment method for use in epidemiological studies in children. Community Dent Oral Epidemiol. 2013;41:526–33.
6. Boye U, Walsh T, Pretty IA, Tickle M. Comparison of photographic and visual assessment of occlusal caries with histology as the reference standard. BMC Oral Health. 2012;12:10.
7. Richter AE, Arruda AO, Peters MC, Sohn W. Incidence of caries lesions among patients treated with comprehensive orthodontics. Am J Orthod Dentofac Orthop. 2011;139:657–64.
8. Van Hilsen Z, Jones RS. Comparing potential early caries assessment methods for teledentistry. BMC Oral Health. 2013;13:16.
9. Cochran JA, Ketley CE, Sanchez L, Mamai-Homata E, Oila A-M, Árnadóttir IB. A standardized photographic method for evaluating enamel opacities including fluorosis. Community Dent Oral Epidemiol. 2004;32 Suppl 1:19–27.
10. Declerck D, Bottenberg P, Carvalho J, Declerck C, De Vos E, Vanden Abbeele A, Vannieuwenhuysen JP, Vannobbergen J, Bogaerts K. Development and Implementation of an Oral Health Data Registration and Evaluation System for the Belgian Population. J Dent Oral Craniofac Epidemiol. 2013;1:45–54.
11. Boye U, Foster GRK, Pretty IA, Tickle M. Children's views on the experience of a visual examination and inta-oral photographs to detect dental caries in epidemiological studies. Community Dent Health. 2011;20:1–5.
12. Gomez J, Zakhian C, Salsone S, Pinto SCS, Taylor A, Pretty IA, Ellwood R. In vitro performance of different methods in detecting occlusal caries lesions. J Dent. 2013;41:180–6.
13. International Caries Detection and Assessment System (ICDAS) Coordinating Committee. Criteria Manual. Bogota, Colombia and Budapest, Hungary, 2009. Available from http://www.icdas.org/ (Accessed 18 Nov 2015).
14. Downer MC. Concurrent validity of an epidemiological diagnostic system for caries with the histological appearance of extracted teeth as validating criterion. Caries Res. 1975;9:231–46.
15. Diniz MB, Monti Lima L, Santos-Pinto L, Eckert GJ, Ferreira-Zandoná AG, De Cássia Loiola Cordeiro R. Influence of the ICDAS E-learning program for occlusal caries detection on dental students. J Dent Educ. 2010;74:862–8.
16. Robin X, Turck N, Hainard A, Tiberti N, Lisacek F, Sanchez JC, Müller M. pROC: an open-source package for R and S+ to analyze and compare ROC curves. BMC Bioinformatics. 2011;12:77.
17. Altarakemah Y, Al-Sane M, Lim S, Kingman A, Ismail AI. A new approach to reliability assessment of dental caries examinations. Community Dent Oral Epidemiol. 2013;41:309–16.
18. Hintze H, Frydenberg M, Wenzel A. Influence of number of surfaces and observers on statistical power in a multiobserver ROC radiographic caries detection study. Caries Res. 2003;37:200–5.
19. Qudeimat MA, Alomari QD, Altarakemah Y, Alshawaf N, Honkala EJ. Variables affecting the inter- and intra-examiner reliability of ICDAS for occlusal caries diagnosis in permanent molars. J Public Health Dent. 2016;76:9–17.
20. Diniz MB, Rodriguez JA, Hug I, Cordeiro RCL, Lussi A. Reproducibility and accuracy of the ICDAS-II for occlusal caries detection. Community Dent Oral Epidemiol. 2009;37:399–404.
21. Knibbs PJ. Methods of clinical evaluation of dental restorative materials. J Oral Rehab. 1997;24:109–23.
22. Bengel WM. Digital photography and the assessment of therapeutic results after bleaching. J Esthet Restor Dent. 2003;15 Suppl 1:S21–32.
23. Jablonski-Momeni A, Hoppe R, Stachniss V. Use of digitally optimized images of ICDAS caries codes by undergraduate dental students. In: Méndez-Villas, editor. Microscopy Microscopy: advances in scientific research and education, vol. 2. Badajoz: Formatex, Research Center; 2014. p. 1203–9.
24. Jablonski-Momeni A, Hoppe R, Stachniss V. Einfluss der digitalen Bildbearbeitung auf das Beurteilungsergebnis des visuellen

Kariesdetektionsverfahrens ICDAS durch Studenten. Dtsch Zahnarztl Z. 2014; 69:196–206.
25. Pitts NB, Ismail AI, Martignon S, Ekstrand K, Douglas GVA, Longbottom C. ICCMS™ Guide for Practitioners and Educators. 2014. www.icdas.org (Accessed April 2016).
26. Haak R, Wicht MJ, Hellmich M, Nowak G, Noack MJ. Influence of room lighting on grey-scale perception with a CRT and a TFT monitor display. Dentomaxillofac Radiol. 2002;31:193–7.

11

Utilization of dental care among patients with severe mental illness: a study of a National Health Insurance database

Po-Ren Teng[1†], Miao-Jean Lin[1†] and Ling-Ling Yeh[2*]

Abstract

Background: The oral health of patients with severe mental illness is poor, in general, and this may be attributed, in part, to inadequate dental care. This study investigated dental care utilization among patients with severe mental illness using a national representative sample.

Methods: This study used Taiwan's National Health Insurance Research Dataset for 2009. Patients with the diagnosis of severe mental illness (ICD-9-CM: 290–298) were recruited as the study sample, and others comprised the control. Any visit to a dentist was defined as positive in terms of dental care utilization. Regression analyses were applied to determine the odds of dental care utilization for each diagnostic entity of severe mental illness, compared with the general population and controlling for potential covariates.

Results: Only 40 % of 19,609 patients with severe mental illness visited the dentist within 12 months. This was significantly lower than the dental visit rate of 48.3 % for the control population (odds ratio [OR] = .72, 95 % confidence interval [CI] = .69–.74; *P* <0.0001). The odds of dental care utilization differed among the severe mental illness diagnostic categories; e.g., the odds were lowest among those with alcohol psychoses (OR = .54, CI = .43–.68), senile dementia (OR = .55, CI = .52–.59) and other organic psychoses (OR = .58, CI = .52–.65), and highest among those with mood disorder (OR = .89, CI = .85–.94), with schizophrenic patients occupying a mid-level position (OR = .63, CI = .59–.67).

Conclusions: Patients with severe mental illness received less dental care than the general population. Health care providers and caregivers of patients with severe mental illness should encourage them to visit the dentist regularly, in order to improve the oral health of these vulnerable patient groups.

Keywords: Mental illness, Dental care utilization, Oral health, Health-care surveys

Abbreviations: ICD, International classification of diseases; NHI, National Health Insurance; NHIRD, National Health Insurance Research Database; NHRI, National Health Research Institute; SES, Socioeconomic status; SPSS, Statistical package for the social sciences

Background

The significance of oral health is becoming more and more apparent. Published reports have indicated a relationship between poor oral health and many systemic diseases, including cardiovascular and respiratory diseases [1–7]. Poor oral health also has physical and psychological effects related to eating, nutrition, speech, quality of life, self-esteem and self-image. Even so, oral health is often overlooked by psychiatric personnel and neglected by the patients themselves. Poor oral health has been found among psychiatric patients in hospitals and in the community [8–16]. Studies have reported that certain factors, including amotivation, the decrease in salivary flow due to drug use, poor oral hygiene, specific dental phobias, the costs of dental visits, lack of accessible dental care facilities and infrequent dental visits, may account for this [14, 17].

Although the treatment need is huge, it has been suggested that the difficulty patients with major psychiatric

* Correspondence: yehll@asia.edu.tw
[†]Equal contributors
[2]Department of Healthcare Administration, Asia University, No. 500, Lioufong RdWufeng, Taichung 41354, Taiwan
Full list of author information is available at the end of the article

diseases have in receiving dental care is due to a lack of motivation, inadequate cooperation and poor communication [18]. Many patients lack awareness of the importance of dental care [15]. They neglect making appointments for routine dental checkups and are more likely to seek dental help only when they experience pain [15]. Besides, prolonged stay in institutions may limit psychiatric patients' ability to access dental care [19].

There have been only a few small surveys investigating dental care utilization among patients with severe mental illness [8, 12, 20, 21]. Moreover, the subjects in those studies were probably biased samples, in that they came from institutions or local outpatient clinics. Using the Danish National Patient Registry, Nielsen et al. found that only 43 % of patients with schizophrenia received dental services within 1 year [22]. To our knowledge, there are no studies that have examined simultaneously dental care utilization among patients with different diagnoses of severe mental illness, using national data.

The aims of this study were to investigate the use of dental care by patients with severe mental diseases within a 12-month period, and to compare this with dental care utilization in the general population. We hypothesized that, first, patients with severe mental diseases would receive dental services less frequently, and second, the rate of dental service utilization would differ among those disease diagnostic entities.

Methods

Sample

Taiwan's National Health Insurance (NHI) program is a single-payer compulsory health insurance plan for all Taiwan residents that guarantees equal access to healthcare for all citizens. In 2003, 21,869,478 residents were enrolled in the NHI, with a coverage rate of 96 %. The Bureau of NHI (BNHI) has contracted with 17,022 medical institutions, constituting 93.8 % of medical institutions nationwide. Nearly all dental services providers are contracted with the BNHI and provide basic dental services with inexpensive co-payments. Over 90 % of dentists are private practitioners. Although patients need to make appointments with the dentists, they could register on-site if there were relatively urgent needs. By the end of 2005, approximately 22.7 million residents were enrolled in Taiwan's NHI program, with a coverage rate of 98 %. Taiwan's NHI program includes the National Health Insurance Research Database (NHIRD), which has collected data on the healthcare utilization of insured residents, including expenditures, medical procedures/treatments, dental services, and basic characteristics of patients, providers and physicians. Using a systematic random sampling method, the National Health Research Institute (NHRI) extracted a representative database of 1,000,000 people from the registry of all NHI enrollees to be used for research purposes; there were no statistically significant differences between this sample and all enrollees. The NHIRD uses the International Classification of Diseases, 9th revision, clinical modification diagnoses (ICD-9-CM). The data for 2009 were used for the current analysis.

All subjects in the NHIRD that met the following criteria were defined as having severe mental illness:

1. Having an inpatient diagnosis of psychoses (ICD-9-CM: 290–298) and/or at least a one-year diagnosis of same in an outpatient service. The childhood psychoses (ICD-9-CM: 299) sample was too small and was excluded from analysis.
2. Having data available for a minimum of 12 months before and after the index date.
3. Aged 18 years or older on the index date.

Data on the use of dental care was obtained from the NHIRD. Visiting any dentist within the study period for whatever reason was defined as having received dental care. For the management of covariates, age was regrouped as follows: 18–35, 35–50, 50–65 and over 65 years, respectively. The income-related insurance payment amount of our study subjects was used as a proxy measure of individual socioeconomic status (SES). SES is recognized as an important factor for dental care utilization. The study subjects were categorized into three groups: (1) low SES, lower than US$528 per month, (2) moderate SES, between US$528 and $833 per month, and (3) high SES, US$833 per month or more [23]. Subjects who received a social welfare reimbursement from the government due to lack of regular income and who self-owned their household were classified as low income. We used a dentist-to-population ratio to represent dental care accessibility. The ratio was regrouped as low (fewer than 3.42 dentists per 10,000 residents), middle (3.43 to 6.5 dentists per 10,000 residents) and high (more than 6.51 dentists per 10,000 residents), based on a lower quartile, middle half and upper quartile division. The number of outpatient visits was used as a proxy for health care utilization, and was categorized as low (fewer than 6 outpatient visits per year), middle (7–23 visits) and high use (24 visits or more). However, since patients with severe mental illness visited doctors significantly more than the control population, when exploring predictors of dental care in this group, the covariates were re-categorized as low (fewer than 18 outpatient visits per year), middle (19–48 visits) and high use (49 visits or more). In addition, hospitalization with at least 30 bed days in a year was used as a proxy for poorer health status.

Statistical analyses

The data were processed using SPSS version 17. Logistic regression was used to determine the odds of dental visits among patients with severe mental illness and the general population. The multiple logistic regression model was further used to determine the odds of dental visits of patients in different diagnostic groups compared with the general population, controlling the following variables: gender, age group (age 18–35, 35–50, 50–65 and over 65 years), hospitalization with at least 30 bed days, socioeconomic status, dentist population density, low income status and outpatient visit frequency. The significance level was set at 0.05.

Results

Basic demographics

A total of 642,784 subjects were recruited for the study. Of this group, 19,609 (3.1 % of the whole group) were diagnosed as having severe mental illness. The patients with severe mental illness were significantly older than the control group (56.1 vs. 44 years; $P < 0.001$). Females were predominant among the subjects with severe mental illness (56.1 % vs. 52.8 %; $P < 0.001$) (Table 1).

In the severe mental illness group, 7625 patients (38.9 %) had mood disorders, followed by 4772 patients (24.3 %) with senile dementia, 4023 (20.5 %) with schizophrenic disorders, 1589 (8.1 %) with other organic psychoses, 542 (2.8 %) with other nonorganic psychoses, 335 (1.7 %) with alcoholic psychoses, 305 (1.6 %) with transient organic psychoses, 275 (1.4 %) with delusional disorders and 127 with drug psychoses (0.6 %).

Dental care utilization

Overall, only 40 % of patients with severe mental illness visited the dentist within 12 months. This is significantly lower than the dental visit rate of 48.3 % in the control population (OR, 0.72, 95 % CI, 0.69–0.74; $P < 0.001$). Of note, the dental visit rates differed significantly among the various diagnostic groups (Table 2). The dental visit rates were 27.2 % among patients with senile dementia, 32.8 % among patients with other organic psychoses, 33.4 % among patients with transient organic psychoses, 34.6 % among patients with alcoholic psychoses, 39.4 % among patients with schizophrenic disorders, 41.1 % among patients with other nonorganic psychoses, 42.5 % among patients with delusional disorders and 44.9 % among patients with drug psychoses, respectively. However, over half (50.1 %) of subjects with mood disorders visited dentists during the study period, which was a significantly higher rate than for patients with other diagnostic entities ($P < 0.001$). The rate of dental care utilization by patients with senile dementia was also lower than that of age-matched (over 60 years old) counterparts (27.2 % vs. 39.3 %).

Table 1 Characteristics of patients with severe mental illness and the controls

Characteristic	Mental illness		Control		*P* value[a]
	N	%	*N*	%	
Gender					
Male	8606	43.9	294,036	47.2	<0.001
Female	11,003	56.1	329,139	52.8	
Age group					
18–34	3256	16.6	220,215	35.3	<0.001
35–49	5131	26.2	190,390	30.6	
50–64	4168	21.3	133,643	21.4	
65+	7054	36	78,927	12.7	
Insurance premium					
Less than US$ 528	11,631	59.3	207,414	33.3	<0.001
US$ 528–833	5830	29.7	220,778	35.4	
US$ 834 or more	2148	11	194,983	31.3	
Dentist no. per 10,000 residents					
Less than 3.43	4968	25.3	153,061	24.6	<0.001
3.43–6.50	7494	38.2	293,535	47.1	
6.61 or more	7147	36.4	176,579	28.3	
Hospitalization bed days					
Less than 30 days	17,746	90.5	618,760	99.3	<0.001
30 days or more	1863	9.5	4415	0.7	
Low income					
Yes	1196	6.1	5368	0.9	<0.001
No	18,413	93.9	617,807	99.1	
Outpatient visit no.					
0–6	889	4.5	158,353	25.4	<0.001
7–23	6083	31.1	315,280	50.6	
24 or more	12,637	64.4	149,542	24	

[a]Chi-square test

Multiple logistic regression

In the multiple logistic regression model, after controlling for potential confounding covariates, patients with severe mental illness had only a 70 % probability of dental care utilization compared with the control group (OR, 0.70; 95 % CI, 0.68–0.72; $P < 0.001$).

All patients with severe mental illness, except delusional disorder and drug psychoses, had a lower likelihood of visiting dentists than did the control subjects (Table 2). Although patients with mood disorders consulted dentists no less frequently than the control group in the crude analysis, they still had a lower likelihood of dental care utilization after controlling confounding factors (OR, 0.89; 95 % CI, 0.85–0.94; $P < 0.001$).

We did a logistic regression analysis limited to patients with severe mental illness only, to determine the predictors for dental care utilization. Older persons, hospitalization for

Table 2 Rates and odds of dental care utilization among patients with severe mental illness

Group	Rate of dental care	No. with dental care /total No.	Adjusted odds ratio[a] (95 % CI[b])
General population	48.3 %	300,937/623,175	Reference
Senile dementia	27.2 %	1298/4772	0.55 (0.52–0.59)*
Alcohol psychoses	34.6 %	116/335	0.54 (0.43–0.68)*
Drug psychoses	44.9 %	57/127	0.75 (0.53–1.08)
Transient organic psychoses	33.4 %	102/305	0.60 (0.47–0.77)*
Other organic psychoses	32.8 %	521/1589	0.58 (0.52–0.65)*
Schizophrenia	39.4 %	1585/4023	0.63 (0.59–0.67)*
Mood disorders	50.1 %	3823/7625	0.89 (0.85–0.94)*
Delusional disorders	42.5 %	117/275	0.83 (0.65–1.06)
Other nonorganic psychoses	41.1 %	223/542	0.67 (0.56–0.80)*

[a]Multiple logistic regression controlling for gender, age, socioeconomic status, dentist/population ratio, hospitalization with 30 or more bed days, low income and outpatient visit numbers
[b]Confidence interval
*$P < 0.001$

more than one month, and subjects with low income were less likely to visit dentists. However, subjects residing in areas with more dentists received more dental care. Those who visited more outpatient clinics also had a higher likelihood of visiting dentists. Patients with a high SES visited dentists more frequently than those with a low SES (Table 3).

Discussion

To the best of our knowledge, this is the first report on the dental care utilization of patients with severe mental illness compared with the general population using Taiwan's NHI database. The main results of this study indicate that, compared with the general population, patients with severe mental illness were less likely to receive dental care within 12 months. In addition, the annual rates of dental visits differed among the groups of different diagnosed psychoses.

Our results are in agreement with the literature, in that some factors, including older age [24], low income [25, 26], poorer health status [27] and lower SES [26], were associated with lower use of dental care. Furthermore, people residing in areas with few dentists had less access to dental care. Extra effort should be put forth to enhance the oral health of patients with severe mental illness and with the abovementioned factors.

Although patients with severe mental illness received more medical care services than the general population, they were less likely to receive routine dental care. Dickerson et al. reported similar findings, but they attributed this to limited dental care insurance coverage [28]. However, in Taiwan, dental care for all residents is covered by the NHI, so cost may not be the principal barrier to receiving dental care of Taiwanese patients with severe mental illness. Other factors, including the subjects' lack of awareness of the importance of dental care, their low levels of perceived need, anxiety about visiting the dentist, difficulty in assessing the dental care needs of institutionalized patients [15], the reluctance of dentists to provide dental care, and possibly negative dental staff attitudes toward the subjects, may account for the under-utilization of the already-insured dental care services [29].

We found discrepancies in dental visiting rates among patients with different severe mental illness diagnoses. The possible causes of this are discussed below.

Teng et al. and Farnam et al. both indicated that schizophrenic patients may not have recognized the necessity of routine dental check-ups and visited the dentist only to seek help for a painful condition [15, 30]. In this regard, those patients probably suffered from prominent negative symptoms that contributed to their neglect of oral health and arranging dental visits. Moreover, even if they worried about their teeth, they may not visit a dentist due to anxiety about the treatment or a lack of trust in the dentist [31]. Also, the mental health staff in institutions may not be aware of patient dental care needs [13], and therefore offer limited access to annual dental check-ups [22]. And last, some dentists were hesitant about treating people with severe psychotic symptoms [32].

Our findings support the work of Mago and Thyvalikakath, which indicated that those who had mood disorders visited dentists less frequently [33]. Reports from individuals with mood disorders indicated that they had unmet dental care needs [34]. There are several explanations that may account for this phenomenon. First, patients with mood disorder were more likely to be irritable or uncooperative during dental visits and to have complaints related to dental care that were inconsistent with objective findings [35, 36]. Second, the patients more commonly reported a high level of dental fear that would

Table 3 Predictors of dental care utilization among patients with severe mental illness

Variable	Unadjusted odds ratio		Adjusted odds ratio	P value
	Estimate (95 % CI)	P value	Estimate (95 % CI)	
Gender				
Female	1		1	
Male	0.89 (0.84–0.94)	<0.001	0.96 (0.91–1.02)	0.207
Age group				
18–34	1		1	
35–49	0.81 (0.74–0.89)	<0.001	0.75 (0.68–0.82)	<0.001
50–64	0.86 (0.78–0.94)	0.001	0.67 (0.61–0.74)	<0.001
65+	0.49 (0.45–0.54)	<0.001	0.36 (0.33–0.40)	<0.001
Socioeconomic status				
Low	1		1	
Middle	0.97 (0.91–1.04)	0.378	0.93 (0.87–1.00)	0.053
High	1.69 (1.54–1.85)	<0.001	1.34 (1.21–1.48)	<0.001
Dentist/population ratio[a]				
Low	1		1	
Middle	1.29 (1.20–1.39)	<0.001	1.27 (1.18–1.38)	<0.001
High	1.62 (1.50–1.75)	<0.001	1.60 (1.48–1.73)	<0.001
Hospitalization bed days				
Less than 30 days	1		1	
30 days or more	0.75 (0.68–0.83)	<0.001	0.82 (0.73–0.91)	<0.001
Low income				
No	1		1	
Yes	0.85 (0.75–0.95)	0.006	0.73 (0.64–0.83)	<0.001
Health care utilization[b]				
Low	1		1	
Middle	2.08 (1.93–2.24)	<0.001	2.41 (2.23–2.61)	<0.001
High	2.82 (2.59–3.07)	<0.001	3.83 (3.50–4.19)	<0.001

[a]Low: less than 3.43, middle: 3.43–6.5, high: 6.51 or more (per 10,000 residents)
[b]umbers of outpatient visits in the year 2009; low: less than 18, middle: 19–48, high: 49 or more

deter them from receiving dental care earlier [37, 38]. Third, the lack of formal or informal support for patients with mood disorder would render them less likely to visit dentists when oral care is needed [33].

Although the risk of poor oral health is increased among patients with dementia, compared to their counterparts [39, 40], the likelihood of their visiting a dentist regularly is lower [41]. Dementia patients might not be able to verbalize their dental needs as a result of cognitive deficits [42]. Moreover, caregivers of persons with dementia may be hesitant to take dementia patients to visit the dentist [43]. Given that patients with dementia may be unable to express their dental discomfort, formal and informal caregivers should be educated on the benefits of regular dental check-ups in facilitating the dental health of dementia patients [41, 44].

The literature has shown that the risk of oral diseases is increased in individuals with alcohol dependence and substance use disorder [45–47]. We recruited patients with alcohol and drug psychoses whose oral health was presumably worse than that of those with substance use disorder alone. Despite the higher rates of dental problems among people with alcohol/drug use disorder, they receive less dental care [48]. Potential contributing factors to this dental care under-utilization include: the lifestyle of people with alcohol/drug use disorder is chaotic, which makes scheduling and adhering to regularly scheduled dental check-ups difficult [49]; those who use some illicit drugs (such as opiates) may feel no pain related to the dental problem, and so delay visiting the dentist; dental treatment is given a low priority due to the lack of expendable income [48]; dentists may be hesitant about providing services to those with substance use disorder [50].

Patients with severe mental illness generally had lower odds of utilizing dental services, and patients with dementia and organic mental disorder had the lowest dentist visiting rate. However, patients with mood disorder received dental care nearly as often as the control population. We postulated that the underlying cognitive function of patients may play a critical role in dentist-seeking behavior. Schizophrenia, as an example, is well-known for causing deterioration of patients' cognitive functions, and one study reported that schizophrenic patients with worse executive cognitive functioning received less regular dental care [51]. Mood disorders, however, do not impair an individual's cognitive functions, except in acute illness phases, and therefore the dental visit rate is close to that of the general population.

The strengths of this study include the representative national health data sample and that dental services are covered by the NHI, so cost is not the primary barrier to dental care access of patients with severe mental illness. However, there are limitations to this study that warrant consideration. First, the validity of the diagnosis of severe mental illness was uncertain, as this was derived from administrative data rather than standardized research interviews. Nevertheless, we further analyzed the data of a sub-sample of individuals who were diagnosed as having severe mental illness by psychiatric specialists, and yielded similar results. Second, information on the psychopathology and illness severity of patients was not available, so the relationship among the period of acute illness, cognitive functions, personal functionality and dental care utilization warrants further investigation. Third, some uncontrollable covariates such as educational level could confound the results, even though the proxy SES was put into consideration. Fourth, the study investigated a dataset for 1 year only; a sampling period of several years might yield more insight into the discrepancy in dental care utilization between patients with severe mental illnesses and the general population. Finally, the present analyses did not explore types of dental care, which could be preventive, restorative or emergency-based.

Conclusions

In summary, patients with severe mental illness visit dentists much less frequently than the general population in Taiwan. Given the discrepancy in the rates of visiting dentists noticed among the different diagnoses of psychosis, the underlying reasons for under-utilization of dental services among patients in each severe mental illness category warrant further exploration. Changing patient care-seeking behavior in the short term would be difficult; therefore, healthcare authorities should organize dental care systems to facilitate meeting the dental needs of patients with psychiatric illnesses. Health care providers, including psychiatrists, dentists, nursing staffs in institutions, and caregivers should encourage patients with severe mental illness to regularly visit the dentist, so as to improve the oral health of these vulnerable patient groups.

Acknowledgments

We thank Miss Chen Yu-Pai for her excellent assistance in data management.

Funding

This study received grant from Department of Medical Research of Chang Bing Show Chwan Memorial Hospital (RD-102029). The funders had no role in study design, data collection, analysis, decision to publish, or preparation of the manuscript.

Authors' contributions

Conceived and designed the experiments: P-RT, M-JL, L-LY. Performed the experiments and analyzed the data: P-RT, M-JL, L-LY. Wrote the paper: P-RT, M-JL. All authors read and approved the final manuscript.

Competing interests

The authors declare that they have no competing interests.

Consent for publication

Not applicable.

Ethics approval and consent to participate

This study was approved by the institutional review board of Show Chwan Memorial Hospital, Taiwan (No. 1011103). Since the NHIRD files contain only de-identified secondary data, the review board waived the requirement for obtaining informed consent from the subjects.

Author details

[1]Department of Psychiatry, Chang Bing Show Chwan Memorial Hospital, No. 6, Lu-Gong Road, Lu-Gang Township, Changhwa County, Taiwan.
[2]Department of Healthcare Administration, Asia University, No. 500, Lioufong RdWufeng, Taichung 41354, Taiwan.

References

1. Williams RC, Barnett AH, Claffey N, Davis M, Gadsby R, Kellett M, Lip GY, Thackray S. The potential impact of periodontal disease on general health: a consensus view. Curr Med Res Opin. 2008;24:1635–43.
2. Chapple IL. The impact of oral disease upon systemic health-symposium overview. J Dent. 2009;37:S568–571.
3. Cullinan MP, Ford PJ, Seymour GJ. Periodontal disease and systemic health: current status. Aust Dent J. 2009;54 suppl 1:S62–69.
4. Humphrey LL, Fu R, Buckley DI, Freeman M, Helfand M. Periodontal disease and coronary heart disease incidence: a systemic review and meta-analysis. J Gen Intern Med. 2008;23:2079–86.
5. Bahekar AA, Singh S, Saha S, Molnar J, Arora R. The prevalence and incidence of coronary heart disease is significantly increased in periodontitis: a meta-analysis. Am Heart J. 2007;154:830–7.
6. Shultis WA, Weil EJ, Looker HC, Curtis JM, Shlossman M, Genco RJ, Knowler WC, Nelson RG. Effect of periodontitis on overt nephropathy and end-stage renal disease in type 2 diabetes. Diabetes Care. 2007;30:306–11.
7. Azarpazhooh A, Leake JL. Systemic review of the association between respiratory diseases and oral health. J Periodontol. 2006;77:1465–82.
8. Hede B. Oral health in Danish hospitalized psychiatric patients. Community Dent Oral Epidemiol. 1995;23:44–8.
9. Angelillo IF, Nobile CG, Pavia M, De Fazio P, Puca M, Amati A. Dental health and treatment needs in institutionalized psychiatric patients in Italy. Community Dent Oral Epidemiol. 1995;23:360–4.
10. Persson K, Axtelius B, Söderfeldt B, Östman M. Monitoring oral health and dental attendance in an outpatient psychiatric population. J Psychiatr Ment Health Nurs. 2009;16:263–71.
11. McCreadie RG, Stevens H, Henderson J, Hall D, McCaul R, Filik R, Young G, Sutch G, Kanagaratnam G, Perrington S, McKendrick J, Stephenson D, Burns

T. The dental health of people with schizophrenia. Acta Psychiatr Scand. 2004;110:306–10.
12. Stiefel DJ, Truelove EL, Menard TW, Anderson VK, Doyle PE, Mandel LS. A comparison of the oral health of persons with and without chronic mental illness in community settings. Spec Care Dentist. 1990;10:6–12.
13. Bertaud-Gounot V, Kovess-Masfety V, Perrus C, Trohel G, Richard F. Oral health status and treatment needs among psychiatric inpatients in Rennes, France: a cross-sectional study. BMC Psychiatry. 2013;13:227.
14. Kisely S, Quek LH, Pais J, Lalloo R, Johnson NW, Lawrence D. Advanced dental disease in people with severe mental illness: systematic review and meta-analysis. Br J Psychiatry. 2011;199:187–93.
15. Teng PR, Su JM, Chang WH, Lai TJ. Oral health of psychiatric inpatients: a survey of central Taiwan hospitals. Gen Hosp Psychiatry. 2011;33:253–9.
16. Gurbuz O, Alatas G, Kurt E, Issever H, Dogan F. Oral health and treatment needs of institutionalized chronic psychiatric patients in Istanbul, Turkey. Community Dent Health. 2010;27:151–7.
17. Jackson E. Psychiatry and dentistry. In: Kaplan HI, Freeman AM, Saddock BJ, editors. Comprehensive textbook of psychiatry, II. Baltimore: Williams and Wilkins; 1980. p. 2069–77.
18. Ramon T, Grinshpoon A, Zusman SP, Weizman A. Oral health and treatment needs of institutionalized chronic psychiatric patients in Israel. Eur Psychiatry. 2003;18:101–5.
19. Chu KY, Yang NP, Chou P, Chiu HJ, Chi LY. Factors associated with dental caries among institutionalized residents with schizophrenia in Taiwan: a cross-sectional study. BMC Public Health. 2010;10:482.
20. Roca RP, Breakey WR, Fischer PJ. Medical care of chronic psychiatric outpatients. Hosp Community Psychiatry. 1987;38:741–5.
21. Velasco E, Machuca G, Martinez-Sahuquillo A, Rios V, Lacalle J, Bullón P. Dental health among institutionalized psychiatric patients in Spain. Spec Care Dentist. 1997;17:203–6.
22. Nielsen J, Munk-Jørgensen P, Skadhede S, Correll CU. Determinants of poor dental care in patients with schizophrenia: a historical, prospective database study. J Clin Psychiatry. 2011;72:140–3.
23. Chang CM, Yin WY, Wei CK, Lin CH, Huang KY, Lin SP, Lee CH, Chou P, Lee CC. The association of socioeconomic status and access to low-volume service providers in breast cancer. PLoS One. 2013;8(12):e81801.
24. Woolfolk MW, Lang WP, Borgnakke WS, Taylor GW, Ronis DL, Nyquist LV. Determining dental checkup frequency. J Am Dent Assoc. 1999;130:715–23.
25. Qiu Y, Ni H. Utilization of dental care services by Asian and native Hawaiian or other Pacific Islanders: United States, 1997-2000. Adv Data. 2003;336:1–11.
26. Manski RJ, Macek MD, Moeller JF. Private dental coverage: who has it and how does it influence dental visits and expenditures? J Am Dent Assoc. 2002;133:1551–9.
27. Mueller CD, Schur CL, Paramore LC. Access to dental care in the United States. J Am Dent Assoc. 1998;129:429–37.
28. Dickerson FB, McNary SW, Brown CH, Kreyenbuhl J, Goldberg RW, Dixon LB. Somatic healthcare utilization among adults with serious mental illness who are receiving community psychiatric services. Med Care. 2003;41:560–70.
29. Patel R, Gamboa A. Prevalence of oral diseases and oral-health-related quality of life in people with severe mental illness undertaking community-based psychiatric care. Br Dent J. 2012;213:E16.
30. Farnam CR, Zipple AM, Tyrrell W, Chittinanda P. Health status risk factors of people with severe and persistent mental illness. J Psychosoc Nurs Ment Health Serv. 1999;37:16–21.
31. Mirza I, Day R, Phelan M, Wulff-Cochrane V. Oral health of psychiatric in-patients. Psychiatric Bull. 2001;25:143–5.
32. Friedlander AH, Marder SR. The psychopathology, medical management and dental implications of schizophrenia. J Am Dent Assoc. 2002;133:603–10.
33. Mago A, Thyvalikakath TP. A population-based study of the impact of mood disorders on oral health-care utilization among middle aged and older adults in Canada. Community Dent Oral Epidemiol. 2014;42:451–9.
34. Heaton LJ, Mancl LA, Grembowski D, Armfield JM, Milgrom P. Unmet dental need in community-dwelling adults with mental illness: Results from the 2007 Medical Expenditure Panel Survey. J Am Dent Assoc. 2013;144:e16–23.
35. Friedlander AH, Mahler ME. Major depressive disorder: psychopathology, medical management and dental implications. J Am Dent Assoc. 2001;132:629–38.
36. Friedlander AH, Friedlander IK, Marder SR. Bipolar I disorder: psychopathology, medical management and dental implications. J Am Dent Assoc. 2002;133:1209–17.
37. Locker D, Poulton R, Thomson WM. Psychological disorders and dental anxiety in a young adult population. Community Dent Oral Epidemiol. 2001;29:456–63.
38. Pohjola V, Mattila AK, Joukamaa M, Lahti S. Anxiety and depressive disorders and dental fear among adults in Finland. Eur J Oral Sci. 2011;119:55–60.
39. Syrjälä A-M H, Ylöstalo P, Sulkava R, Knuuttila M. Relationship between cognitive impairment and oral health: results of the Health 2000 Health Examination Survey in Finland. Acta Odontol Scand. 2007;65:103–8.
40. Syrjälä A-M H, Ylöstalo P, Ruoppi P, Komulainen K, Hartikainen S, Sulkava R, Knuuttila M. Dementia and oral health among subjects aged 75 years or older. Gerodontology. 2012;29:36–42.
41. Lee KH, Wu B, Plassman BL. Dental care utilization among older adults with cognitive impairment in the USA. Geriatr Gerontol Int. 2015;15:255–60.
42. Abbott A. Dementia: a problem for our age. Nature. 2011;475(7355):S2–4.
43. Hilton C, Simons B. Dental surgery attendance amongst patients with moderately advanced dementia attending a day unit: a survey of caregivers' views. Br Dent J. 2003;195:39–40.
44. Chalmers JM, Pearson A. A systematic review of oral health assessment by nurses and carers for residents with dementia in residential care facilities. Spec Care Dentist. 2005;25:227–33.
45. Hede B. Determinants of oral health in a group of Danish alcoholics. Eur J Oral Sci. 1996;104:403–8.
46. Molendijk B, Horst GT, Kasbergen M, Truin GJ, Mulder J. Dental health in Dutch drug addicts. Community Dent Oral Epidemiol. 1996;24:117–9.
47. Khocht A, Janal M, Schleifer S, Keller S. The influence of gingival margin recession on loss of clinical attachment in alcohol-dependent patients without medical disorders. J Periodontol. 2003;74:485–93.
48. Sheridan J, Aggleton M, Carson T. Dental health and access to dental treatment: a comparison of drug users and non-drug users attending community pharmacies. Br Dent J. 2001;191:453–7.
49. Scheutz F. Five-year evaluation of a dental care delivery system for drug addicts in Denmark. Community Dent Oral Epidemiol. 1984;12:29–34.
50. Dawkes M, Sparkes S, Smith M. Dentists' responses to drug misusers. Health Trends. 1995;27:12–4.
51. Janardhanan T, Cohen CI, Kim S, Rizvi BF. Dental care and associated factors among older adults with schizophrenia. J Am Dent Assoc. 2011;142:57–65.

12

Relationship between risk assessment and payment models in Swedish Public Dental Service

Gunnel Hänsel Petersson[1*] and Svante Twetman[2]

Abstract

Background: To a) compare risk categories in patients selecting a capitation payment (CP) model with those in fee-for-service (FFS), b) determine the 3-year caries increment in the two groups, and c) compare the amount of delivered preventive care in the two groups.

Methods: A comprehensive risk assessment was carried out in 1295 young adults attending eight Public Dental Clinics in the Scania region and 75% could be re-examined after 3 years; 615 had selected the CP model and 310 the traditional FFS. Caries was scored according to WHO and data concerning preventive care was extracted from the dental records.

Results: More patients in the low risk category preferred the CP model (74% vs. 26%) while >80% with high risk selected FFS. The baseline caries level was significantly higher in the FFS group as well as the 3-year caries increment (1.6 vs. 0.8 DFS: $p < 0.05$). The amount of additional preventive care delivered to each patient was generally lower in the FFS model; it was most frequent among patients with "some" risk in the CP model (83.8%) while the lowest delivery rates were found among low risk patients in the FFS system (32.4%).

Conclusions: Young adults in public dental care with low risk preferred the prepaid model while those in the higher risk categories selected fee-for-service. As more additional preventive care was delivered to patients in the subscribed care, oral health planners and decision makers should be aware of the fact that capitation payment models may enhance inequalities in dental health over time.

Keywords: Caries prevention, Dental care models, Risk assessment, Young adults, Sweden

Background

Dental care in Sweden is provided by the Public Dental Service or by private practitioners free of charge for the patients younger than 20 years of age. The costs are covered by a National Dental Insurance through a capitation system constructed to promote health and encourage preventive care. At the age of 20 years, all patients that wish to remain in the Public Dental Service have the opportunity to choose one of two payment systems, a) a monthly fixed payment (capitation payment, CP) or, b) a traditional fee-for-service system (FFS) with payments for each treatment that is carried out. In the former payment model, the patient signs a 3-year contract with the clinic at a fixed fee covering all necessary basic dental care over the time period. A subscription agreement for dental care includes check-ups, preventive procedures, treatment of the disease and restorative care (fillings and single crowns). For example orthodontics, aesthetic dental care and implants are excluded from the basic care. The CP fee is based on a comprehensive risk assessment and the higher the risk, the higher the fee. The methodology for the risk assessment, as well as the size of the fee, varies however somewhat across different regions in Sweden and also over time. So does the share of patients over 19 years of age preferring the CP model, varying from a few percent in more rural areas to up to more than 50% subscribers in other regions.

* Correspondence: gunnel.hansel-petersson@mah.se
[1]Department of Cariology, Faculty of Odontology, Malmö University, SE-205 06 Malmö, Sweden
Full list of author information is available at the end of the article

Although the CP model was introduced more than 10 years ago, few studies have been published on its effect on oral health and whether or not this is beneficial for the patients and/or the organisation [1, 2]. There are some international low-quality evidence to suggest that the payment method does influence the behaviour of dentists in child dental care with a tendency to higher activity and more preventive advice in the capitation system [2]. Among adults, it has been shown that patients selecting the CP model had healthier habits and were more motivated to follow self-care advice than those adhering to FFS system [3]. As a consequence, fewer fillings were carried out among the patients in the pre-payment scheme [4]. Furthermore, the CP patients received more emergency and preventive treatments and were more frequently examined by dental hygienists than the FFS patients [5].

We have previously validated a risk assessment model in a population of young adults living in the Scania region in southern Sweden over a period of 3 years [6]. After the assessment, the patients had to choose the CP model for the next 3 years. Those who not selected the CP model were offered continues care based on FFS. This gave us an opportunity for a pragmatic comparison of the two payment models with respect to caries risk and caries development. The aims of the study were a) to compare risk categories in patients selecting the CP or FFS model, b) to determine the 3-year caries increment in the two groups, and c) to compare the amount of delivered preventive care in the two groups.

Methods

The selection and enrolment of the study cohort has been described before [6]. In brief, 1699 19-year-olds were invited from eight different Public Dental Clinics (PDC's) across the region to form a representative sample of this age group. At baseline, 1295 patients were examined and risk assessed according to the regional guidelines. After 3 years, 925 patients who remained at the PDC could be re-examined; 615 with a CP payment scheme and 310 with FFS payments. A flowchart with the sex distribution and reasons for exclusion and drop out is provided in Fig. 1. All the participants were residents in areas with low natural fluoride content in the drinking water supply but were strongly encouraged to use of fluoridated dentifrice on daily basis. The study design was approved by the Ethical Committee, Lund University, Sweden.

Study design and risk assessment

The study had a 3-year prospective observational design. At baseline, the risk category of each patient was assessed by the patient's regular dental team (dentist and/or dental hygienist) according to the "adult guidelines for risk assessment of oral diseases" issued by the regional Public Dental Service. Based on clinical and radiographic findings, the risk grouping relied on past and present caries, periodontal conditions, general risk and technical risk as previously described [6]. Four risk categories were used and each patient was classified into one of the following risk groups; "low risk" (42.7%), "some risk" (45.4%), "high risk" (10.4%) and "very high risk" (1.5%). The patient was informed on the outcome of risk assessment and asked to choose payment model. All decisions on preventive and restorative dental care were solely the responsibility of the patient's regular dental team during the entire study period. All patients, irrespective of payment model,

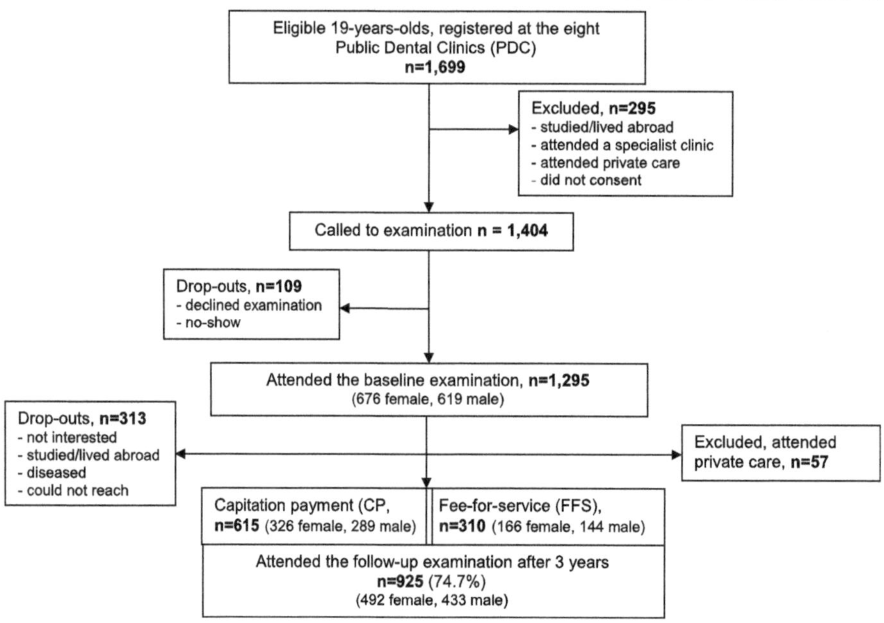

Fig. 1 Flow-chart indicating attrition and reason for drop-outs

were regularly attending the Public Dental Service for check-ups.

Clinical examination

Prior to baseline, each of the eight selected public dental clinics was visited by the principal investigator (GHP). The staff was trained and calibrated on caries detection and different stages of lesions were discussed. The clinical visual-tactile examination, including bitewing radiographs, was carried out by the regular dentist, or a dental hygienist, under optimal light and cleaned, air-dried teeth. Caries prevalence and experience was registered at manifest dentin level according to the WHO-criteria [7] and expressed as DFT/DFS. Information concerning general health and medication, diet and oral hygiene habits including tooth brushing frequency and the use of fluoride and tobacco was collected through a structured questionnaire and these data were incorporated in the risk assessment model. The caries increment was calculated by counting the number of teeth/surfaces that changed from sound to decayed or filled over the study period. Possible caries reversals were not considered.

Preventive measures

Data on the delivered preventive care to each patient over the 3-year study period was extracted from the digital dental records by one of the authors as previously described [8]. In brief, the frequency of activities within three domains was scored 0–3: "oral health information" (i.e. current disease situation, diet information and counselling), "extra fluoride therapy" (i.e. fluoride varnish application, additional fluoride supplements), and "professional tooth cleaning and oral hygiene instructions". The scores of the three domains were then added to reflect the total preventive care delivered to each patient with a maximal cumulative score of nine. A cumulative score between 0 and 3 was regarded as "basic prevention" while 4–9 was considered as "additional prevention".

Statistical methods

All data were processed with the IBM-SPSS software (version 23.0, Chicago, IL, USA). Descriptive statistics were employed and differences between the groups and were compared with chi-square test for proportions and non-parametric two-tailed tests for continuous data. P-values less than 0.05 were considered statistically significant.

Results

At follow-up there were an equal proportion of females in the CP and FFS groups, 53.0 and 53.5% respectively. The distribution of the risk categories at baseline is shown in Fig. 2. Significantly more patients in the "low" or "some" risk categories selected the prepaid model while all those assessed with "very high" risk preferred the FFS system ($p < 0.05$). The mean caries frequency at baseline and the 3-year caries increment is shown in Table 1. The patients in the FFS group had significantly more caries at baseline compared with the CP group ($p < 0.05$) and the mean 3-year increment was also significantly higher, 1.6 vs. 0.8 DFS. The additional delivered preventive care in the two groups in relation to the baseline risk category is shown in Fig. 3. The proportion of patients that received "additional preventive care" was significantly higher in the CP group ($p < 0.05$). Additional prevention was most frequent in patients with "some" risk in the CP model (83.8%). The lowest frequency was seen in the low risk FFS group (32.4%).

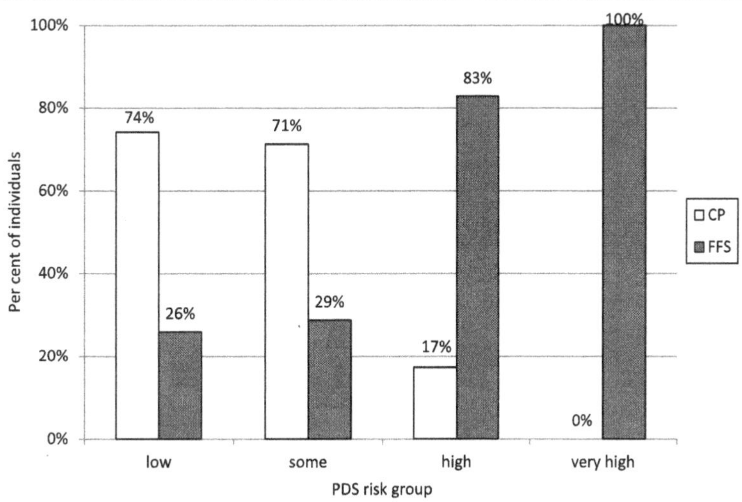

Fig. 2 Distribution of individuals (%) in the different Public Dental Service risk categories at baseline in the capitation payment group (CP) and fee-for-service group (FFS)

Table 1 Mean (SD) caries prevalence at baseline and mean (SD) caries prevalence and increment after 3 years in the CP ($n = 615$) and FFS ($n = 310$) groups

Group	DFT	DFS	DFSa
CP - baseline	2.74 (2.70)	3.64 (4.16)	0.70 (1.59)
CP - after 3 years	3.23 (3.05)	4.44 (4.85)	0.98 (2.00)
CP - increment	0.48 (0.90)	0.77 (1.53)	0.29 (0.74)
FFS – baseline	3.75 (3.55)	5.39 (6.05)	1.41 (2.65)
FFS - after 3 years	4.55 (4.05)	6.96 (7.54)	2.19 (3.57)
FFS - increment	0.80 (1.33)	1.57 (2.69)	0.78 (1.54)

CP capitation payment, *FFS* fee-for-service, *DFT* Decayed Filled Teeth, *DFS* Decayed Filled Surfaces, *DFSa* Decayed Filled approximal Surfaces

Discussion

In this material of young adults, 66.5% utilized the capitation model at the 3-year follow-up and this proportion was substantially higher than the national average. However, according Andrén Andås and Hakeberg [3] and a national social insurance report [9], young adults (20–29 years) were clearly overrepresented among subscription dental care patients and they were more often females. Interestingly, this gender difference was not unveiled in our present material. One should however keep in mind that there was a possible risk for selection bias since 28.5% of the patients examined at baseline was lost to follow-up. It seemed to be no apparent reason for dropping out although lack of interest and migration were most commonly registered. Interestingly, only 4.4% of the originally enrolled subjects had moved to private practitioners after 3 years. Although data on caries frequency was available, the private patients were excluded due to lack of information concerning the delivered preventive care. Furthermore, patient's attending private care did not have the opportunity to select the capitation model since this is not available in private dental care.

The main finding of this study was that young adults assessed with low risk for caries development, periodontal disease or technical problems, were more likely to adopt the capitation model. Over 70% in the "low" and "some" risk groups preferred to pay a fixed rate and it seemed clear that the subscription dental care largely attracted those with good oral health and presumably, small dental care needs. Only 17% of those assessed with high risk, and thereby likely to have more extensive treatment needs and unforeseen costs, signed the agreement. No one in the very high risk group selected the CP model, which was notable. An explanation for this could be that the annual fee was seven times higher in the very high risk group compared to the lowest risk category, indicating that the economical factor had a pivoting influence the patients' choice of payment model. Our findings were therefore basically in support of the observations made by Andren Andås and Hakeberg [3] who suggested that patients choosing prepaid care were young, educated people that judged their oral health to be good or very good.

As could be expected from the distribution of the risk categories, the patients in the FFS group had more caries at baseline and displayed a significantly higher DFS increment over the 3-year study period. Similar observations have been made in children [10] and in adults [5]. The latter research team showed also that subscription patients received significantly more prevention and fewer fillings than FFS patients. We were however unable to fully disseminate the reasons for this difference in caries burden in our material. First of all, the patients in the CP group received more additional prevention than those selecting the FFS model. A paradox was that more prevention actually was delivered to the "low risk" and "some risk" groups than the high risk group over a 3-year period [8]. This is however not a unique observation from dentistry but well-known from general health care as the "inverse care

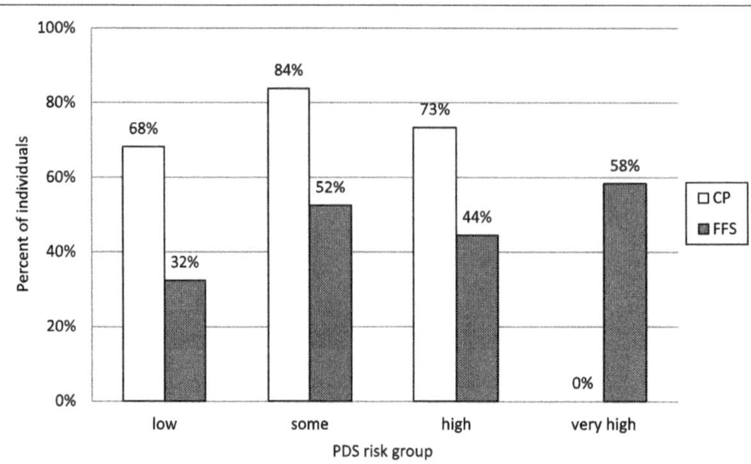

Fig. 3 Percentage received "additional preventive care" in the capitation payment group (CP) and the fee-for-service group (FFS), in relation to the baseline risk categories

law" [11]. The primary method of choice was professional fluorides which are in systematic reviews proven to be effective for both primary and secondary prevention [12, 13]. A second reason could be that dentists in the CP model restored lesions at later stages [14]. Subscription patients are more likely to return on a regular basis [9] and this fact can promote a tendency towards watchful waiting and more preventive care. In a wider perspective, this is an obvious ethical dilemma. The overarching goal of subscription dental care is to encourage regular preventive-oriented measures and to retain customer loyalty. The economical outcome seems also positive; a recent study has shown that the revenue from the prepaid fees is exceeding the costs for the provided care over time [5]. There is however an obvious risk that the inequality gaps in caries burden across the population will become wider with time. The occurrence of caries has a strong socioeconomic gradient in all age groups [15, 16] and the disadvantaged socioeconomic groups are generally found in the FFS system [17]. Moreover, displacement effects cannot be excluded if low risk subscription patients are crowding out patients with more extensive needs. Theses aspects must be considered and addressed by regional chief dental officers and oral health planners.

In this study, we did not have the possibility to investigate the patient's perspective on the different payment systems. Previous reports indicate however that patients generally were in favour of the capitation payment system [18] and that the individual's relation to the public dental clinics together with his/her health-related attitudes and perceptions were the main factors impacting the choice of payment system [19]. In addition, Johansson and co-workers have shown that patients in prepaid care had better general health [17] and a better oral health related quality in life than those in FFS [20]. Thus, it is a future challenge to communicate the benefits of subscribed prepaid care also to patients with high risk and increased treatment needs. With an enhanced preventive approach, individual patients may lower their risk category and spread the costs for dental care out over time.

Conclusions

Within the limitations of the present study, our findings displayed that young adults in public dental care assessed with low risk preferred a prepaid capitation model while those with higher risk categories selected the traditional fee-for-service. The mean caries increment among the fee-for-service patients were significantly higher compared with the prepaid group over a 3-year period and more additional preventive care was delivered to patients in the subscribed group. Thus, oral health planners and decision makers should be aware of, and deal with, the fact that capitation care may increase inequalities in dental health over time.

Abbreviations

CP: Capitation payment; DFS: Decayed filled surfaces; DFSa: Decayed filled approximal surfaces; DFT: Decayed filled teeth; FFS: Fee-for-service; PDC: Public dental clinic; WHO: World Health Organisation

Acknowledgements

The authors would like thank the staff at all participating Public Dental Clinics for their collaboration.

Funding

The study was supported by grants from the Skåne Region and from the Swedish Patent Revenue Research Fund for Preventive Odontology.

Authors' contributions

GHP participated in data retrieval. Both authors have substantially contributed to all part of the study, read and approved the manuscript.

Competing interests

The authors declare that they have no competing interests. The authors alone are responsible for the content and writing of the paper.

Consent for publication

Not applicable.

Ethics approval and consent to participate

The study design was approved by the Ethical Board at the University of Lund, Sweden. Patients were informed about the survey and signed a written consent.

Author details

[1]Department of Cariology, Faculty of Odontology, Malmö University, SE-205 06 Malmö, Sweden. [2]Department of Odontology, Faculty of Health and Medical Sciences, University of Copenhagen, Copenhagen, Denmark.

References

1. Zickert I, Jonson A, Klock B, Krasse B. Disease activity and need for dental care in a capitation plan based on risk assessment. Br Dent J. 2000;189:480–6.
2. Brocklehurst P, Price J, Glenny AM, Tickle M, Birch S, Mertz E, Grytten J. The effect of different methods of remuneration on the behaviour of primary care dentists. Cochrane Database Syst Rev. 2013;6:CD009853.
3. Andås CA, Hakeberg M. Who chooses prepaid dental care? A baseline report of a prospective observational study. BMC Oral Health. 2014;14:146.
4. Andrén Andås C. PhD thesis. A new payment model in Swedish dental care. Institute of odontology at Sahlgrenska Academy University of Gothenburg. p. 55–57. https://gupea.ub.gu.se/handle/2077/39557.
5. Andås CA, Ostberg AL, Berggren P, Hakeberg M. A new dental insurance scheme-effects on the treatment provided and costs. Swed Dent J. 2014;38:57–66.
6. Hänsel Petersson G, Ericson E, Isberg PE, Twetman S. Caries risk assessment in young adults: a 3-year validation of clinical guidelines used in public dental service. Acta Odontol Scand. 2013;71:1645–50.
7. World Health Organisation, WHO. Oral health surveys: basic methods. 3rd ed. Geneva: WHO; 1987.
8. Hänsel Petersson G, Ericson E, Twetman S. Preventive care delivered within Public Dental Service after caries risk assessment of young adults. Int J Dent Hyg. 2015. doi: 10.1111/idh.12135
9. Social Insurance Report. Abonnemangstandvård. En beskrivning av abonnemangstandvården och de patienter som tecknar avtal. Sweden: Försäkringskassan; 2012:2. ISSN 1654-8574. https://www.forsakringskassan.se/statistik/statistik_och_analys2/publikationer/socialrapporter.
10. Coventry P, Holloway PJ, Lennon M, Mellor AC, Worthington HV. A trial of a capitation system of payment for the treatment of children in the General Dental Service. Final report. Dental Health Services Research Unit, University of Manchester. Community Dent Health. 1989;6:1–63.

11. Hart JT. The inverse care law. Lancet. 1971;1:405–12.
12. Marinho VC, Worthington HV, Walsh T, Clarkson JE. Fluoride varnishes for preventing dental caries in children and adolescents. Cochrane Database Syst Rev. 2013;7:CD002279.
13. Lenzi L, Montagner AF, Soares FZ, de Oliveira Rocha R. Are topical fluorides effective for treating incipient carious lesions?: A systematic review and meta-analysis. J Am Dent Assoc. 2016;147:84–91.
14. Malone A, Conway DI. Payment methods may influence behaviour of primary care dentists. Evid Based Dent. 2015;16:4–5.
15. Bernabé E, Sheiham A. Tooth loss in the United Kingdom–trends in social inequalities: an age-period-and-cohort analysis. PLoS One. 2014;9:104808.
16. Schwendicke F, Dörfer CE, Schlattmann P, Foster Page L, Thomson WM, Paris S. Socioeconomic inequality and caries: a systematic review and meta-analysis. J Dent Res. 2015;91:10–8.
17. Johansson V, Axtelius B, Söderfeldt B, Sampogna F, Paulander J, Sondell K. Patients' health in contract and fee-for-service care. I. A descriptive comparison. Swed Dent J. 2007;31:27–34.
18. Strand J, Andås AC, Boman UW, Hakeberg M, Tidefors I. A new capitation payment system in dentistry: the patients' perspective. Community Dent Health. 2015;32:83–8.
19. Ostberg AL, Ahlström B, Hakeberg M. Patients' choice of payment system in the Swedish Public Dental Service-views on dental care and oral health. Swed Dent J. 2013;37:131–42.
20. Johansson V, Axtelius B, Söderfeldt B, Sampogna F, Paulander J, Sondell K. Multivariate analyses of patient financial systems and oral health-related quality of life. Community Dent Oral Epidemiol. 2010;38:436–44.

13

Human cathelicidin LL-37 enhance the antibiofilm effect of EGCG on *Streptococcus mutans*

Yi-jie Guo[1,3*†], Bo Zhang[1,2†], Xue-song Feng[1,3], Hui-xun Ren[1,3] and Ji-ru Xu[1,3*]

Abstract

Background: *Streptococcus mutans* forms biofilms as a resistance mechanism against antimicrobial agents in the human oral cavity. We recently showed that human cathelicidin LL-37 exhibits inhibitory effects on biofilm formation of *S. mutans* through interaction with lipoteichoic acid (LTA), but without antibacterial or biofilm dispersal abilities. (−)-Epigallocatechin gallate (EGCG) is the most abundant constituent of tea catechins that has the greatest anti-infective potential to inhibit the growth of various microorganisms and biofilm formation. Therefore, in this study, we evaluated whether LL-37 interacts with EGCG to enhance the antibiofilm effect of EGCG on *S. mutans* biofilm formation.

Methods: Clinical *S. mutans* strains ($n = 10$) isolated from children's saliva were tested in a biofilm formation assay. The antibiofilm effect of EGCG with and without LL-37 was analyzed by the minimum biofilm eradication concentration assay and confirmed using field emission-scanning electron microscopy. In addition, the interaction among EGCG, LL-37, and LTA of *S. mutans* was determined using quartz crystal microbalance analysis.

Results: EGCG killed 100 % of planktonic *S. mutans* within 5 h, inhibited biofilm formation within 24 h, and reduced bacteria cells in preformed biofilms within 3 h at a concentration of 0.2 mg/mL. However, EGCG did not appear to interact with LTA. LL-37 effectively enhanced the bactericidal activity of EGCG against biofilm formation and preformed biofilms as determined by quantitative crystal violet staining and field emission-scanning electron microscopy. In addition, quartz crystal microbalance analysis revealed that LL-37 interacted with EGCG and promoted binding between EGCG and LTA of *S. mutans*.

Conclusions: We show that LL-37 enhances the antibiofilm effect of EGCG on *S. mutans*. This finding provides new knowledge for dental treatment by using LL-37 as a potential antibiofilm compound.

Keywords: LL-37, EGCG, *Streptococcus mutans*, Biofilm

Background

Pathogenic bacteria can form biofilms that cause much infectious disease in the human oral cavity. Among these diseases, dental caries is one of the most ubiquitous biofilm-dependent oral diseases worldwide, which frequently occurs in both children and adults [1]. Oral streptococci, including *Streptococcus mutans* and *Streptococcus sobrinus*, are generally considered the primary etiologic agents of dental caries [2, 3]. One of the most well-documented virulence characteristics of *S. mutans* is its ability to establish cariogenic biofilms on tooth surfaces as an assembled extracellular matrix [4, 5]. Extracellular polymeric substances, especially water-insoluble glucans, are the main constituents of the matrix and can mediate *S. mutans* adherence [6, 7]. Other constituents such as extracellular DNA [8] and lipoteichoic acids (LTA) have also been found in high concentrations in the matrix of cariogenic biofilms [9, 10].

Tea is the most frequently consumed beverage in the world after water [11]. The antimicrobial activity of tea was first demonstrated almost 100 years ago by

* Correspondence: yijie_guo@mail.xjtu.edu.cn; xujiru@mail.xjtu.edu.cn
†Equal contributors
[1]Department of Pathogenic Microbiology and Immunology, School of Basic Medical Sciences, Xi'an Jiaotong University, Yanta West Road No.76, Xi'an 710061, ShaanXi, China
Full list of author information is available at the end of the article

McNaught [12]. Green tea (*Camellia sinensis*) is a non-fermented tea that has more beneficial effects than black tea or oolong tea [13]. It has been observed that catechin components of green tea are responsible for its antibacterial activity, and (−)-epicatechin gallate, (−)-epigallocatechin (EGC), and (−)-epigallocatechin gallate (EGCG) constitute the most important antibacterial agents of tea catechins [14, 15].

EGCG is the most abundant constituent of tea catechins that has the greatest anti-infective ability by inhibiting the growth of various microorganisms [16], biofilm formation [17], and quorum sensing [18, 19]. Xu et al. reported that EGCG inhibits the growth of *S. mutans*, decreases glucosyltransferases activity, and suppresses *gtf* genes, which are associated with bacterial biofilm formation [20, 21]. However, the effects of EGCG on biofilm and cariogenic virulence factors of oral streptococci other than glucosyltransferases have not been well documented, especially regarding its potential interaction with LTA.

The antibacterial peptide LL-37 is the only member of the cathelicidin family found in humans. LL-37 is an 18-kDa peptide [22] with 37 amino acid residues that start with two leucines [23]. LL-37 is expressed in many tissues and body fluids, such as saliva, gingiva, sweat, amniotic fluids, and seminal plasma [24]. It has been reported that the intravital concentration of LL-37 is about 86 μg/mL in seminal plasma of healthy donors [25], and ranges from less than 1.2 to more than 80 μg/mL in unstimulated and nonpurulent nasal secretions [26], respectively. Cariogenic species, such as *S. sobrinus*, *Lactobacillus paracasei*, and *Actinomyces viscosus* have been reported to be resistant to LL-37 through growth inhibition and bactericidal tests [27], especially when biofilm formation occurred. We recently showed that LL-37 has the ability to bind to LTA of *S. mutans*, inhibiting biofilm formation [28]. Therefore, in this study, we evaluated whether LL-37 could be used as a binding agent to enhance the interaction between EGCG and LTA of *S. mutans* to increase the antibiofilm effect of EGCG.

Methods

Bacterial strains and culture conditions

Ten clinical *S. mutans* strains isolated from children's saliva were kindly provided by Dr. E. Isogai [29]. Bacteria were grown in brain heart infusion (BHI) broth (Merck KGaA, Darmstadt, Germany) for 24 h at 37 °C. The present study was approved by the Ethics Committee of Xi'an Jiaotong University Faculty of Medicine (XJTU2014-014).

Catechin and antimicrobial peptide

EGCG (NH020403) was purchased from Nagara Science Co. Ltd. (Gifu, Japan). EGCG was dissolved in absolute ethyl alcohol at a concentration of 10 mg/mL. Then, EGCG/ethanol was used a concentration of 2 % to yield a maximum concentration of 0.2 mg/mL. LL-37 (sequence: LLGDF FRKSK EKIGK EFKRI VQRIK DFLRN LVPRT ES) powder was synthesized as described previously using the solid-phase method [30]. Briefly, the peptide was purified (>99.9 %) by reverse-phase high-performance liquid chromatography (Model LC-8A; Shimadzu Corporation, Kyoto, Japan) on a YMC-A 302 column (YMC Co. Ltd., Kyoto, Japan). The final product was confirmed by electrospray ionization mass spectrometry and conserved by suspension in Hank's balanced salt solution (HBSS, pH 7.4; Gibco, Grand Island, NY, USA).

Growth inhibition test

Precultured bacteria were measured at an optical density (OD) of 660 nm using an ultraviolet/visible spectrophotometer (Ubest-35; JASCO Corporation, Tokyo, Japan). Samples were adjusted to $OD_{660} = 0.5$ using BHI broth. Then, bacteria were diluted to a final concentration of 10^3–10^4 Colony-forming unit (CFU)/mL with BHI broth, and 1 mL of adjusted culture and 1 mL of EGCG solution were mixed together [28, 31]. The EGCG solution was prepared by two-fold serial dilution in BHI broth. Each mixture solution was incubated at 37 °C. The bactericidal activity of EGCG was estimated by measuring the minimum inhibitory concentration (MIC) and minimum bactericidal concentration (MBC) at 3, 5, and 24 h of incubation according to Clinical and Laboratory Standards Institute 2014 (CLSI) guidelines. After each incubation, 100 μL of EGCG–cell suspension was removed and inoculated on BHI agar plates. The plates were incubated for 48 h at 37 °C, followed by colony counting (CFU/mL). Control samples were prepared by mixing 1 mL of bacterial suspension with 0.9 mL of BHI broth and 0.1 mL of HBSS. The MIC was defined as the lowest concentration of EGCG that inhibited visible bacterial growth after overnight incubation. The MBC was defined as the lowest concentration of EGCG that killed 99.9 % of the initial inoculum.

Biofilm formation assays

Biofilm formation was measured under two static conditions using a quantitative crystal violet assay on a polystyrene 96-well, minimum biofilm eradication concentration plate (MBEC; Biosurface Technologies, Bozeman, MT, USA) as described previously [32]. The MBEC biofilm assay used 96 polystyrene pegs that fit the wells of a conventional plate. Briefly, overnight cultures of S. mutans were diluted to $OD_{660} = 0.5$ (1×10^7 CFU/mL) in fresh BHI. Two hundred microliters of bacterial suspensions were transferred to a 96-well microtiter plate with 20 μL of varying concentrations of

EGCG in the presence or absence of LL-37 (final concentration of 80 μL/mL). The microtiter plates were then incubated at 37 °C with shaking for 12, 24, and 36 h. After incubation, the pegs were washed several times with phosphate buffered solution (PBS) and then fixed with 200 μL of 100 % ethanol prior to staining for 2 min with 200 μL of 0.41 % (wt/vol) crystal violet in 12 % ethanol (Bio Chemical Sciences, Swedesboro, NJ, USA). The pegs were washed several times with PBS to remove excess stain. Quantitative assessment of biofilm formation was performed by the immersion of pegs in a sterile microtiter plate containing 200 μL of 100 % ethanol and incubation at room temperature for 10 min. The absorbance at 550 nm was then determined. Three independent experiments were performed for each abovementioned assay.

Biofilm susceptibility assays

To measure the antimicrobial susceptibility of *S. mutans* growing in biofilms, the MBEC High-throughput (HTP) Assay (Innovotech Inc., Edmonton, Alberta, Canada) was performed [33]. Briefly, overnight cultures of *S. mutans* were diluted to $OD_{660} = 0.5$ (1×10^7 CFU/mL) in fresh BHI. Then, 200 μL of bacterial suspensions was transferred to the wells of a MBEC microtiter plate and the MBEC lid was placed on top of the wells. Biofilms were grown on the MBEC pegs at 37 °C under shaking conditions for 24 h. The lid was removed and transferred to a new plate with wells filled with varying concentrations of EGCG in the presence or absence of LL-37 (final concentration of 80 μL/mL), and incubated for 3 and 5 h at 37 °C. After each incubation, the lid was gently washed twice with 200 μL of PBS to remove non-adherent cells. Adherent biofilms were fixed with 200 μL of 100 % ethanol prior to staining for 2 min with 200 μL of 0.41 % (wt/vol) crystal violet in 12 % ethanol. The pegs were washed several times with PBS to remove excess stain. Quantitative assessment of biofilm formation was performed by the immersion of pegs in a sterile polystyrene microtiter plate which contained 200 μL of 100 % ethanol. The plate was incubated at room temperature for 10 min, then the absorbance at 550 nm was determined using a microplate spectrophotometer. Three independent experiments were performed for each assay.

Field emission-scanning electron microscopy (FE-SEM)

To visualize the effects of EGCG on planktonic bacteria [28, 31], 10 μL of EGCG solution (0.2 mg/mL) was plated on a glass slide followed by 10 μL of bacteria mixed with the solution. This cell suspension was then incubated at 37 °C for 24 h and dried. Saturated 70 % ethanol was then applied for 5 min, followed by saturated 100 % ethanol for 5 min, and then the sample was dried. The sample was then coated with palladium alloy and examined using FE-SEM (SU8000; Hitachi High-Technologies Corporation, Tokyo, Japan).

To visualize the effect of EGCG on biofilms, the MBEC HTP Assay (Innovotech Inc.) was used [28]. Pegs with adherent biofilms were removed from the MBEC biofilm assay and rinsed in 0.9 % saline for 1 min to remove non-adherent bacteria. The samples were then fixed with 2.5 % glutaraldehyde (Kanto Chemical Co., Inc., Tokyo, Japan) in 0.1 M cacodylic acid (Wako Pure Chemical Industries, Ltd., Miyagi, Japan) at 4 °C for 16 h. The pegs were washed in 0.1 M cacodylic acid and then washed once in distilled water for approximately 10 min. Saturated 70 % ethanol was applied for 15–20 min and then the sample was air dried for a minimum of 24 h. Specimens were finally mounted and examined using FE-SEM.

EGCG, LL-37 and LTA interaction analysis using quartz crystal microbalance (QCM)

QCM was used to analyze the potential enhancement effect of LL-37 on binding between EGCG and bacterial LTA. EGCG was used as a ligand and LTA from *S. mutans* (L4152; Sigma-Aldrich, St. Louis, MO, USA) was used as an analyst. QCM measurements were performed using AFFINIX QN μ (INITIUM Inc., Kanagawa, Japan). This instrument has a 500-μL cell equipped with a 27-MHz QCM plate at the bottom of the cell, in addition to a stirring bar and temperature control system. Gold-coated quartz crystal sensor surfaces were washed twice by mounting 3:1 mixture of concentrated sulfuric acid and hydrogen peroxide solution for 5 min. An AFFINIX immobilization kit was then used following the manufacturer's instruction. Briefly, the surfaces of the sensors were coated with carboxylic acid-terminated thiol and carboxylic acids were activated as N-hydroxysuccinimidyl esters as previously described [34]. Activated carboxyl groups reacted with EGCG (0.2 mg/mL). After the binding of EGCG to the sensor, unreacted esters were deactivated using 1 mol ethanolamine solution. The amount of LTA solution (10 μg/mL) and/or LL-37 (80 μg/mL) injected each time was 5 μL each. HBSS was used as a measurement buffer. The stirring speed was set at 1000 rpm, and experiments were conducted at 25 °C. Frequency changes in response to the addition of LTA solution were monitored in real time. As a control, 10 μg/mL of LTA was injected without initially binding EGCG on the sensor.

Statistical analysis

Data are presented as the means and standard deviations. Significant differences were determined by the *t*-test using Microsoft Excel 2007 (Microsoft Corporation).

Values were considered to be statistically significant at $p < 0.05$.

Results

Short-term antibacterial effect of EGCG on the growth of *S. mutans*

In growth inhibition tests, MICs of EGCG for *S. mutans* planktonic cells ($n = 10$) ranged from 0.025 to 0.1 mg/mL; MBCs ranged from 0.1 to 0.4 mg/mL (Additional file 1: Table S1). To determine the kinetics of the antimicrobial activity of EGCG, bacterial suspensions were incubated with varying concentrations of EGCG for 3 and 5 h. The percentage of viable bacteria clearly decreased from 64.7 to 4.0 % and 45.3 to 0 % with the treatment of 0.0125–0.2 mg/mL EGCG after incubation for 3 and 5 h, respectively (Fig. 1). These results show EGCG has a short-term bactericidal effect on *S. mutans*.

Inhibitory effect of EGCG on biofilm formation in the presence and absence of LL-37

The inhibitory effect of EGCG with or without LL-37 on biofilm formation of *S. mutans* was measured by crystal violet staining of pegs in MBEC assays. The number of biofilm cells on 0.2 mg/mL EGCG with or without 80 μg/mL LL-37-treated pegs were slightly less than untreated pegs at 12 h and showed a significantly decrease after 24- and 36-h incubation ($p < 0.05$) (Fig. 2). Moreover, EGCG treatment with LL-37 resulted in less adherent bacteria than EGCG treatment alone. These results indicate that the inhibitory effect of EGCG on *S. mutans* biofilm formation could be enhanced by the addition of LL-37.

Inhibitory effect of EGCG on preformed *S. mutans* biofilms in the presence and absence of LL-37

The dispersion of preformed biofilms treated with EGCG was then evaluated using biofilm susceptibility assays. *Streptococcus mutans* biofilms were grown on MBEC pegs and then exposed to 0.2 mg/mL EGCG with or without the addition of 80 μg/mL LL-37 in fresh media for 3 and 5 h. After removal of the pegs, the number of viabel bacteria that remained on the pegs was determined using quantitative crystal violet staining. Compared with the control group, *S. mutans* preformed biofilms showed sensitivity to 0.2 mg/mL EGCG treatment, with the highest sensitivity to EGCG in the presence of 80 μg/mL LL-37 at 5 h (Fig. 3).

Effect of EGCG on *S. mutans* cell morphology and biofilm formation

FE-SEM was used to observe the effect of EGCG on *S. mutans* cell morphology and preformed biofilms. As shown in Fig. 4a, the surface of 0.2 mg/mL EGCG-treated cells became rough and exhibited broken membranes with leaked cytoplasm, whereas untreated *S. mutans* cells were smooth (Fig. 4b). Microscopic images of *S. mutans* preformed biofilms on MBEC pegs are shown in Fig. 4c–e, and whole-cell images of treated cells are shown in Additional file 2: Figure S1. EGCG-treated samples had decreased numbers of adherent bacteria and cell membranes were rough. Moreover, the antibiofilm activity of EGCG was more effective in the presence of LL-37.

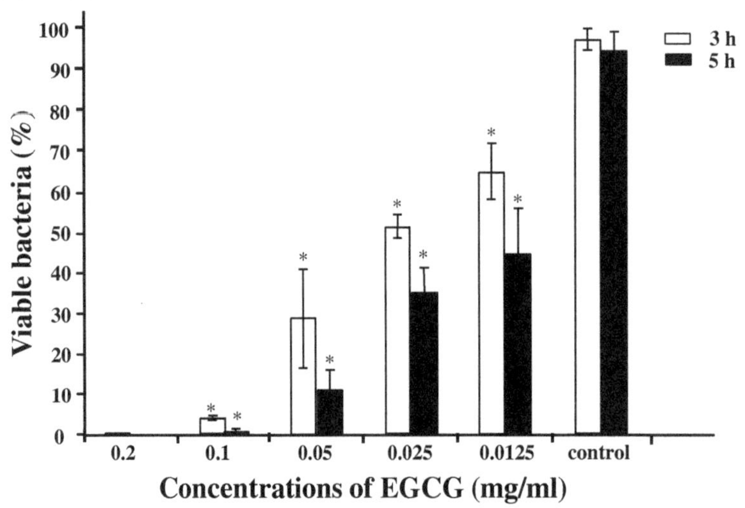

Fig. 1 Short-term killing assays for EGCG against *S. mutans* ($n = 10$). Standardized overnight cultures of *S. mutans* strains (3000 CFU/mL) were seeded in a 96-well microtiter plate with varying concentrations of EGCG and incubated for 3 and 5 h at 37 °C. Data are presented as the mean ± SEM from three independent experiments. *, significant difference compared with untreated control ($p < 0.05$)

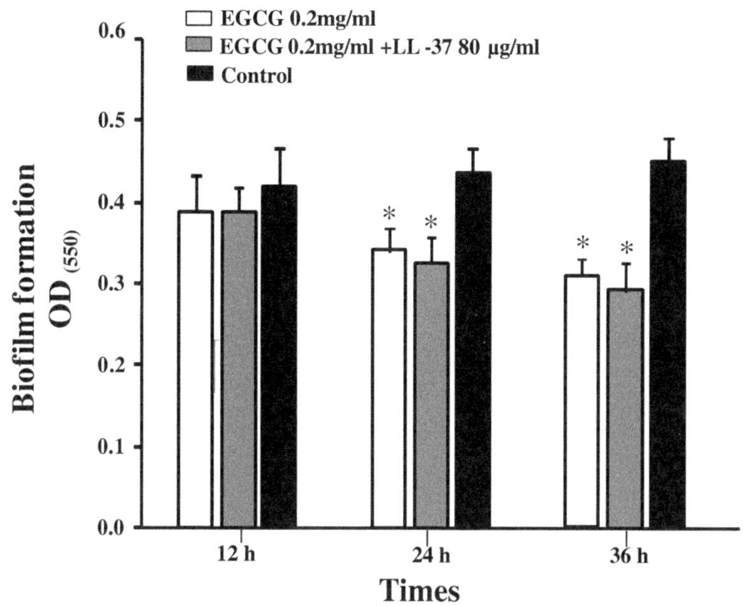

Fig. 2 Biofilm inhibition assay. Standardized overnight cultures of *S. mutans* strains ($n = 10$) were grown on MBEC pegs incubated with 0.2 mg/mL EGCG in the presence or absence of 80 μg/mL LL-37 for 12, 24, or 36 h at 37 °C. Adherent cells were then fixed with ethanol, stained with crystal violet, eluted with ethanol, and the absorbance was measured. Data are presented as the mean ± SD from three independent experiments. *, significant difference compared with untreated control ($p < 0.05$)

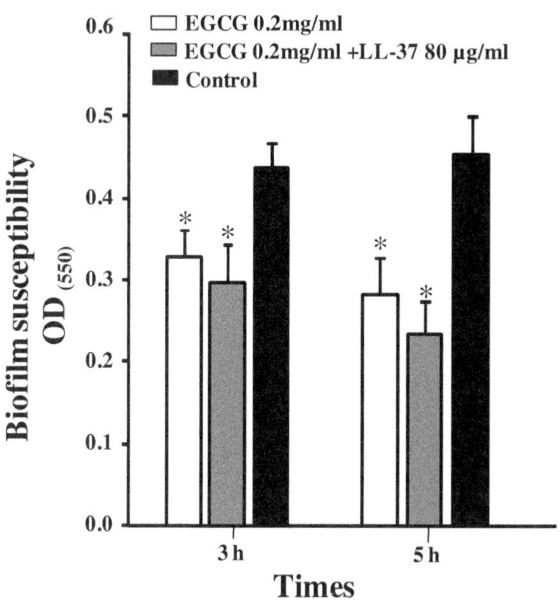

Fig. 3 Biofilm susceptibility assays. Standardized overnight cultures of *S. mutans* strains grown on MBEC pegs and incubated overnight at 37 °C to form mature biofilms. The pegs were immersed in wells containing 0.2 mg/mL EGCG in the presence or absence of 80 μg/mL LL-37 for 3 and 5 h to allow the biofilm to disperse from the pegs to the wells below, and the absorbance was measured. Data are presented as the mean ± SD from three independent experiments. *, significant difference compared with untreated control ($p < 0.05$)

Intermolecular interactions with LTA

The preceding experiments indicated that EGCG likely binds to a component in the bacterial membrane, and this interaction could be enhanced by LL-37. Therefore, we conducted a QCM analysis to determine the precise interaction(s) between EGCG, LL-37, and LTA. In the control experiment, the frequency decreased to below the significance level. The level of decrease caused by non-specific binding between LTA and the blocking agent was 12 Hz. When 1 mg/mL LTA was added, the frequency decreased by 162 Hz, indicating disruption of the interaction between EGCG and LTA. When 80 μg/mL of LL-37 was added, the frequency decreased by 313 Hz, indicating an intermolecular interaction between EGCG and LL-37. After the addition of 1 mg/mL LTA and 80 μg/mL LL-37, the frequency decreased by 524 Hz. These results suggest that EGCG interacts with LTA through binding of LL-37.

Discussion

Catechins have a broad spectrum of antimicrobial activity against both Gram-positive and Gram-negative bacteria, especially galloylated derivatives such as EGCG, which have been documented to possess antimicrobial effects against oral streptococci [11]. According to our early study, EGCG demonstrates the highest activity against *S. mutans* [28], which also supported by other researches [20, 21, 31, 35].

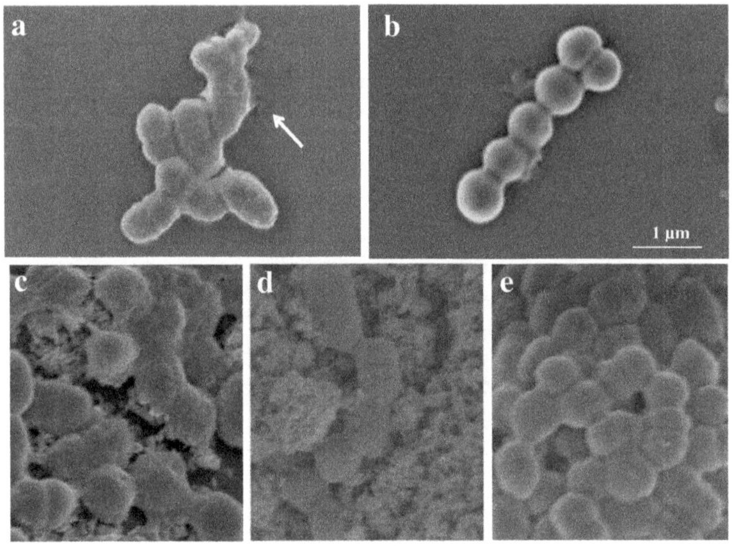

Fig. 4 Changes in number of planktonic cells and preformed biofilms following incubation of EGCG with/without LL-37. Representative images of bacterial cells observed by field emission-scanning electron microscope (working distance: 10 mm, field width: 5 μm) are shown. *Streptococcus mutans* suspensions incubated in the presence (**a**) or absence (**b**) of 0.2 mg/mL EGCG for 24 h. *Streptococcus mutans* biofilms on MBEC pegs incubated with 0.2 mg/mL EGCG (**c**), 0.2 mg/mL EGCG, and 80 μg/mL LL-37 (**d**), or BHI medium (**e**) for 24 h. The white arrow indicates the "ring" phenomena around damaged cells

Biofilms increase the ability of bacteria to resist most antibiotics and therapeutic agents [36]. Stable biofilm formation is also considered one of the key factors of caries pathogenesis. In this study, the inhibitory effect of EGCG on *S. mutans* planktonic cells, biofilm formation, and mature biofilms was examined. EGCG was found to inhibit visible bacterial growth at 0.1 mg/mL, decrease biofilm formation, and exhibit a bactericidal effect on preformed biofilms at 0.2 mg/mL (data not shown). *Streptococcus mutans* in biofilms displayed

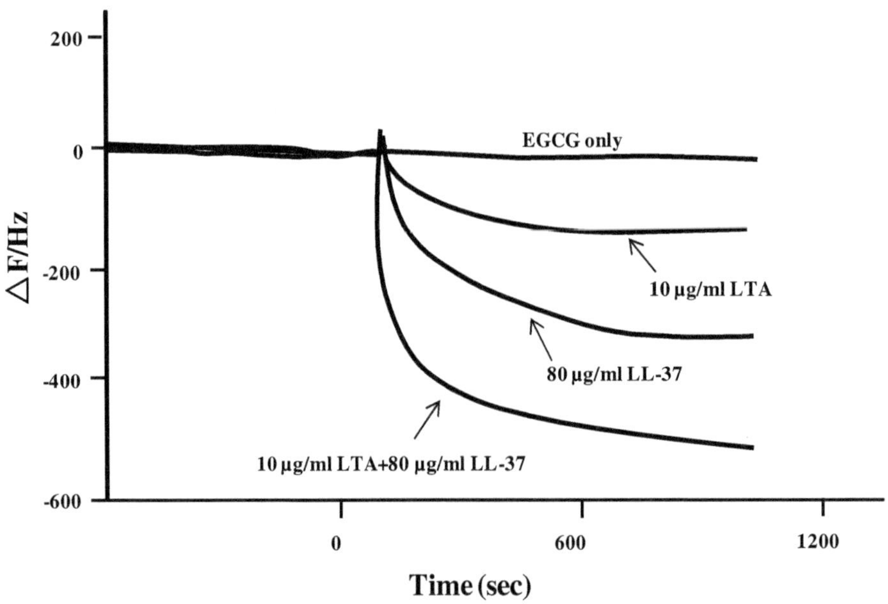

Fig. 5 Interaction among EGCG, LL-37, and LTA of *S. mutans*. Graphs show the change in delta frequency after injecting LTA and/or LL-37 on the sensor of quartz crystal microbalance. Five microliters of LTA (1 mg/mL) and/or LL-37 (8 mg/mL) were injected. The final concentrations of LTA and LL-37 were 10 and 80 μg/mL, respectively. LTA without initially binding EGCG was injected on the sensor as a control. Data presented are representative of three independent experiments with similar results

lower susceptibility to EGCG compared with planktonic bacteria [20]. We also observed that EGCG treatment reduced attachment of *S. mutans*, as previously shown [21], and caused changes in the cell membrane. Based on these results, the antimicrobial mechanism of EGCG is likely attributable to irreversible damage of the microbial cytoplasmic membrane, as previously described [37].

LL-37, which is expressed in many tissues and body fluids, has a broad spectrum of antimicrobial activity against both Gram-positive and Gram-negative bacteria, including *Staphylococcus aureus* and *Pseudomonas aeruginosa*. In our previous study, we showed that *S. mutans* was resistant to LL-37 in growth inhibition and bactericidal tests, but sensitive to LL-37 during biofilm formation, which was partly because of binding to LTA [28]. In this study, we observed that EGCG had an inhibitory effect on *S. mutans* biofilm formation and reduced the viability of preformed biofilms, without interacting with LTA. Therefore, we analyzed the potential cooperative antibacterial effect of EGCG and LL-37. Our results showed that LL-37 has no effect on the antibacterial effect of EGCG on *S. mutans* planktonic cells (data not shown), whereas it plays an enhancer role in the inhibition ability of EGCG on preformed biofilms. The number of bacteria in preformed biofilms was decreased in the presence of LL-37 compared with EGCG treatment alone, which was confirmed by FE-SEM. This indicates that LL-37 may enhance the antibiofilm effect of EGCG on *S. mutans*.

To understand the LL-37 enhancement effect on the antibiofilm activity of EGCG, we subsequently analyzed the interaction among EGCG, LL-37, and LTA of *S. mutans*. EGCG lacked direct interaction with LTA of *S. mutans*. In our previous study, we demonstrated that LL-37 can interact with LTA on *S. mutans* [28]. In this study, EGCG and LL-37 exhibited a synergistic antibiofilm effect on *S. mutans* (Fig. 5). We hypothesize the two following mechanisms: 1) LL-37 binds to LTA of *S. mutans*, enhancing the attachment site of EGCG; or 2) LL-37 interacts with EGCG, raising the cations on EGCG and increasing the affinity between EGCG and LTA, which is supported by Heptinstall et al. [38]. Further studies on the precise mechanism(s) by which LL-37 enhances the antibiofilm effect of EGCG on *S. mutans* are necessary.

Conclusions

Our results indicated that LL-37 can enhance the antibiofilm effect of EGCG on *S. mutans* biofilms. This finding provides new knowledge for dental treatment by using LL-37 as a potential antibiofilm compound.

Abbreviations

BHI: Brain heart infusion; CFU: Colony-forming unit; CLSI: Clinical and laboratory standards institute; EGC: (−)-epigallocatechin; EGCG: (−)-epigallocatechin gallate; FE-SEM: Field emission-scanning electron microscopy; HBSS: Hank's balanced salt solution; HTP: High-throughput; LL-37: Human cathelidicin; LTA: Lipoteichoic acids; MBC: Minimum bactericidal concentration; MBEC: Minimum biofilm eradication concentration; MIC: Minimum inhibitory concentration; PBS: Phosphate buffered solution; QCM: Quartz crystal microbalance

Acknowledgements

We are grateful to Prof. E. Isogai (Graduate School of Agriculture Science, Tohoku University, Japan) and Dr. Lanlan Bai for providing clinical isolate *Streptococcus mutans* strains and Dr. Hafiz Muhammad Ishaq (School of Basic Medical Sciences, Xi'an Jiaotong University, China) for critically reading the manuscript.

Funding

This study was supported by the China Postdoctoral Science Foundation (No. 2015 M582672) and Natural Science Basic Research Plan in Shaanxi Province, China (No. 2016JQ8051).

Authors' contributions

YJG participated in the microbiological analysis and drafted the manuscript. XSF and HXR participated in the FE-SEM. BZ performed the bacterial culture and storage. JRX participated in study design. All authors read and approved the final manuscript.

Competing interests

The authors declare that they have no competing interests.

Consent for publication

Not applicable.

Ethics approval and consent to participate

The present study was approved by the Ethics Committee of Xi'an Jiaotong University Faculty of Medicine (XJTU2014-014) and written informed consent was obtained from Committee of Xi'an Jiaotong University Faculty of Medicine before recruitment.

Author details

[1]Department of Pathogenic Microbiology and Immunology, School of Basic Medical Sciences, Xi'an Jiaotong University, Yanta West Road No.76, Xi'an 710061, ShaanXi, China. [2]Clinical Laboratory, AnKang City Central Hospital, Jinzhou South Road No.85, AnKang 725000, ShaanXi, China. [3]Key Laboratory of Environment and Genes Related to Diseases, Ministry of Education of China, Xi'an Jiaotong University, Yanta West Road No.76, Xi'an 710061, ShaanXi, China.

References

1. Marcenes W, Kassebaum NJ, Bernabe E, Flaxman A, Naghavi M, Lopez A, Murray CJ. Global burden of oral conditions in 1990–2010: a systematic analysis. J Dent Res. 2013;92(7):592–7.
2. Loesche WJ. Role of *Streptococcus mutans* in human dental decay. Microbiol Rev. 1986;50(4):353–80.
3. Beighton D. The complex oral microflora of high-risk individuals and groups and its role in the caries process. Community Dent Oral Epidemiol. 2005; 33(4):248–55.

4. Hamada S, Slade HD. Biology, immunology, and cariogenicity of *Streptococcus mutans*. Microbiol Rev. 1980;44(2):331–84.
5. Bowen WH, Koo H. Biology of *Streptococcus mutans*-derived glucosyltransferases: role in extracellular matrix formation of cariogenic biofilms. Caries Res. 2011;45(1):69–86.
6. Mattos-Graner RO, Smith DJ, King WF, Mayer MP. Water-insoluble glucan synthesis by mutans streptococcal strains correlates with caries incidence in 12- to 30-month-old children. J Dent Res. 2000;79(6):1371–7.
7. Vacca SAM, Scott-Anne KM, Whelehan MT, Berkowitz RJ, Feng C, Bowen WH. Salivary glucosyltransferase B as a possible marker for caries activity. Caries Res. 2007;41(6):445–50.
8. Perry JA, Cvitkovitch DG, Levesque CM. Cell death in *Streptococcus mutans* biofilms: a link between CSP and extracellular DNA. FEMS Microbiol Lett. 2009;299(2):261–6.
9. Rolla G, Oppermann RV, Bowen WH, Ciardi JE, Knox KW. High amounts of lipoteichoic acid in sucrose-induced plaque in vivo. Caries Res. 1980;14(4): 235–8.
10. Denapaite D, Bruckner R, Hakenbeck R, Vollmer W. Biosynthesis of teichoic acids in *Streptococcus pneumoniae* and closely related species: lessons from genomes. Microb Drug Resist. 2012;18(3):344–58.
11. Sannella AR, Messori L, Casini A, Francesco VF, Bilia AR, Majori G, Severini C. Antimalarial properties of green tea. Biochem Biophys Res Commun. 2007; 353(1):177–81.
12. McNaught JG. On the action of cold or lukewarm tea on Bacillus typhosus. J R Army Med Corps. 1906;7:372–3.
13. Jazani NH, Sh S, Ali AA. Antibacterial effects of water soluble green tea extracts on multi-antibiotic resistant isolates of *Pseudomonas aeruginosa*. Pak J Biol Sci. 2007;10(9):1544–6.
14. Yam TS, Hamilton-Miller JM, Shah S. The effect of a component of tea (Camellia sinensis) on methicillin resistance, PBP2' synthesis, and beta-lactamase production in *Staphylococcus aureus*. J Antimicrob Chemother. 1998;42(2):211–6.
15. Bidlack WR. Green Tea: Health Benefits and Applications. J Am Coll Nutr. 2001;20(6):656–8.
16. Kohda C, Yanagawa Y, Shimamura T. Epigallocatechin gallate inhibits intracellular survival of *Listeria monocytogenes* in macrophages. Biochem Biophys Res Commun. 2008;365(2):310–5.
17. Blanco AR, Sudano-Roccaro A, Spoto GC, Nostro A, Rusciano D. Epigallocatechin gallate inhibits biofilm formation by ocular staphylococcal isolates. Antimicrob Agents Chemother. 2005;49(10):4339–43.
18. Huber B, Eberl L, Feucht W, Polster J. Influence of polyphenols on bacterial biofilm formation and quorum-sensing. Z Naturforsch C. 2003;58(11–12): 879–84.
19. Lee KM, Kim WS, Lim J, Nam S, Youn M, Nam SW, Kim Y, Kim SH, Park W, Park S. Antipathogenic properties of green tea polyphenol epigallocatechin gallate at concentrations below the MIC against enterohemorrhagic *Escherichia coli* O157:H7. J Food Prot. 2009;72(2):325–31.
20. Xu X, Zhou XD, Wu CD. The tea catechin epigallocatechin gallate suppresses cariogenic virulence factors of *Streptococcus mutans*. Antimicrob Agents Chemother. 2011;55(3):1229–36.
21. Xu X, Zhou XD, Wu CD. Tea catechin epigallocatechin gallate inhibits *Streptococcus mutans* biofilm formation by suppressing gtf genes. Arch Oral Biol. 2012;57(6):678–83.
22. Agerberth B, Gunne H, Odeberg J, Kogner P, Boman HG, Gudmundsson GH. FALL-39, a putative human peptide antibiotic, is cysteine-free and expressed in bone marrow and testis. Proc Natl Acad Sci. 1995;92(1):195–9.
23. Ramos LD R, Gama M. LL37, a human antimicrobial peptide with immunomodulatory properties. Sci Against Microb Pathogens. 2011;9: 915–25.
24. Johansson J, Gudmundsson GH, Rottenberg ME, Berndt KD, Agerberth B. Conformation-dependent antibacterial activity of the naturally occurring human peptide LL-37. J Biol Chem. 1998;273(6):3718–24.
25. Malm J, Sorensen O, Persson T, Frohm-Nilsson M, Johansson B, Bjartell A, Lilja H, Stahle-Backdahl M, Borregaard N, Egesten A. The human cationic antimicrobial protein (hCAP-18) is expressed in the epithelium of human epididymis, is present in seminal plasma at high concentrations, and is attached to spermatozoa. Infect Immun. 2000;68(7):4297–302.
26. Lysenko ES, Gould J, Bals R, Wilson JM, Weiser JN. Bacterial phosphorylcholine decreases susceptibility to the antimicrobial peptide LL-37/hCAP18 expressed in the upper respiratory tract. Infect Immun. 2000; 68(3):1664–71.
27. Altman H, Steinberg D, Porat Y, Mor A, Fridman D, Friedman M, Bachrach G. In vitro assessment of antimicrobial peptides as potential agents against several oral bacteria. J Antimicrob Chemother. 2006;58(1):198–201.
28. Bai LL, Takagi S, Guo YJ, Kuroda K, Ando T, Yoneyama H, Ito K, Isogai E. Inhibition of *Streptococcus mutans* Biofilm by LL-37. IntJ Med Sci Biotech. 2013;l(l):56–64.
29. Hirose H, Hirose K, Isogai E, Miura H, Ueda I. Close association between *Streptococcus sobrinus* in the saliva of young children and smooth-surface caries increment. Caries Res. 1993;27(4):292–7.
30. Isogai E, Isogai H, Matuo K, Hirose K, Kowashi Y, Okumuara K, Hirata M. Sensitivity of genera Porphyromonas and Prevotella to the bactericidal action of C-terminal domain of human CAP18 and its analogues. Oral Microbiol Immunol. 2003;18(5):329–32.
31. Takagi S, Hayashi S, Takahashi K, Isogai H, Bai L, Yoneyama H, Ando T, Ito K, Isogai E. Antimicrobial activity of a bovine myeloid antimicrobial peptide (BMAP-28) against methicillin-susceptible and methicillin-resistant *Staphylococcus aureus*. Anim Sci J. 2012;83(6):482–6.
32. Wei GX, Campagna AN, Bobek LA. Effect of MUC7 peptides on the growth of bacteria and on *Streptococcus mutans* biofilm. J Antimicrob Chemother. 2006;57(6):1100–9.
33. Coraca-Huber DC, Fille M, Hausdorfer J, Pfaller K, Nogler M. Evaluation of MBEC-HTP biofilm model for studies of implant associated infections. J Orthop Res. 2012;30(7):1176–80.
34. Lahiri J, Isaacs L, Tien J, Whitesides GM. A strategy for the generation of surfaces presenting ligands for studies of binding based on an active ester as a common reactive intermediate: a surface plasmon resonance study. Anal Chem. 1999;71(4):777–90.
35. Sasaki H, Matsumoto M, Tanaka T, Maeda M, Nakai M, Hamada S, Ooshima T. Antibacterial activity of polyphenol components in oolong tea extract against *Streptococcus mutans*. Caries Res. 2004;38(1):2–8.
36. Costerton JW, Stewart PS, Greenberg EP. Bacterial biofilms: a common cause of persistent infections. Science. 1999;284(5418):1318–22.
37. Taylor PW, Hamilton-Miller JM, Stapleton PD. Antimicrobial properties of green tea catechins. Food Sci Technol Bull. 2005;2:71–81.
38. Heptinstall S, Archibald AR, Baddiley J. Teichoic acids and membrane function in bacteria. Nature. 1970;225(5232):519–21.

14

Current stress and poor oral health

A. Vasiliou[1], K. Shankardass[2,3,4*], R. Nisenbaum[3,4] and C. Quiñonez[1,4]

Abstract

Background: Psychological stress appears to contribute to poor oral health systemically in combination with other chronic diseases. Few studies directly examine this relationship.

Methods: Data from a cross-sectional study of 2,412 participants between the ages of 25–64 years old living in the City of Toronto between 2009 and 2012 were used to examine the relationship between current stress and two self-rated oral health outcomes (general oral health and oral pain). Dental care utilization and access to dental insurance were examined as effect modifiers.

Results: A positive relationship between current stress and poor oral health was observed for both outcomes (oral pain coefficient 0.32, 95 % CI 0.26–0.38; general oral health coefficient 0.28, 95 % CI 0.19–0.36). Effects on oral pain were stronger for the uninsured, while effects on general oral health were stronger with decreasing socioeconomic position.

Conclusions: Our findings suggest that individuals with greater perceived stress also report poorer oral health, and that this relationship is modified by dental insurance and socioeconomic position. These findings warrant a greater focus on the role of psychological stress in the development of oral disease, including how perceived stress contributes to health inequities in self-reported oral health status. Patients experiencing stressful lives may differentially require closer monitoring and more vigilant maintenance of their oral health, above and beyond that which is needed to achieve a state of health in the oral environment of less stressed individuals. There may be health promoting effects of addressing psychosocial concerns related to dental care - particularly for the poor and uninsured.

Keywords: Stress, Oral pain, General oral health, Dental insurance

Abbreviations: NEHW, Neighbourhood effects on health and well-being; SEP, Socioeconomic position

Background

In the absence of policy changes to fully include dental health services in the Ontario Health Insurance Plan (OHIP), or through other social welfare programs, (such as Healthy Smiles Ontario) [1], more effective approaches to prevention are needed to maintain oral health status in some populations and to improve status in the general population. Whereas policy strategies to improve oral health in the population have traditionally targeted behavior change at the individual level by promoting brushing and flossing practices [2], more research is needed to understand the more distal and structural determinants of oral health.

The prevalence of poor dental health outcomes is usually markedly increased in populations of lower socio-economic position relative to those of higher socio-economic position, even after accounting for differences in access to care [3]. This has inspired growing interest in understanding the role of psychosocial factors in the development of diminished oral health status [4], including chronic stress (e.g., [5–8]).

A systemic view of oral health and stress

In fact, poor oral health has long been theorized to cause the dysfunction of other critical physiologic systems [9]. A growing body of evidence has come to support the existence of such an "oral-systemic" relationship [10–12]. This relationship has been demonstrated for some diseases

* Correspondence: kshankardass@wlu.ca
[2]Department of Health Sciences, Wilfrid Laurier University, 75 University Ave West, Waterloo, ON N2L 3C5, Canada
[3]Centre for Urban Health Solutions, Li Ka Shing Knowledge Institute, St Michael's Hospital, Toronto, ON, Canada
Full list of author information is available at the end of the article

more so than others, including respiratory infections, osteoporosis, childhood obesity, cardiovascular disease, and type II diabetes [13–16]. A shared impetus for the development of both oral and systemic disease may be the presence of stress. As a common risk factor for both diseases of the oral cavity as well as for non-communicable diseases (e.g. cancer, cardiovascular disease, diabetes, and respiratory disease), the minimization of stress has become an integral component of novel systemic healthcare promotion techniques, such as the common risk factor approach [17].

Chronic stress is likely to contribute to the progressive, long-term development of oral disease through at least two distinguishable pathways. First, stress can motivate individuals to cope in unhealthy ways that foster oral disease (e.g., substance use, including illicit drugs, alcohol and tobacco, poor diet, and sedentary behavior). Second, chronic stress contributes to high allostatic load that can lead to the dysfunction of physiological systems critical to homeostasis, and thus, affect the underlying mechanisms of disease progression, more generally [18].

Our conceptual framework is described below and in Fig. 1, and many elements are elaborated on in Shankardass [18]. While stress is a concern of an array of disciplines, including psychology, sociology, psychoneuroimmunology, we adopt a transdisciplinary approach to defining chronic stress based on the stress process paradigm of Pearlin et al. [19]. They conceptualized stress as a process "in which demands strain on an individual's ability to adapt - physiologically and emotionally - with implications for physiological and behavioural pathways" [19].

Individuals may experience potential *sources* of current stress, including people (such as children in the case of parents), places (such as densely populated intersections), and things (such as a paucity of money, food, and shelter). Typically, stressors can be categorized into one of four types: major life events (such as a death in the family), ambient strains (such as a concern for safety in the neighbourhood you live in), role strains (such as stress related to workplace hierarchy), and quotidian nature strains (stresses that result from activities of a repeated nature, such as a daily commute to work) [19].

Some factors may mediate whether or not the experience of stress currently translates into more chronic stress over time (*manifestations*), including whether or not they perceive certain stressors as threatening, and if so, manageable given resources at hand [19]. Then, where perceived current stress occurs, the coping behaviours used to deal with stressors mediate whether chronic stress manifests and harms oral health and general well-being in two main ways. First, if stressors associated with perceived current stress are not coped with in an effective manner, then chronic stress is more likely to occur. Allostatic load, a cumulative physiological impact of chronic stress, has been associated with periodontal disease [20], and some evidence indicates that this occurs due to increased inflammation [21]. However, the precise causal mechanisms remain somewhat unclear [22]. Second, regardless of how effective coping behaviours are, they may manifest as habits that are either healthy (e.g., exercise and relaxation, problem solving) or unhealthy (e.g., tobacco, alcohol and

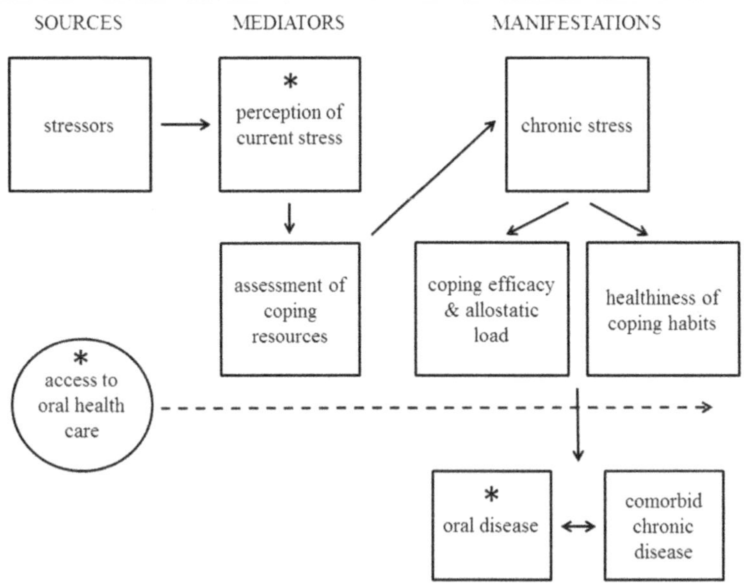

Fig. 1 Conceptual framework of causal and moderating pathways linking the stress process to oral health practices and outcomes. Boxes indicate factors involved in the stress process (i.e., sources, mediators and manifestations). Straight lines indicate main causal relationships of interest. Circle with dashed line indicates a moderating effect of oral health practices

other drug use, poor oral maintenance) with respect to oral disease.

In this analysis we consider the general salience of our framework by investigating whether or not the perception of current stress is associated with self-reported poor oral health status among residents of Toronto, Ontario's most populous city. We also examine whether this relationship is moderated by dental insurance and dental care utilization, since having greater access to oral health care (e.g., because of dental insurance or as reflected by actual visits to the dentist) may help to buffer the impact of chronic stress on poor oral health and other social and health outcomes.

Methods

Study design and instruments

We conducted a secondary analysis of the cross-sectional Neighbourhood Effects on Health and Well-Being (NEHW) study. The Research Board at St. Michael's Hospital in Toronto, Canada provided ethics approval for this study. All participants provided written informed consent at the time of their interview and were compensated $50 for their participation. As described elsewhere in more detail, a three stage sampling strategy was employed to randomly sample households within a random sample of census tracts and neighbourhood planning areas in the City of Toronto [23].

Participants of the study were recruited between 2009 and 2012. Participants were eligible for the study if they were able to communicate in English, were between the ages of 25–64 years old, lived in their neighbourhood for at least 6 months, and were a resident of the home. Further details on study procedures can be obtained elsewhere [23].

The NEHW study collected data on neighbourhood and individual level factors that promote or diminish mental health using same-room face-to-face surveys in a total of 2,412 participants (response rate of 72 %; [24]) living in a random sample of 47 neighbourhoods throughout Toronto [23]. The survey included two self-rated oral health questions utilized as dependent variables in this analysis. General oral health was assessed using the question, "In general, would you say the health of your teeth and mouth is...?" (5-point Likert scale from 1 = "excellent" to 5 = "poor" health), while oral pain was assessed using the question, "In the past month, how often have you had any pain or discomfort in your teeth or gums? (4-point Likert scale from 1 = "often" to 4 = "never"). Therefore, higher scores indicate poorer oral health for both outcomes. Although not a direct measure of oral disease (see: [25]), self-reported oral health has been associated with greater chronic stress, depressive symptoms, and material hardship [26], so we expected it to be sensitive to perceived current stress.

Recency of dental care utilization was assessed using the question, "How long has it been since your last dentist visit?" (<1 year, 1- < 2 year, 2+ years), and access to dental insurance was assessed using the question, "Do you have insurance that covers all or part of your dental expenses?" (yes versus no).

Data were also available for several stress items, including some items from the Cumulative Adversity Interview (CAI) [27]. Higher levels of subjective stress based on the CAI have been associated with smaller grey matter volumes in parts of the brain [27]. Three items from the CAI were used in this study to capture a general index of whether or not participants perceived their lives as generally stressful at the time of the study (i.e., currently): "You're trying to take on too many things at once", "There is too much pressure on you to be like other people", "Too much is expected of you by others". We viewed the first item as indicating personal or work-related stress, and the other two as indicators of social stress. Each item was rated on a 3-point Likert scale (0 = "Not true", 1 = "Somewhat true", 2 = "Very true") and an index was calculated by taking the average of the three items. Although this index has not been previously validated, we viewed it as measuring the level that participants perceived their lives as generally stressful at the time of the study (i.e., currently).

Other questions included in this analysis are age (years), sex (male or female), total household income (>$10,000, $10,000–$14,999, $15,000–$19,999, $20,000–$29,999, $30,000–$39,999, $40,000–$49,999, $50,000–$74,999, >$75,000), current employment status (indicator of any current employment), immigration status (Canadian born, immigrated ≤10 years ago, immigrated >10 years ago), high educational attainment (indicator of education beyond high school diploma). We also identified participants who were foreign born immigrants to Canada, i.e., not including those who were citizens through birth or parental descent. To parsimoniously test for the effect of these factors as confounders and moderators of the relationship between stress and oral health, an index of socioeconomic position was constructed by summing three indicator variables for high educational attainment, current employment, and high total household income (i.e., greater than or equal to $30,000); this resulted in an index with possible values ranging from 0 to 3.

Data analysis

The crude and adjusted associations between perceived current stress and poor oral health outcomes were examined using univariate and multivariate linear regression models, respectively. All analyses were performed using IBM SPSS Statistics 22. The selection of confounders began with the use of theory to identify a list of candidates, including age, sex, socioeconomic position, foreign born, immigrant status, recency of dental care utilization and presence of dental insurance. Potential confounders were deemed appropriate for inclusion in the model building process if there was a statistically significant association with the oral health outcomes (alpha = 0.05). The final model was developed using a forward stepwise process using a cut-off for inclusion of a 10 % change in the coefficient for stress.

Moderation of the relationship between stress and oral health was examined by testing for statistical significance of multiplicative interaction terms in the final models. Given the exploratory nature of this analysis, we adopted a relatively broad alpha level for these tests of 0.10. Factors examined as potential moderators included age, sex, socioeconomic position, foreign born immigrant status, recency of dental care utilization and presence of dental insurance.

The assumption of a linear effect of stress on oral health status was tested by including dummy variables for quarter-point increase in the perceived current stress index (i.e., allowing a non-linear relationship to take shape). Plots of these models compared to a line of best fit (i.e., linear trend) did not indicate deviation from a linear trend (data not shown), and adjusted R-square values were also largely similar when the effect of stress was modeled as an exponential or cubic factor compared with linear models (data not shown).

Both rudimentary (via visual inspections of lines of best fit) and statistical (via R-square values) assessments of linearity were performed in an effort to detect whether the assumption of linearity was appropriate for the relationship between perceived current stress and oral health outcomes.

Sampling weights were derived previously [23] and utilized in all analyses to correct for any selection biases by comparing the distribution of sample characteristics using 2006 Census data for the City of Toronto.

Results

Survey participants were 44 years of age on average (standard deviation of 11 years) and 48 % were male (Table 1). In general, participants were well educated (77.2 % had more than a high school education), wealthy (45.7 % had a total combined household income of greater than $75,000), and employed (71.6 % were currently employed). Almost 40 % of participants were born in Canada, while 15 % were recent immigrants and 46 % were long-term immigrants. Of all immigrant participants, 38 % were of a minority race/ethnicity. Almost 65 % of participants had some dental care insurance, while most participants (74 %) had visited the dentist within the previous year.

Table 1 Study participant characteristics

Characteristics	n (%)	Mean (SD)
Age (Years)		44.4 (10.7)
Male Sex	1163 (48.2)	
Reports of Pain or Discomfort in Teeth or Gums Over Past Month (1–4; 1 = Never, 4 = Often)		1.6 (0.86)
General Health of Teeth and Mouth (1–5; 1 = Excellent, 5 = Poor)		2.6 (1.1)
Perceived Current Stress Index (average of a - c)		0.67 (0.55)
a. You are trying to take on too many things at once (0–2; 0 = Not True, 2 = Very True)		0.89 (0.74)
b. There is too much pressure on you to be like other people (0–2; 0 = Not True, 2 = Very True)		0.41 (0.65)
c. Too much is expected of you by others (0–2; 0 = Not True, 2 = Very True)		0.69 (0.73)
Total Combined Household Income		
<$10,000	22 (1.0)	
$10,000–$14,999	87 (3.9)	
$15,000–$19,999	60 (2.7)	
$20,000–$29,999	231 (10.3)	
$30,000–$39,999	180 (8.0)	
$40,000–$49,999	188 (8.4)	
$50,000–$74,999	450 (20.1)	
>$75,000	1023 (45.7)	
Educational Attainment Greater Than High School Diploma? (Yes vs No)	1859 (77.2)	
Currently Employed? (Yes vs No)	2099 (87.2)	
Socioeconomic Position Index? (0–3)		2.4 (0.79)
Citizenship Status		
Canadian Born	947 (39.4)	
Non-Recent Immigrant	1106 (46.0)	
Recent Immigrant (≤10 Years in Canada)	351 (14.6)	
Has Dental Insurance That Covers All or Part of Dental Expenses? (Yes vs No)	1549 (64.3)	
Length Of Time Since Last Visit to the Dentist?		
<1 Year Ago	1782 (74.0)	
1–2 Years Ago	318 (13.2)	
>2 Years Ago	308 (12.8)	

The crude association between perceived stress and both perceived oral pain and perceived general oral health yielded similar positive and statistically significant ($\alpha = 0.05$) beta coefficients (0.33 and 0.31, respectively) [Table 2, Model 1]. Age and sex were identified as confounders in the final model for both oral health outcomes, while household income was also a confounder of general oral health. While the effect of stress remained positive and statistically significant after adjusting for confounders,

Table 2 Coefficients for perceived current stress index with oral health outcomes

	Model 1	Model 2
Oral Health Outcomes	Crude Current Stress Beta Coefficient (95 % CI)	Adjusted Current Stress and Oral Health Beta Coefficient (95 % CI)
Pain or discomfort in teeth or gums over past month	0.33 (0.27–0.39)	0.32 (0.26–0.38)
General health of teeth and mouth	0.31 (0.23–0.39)	0.28 (0.19–0.36)

Model 1 models the crude effect of the perceived current stress index. Model 2 is further adjusted age and sex for oral pain, and for age, sex and household income for general oral health

the coefficient was reduced by 10 % in the case of general oral health; whereas the effect on oral pain was relatively stable (3 % reduction) [Table 2, Model 2].

Table 3 examines whether the effect of the perceived current stress index was driven by any particular item. Coefficients for personal/work stress items were generally weaker than those for social stress.

There was a statistically significant interaction between perceived current stress and dental insurance on oral pain ($p = 0.09$), where the effect of perceived current stress was slightly stronger for participants without dental insurance compared to the insured. Figure 2 describes the predicted levels of oral pain across levels of perceived current stress for insured and uninsured 44 year-old females who have a total household income of $40,000-$49,999. This model predicted a difference in oral pain of 0.31 where these insured and uninsured individuals are experiencing high perceived current stress.

We also observed a statistically significant interaction between perceived current stress and socioeconomic position on oral pain ($p = 0.06$), where the effect of perceived current stress was stronger for participants of lower socioeconomic position. Figure 3 describes the predicted levels of oral pain across levels of perceived current oral stress for participants across four levels of socioeconomic position who are 44 year-old females with a total household income of $40,000–$49,999. This model predicted a difference in oral pain of 0.64 between individuals experiencing high perceived current stress with highest and lowest socioeconomic position.

Discussion

We found that Toronto participants who reported greater perceived current stress in their lives also self-reported progressively poorer oral health and greater oral pain compared to those with lesser stress. The association with oral pain is novel, while our findings generally support other studies indicating a positive association between stress and poor oral health. Segura and Sheiham (1992) found a positive association between work-related demands and periodontal illness indicated by bleeding or pockets in a clinical exam [5]. Finlayson et al (2010) found positive associations between chronic stress and poorer self-rated oral health [26]; as did Armfield et al (2013), including a positive significant associated between chronic stress and untreated decayed teeth [8]. These findings indicate the salience of our framework linking perceived current stress to chronic disease, including oral disease (Fig. 1).

Some other studies have not observed associations between measures of stress and poor oral health (e.g., [7]). One explanation for inconsistent findings is that studies about stress are not properly accounting for the stress process and potential moderators of effects on oral health in the analysis of data. For example, associations observed in the study by Armfield et al (2013) were diminished in size and rendered non-significant in the case of untreated decayed teeth when models were adjusted for oral maintenance behaviours (i.e., tooth brushing) [8]. We argue that such factors may be on the causal pathway (e.g., [6]) as part of the response to perceived stress, and therefore should not be included in statistical models as potential confounders of effects of stress on oral health. Dental care utilization was also included as a confounder in that analysis and contributed to the diminished effect of stress on poor oral health [8]; whereas our findings suggest that this factor may actually moderate this association.

We were not able to clarify whether current stress (i.e., at the time of the study) reflected generally more stressful lives, (i.e., chronic stress); nor could we measure much of the inherent behavioural and physiological process that ultimately contribute to oral disease pathology (as indicated by Fig. 1). Future studies should test hypotheses that involve more components of our framework, including the efficacy and healthfulness of coping behaviours, the experience of chronic stress and biomarkers of allostatic

Table 3 Comparison of coefficients for stress index components against oral health outcomes

	You are trying to take on too many things at once	There is too much pressure on you to be like other people	Too much is expected of you by others
Oral health outcomes	Coefficient (95 % CI)	Coefficient (95 % CI)	Coefficient (95 % CI)
Pain or discomfort in teeth or gums over past month	0.15 (0.10–0.19)	0.29 (0.22–0.32)	0.17 (0.13–0.22)
General health of teeth and mouth	0.13 (0.07–0.19)	0.17 (0.10–0.24)	0.19 (0.13–0.25)

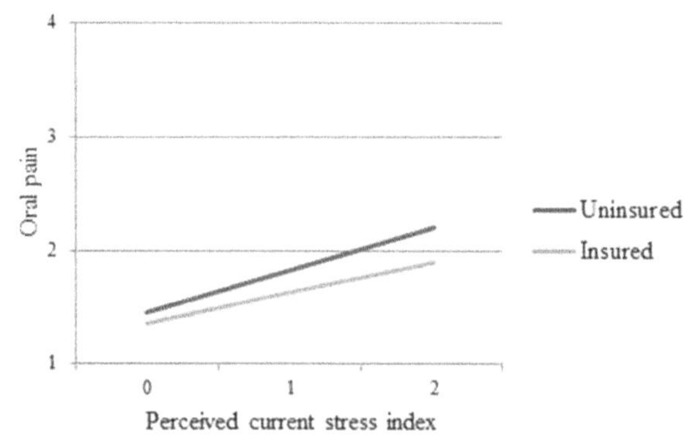

Fig. 2 Predicted oral pain by perceived current stress for levels of dental insurance. Oral pain (1 – 4; 1 = Never, 4 = Often)

load, and comorbid chronic disease outcomes. While subjective measures of stress are likely to be good indicators of manifestations on health and well-being [27], future studies should examine effects on a wider range of specific oral disease end-points to help further clarify the precise mechanism that links stress to oral health.

The harmful effect of perceived current stress on oral pain was more pronounced for participants without dental insurance and of lower socioeconomic position. It is not unexpected that dental insurance conditioned the relationship between perceived current stress and oral pain since dental services are not publicly insured for residents of Toronto under Canada's Medicare program. This pattern could indicate that those without insurance are not receiving adequate dental care (i.e., have unmet needs); for example, because they cannot afford to pay for service out-of-pocket [28–31].

The moderating effect of socioeconomic position was stronger than that observed for dental insurance. This relative difference could be explained if individuals of lower socioeconomic position experience a multitude of barriers to health. For example, this population may experience: 1) poorer access to adequate dental care given unemployment or employment in a position with miserly health benefits [32, 33]; 2) greater chronic stress and coping in ways that are more damaging to their oral health (e.g., tobacco use, alcohol use, consumption of junk food); and 3) greater risk of other chronic diseases, which may impact oral disease via the oral-systemic relationship.

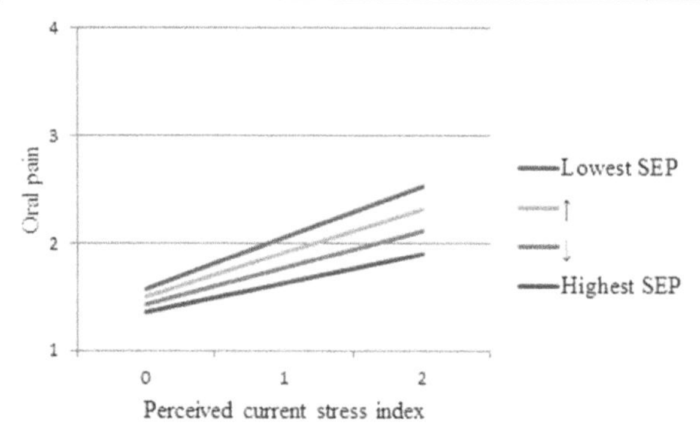

Fig. 3 Predicted oral pain by perceived current stress for levels of socioeconomic position (SEP). Oral pain (1–4; 1 = Never, 4 = Often)

In addition to water fluoridation, current preventative measures for oral health rely largely on the agency of individuals to maintain oral health practices and on education and early screening in clinical and other settings. For example, the Toronto Public Health Unit implements free dental screening in both public and non-public schools for children from Junior Kindergarten to Grade 8, as well as provides educational programs such as the Community Oral Health Outreach Program in an effort to teach individuals about dental health and disease prevention strategies [33]. Our findings may motivate future studies to investigate the impact of stress, dental insurance, and socioeconomic position on dental health outcomes - if a strong link is established, these current interventions are unlikely to be sufficient to prevent oral disease. To the extent that the relationships between stress, oral pain, dental insurance and socioeconomic position are causal, strategies to improve prevention include greater promotion of psychosocial health, broadened accessibility of dental care and greater promotion of social (read: income) equality.

The apparent importance of psychosocial causes of oral disease suggests that the Canadian status quo of excluding dental care services from Medicare simply because the causes of oral disease are easy to prevent (e.g., by large-scale treatment interventions such as fluoridation, and individuals practicing oral health promotion, such as brushing and flossing) [32] is not defensible. Thus, efforts to improve access to dental care as a way of buffering the impact of stress on oral health may be needed; particularly for the uninsured and those of lower socioeconomic position. In lieu of the Federal Government requiring dental care services to be insured under Medicare, other incentives for dentists in Toronto, Ontario to provide affordable care for the uninsured are needed. In addition, social welfare programs could be introduced to broaden access to dental services. For example, the Provincial Government recently introduced the Healthy Smiles Ontario program to provide dental insurance to children of lower income families, and this program could be expanded to cover all lower income Ontarians.

Our study participants were drawn from a random sample of neighbourhoods in Toronto, which strengthens the generalizability of our findings to adults living in the city. While psychological stress can be challenging to measure accurately, our findings are based on an index based on diverse types of stress, which strengthens the internal validity of the findings. Our study was limited by its reliance on self-reported measures of perceived oral health and current stress, making the results subject to recall and social desirability biases. Our study was also limited by cross-sectional data collection; although it could be argued that poorer oral health status is not likely to lead participants to report higher levels of the indicators used to measure stress in this study. Still, in order to better understand the mechanisms linking psychological stress to oral disease, longitudinal study designs should be employed in future studies.

Conclusions

Our findings suggest that individuals with greater perceived stress also report poorer oral health, and that this relationship is modified by dental insurance and socioeconomic position. These findings may warrant greater attention be paid to the role of psychological stress in the development of oral disease, including as a cause of social inequalities in oral health, and health inequity, more generally. More research is needed to explain the relationship between perceived current stress and oral health and to inform the design of interventions for the uninsured and those disadvantaged in other ways.

Acknowledgements

We would like to acknowledge the Neighbourhood Effects on Health and Well-Being study that was funded by the Canadian Institute for Health Research Grant MOP-84439 and the Social Science and Health Research Council Grant 410-2007-1499.

Funding

Although this analysis was not supported by any funding sources, the NEHW study was originally funded by the Canadian Institute for Health Research grant MOP-84439 and the Social Science and Health Research Grant Council grant 410-2007-1499.

Authors' contributions

AV participated in study design and led data analysis, and the writing of this manuscript was part of his senior undergraduate thesis project. KS supervised AV and participated in study design, data analysis, and the writing of the manuscript. CQ and RN participated in the data analysis and writing of the manuscript. All authors read and approved the final manuscript.

Competing interests

The authors declare that they have no competing interests.

Consent for publication

Not applicable.

Ethics approval and consent to participate

This study has conducted a secondary data analysis of the cross-sectional Neighbourhood Effects on Health and Well-Being (NEHW) study. The Research Ethics Board at St. Michael's Hospital in Toronto, Canada provided ethics approval for this study. All participants provided written informed consent at the time of their interview and were compensated $50 for their participation.

Author details

[1]Faculty of Dentistry, University of Toronto, Toronto, ON, Canada. [2]Department of Health Sciences, Wilfrid Laurier University, 75 University Ave West, Waterloo, ON N2L 3C5, Canada. [3]Centre for Urban Health Solutions, Li Ka Shing Knowledge Institute, St Michael's Hospital, Toronto, ON, Canada. [4]Dalla Lana School of Public Health, University of Toronto, Toronto, ON, Canada.

References

1. Government of Ontario. Get dental care: How to receive government-funded dental care. 2015. http://www.ontario.ca/page/get-dental-care. Accessed 4 Sept 2015.
2. Graves R, Disney J, Stamm J. Comparative effectiveness of flossing and brushing in reducing interproximal bleeding*. J Periodontol. 1989;60(5):243–7.
3. World Health Organization. World health organization oral health fact sheet. 2015. http://www.who.int/mediacentre/factsheets/fs318/en/index.html. Accessed 6 Sept 2015.
4. Lencová E, Broukal Z, Dusková J. Psychosocial, behavioural and oral health indicators–review of the literature. Prague Med Rep. 2006;107(3):305–16.
5. Segura Marcenes W, Sheiham A. The relationship between work stress and oral health status. Soc Sci Med. 1992;35(12):1511–20.
6. Deinzer R, Granrath N, Spahl M, Linz S, Waschul B, Herforth A. Stress, oral health behaviour and clinical outcome. Br J Health Psychol. 2005;10(2):269–83.
7. Wennström A, Boman UW, Ahlqwist M, Björkelund C, Hakeberg M. Perceived mental stress in relation to oral health over time in middle-aged Swedish women. Community Dent Health. 2015;32(4):241–6.
8. Armfield JM, Mejía GC, Jamieson LM. Socioeconomic and psychosocial correlates of oral health. Int Dent J. 2013;63(4):202–9.
9. Hunter W. Oral sepsis as a cause of disease. Br Med J. 1900;2(2065):215–6.
10. Li X, Kolltveit KM, Tronstad L, Olsen I. Systemic diseases caused by oral infection. Clin Microbiol Rev. 2000;13(4):547–58.
11. Barnett ML. The oral-systemic disease connection An update for the practicing dentist. J Am Dent Assoc. 2006;137 suppl 2:5S–6S.
12. Bansal M, Rastogi S, Vineeth NS. Influence of periodontal disease on systemic disease: inversion of a paradigm: a review. J Med Life. 2013;6(2):126.
13. U.S. National Institutes of Health. Chapter 5: Linkages with General Health. US National Institutes of Health, National Institute of Dental and Craniofacial Research. 2015. http://www.nidcr.nih.gov/datastatistics/surgeongeneral/sgr/chap5.htm. Accessed 6 Sept 2015.
14. Rodrigues PH, Progulske-Fox A. Gene expression profile analysis of Porphyromonas gingivalis during invasion of human coronary artery endothelial cells. Infect Immun. 2005;73(9):6169–73.
15. Hahn CL, Schenkein HA, Tew JG. Endocarditis-associated oral streptococci promote rapid differentiation of monocytes into mature dendritic cells. Infect Immun. 2005;73(8):5015–21.
16. Beck JD, Eke P, Heiss G, Madianos P, Couper D, Lin D, Offenbacher S. Periodontal disease and coronary heart disease a reappraisal of the exposure. Circulation. 2005;112(1):19–24.
17. Sheiham A, Watt RG. The common risk factor approach: a rational basis for promoting oral health. Community Dent Oral Epidemiol. 2000;28(6):399–406.
18. Shankardass K. Place-based stress and chronic disease: A systems view of environmental determinants. In: O'Campo P, Dunn JR, editors. Rethinking social epidemiology: towards a science of change. New York: Springer Publishing Company; 2012. p. 117–8.
19. Pearlin LI, Menaghan EG, Lieberman MA, Mullan JT. The stress process. J Health Soc Behav. 1981;22(4):337–56.
20. Sabbah W, Watt RG, Sheiham A, Tsakos G. Effects of allostatic load on the social gradient in ischaemic heart disease and periodontal disease: evidence from the Third National Health and Nutrition Examination Survey. J Epidemiol Community Health. 2008;62(5):415–20.
21. Buchwald S, Kocher T, Biffar R, Harb A, Holtfreter B, Meisel P. Tooth loss and periodontitis by socio-economic status and inflammation in a longitudinal population-based study. J Clin Periodontol. 2013;40(3):203–11.
22. Gomaa N, Glogauer M, Tenenbaum H, Siddiqi A, Quiñonez C. Social-Biological Interactions in Oral Disease: A 'Cells to Society' View. PLoS One. 2016;11(1):e0146218.
23. O'Campo P, Wheaton B, Nisenbaum R, Glazier RH, Dunn JR, Chambers C. The Neighbourhood Effects on Health and Well-being (NEHW) study. Health Place. 2015;31:65–74.

24. Borenstein H, Renahy E, Quiñonez C, O'Campo P. Oral health, oral pain, and visits to the dentist: neighborhood influences among a large diverse urban sample of adults. J Urban Health. 2013;90(6):1064–78.
25. Locker D. Issues in measuring change in self-perceived oral health status. Community Dent Oral Epidemiol. 1998;26(1):41. doi:10.1111/j.1600-0528.1998.tb01923.x.
26. Finlayson TL, Williams DR, Siefert K, Jackson JS, Nowjack-Raymer R. Oral health disparities and psychosocial correlates of self-rated oral health in the National Survey of American Life. Am J Public Health. 2010;100(S1):S246–55.
27. Ansell EB, Rando K, Tuit K, Guarnaccia J, Sinha R. Cumulative adversity and smaller gray matter volume in medial prefrontal, anterior cingulate, and insula regions. Biol Psychiatry. 2012;72(1):57–64.
28. Ramraj C, Quiñonez C. Self-reported cost-prohibitive dental care needs among Canadians. Int J Dent Hyg. 2013;11(2):115–20.
29. Thompson B, Cooney P, Lawrence H, Ravaghi V, Quiñonez C. Cost as a barrier to accessing dental care: findings from a Canadian population-based study. J Public Health Dent. 2014;74(3):210–8.
30. Thompson B, Cooney P, Lawrence H, Ravaghi V, Quiñonez C. The potential oral health impact of cost barriers to dental care: findings from a Canadian population-based study. BMC Oral Health. 2014;14(1):78. doi:10.1186/1472-6831-14-78.
31. Health Canada. Report On The findings Of The oral health component Of The Canadian health measures survey 2007-2009. 1st ed. 2010. http://www.fptdwg.ca/index_htm_files/CHMS-E-summ.pdf. Accessed 6 Sept 2015.
32. Quiñonez C. Why was dental care excluded from Canadian Medicare? Network for Canadian Oral Health Services. 2013. http://ncohr-rcrsb.ca/knowledge-sharing/working-paper-series/content/quinonez.pdf. Accessed 6 Sept 2015.
33. City of Toronto. Dental and oral health services - children and youth. Www1torontoca. 2013. http://www1.toronto.ca/wps/portal/contentonly?vgnextoid=29574485d1210410VgnVCM10000071d60f89RCRD&vgnextfmt=default. Accessed 5 Sept 2015.

15

Dental anxiety in patients with borderline intellectual functioning and patients with intellectual disabilities

Antonio Fallea[1*†], Rosa Zuccarello[2†] and Francesco Calì[3]

Abstract

Background: This study was aimed to investigate the prevalence of dental anxiety in a population of patients with Borderline Intellectual Functioning (BIF) and patients with mild and moderate intellectual disability (ID), and how dental anxiety correlated with their age and gender.

Methods: The sample was made of 700 patients, 287 females and 413 males, 6-to-47 years old, either with borderline intellectual functioning or mild/moderate intellectual disabilities. All patients were administered the Dental Anxiety Scale to assess their level of dental anxiety.

Results: Moderate Anxiety was the most prevalent dental anxiety category for patients with intellectual borderline functioning (15.56 %) and mild intellectual disabilities(18.79 %), while Severe Anxiety was the most prevalent category for patients with moderate intellectual disabilities(21 %). Overall, a statistically significant difference ($p < 0.001$) between the three groups (BIF, Mild-ID and Moderate-ID) was found. Also, the correlation analysis between participants' age and dental anxiety was statistically significant ($p < 0.001$); indeed, dental anxiety turned out to decrease with the increasing of the age. Moreover, the analysis between gender and dental anxiety was found to be significant as well ($p < 0.001$), where higher prevalence of dental anxiety was found in females.

Conclusions: To our knowledge, this is the first study on dental anxiety carried out in the field of intellectual disability. Results show that the higher the level of intellectual disability – and consequently the lower the cognitive functioning – the higher the percentage and the severity of dental anxiety.

Keywords: Dental anxiety scale, Dental fear, Intellectual disabilities

Background

Despite the continuous evolution of dental technologies, dental anxiety has been consistently reported for long time [1]. Dental anxiety, fear and phobia are subcategories of overall anxiety [2].

The level of anxiety and fear when undergoing dental treatments in the general population has been investigated in many countries. In France, Nicolas et al. [3] studied the percentage and severity of dental anxiety in the adult population, using a French version of the Dental Anxiety Scale (DAS). Other countries have also performed studies on dental anxiety, such as Denmark [4], England [5], Finland [6], Saudi Arabia [7], Hungary [8], and Sri Lanka [9]. Several studies have attempted to determine a correlation between fear of the dentist and other factors, in order to prevent some anxiety causes, to recognize anxious subjects and design customized treatments. The variables most often considered to be associated to anxiety were: gender, age, level of education, past dental experiences, fear of pain, parents' attitudes and influence. Results from the previous literature have not always been consistent, albeit the majority of authors agree that anxiety toward dental care is one of the major causes of renouncing dental treatment, thus impacting on social and economic aspects.

A higher prevalence of anxiety in females was found in Turkey, in the studies by Firat et al. [10] and Tunc et al.

* Correspondence: afallea@oasi.en.it
†Equal contributors
[1]Unit of Dentistry, IRCCS Associazione Oasi Maria SS, Troina (EN), Italy
Full list of author information is available at the end of the article

[11], and in India in the study by Mohammed et al. [1]. In Australia as well, Armfield et al. [12] found that the fear of the dentist was prevalent in females and correlated with the age of the sample. Nevertheless, Erten at al. [13] found no statistically significant differences between genders and no meaningful effects of the age on the final results, while a significant correlation with the level of education and the frequency of dental care sessions was reported.

In India, Appukuttan et al. [14] reported a correlation between dental anxiety and painful dental care experiences. In Brazil, the study by Soares et al. [15] aimed to determine anxiety prevalence in dentistry practice by analyzing correlations between previous experiences and history of pain. Honkala et al. [16] measured dental anxiety prevalence in adolescents from Kuwait using the Modified Dental Anxiety Scale (MDAS), whereas Majstorovic et al. [17] compared children's and parents' fears.

Finally, other authors, such as Liddel and Locker [18], in 1997, reported a higher level of dental anxiety in females and young persons than in males and older persons. The same authors, however, stated that the main factor playing a role in determining dental anxiety was the fear of pain, which seems to be more prevalent in males than in females.

Different studies (e.g. Reid et al.) [19], have observed that intellectual disabilities relate with anxiety disorders, therefore, our aim was to investigate how specific anxiety (dental anxiety) relates to ID. In the field of intellectual disabilities (ID), because of the high prevalence of marked functional impairments and psychiatric disorders, the fear of the dentist makes the dental treatment more difficult.

Not many studies have dealt with dental anxiety rehabilitation interventions in the ID population and, to our knowledge, there are no available estimates of its prevalence in this population.

The aim of this study is to investigate dental anxiety and its correlation with age and gender of patients with Borderline Intellectual Functioning (BIF) as well as patients with mild and moderate Intellectual Disabilities (Mild-ID; Moderate-ID respectively). See Table 1 for a detailed description of the different kinds of ID.

Table 1 Borderline Intellectual Functioning and mild/moderate intellectual disabilities

Borderline Intellectual Functioning (BIF)
Borderline Intellectual Functioning is the result of different causes. In the DSM-5, IQ boundaries are no longer part of the classification: a careful assessment of intellectual and adaptive functions and their discrepancies is required, although a clear definition of the disorder is not provided. In the previous versions of the DSM, intellectual functions were measured with IQ testing procedures and cognitive functioning was defined as an IQ range that is higher than that for mental retardation – cut-off value: 1–2 standard deviations from the mean (IQ 71–84).
Mild Intellectual Disability (Mild-ID)
Individuals with Mild intellectual disability present with difficulties in conceptual domains such as, learning academic skills, time and money, with support needed in one or more areas to meet age-related expectations. In adults, abstract thinking, executive function and short-term memory are impaired. In the social domain, individuals are immature in social interactions. Communication, conversation and language are more concrete than expected for age. In the practical domain, individuals need some support with complex daily living tasks. In the previous versions of DSM, the IQ fell between 50–55 and 70.
Moderate Intellectual Disability (Moderate-ID)
In Moderate intellectual disability, progress in conceptual skills occurs slowly especially in language development, academic skills, understanding of time and money, which result markedly limited compared with that of peers and thus requiring continuous support. In the social domain, despite a certain capacity for relationships, social judgment and decision-making abilities are limited. In the practical domain, individuals can care for personal needs; independent employment can be achieved only in jobs that require limited conceptual and communication skills. Maladaptive behaviour is present in a significant minority and causes social problems. In the previous versions of the DSM, the IQ ranged from 35–40 through 50–55.

Methods

Sample

The study was approved by the Ethical Committee of the Research Institute "IRCCS Associazione Oasi Maria SS.", Troina (EN), Italy. Written informed consent was obtained for all participants. The subjects were recruited among 734 consecutive patients referring to diagnostic and rehabilitation services of the IRCCS Associazione Oasi Maria SS. (Troina – EN – Italy), a research institute dealing with treatment and rehabilitation in the field of intellectual disabilities. All participants with BIF and ID were diagnosed by expert qualified psychologists, following the DSM-5 (2014) criteria [20] (See also Table 1). Thirty-four subjects were unable to complete the questionnaire because of their low intellectual level; thus, the final sample consisted of 700 Italian patients, 287 females and 413 males. Their age ranged from 6 to 47 years. The sample was divided into three subgroups: 270 patients with BIF, 330 with Mild-ID, and 100 with Moderate-ID.

Questionnaire

Dental anxiety was assessed using Corah's DAS, 1978 [21]. It's a four-item scale with 5 multiple-choice answers, tapping on dental practice-related situations and assessing anticipatory anxiety as well as assumed anxiety during treatment (Table 2). Answers were scored from 4 to 20 and grouped in 5 categories: No Anxiety (NA, score = 4); Slight Anxiety (SLA, score = 5 to 8); Moderate Anxiety (MA, score = 9 to 12); High Anxiety (HA, score = 13 to 14); Severe Anxiety (SA, score = 15 to 20). Personal data were collected and integrated to the information derived from the scale. Corah's scale was administered through interviews either to patients. Data were collected

Table 2 Dental Anxiety Scale questionnaire (by Corah et al. 1978) [21]

1. If you had to go to the dentist tomorrow, how would you feel about it?

✓I would look forward to it as a reasonably enjoyable experience.

✓I wouldn't care one way or the other.

✓I would be a little uneasy about it.

✓I would be afraid that it would be unpleasant and painful.

✓So anxious, that I sometimes break out in a sweat or almost feel physically sick.

2. When you are waiting in the dentist's office for your turn in the chair, how do you feel?

✓Relaxed.

✓A little uneasy.

✓Tense.

✓Anxious

✓So anxious, that I sometimes break out in a sweat or almost feel physically sick.

3. When you are in the dentist's chair waiting while he gets his drill ready to begin work on your teeth, how do you feel?

✓Relaxed.

✓A little uneasy.

✓Tense.

✓Anxious

✓So anxious, that I sometimes break out in a sweat or almost feel physically sick.

4. You are in the dentist's chair to have your teeth cleaned. While you are waiting and the dentist is getting out the instruments which he will use to scrape your teeth around the gums, how do you feel?

✓Relaxed.

✓A little uneasy.

✓Tense.

✓Anxious.

✓So anxious, that I sometimes break out in a sweat or almost feel physically sick

between January 2014 and May 2015. Our a priori hypotheses were that, in our ID sample, anxiety levels would show differences depending on the gender and age variables.

Statistical analyses

For the statistical analyses, the *chi-square* and Pearson's correlation tests were used. p values less than 0.05 were considered to be statistically significant. The statistical appropriateness of the chi-square tests used in this study was assessed *"a posteriori"* by calculating first the effect size of each test carried-out and then calculating the corresponding sample size required with $\alpha = 0.05$, resulting in an actual power of 98 % and a required sample size of 399 for the 5 × 3 matrix (Table 3) and of 202 for the 5 × 2 matrix (Fig. 1).

Table 3 Anxiety rating in patients with Borderline Intellectual Functioning (BIF) and patients with Intellectual Disabilities (IDs)

	BIF		Mild-ID		Moderate-ID	
Anxiety Rating	N	%	N	%	N	%
No Anxiety (NA)	26	9.63	40	12.12	11	11
Slight Anxiety (SLA)	168	62.22	134	40.61	34	34
Moderate Anxiety (MA)	42	15.56	62	18.79	15	15
High Anxiety (HA)	21	7.78	58	17.58	19	19
Severe Anxiety (SA)	13	4.81	36	10.91	21	21
Total	270	100	330	100	100	100

N Number of patients

Results

Seven hundred Italian participants were analyzed for this study, 287 females and 413 males, with an age range of 6-to-45 years for females (mean age: 18.51, +/− 9.84 SD) and 6-to-47 for males (mean age: 16.93, +/− 8.99 SD). Results obtained from the three subgroups (BIF, Mild-ID and Moderate-ID) are shown in the Table 3.

The highest percentages of the three sample subgroups fell within the SLA range. These percentages decreased with the increase in severity level of IDs. As far as the BIF group is concerned, 15.56 % of patients fell within the MA range, 7.78 % within the HA range and 4.81 % within the SA range. As for the Mild-ID group, the highest percentage was found in the MA range (18.79 %, higher than in BIF); 17.58 % (doubling the BIF) fell within the range of HA range. Finally, the percentage peak for the group with Moderate-ID fell within the SA range (21 %), followed by the HA range (19 %).

Overall, a statistically significant difference (*chi-square* = 53.14, $p < 0.001$) between the three groups (BIF, Mild-ID and Moderate-ID) was found using chi-square test. The correlation analysis (Pearson's *coefficient*) between participants' age and dental anxiety was statistically significant ($r = -0.166$, $p < 0.001$). When the data were analyzed separately by gender it was statistically significant (males: $r = -0.145$, $p < 0.002$; females: $r = -0.209$, $p < 0.001$; see Fig. 2). Fig. 1 shows results from DAS, comparing data obtained by gender, which were found to be significant (*chi-square* = 36.044, $p < 0.001$) using chi-square test. Within the NA range, male patients turned out to be the most numerous. Within the HA, the chart shows how the female percentage was higher than that of males.

Discussion

The higher the ID, as shown in Table 3, the lower the cognitive functioning and the higher the percentage of severity of dental anxiety.

To our knowledge, this is the first epidemiological study on dental anxiety in a population with intellectual disabilities, hence the incomparability of our data with

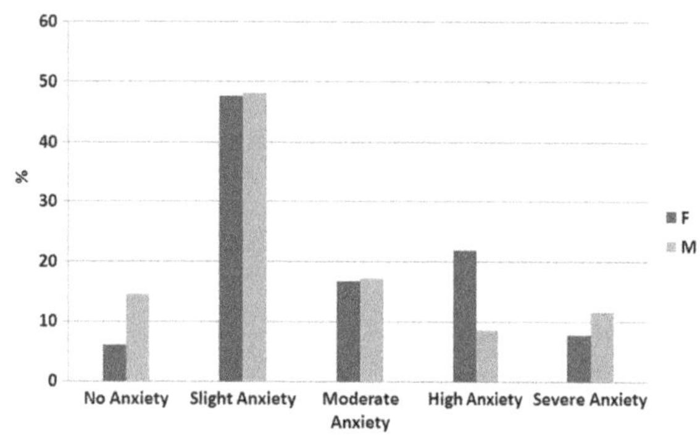

Fig. 1 Anxiety rating (DAS scale) in males/females comparison

those obtained from other authors. However, we have estimated that the increase in dental anxiety, directly proportional to higher levels of intellectual disability, might correlate with the fact that this population has lower psychological resources available to effectively face stressing events, is deprived of several cognitive abilities such as memory, problem-solving and planning skills [22]. As far as phobias are concerned, they seem to be prevalent in individuals with ID. Moreover, a number of phobias are physiologically related to age, therefore some kind of fears in ID individuals might be relating to their developmental levels [23, 24].

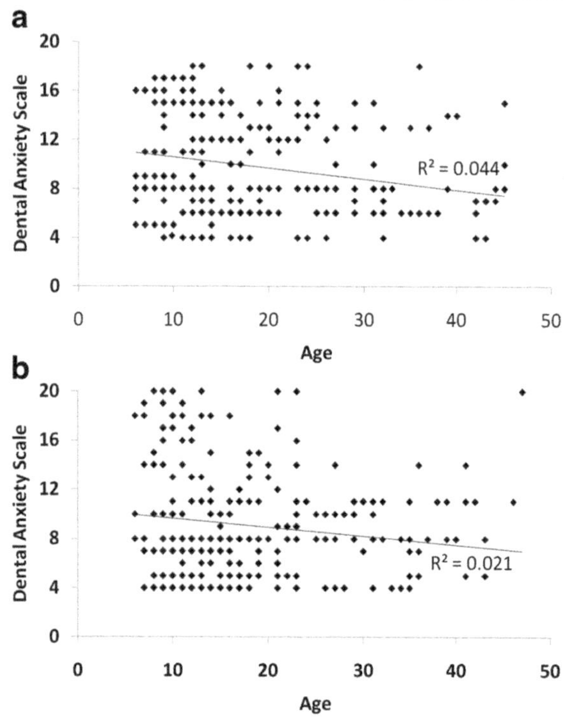

Fig. 2 Scatterplot of the relationship between Dental Anxiety Scale and Age in females (**a**) and males (**b**). Trend line and R^2 values are shown

The significant correlation that was found in this study between the age of the sample and dental anxiety highlights that decreased levels of dental anxiety can be detected more in the older than the younger population. Note that significant correlation didn't change when analysis was performed separately by gender (Fig. 2). In Australia, Armfield et al. [12] carried out a telephone survey with a sample of 7,312 individuals 5 to over 80 years old. The highest prevalence of fear was found in the adult population 40–64 years old, while the lowest in the over-80. These results seem also to confirm a correlation between age and dental anxiety, but are inconsistent with our findings. However, it's worth noting that our sample's age ranges largely differed from Armfield's.Erten et al. [13] administered the DAS questionnaire and the Dental Fear Scale (DFS) to 1,437 patients, divided into 5 groups by age. Authors reported no statistically significant difference between genders and the correlation between dental anxiety and the age of patients did not significantly affected final results; on the other hand, a significant correlation was found with the level of education and frequency of dental treatments of patients.

Further investigations focusing on the frequency of dental treatments and their correlation with age are strongly recommended in future studies, in order to confirm our hypothesis that the older the sample, the higher the frequency of dental treatments and the lower the dental anxiety.

In their Indian study, Mohammed et al. [1] examined a sample of 340 individuals, 180 females and 160 males, 15–65 years old. Results from DAS questionnaire showed high levels of anxiety in the age range 25–35, and low levels of anxiety in the age range 55–65. This finding is consistent with our results. Appukuttan et al. [14] examined a sample of 1,148 patients 18–70 years old, who were administered the MDAS questionnaire to assess their level of anxiety. Younger patients turned out to be more anxious, while dental anxiety seemed to decrease with the age.

Locker and Liddel in 1991 [25] reported the capability of facing certain events based on previous experiences, and the capability of adapting to unavoidable conditions, as relevant factors in reducing dental anxiety; in 1997, these authors [18] also stated that gender and age ranges seemed to be reflected into attitudes towards pain.

Another important finding in our study was that anxiety seemed to be more prevalent in females than in males. Male patients turned out to be the most numerous within the NA range, while within the HA the female percentage was higher than that of males. (see Fig. 1). These statistically significant data are consistently with findings by Armfield et al. [12], Firat et al. [10], Tunc et al. [11], Liddel et al. [18], Mohammed et al. [1], Majstorovic et al. [17], and Appukuttan et al. [14].

The samples recruited in the studies above are largely variable as for the number of participants and the age ranges; nevertheless, the majority of them seem to indicate a prevalence of dental anxiety in female samples.

Honkala et al. [16] in Kuwait found that, in a sample of 757 students 13–15 years old, one third of the girls and 6 % of the boys were afraid of visiting a dentist.

Soares et al. [15] in Brazil, in a sample of 101 children 6–16 years old, found that female children turned out to be three times more anxious than male children.

It might be that the higher prevalence of dental anxiety in female samples is due to women's willingness to overtly admit their fears. Our hypothesis of a prevalence of dental anxiety in female samples is also corroborated by other authors [26–29]. A potential variable for further investigate would be personality styles. Since a correlation exists between personality styles and anxiety levels [30], in future studies, it would be interesting to analyze how specific anxiety (dental anxiety) relates to personality styles.

Conclusions

To our knowledge, this is the first study on dental anxiety carried out in the field of ID. Based on our results, the higher the ID – and therefore the lower the cognitive functioning – and the higher the percentage and severity of dental anxiety. Moreover, the age of the sample significantly correlated with patients' dental anxiety levels. Finally, higher percentages of dental anxiety were found in the female portion of the sample.

Based on our findings, further investigations might include other variables, such as past traumatic dental experiences, and the number of exposures to dental treatments.

Abbreviations

BIF: Borderline intellectual functioning; DAS: Dental anxiety scale; DFS: Dental fear scale; HA: High anxiety; ID: Intellectual disabilities; MA: Moderate anxiety; MDAS: Modified dental anxiety scale; Mild-ID: Mild intellectual disabilities; Moderate-ID: Moderate intellectual disabilities; NA: No anxiety; SA: Severe anxiety; SLA: Slight anxiety

Acknowledgements

We thank Mrs. Rosi Di Giorgio for her editorial support.

Funding

This research study was funded by the Italian Ministry of Health.

Authors' contributions

AF, RZ conceived of the study, and participated in its design and coordination and helped to draft the manuscript. FC performed the statistical analysis. All authors read and approved the final manuscript.

Competing interests

The authors declare that they have no competing interests.

Consent for publication

Not applicable.

Ethics approval and consent to participate

This study has been approved by the Local Ethical Committee of the Associazione Oasi Maria SS. (Troina, EN, Italy) on June 17, 2013 under the reference number CE17/06/2013OASI. Permission to collect data was obtained from the parents or the legal tutor prior to entering the study.

Author details

[1]Unit of Dentistry, IRCCS Associazione Oasi Maria SS, Troina (EN), Italy. [2]Unit of Pedagogy, IRCCS Associazione Oasi Maria SS, Troina (EN), Italy. [3]Laboratory of Molecular Genetics, Unit of Medical Genetics, IRCCS AssociazioneOasi Maria SS, Troina (EN), Italy.

References

1. Mohammed RB, Lalithamma T, Varma DM, Sudhakar KN, Srinivas B, Krishnamraju PV, et al. Prevalence of dental anxiety and its relation to age and gender in coastal Andhra (Visakhapatnam) population. India J Nat SciBiol Med. 2014;5:409–14.
2. Mehrstedt M, John MT, Tönnies S, Micheelis W. Oral health-related quality of life in patients with dental anxiety. Community Dent Oral Epidemiol. 2007;35:357–63.
3. Nicolas E, Collado V, Faulks D, Bullier B, Hennequin M. A national cross-sectional survey of dental anxiety in the French adult population. BMC Oral Health. 2007;10(7):12.
4. Moore R, Birn H, Kirkegaard E, Brødsgaard I, Scheutz F. Prevalence and characteristics of dental anxiety in Danish adults. Community Dent Oral Epidemiol. 1993;21:292–6.
5. Mellor AC. Dental anxiety and attendance in the north-west of England. J Dent. 1992;20:207–10.
6. Lahti S, Vehkalahti MM, Nordblad A, Hausen H. Dental fear among population aged 30 years and older in Finland. Acta Odontol Scand. 2007;65:97–102.
7. Al-Madi EM, AbdelLatif H. Assessment of dental fear and anxiety among adolescent females in Riyadh, Saudi Arabia. Saudi Dent J. 2002;14:77–81.
8. Gáspár J, Tóth Z, Fejérdy L, Kaán B, Fábián TK. Some background data about the high dental anxiety of the Hungarian population. Fogorv Sz. 2004;97:85–9.
9. Ekanayake L, Dharmawardena D. Dental anxiety in patients seeking care at the University Dental Hospital in Sri Lanka. Community Dent Health. 2003;20:112–6.
10. Firat D, Tunc EP, Sar V. Dental anxiety among adults in Turkey. J Contemp Dent Pract. 2006;7:75–82.
11. Tunc EP, Firat D, Onur OD, Sar V. Reliability and validity of the Modified Dental Anxiety Scale (MDAS) in a Turkish population. Community Dent Oral Epidemiol. 2005;33:357–62.
12. Armfield JM, Spencer AJ, Stewart JF. Dental fear in Australia: who's afraid of the dentist? Aust Dent J. 2006;51:78–85.
13. Erten H, Akarslan ZZ, Bodrumlu E. Dental fear and anxiety levels of patients attending a dental clinic. Quintessence Int. 2006;37:304–10.
14. Appukuttan D, Subramanian S, Tadepalli A, Damodaran LK. Dental anxiety among adults: an epidemiological study in South India. N Am J Med Sci. 2015;7:13–8.
15. Soares FC, Souto G, Lofrano M, Colares V. Anxiety related to dental care in children and adolescents in a low-income Brazilian community. Eur Arch Paediatr Dent. 2015;16:149–52.
16. Honkala S, Al-Yahya H, Honkala E, Freeman R, Humphris G. Validating a measure of the prevalence of dental anxiety as applied to Kuwaiti adolescents. Community Dent Health. 2014;31:251–6.
17. Majstorovic M, Morse DE, Do D, Lim LI, Herman NG, Moursi AM. Indicators of dental anxiety in children just prior to treatment. J Clin Pediatr Dent. 2014;39:12–7.
18. Liddell A, Locker D. Gender and age differences in attitudes to dental pain and dental control. Community Dent Oral Epidemiol. 1997;25:314–8.
19. Reid KA, Smiley E, Cooper SA. Prevalence and associations of anxiety disorders in adults with intellectual disabilities. J Intellect Disabil Res. 2011;55:172–81.

20. American Psychiatric Association. Diagnostic and Statistical Manual of Mental Disorders, Fifth Edition (DSM-5). Washington, D.C: APA; 2013. Italian Transl.: American Psychiatric Association. Manuale diagnostico e statistico dei disturbi mentali. Quinta edizione – DSM-5. Milano: Raffaello Cortina, 2014.
21. Corah NL, Gale EN, Illig SJ. Assessment of a dental anxiety scale. J Am Dent Assoc. 1978;97:816–9.
22. Taylor JL, Lindsay WR, Willner P. CBT for people with intellectual disabilities: emerging evidence, cognitive ability and IQ effects. Behav Cogn Psychoth. 2008;36:723–33.
23. Pruijssers, AC, van Meijel B, Maaskant M, Nijssen W, van Achterberg T. The relationship between challenging behaviour and anxiety in adults with intellectual disabilities: a literature review. J Intellect Disabil Res. 2014;58:162–71.
24. Reardon TC, Gray KM, Melvin GA. Anxiety disorders in children and adolescents with intellectual disability: prevalence and assessment. Res Dev Disabil. 2014;36C:175–90.
25. Locker D, Liddell AM. Correlates of dental anxiety among older adults. J Dent Res. 1991;70:198–203.
26. Malvania EA, Ajithkrishnan CG. Prevalence and socio-demographic correlates of dental anxiety among a group of adult patients attending a dental institution in Vadodara city, Gujarat. India Indian J Dent Res. 2011;22:179–80.
27. Marya CM, Grover S, Jnaneshwar A, Pruthi N. Dental anxiety among patients visiting a dental institute in Faridabad. India West Indian Med J. 2012;6:187–90.
28. Nair MA, Shankarapillai R, Chouhan V. The dental anxiety levels associated with surgical extraction of tooth. Int J Dent Clin. 2009;1:17–9.
29. Sanikop S, Agrawal P, Patil S. Relationship between dental anxiety and pain perception during scaling. J Oral Sci. 2011;53:341–8.
30. Bienvenu OJ, Stein MB. Personality and anxiety disorders: a review. J Pers Disord. 2003;17:139–51.

16

Utilising daily diaries to examine oral health experiences associated with dentine hypersensitivity

Jenny M. Porritt[1*], Farzana Sufi[2] and Sarah R. Baker[3]

Abstract

Background: The current investigation examined the determinants of oral health experiences associated with dentine hypersensitivity using prospective diary methodology.

Methods: Staff and students from a large UK university who had self-diagnosed dentine hypersensitivity completed an online daily diary and text survey for 2 weeks recording their mood, oral health-related coping behaviours, coping and pain appraisals, pain experiences and functional limitations. Cross sectional and lagged path analyses were employed to examine relationships.

Results: One hundred one participants took part in the diary study. Participants had a mean age of 26.3 years (range = 18–63) and most were female ($N = 69$). Individuals who used more oral health-related coping behaviours predicted and experienced greater levels of pain on subsequent days. Negative mood also predicted worse pain outcomes. The daily diary method provided a useful avenue for investigating variations in oral health experiences and relationships between variables that can fluctuate daily.

Conclusions: Psychological variables such as coping and mood play an important role in the pain experiences of people with dentine hypersensitivity. The study highlights the benefits of using prospective methods to elucidate the experiences of people with oral conditions.

Keywords: Pain, Dentine hypersensitivity, Coping, Diary, Oral impacts

Background

Dentine hypersensitivity affects approximately half of the population and the pain associated with this condition can limit oral functions such as eating and tooth brushing, which negatively affect individual oral health related quality of life [1–5]. Previous research has revealed that key psychological factors can impact on the quality of life of people with dentine hypersensitivity [6], however, the symptoms of this condition are transient and fluctuate frequently. Moreover, even the self-management of dentine hypersensitivity can vary frequently as people may only use products occasionally. For this reason, study designs that enquire about dentine hypersensitivity need to allow adequate investigation of the everyday experience of the condition and factors that may influence this experience.

Coping may play an important role in an individual's dynamic response to health conditions [7, 8] People may not have consistent styles of coping (e.g. traits) but appear to respond differently in response to specific situations, such as pain [9, 10]. People with dentine hypersensitivity use a number of dentine hypersensitivity-related coping behaviours, which are problem focused (to prevent pain sensations from occurring) such as warming cold food/drinks up before consuming them and the use of toothpaste specially formulated for sensitive teeth [4, 11]. However, there is little research examining how these adaptations are associated with health outcomes in this group of the population. Understanding how well people feel these

* Correspondence: j.porritt@shu.ac.uk
[1]Department of Psychology, Sociology & Politics, Sheffield Hallam University, Collegiate Crescent, Sheffield S10 2BQ, UK
Full list of author information is available at the end of the article

behaviours help them cope with this oral health condition on a daily basis (e.g. perceived coping efficacy) is also extremely important because positive appraisals of coping are associated with less frequent subsequent pain [12, 13]. Such research would require frequent assessments given the specificity of stimuli and responses.

Another possible predictor of daily pain experience is mood [14, 15]. There is convincing evidence that individual mood and pain experience are intrinsically linked. Low mood both predicts future pain experience [16–18] and may be a consequence of prior pain experience [19]. Clearly this is relevant to a condition with recurring symptoms but to date no research has investigated the relationship between mood, oral health-related coping behaviours and the oral health experiences of dentine hypersensitivity, or indeed any other acutely-experienced oral health condition. Research of this nature, which can expose both within and between-person variation in the oral health experiences related to dentine hypersensitivity, could help clinicians and patients develop a better understanding of the impact and effective management of the condition.

Therefore, to deepen our understanding of how pain experiences are associated with a particular health condition it has been proposed that studies should be prospective and provide more reliable data on how psychological variables and health outcomes may be inter-related and the day-to-day impacts of health conditions [14, 20–22]. Clearly such research requires frequent data collection. Daily diaries offer a unique opportunity to capture day-to-day experiences as they occur thus overcoming the recall bias arising when data are collected retrospectively [14]. Therefore, the current investigation had two aims; firstly, to identify the determinants of the daily experiences of oral health in people with dentine hypersensitivity and secondly, to explore how daily diaries can be used to examine the daily impacts caused by this oral condition. The specific research questions were as follows:

- Do oral health-related coping, perceived coping efficacy and pain predictions successfully predict following day health outcomes in individuals with dentine hypersensitivity?
- Are daily mood and oral health behaviours associated with dentine hypersensitivity-related pain experience?
- What are participants' experiences of using daily diary methodology to examine dentine hypersensitivity?

Method

This prospective daily diary study formed part of a larger research project and longitudinal data obtained from a retrospective questionnaire-based study, which examined how key clinical and psychological factors (e.g. illness beliefs) influence the oral health-related and health-related quality of life outcomes in individuals with dentine hypersensitivity, have been published elsewhere [6].

An advertisement for the study was placed on the intranet page of a large UK University available for staff and students to view. Individuals interested in participating in the study completed a pre-study screening questionnaire and a strict exclusion criteria based on Holland et al.'s guidelines [23] were employed. Only those individuals who experienced dentine hypersensitivity on a frequent basis (a minimum of 'several times a week') were invited to participate in the study. Individuals were excluded from participating if they were pregnant/breastfeeding, taking pain medication, experiencing serious and/or painful health conditions, had experience of a dental professional hygiene visit within the past 14 day (or periodontal surgery within the past 6 months), were suffering from xerostomia or if they had a recent history of substance misuse. Individuals who did not regularly access routine dental appointments were also excluded. The screening questionnaire therefore aimed to identify and exclude individuals whose sensitivity could have been caused by alternative factors/clinical pathology.

Participants who met the inclusion criteria were provided with additional study information. Upon obtaining informed consent, participants were asked to complete a text survey at 2 pm every day for 2 weeks. Participants also completed an online daily diary every evening.

The online diary was used to assess dentine hypersensitivity-related coping behaviours, oral health behaviours, perceived coping efficacy, pain predictions and mood on a daily basis.

Dentine hypersensitivity-related coping behaviours were assessed using the mean score from the 12 item 'adaptation' subscale from the revised Dentine Hypersensitivity Experience Questionnaire [11]. An example item is 'Today, when I ate some foods I have made sure they didn't touch certain teeth' (1 = strongly disagree to 7 = strongly agree). The participant's use of sensitivity toothpaste was assessed using the item: 'Have you used sensitivity toothpaste designed for sensitive teeth today (or do you expect to have by the end of the day?' (No = 1, Yes = 2).

Perceived efficacy of pain coping was assessed on a 5-point scale (1 = not at all, 2 = slightly, 3 = somewhat, 4 = moderately, 5 = very much) in response to the item 'Considering all the things you did or thought today to contend with your pain, how much were you able to alleviate your pain by doing or thinking these things?' [14]. Higher scores reflected greater perceived coping efficacy. Pain frequency prediction was assessed via the online diary by asking respondents 'How often do you expect you will experience these sensations tomorrow?'

The Short Positive and Negative Affect Scale (PANAS) assessed daily mood [24] on two primary dimensions:

positive (PANAS-P, 5 items) and negative affect (PANAS-N, 5 items). Items are rated on a 5-point scale (1 = very slightly or not at all to 5 = extremely). Total scores for each mood dimension range from 5 to 25. In the current study state mood was assessed by asking participants to rate how they had felt over the course of the day.

Pain frequency was recorded at two points throughout the day by enquiring 'How many times have you experienced sensations up until 2 pm today?' (text survey) and 'How many times have you experienced sensations since 2 pm today?' (online diary). At the end of each day the online survey assessed overall pain intensity, bothersomeness and tolerability for that day using three visual analogue scales (scored 1–10) (11). Functional limitations were assessed using mean scores from the 4 item 'restrictions' subscale of the DHEQ [11].

On completion of the study participants were asked to provide feedback on their experiences (see Table 1). Items included 'Has taking part in the study changed your experience of sensitivity?' and 'How easy or difficult was it to complete the online daily diaries?'. Participants were paid a small financial incentive for each diary entry submitted.

Models and analysis

Model 1 aimed to examine the relationship between coping, appraisal, pain experience and functional impacts associated with dentine hypersensitivity using lagged analysis (e.g. examining how coping and appraisal from day 1 influenced outcomes on day 2). Model 2 aimed to examine the relationship between mood, coping and pain experience using longitudinal data using a cross sectional method of analysis (mean scores across the 14 days were calculated for each variable). Based on sample size concerns a pre-selection criteria was employed for Model 2 and only significant baseline predictors of pain experience ($p < 0.20$) were entered into the model (pre-selection based on Spearman & Pearson correlations).

The statistical modelling procedure of Path Analysis was used (AMOS 18.0) to test the extent to which the models fitted the dataset. Bootstrapping was conducted and bias corrected 95 % confidence interval (CI) bootstrap percentiles were used to interpret the results. This approach is recommended for sample sizes of less than 20 [25, 26]. Due to the inclusion of a dichotomous variables (use of sensitivity toothpaste: 1 = no; 2 = yes) in both models, the ADF estimation method was used.

Results

Two-hundred and eighty individuals expressed an interest in the study, of whom 101 respondents fulfilled the inclusion criteria. Most were female ($N = 69$) and ranged between 18 years and 63 years (mean age 26.3 years, SD = 8.6).

Scores for the daily variables are summarised in Table 2. Dentine hypersensitivity-related coping behaviours reported most frequently on day one included 'today, when I ate some foods I have made sure they don't touch certain teeth' and 'today, I had to change the way I drank or ate certain things' (54 and 51 %, respectively). Just over a third of participants used sensitivity toothpaste but daily use varied over the 2-week daily diary study (range 34 to 43 %, average across 14 days = 37 %). When asked 'considering all the things you did or thought today to contend with your pain how much were you able to alleviate pain by doing or thinking these things?' 18 % reported 'not at all', 26 % reported 'slightly', 20 % reported 'somewhat', 16 % reported 'moderately' and 19 % reported 'very much' (on day one) revealing a wide variety of responses related to coping efficacy.

The functional limitations reported most frequently on day one of the diary study was 'today, having sensations in my teeth took a lot of pleasure out of eating and drinking' (33 %) and the least frequent limitation reported was 'today, there have been times when I couldn't finish my meal because of the sensations' (7 %). Mean pain frequency over the 2-week diary study was 2.8 (SD = 2.3) and the median pain frequency value ranged between 2 and 3 pain sensations per day. However, the number of pain sensations individuals reported ranged from 0–11 (day 1) to 0–43 (day 8) highlighting the between-person variability in dentine hypersensitivity pain over the 2-week period. Examination of individual trajectories also highlighted considerable within-person variation in pain frequency over the same period (Fig. 1).

Do oral health-related coping, perceived coping efficacy and pain predictions successfully predict following day health outcomes in dentine hypersensitivity?

Model 1: coping strategies, appraisal and following day impacts

The model hypothesised 10 direct pathways based on previous findings from the stress and coping literature. To examine the relationship between oral health coping and outcomes for dentine hypersensitivity, pathways between dentine hypersensitivity-related coping behaviours and the following factors were examined: use of sensitivity toothpaste (path 1); perceived coping efficacy (path 2); pain predictions (path 3) and following day functional limitations and pain frequency (paths 4 & 5). Relationships between use of sensitivity toothpaste and pain predictions (path 6) and the primary outcome of pain were also examined (paths 6 & 7). To examine the role cognitive appraisals play in dentine hypersensitivity relationships between perceived coping efficacy and pain predictions (path 8) and between pain predictions and following day pain frequency (path 9) were examined.

Table 1 Participant methodology feedback

Feedback item within follow-up questionnaire	Number of people ($N = 99$)
Has taking part in the study changed your experience of sensitivity?	
Yes	43
Don't know	20
No	36
How easy or difficult was it to complete the daily text survey?	
Very difficult	0
Difficult	1
Neither easy not difficult	1
Easy	11
Very easy	86
Did completing the text survey mid afternoon help you remember how many times you had experienced sensitive teeth that day?	
Yes	83
Don't know	7
No	9
How easy or difficult was it to complete the onl	
Very difficult	0
Difficult	5
Neither easy not difficult	8
Easy	34
Very easy	52
If, on occasions, you completed the daily diary in the evening how easy or difficult was it to remember the experiences related to your sensitive teeth that day?	
Very difficult	0
Difficult	4
Neither easy not difficult	13
Easy	44
Very Easy	38
If, on occasions, you completed the daily diary following day but before 10 am how easy or difficult was it to remember the experiences related to your sensitive teeth the previous day?	
Very difficult	2
Difficult	10
Neither easy not difficult	15
Easy	37
Very Easy	15
Not applicable	20
If, on occasions, you completed the daily diary after 10 am the following day how easy or difficult was it to remember the experiences related to your sensitive teeth the previous day?	
Very difficult	5
Difficult	7
Neither easy not difficult	17
Easy	18
Very Easy	9
Not applicable	43
How did you feel about the duration of the study?	
I felt the duration of the study was about right	46
I felt two-weeks was too long a period of time to be completing diary entries each day	3
I would have been willing to complete more daily diaries over a longer period of time	50

Finally, the relationship between pain frequency and functional limitations was also investigated to examine whether these health outcomes are inter-related in dentine hypersensitivity sufferers (path 10).

In order to examine whether pathways identified in Model 1 were 'stable' over the 2-week period, seven identical validation models were examined using 'pairings' of discrete daily diary data (e.g. day 1 to 2, days 3 to 4 etc.). Model 1 did not differ significantly from the data across the seven daily pairings ($p > 0.05$), suggesting that the relationships between the key variables remained stable over the study period. Goodness of fit indices were all acceptable (Table 3) and significant pathways for the different days of interest are presented in Table 4. Variables included within the models accounted for between 23 and 66 % of the variance in pain frequency and 30 & 54 % of the variance for functional limitations.

Three significant direct pathways and one indirect pathway remained significant across all daily pairings (Table 4). Individuals using more dentine sensitivity-related coping behaviours were more likely to predict that they would experience more painful sensations the following day and were more likely to experience more functional limitations the following day. The prediction of more sensations was also associated with more pain the following day. Significant total effects, which existed when combining both direct and indirect pathways within the model can be seen in Fig. 2.

Are daily mood and oral health behaviours associated with dentine hypersensitivity-related pain experience?

Model 2: mood, coping and pain experience

Positive mood was unrelated to the other variables so was not entered into the Path Analysis. The nine direct pathways hypothesised within the model were based on previous findings from the stress and coping literature. To examine the relationship between mood, oral health-

Table 2 Daily mean scores

Day	Positive mood mean (SD)	Negative mood mean (SD)	Coping mean (SD)	Efficacy mean (SD)	Pain frequency prediction mean (SD)	Pain frequency mean (SD)	Pain intensity mean (SD)	Pain bothersome-ness mean (SD)	Pain (in) tolerability mean (SD)	Functional limitations mean (SD)
1	15.1 (4.3)	8.4 (4.0)	2.8 (1.0)	2.9 (1.4)	2.8 (2.9)	3.0 (3.0)	3.9 (1.7)	3.4 (1.8)	2.7 (1.7)	2.7 (1.3)
2	14.6 (4.9)	8.3 (4.1)	2.8 (1.3)	2.9 (1.4)	2.5 (1.9)	2.9 (3.2)	3.5 (2.0)	3.3 (2.2)	3.0 (2.1)	2.8 (1.6)
3	14.4 (5.1)	8.3 (4.1)	2.8 (1.2)	2.9 (1.4)	2.3 (1.9)	2.7 (3.5)	3.4 (2.0)	3.1 (2.1)	2.9 (2.1)	2.8 (1.6)
4	14.0 (5.0)	8.8 (4.5)	2.8 (1.2)	3.0 (1.4)	2.3 (1.8)	2.6 (2.6)	3.3 (1.7)	3.0 (1.7)	2.7 (1.7)	2.8 (1.2)
5	13.8 (5.0)	7.4 (3.4)	2.9 (1.5)	3.0 (1.5)	2.3 (1.8)	2.8 (2.6)	3.6 (2.0)	3.3 (2.1)	3.1 (2.0)	3.0 (1.6)
6	14.0 (5.3)	7.1 (3.0)	2.9 (1.2)	3.0 (1.3)	2.3 (1.8)	2.9 (3.7)	3.3 (1.8)	3.1 (1.8)	2.9 (1.7)	3.0 (1.5)
7	14.0 (5.3)	7.8 (3.5)	2.9 (1.2)	3.0 (1.4)	2.3 (1.9)	2.7 (2.7)	3.3 (1.8)	3.0 (1.9)	2.7 (1.7)	3.1 (1.6)
8	14.3 (4.8)	8.0 (4.1)	3.0 (1.4)	3.0 (1.4)	2.5 (2.4)	3.2 (5.0)	3.5 (2.0)	3.1 (2.0)	2.9 (1.9)	3.1 (1.7)
9	14.1 (5.0)	8.0 (4.3)	3.0 (1.4)	2.8 (1.3)	2.4 (1.9)	2.6 (2.3)	3.3 (2.0)	3.3 (2.1)	3.0 (2.0)	3.1 (1.6)
10	14.2 (5.1)	7.7 (4.0)	3.0 (1.4)	2.8 (1.4)	2.3 (1.8)	2.4 (2.4)	3.3 (1.8)	3.0 (1.8)	2.9 (1.8)	2.9 (1.6)
11	15.0 (5.1)	7.4 (3.0)	3.0 (1.4)	3.1 (1.3)	2.4 (2.0)	3.0 (2.6)	3.2 (1.7)	3.0 (1.8)	3.0 (1.9)	2.9 (1.6)
12	15.0 (5.1)	6.9 (3.3)	2.9 (1.4)	2.9 (1.3)	2.2 (1.8)	2.5 (2.7)	3.1 (1.9)	2.9 (1.9)	2.7 (1.4)	2.7 (1.5)
13	13.1 (4.8)	7.3 (3.5)	3.1 (1.3)	2.9 (1.3)	2.4 (1.9)	2.7 (2.9)	3.1 (1.7)	2.8 (1.6)	2.7 (1.6)	2.9 (1.5)
14	13.4 (5.1)	7.7 (4.0)	3.1 (1.3)	2.8 (1.3)	2.4 (1.9)	3.1 (3.2)	3.3 (1.9)	2.9 (1.8)	2.7 (1.9)	3.0 (1.6)
14 day mean	14.2 (3.3)	7.8 (2.5)	2.9 (1.1)	2.9 (1.1)	2.4 (1.7)	2.8 (2.3)	3.3 (1.3)	3.1 (1.4)	2.8 (1.4)	2.9 (1.1)

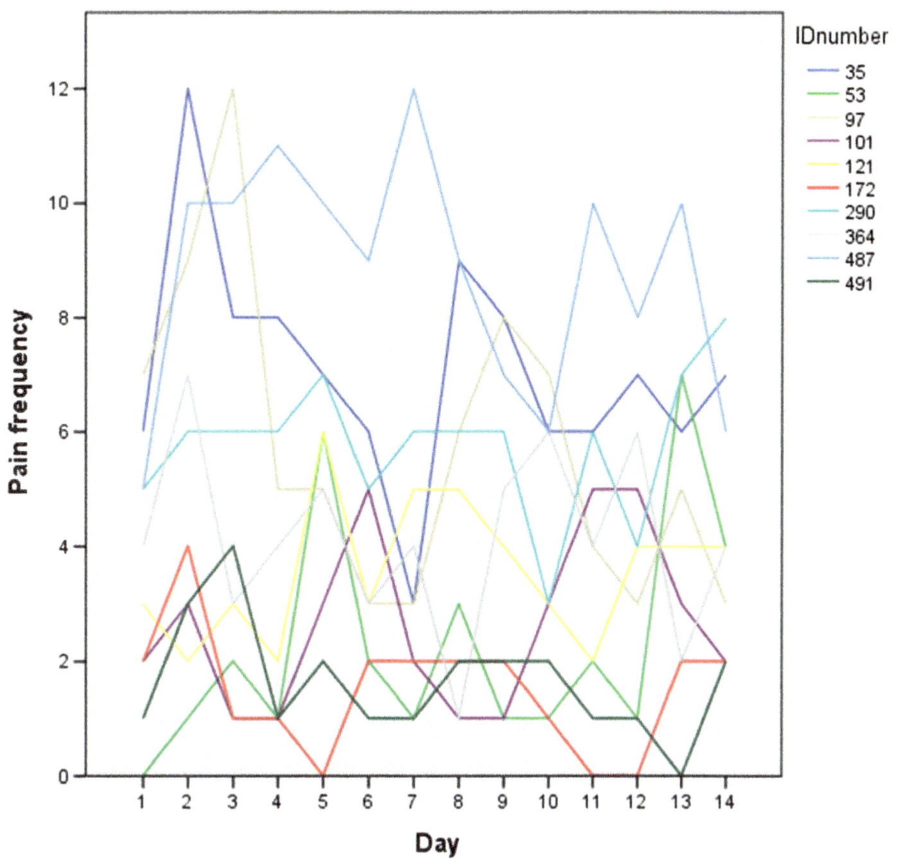

Fig. 1 Random sample (10 %) of individuals' pain frequency trajectories

Table 3 Goodness of fit indices for Model 1 and Model 2

Model 1 ($N = 101$)	Goodness of fit indices					
	X^2/df ($p > .05$)	CMIN/df (<2.0)	IFI (>0.95)	RMSEA (<0.08)	SRMR (<0.08)	Criteria fitted
Day 1–2	**3.93/5 ($p = 0.56$)**	**0.79**	**1.02**	**0.00**	**0.07**	5
Day 3–4	**2.11/5 ($p = 0.83$)**	**0.42**	**1.09**	**0.00**	**0.03**	5
Day5–6	**3.16/5 ($p = 0.68$)**	**0.63**	**1.04**	**0.00**	**0.03**	5
Day7–8	**4.57/5 ($p = 0.47$)**	**0.91**	**1.01**	**0.00**	**0.04**	5
Day9–10	**2.99/5 ($p = 0.70$)**	**0.60**	**1.02**	**0.00**	**0.03**	5
Day 11–12	**6.33/5 ($p = 0.28$)**	**1.26**	**0.99**	**0.05**	**0.06**	5
Day13–14	**4.09/5 ($p = 0.54$)**	**0.82**	**1.02**	**0.00**	**0.05**	5
Model 2 ($N = 101$)	**1.95/3 ($p = 0.58$)**	**0.65**	**1.00**	**0.00**	**0.03**	5

Note: Figures in bold are those which meet the model-fitting criteria

Table 4 Significant pathways between oral health coping, appraisal and following day impacts (Model 1)

Daily models ($N = 101$)	Significant pathways	Total β value (bootstrap bias corrected 95 % CI)	Indirect β value (bootstrap bias corrected 95 % CI)	Direct β value (bootstrap bias corrected 95 % CI)
Days 1–2	D1 coping[a] → D1 perceived efficacy	.27** (.06 to .45)	–	.27** (.06 to .45)
	D1 coping → D1 pain prediction	.27** (.07 to .70)	n/s	.30* (.06 to .72)
	D1 coping → D2 pain frequency	.45** (.24 to .65)	.18* (.05 to .84)	.27* (.03 to .41)
	D1 coping → D2 functional	.53** (.32 to .67)	.18* (.05 to .35)	.35* (.16 to .54)
	D1 pain prediction → D2 pain frequency	.68** (.46 to .83)	–	.68** (.46 to .83)
Days 3–4	D3 coping → D3 pain prediction	.31** (.10 to .50)	–	.31** (.10 to.50)
	D3 coping → D4 pain frequency	.23* (.03 to .41)	.20** (.07 to .34)	n/s
	D3 coping → D4 functional	.32** (.08 to .50)	.10* (.02 to .20)	.22* (.02 to .38)
	D3 pain prediction → D4 pain frequency	.61** (.35 to .76)	–	.61** (.35 to .76)
	D3 pain prediction → D4 functional	.28** (.11 to .44)	.28** (.11 to .44)	-
	D4 pain frequency → D4 functional	.46** (.24 to .62)	–	.46** (.24 to .62)
Days 5–6	D5 coping → D5 pain prediction	.34** (.15 to .50)	n/s	.33** (.13 to .50)
	D5 coping → D6 pain frequency	–	.22** (.06 to .35)	n/s
	D5 coping → D6 functional	.38** (.17 to .54)	n/s	.31** (.14 to .46)
	D5 pain prediction → D6 pain frequency	.63* (.21 to .74)	–	.63** (.21 to .74)
	D5 pain predictions → D6 functional	.35* (.23 to .43)	.35* (.23 to .43*)	–
	D6 pain frequency → D6 functional	.56** (.41 to .65)	–	.56** (.41 to .65)
Days 7–8	D7 coping → D7 pain prediction	.30** (.13 to .46)	–	.29** (.11 to .44)
	D7 coping → D8 functional	.45** (.24 to .60)	–	.42** (.25 to .56)
	D7 coping → pain frequency	–	.15* (.03 to .26)	n/s
	D7 pain prediction → D8 pain frequency	.46* (.33 to .67)	–	.46* (.33 to .67)
	D7 pain predictions → D8 functional	.16* (.06 to .23)	.16* (.06 to .23)	–
	D8 pain frequency → D8 functional	.34** (.15 to .46)	–	.34** (.15 to .46)
Days 9–10	D9 coping → D9 pain prediction	.37** (.18 to .53)	n/s	.34** (.14 to 51)
	D9 coping → D10 pain frequency	.26** (.07 to .42)	.24** (.09 to .38)	n/s
	D9 coping → D10 functional	.40** (.40 to .71)	.06** (.02 to .15)	.52** (.33 to .66)
	D9 pain prediction → D10 pain frequency	.69* (.40 to .80)	–	.69* (.40 to .80)
	D9 pain predictions → D10 functional	.17** (.05 to .28)	.17** (.05 to .28)	–
	D10 pain frequency → D10 functional	.25** (.09 to .41)	–	.25** (.09 to .41)
Days 11–12	D11 coping → D11 pain prediction	.41** (.22 to .56)	n/s	.35** (.18 to .51)
	D11 coping → D12 pain frequency	.36** (.18 to .53)	.31** (.18 to .44)	n/s
	D11 coping → D12 functional	.68** (.42 to .82)	.11* (.02 to .19)	.57** (.31 to .77)
	D11 use of toothpaste → D12 pain frequency	.29** (.09 to .47)	n/s	.19* (.02 to .37)
	D11 use of toothpaste → D12 functional	.09* (.02 to .20)	.09* (.02 to .20)	–
	D11 pain prediction → D12 pain frequency	.62* (.41 to .80)	n/s	.64* (.41 to .80)
	D12 pain frequency → D12 functional	.31* (.01 to .50)	n/s	.31* (.01 to .50)
Days 13–14	D13 coping → D13 pain prediction	.41** (.24 to .57)	n/s	.37** (.18 to .55)
	D13 coping → D14 pain frequency	.40** (.22 to .61)	.28** (.17 to .44)	n/s
	D13 coping → D14 functional	.61** (.40 to .76)	.14* (.00 to .27)	.47** (.24 to .72)
	D13 pain prediction → D14 pain frequency	.69** (.56 to .83)	–	.69** (.56 to .83)

[a]dentine hypersensitivity-related coping behaviours
*$p < 0.05$, **$p < 0.01$

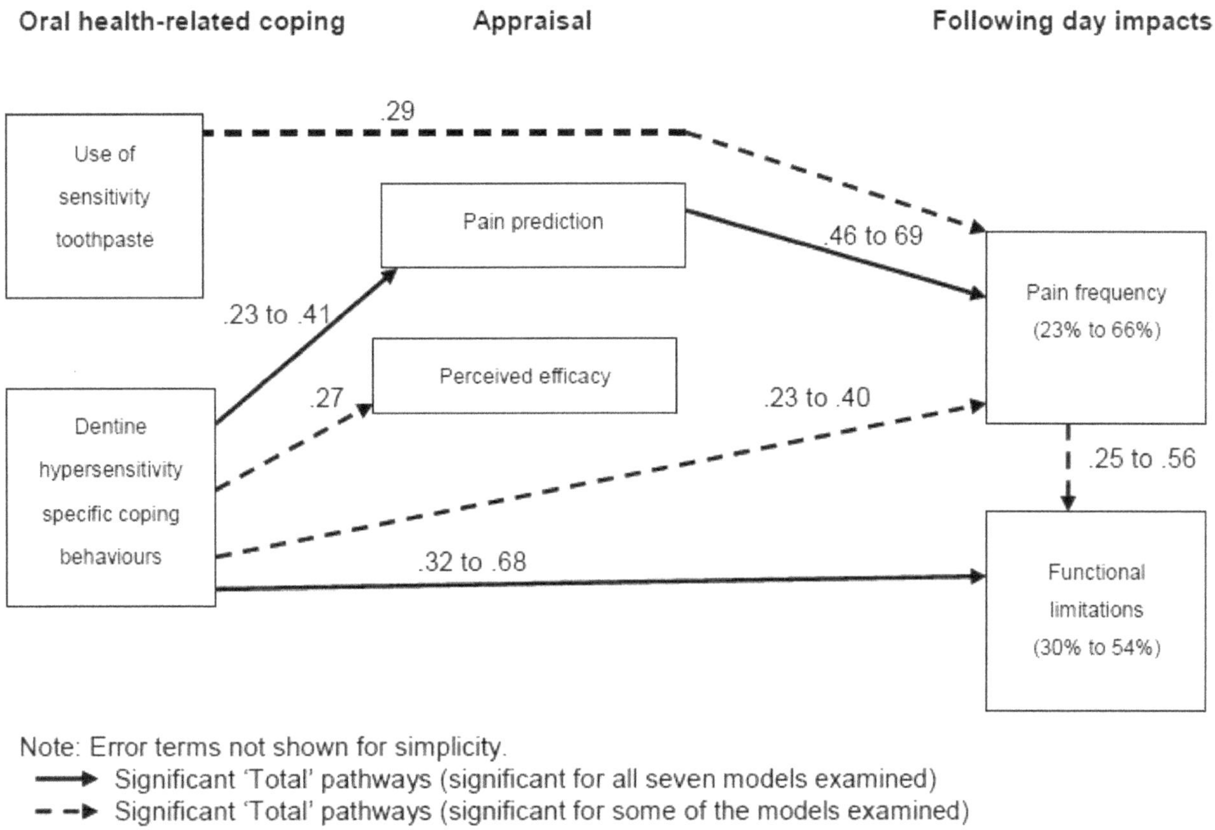

Fig. 2 Significant total pathways between oral health coping behaviours, appraisal and following day impacts proposed within Model 1

related coping and oral health experiences five direct pathways between negative mood and use of sensitive toothpaste (path 1), pain frequency (path 2), pain intensity (path 3), pain tolerability (path 4) and pain bothersomeness (path 5) were examined. The relationship between the use of sensitivity toothpaste and pain was also examined (path 6). Finally, to examine how pain experiences of dentine hypersensitivity are inter-related, relationships between pain frequency and pain intensity (pain 7), bothersomeness (path 8) and tolerability (path 9) were all examined.

Model 2 did not differ significantly from the observed data (x2 = 1.95, df = 3, $p = 0.58$) and the goodness of fit indices were all excellent (Table 3). The variables included within the model accounted for 12 % of variance in pain frequency, 21 % of the variance for pain intensity, 13 % of the variance for pain tolerability and 18 % of the variance in pain bothersomeness.

The model contained five significant direct pathways and six indirect pathways (Table 5). More negative mood throughout the 2-week period was associated with more frequent painful sensations. Frequent sensations were associated with more intense pain, bothersomeness and less tolerability. Individuals who typically used sensitivity toothpaste reported more frequent pain. Significant total effects, which existed when combining both direct and indirect pathways can be seen in Fig. 3.

Participants' experiences of using daily diary methodology to examine dentine hypersensitivity

The number of participants who completed daily diaries on each of the study days ranged from 98 to 101. Almost half of participants felt that taking part in diary study had changed their experience of sensitivity, largely because it changed their awareness of how frequently they experienced their sensations:

> *"It has made me realise that I do not feel sensations as often as I thought"*

> *"I think I notice any sensations in my teeth more, and am probably generally more aware of my oral health as a result"*

Some perceptions and understanding of the oral condition had changed since participating in the study (e.g. understanding the triggers of dentine sensitivity):

> *"I've begun to notice that it varies with my mood, I'm not sure how much one influences the other!"*

Table 5 Significant direct, indirect and total pathways between mood, toothpaste use and pain experience proposed within Model 2

Significant pathways	Direct pathways		Indirect pathways		Total pathways	
	β value	Bootstrap bias corrected 95 % CI	β value	Bootstrap bias corrected 95 % CI	β value	Bootstrap bias corrected 95 % CI
Negative mood → Use of sensitivity toothpaste	-.08	-.29 to .18	–	–	-.08	-.29 to .18
Negative mood → Pain frequency	.24*	.05 to .42	-.02	-.09 to .05	.23*	.02 to .43
Negative mood → Pain intensity	.12	-.06 to .37	.09*	.02 to .20	.21*	.02 to .54
Negative mood → Pain intolerability	.17	-.07 to .45	.06*	.01 to .16	.23	-.02 to .51
Negative mood → Pain bothersomeness	.18	-.00 to .42	.08*	.01 to .17	.26*	.06 to .50
Use of sensitivity toothpaste → Pain frequency	.26*	.04 to .47	–	–	.26*	.04 to .47
Use of sensitivity toothpaste → Pain intensity	–	–	.11**	.02 to .25	.11**	.02 to .25
Use of sensitivity toothpaste → Pain intolerability	–	–	.07**	.01 to .18	.07**	.01 to .18
Use of sensitivity toothpaste → Pain bothersomeness	–	–	.09**	.02 to .20	.09**	.02 to .20
Pain frequency → Pain intensity	.41**	.22 to .58	–	–	.41**	22 to .58
Pain frequency → Pain intolerability	.28*	.07 to .45	–	–	.28*	.07 to .45
Pain frequency → Pain bothersomeness	.35**	.18 to .51	–	–	.35**	.18 to .51

*$p < 0.05$, **$p < 0.01$

For some individuals, participating had helped them develop ways of coping with the pain or accepting their condition:

> *"Made me think about the frequency and methods of dealing with it"*

Most participants felt that receiving the text survey mid-afternoon helped them recall information on their pain experiences and found the daily diary study easy to complete. However, they found it more difficult to complete the following day.

Discussion

This research revealed how psychological factors may play an important role in the day-to-day oral experiences of people with dentine hypersensitivity. These factors, coping strategies and experiences, fluctuated within individuals throughout the study period and thus the daily diary approach allowed sufficient precision to detect associations between these fluctuations.

Previous diary research has found mixed results in relation to the use of coping and subsequent pain levels. For example, the use of cognitive reframing strategies in the morning predicted less evening pain experience, whereas morning use of active problem solving predicted more evening pain [27]. Within the current study, the use of dentine hypersensitivity-related coping behaviours predicted worse pain and functional limitations the following day. However, there was some evidence that greater use of specific coping adaptations were positively associated with higher levels of perceived coping efficacy.

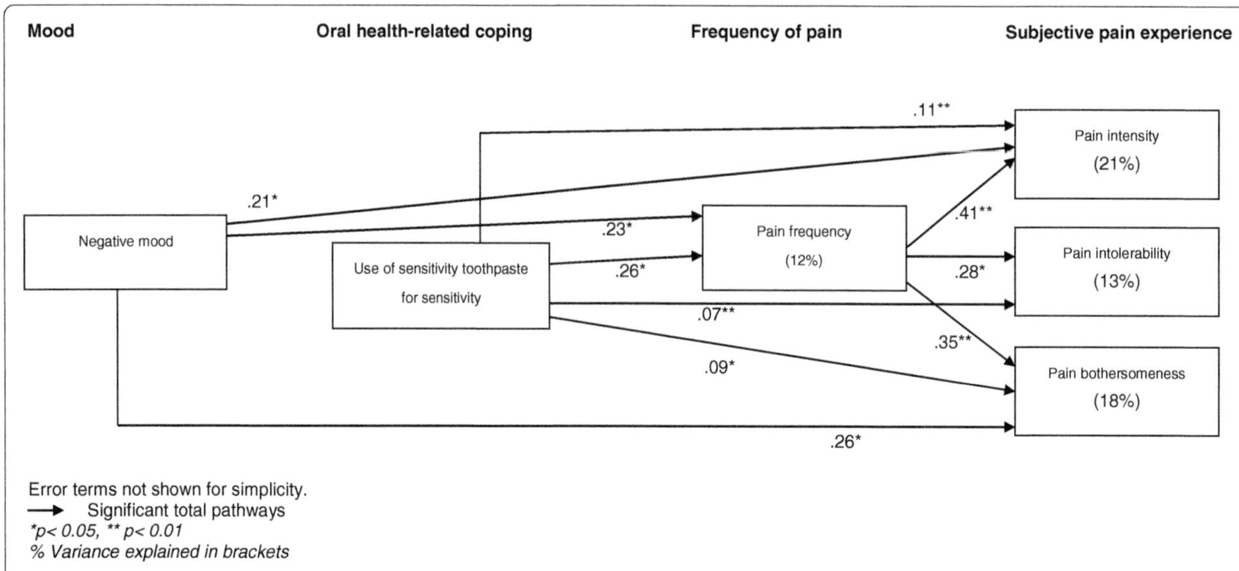

Fig. 3 Significant total pathways between mood, oral health coping behaviours and pain experience in individuals with dentine hypersensitivity (Model 2)

Therefore, an explanation for the relationship between coping and following day pain experience could be that those individuals who felt the need to use dentine sensitivity related-coping behaviours were already experiencing more pain and found the coping adaptations did help them control this pain. This highlights the importance of examining individuals' coping appraisals as a mechanism for aiding our understanding into the complex, and probable bi-directional, nature of the relationship between coping and pain.

Pain predictions were strongly associated with subsequent pain experience, indicating that despite its fluctuating nature, pain is predictable in dentine hypersensitivity. The mechanisms through which pain predictions influence subsequent pain experience warrants further examination [28]. Individuals with worse negative daily mood were also more likely to report more pain, of a higher intensity, less tolerability and greater bothersomeness. This is the first research to highlight the role of mood in individuals' experiences of this specific type of dental pain. These findings are compatible with previous research which has found similar effects in relation to chronic pain [17, 18]. Whilst the causality of the relationship between mood and pain is subject to debate, state negative affect can increase symptom perception and reporting [29, 30].

The explained variance in pain frequency and functional limitations differed considerably across the 2-week period (23–66 % and 30–54 %,respectively). This variation in the explanatory power of coping and appraisal factors on dentine hypersensitivity experiences provides evidence that the factors and processes that influence these daily oral health experiences may also fluctuate on a daily basis. It is also important to recognise that there were only small to moderate associations between pain frequency and the other subjective elements of pain experience reported (intensity, bothersomeness and intolerability). This suggests that only measuring the frequency with which someone experiences pain may fail to provide a reliable and holistic account of the individual's pain experience.

A major strength of the current study was its prospective design of the research with frequent data collection, which is less likely to be subject to recall error or bias. This success was reflected in the high response rate throughout the daily data collection and the positive feedback from participants regarding different aspects of the study's design which is consistent with findings from studies using similar methods [31, 32]. However, participants' response times became increasingly delayed during the study, supporting previous research describing the cumulative burden of completing daily diaries and decreased reliability of responses over time [31]. The data revealed that most individuals felt the text surveys had acted as a useful aid to their pain recall throughout the day, highlighting the usefulness of signal-contingent methods in daily diaries [33]. Incentives were used in the current study and this could have also contributed to the high response rate. The use of incentives are associated with higher levels of engagement levels in research studies which employ diary methods [34].

The potential value of utilising e-diaries (e.g. via a phone app) as a clinical assessment tool could also be examined in future research. Prospective diary methods could be used to collect accurate data on patient's dentine hypersensitivity-related pain and coping, this information could aid the patient's and clinician's understanding of the patient's own unique experience of the condition and the possible factors that may help them effectively manage their symptoms. However, further evaluation of the feasibility and utility of using this type of assessment tool in a clinical setting is required.

Whilst these data start to explain the experience of dentine hypersensitivity, the research was not without limitations. Individuals were university students and staff and may not represent the general population and this could affect the generalisability of the findings. For example, the high response rate and level of engagement with the daily diaries may not be replicated in studies that use different groups of the population. The methods employed (e.g. internet diaries and text surveys) also excluded individuals who did not have daily access to the internet and a mobile phone, which could have further biased the sample.

It is important to recognise that participants self-diagnosed their dentine hypersensitivity and no clinical examinations were undertaken to identify alternative clinical pathologies which could have been responsible for pain experiences. Oral conditions, which have symptoms similar to dental hypersensitivity, should be excluded to ensure an accurate diagnosis of dentine hypersensitivity can be made [23]. Within the current study it is possible that some individuals could have been experiencing oral pain caused by a different pathology. However, a pre-study screening questionnaire and strict exclusion criteria based on Holland et al.'s guidelines [23] were employed. Irregular dental attendance was one of the exclusion criteria employed to minimise the likelihood that individuals with untreated dental disease/conditions (e.g. cavities or trauma) could participate in the study. It is also possible that participants self-monitoring effects could have influenced the data obtained. Self-monitoring is an intervention in its own right and several psychological models highlight the impact selective attention to bodily symptoms can have on the experiencing of symptoms [35, 36]. Therefore, the issues associated with self-monitoring should be recognised by researchers and clinicians who employ daily diary methods.

Conclusions

These data offer unique insights into the experiences of people with dentine hypersensitivity. The study revealed how dentine hypersensitivity experiences fluctuate on a daily basis, which has significant implications for the how these oral health experiences can be measured in a meaningful and reliable way. The use of prospective methods of data collection, such as daily diaries, can develop understanding of the day-to-day impacts caused by oral conditions and the complex relationships that exist between transient states and experiences such as psychological factors and dental pain. This information can place clinicians in a stronger position to manage their patients' oral health conditions.

Abbreviations

ADF: Asymptotically distribution-free; DHEQ: Dentine hypersensitivity experience questionnaire; PANAS: Positive and negative affect scale

Acknowledgements

The authors would like to thank the individuals who shared their time to participate in this study and Professor Peter Robinson for his guidance and feedback that greatly improved the manuscript.

Funding

This research was funded by GlaxoSmithKline Consumer Healthcare (grant number: R/125710-1).

Authors' contributions

SB, JP and FS contributed to the conception and design of the study. JP was responsible for the collection, analysis and interpretation of data. JP and SB were involved in drafting and revising the manuscript. All authors have given approval for the manuscript to be published.

Competing interests

FS is employed by GlaxoSmithKline Consumer Healthcare. JP and SB declare they have no competing interests.

Consent for publication

Not applicable.

Ethics approval and consent to participate

Informed written consent was obtained from participants prior to their involvement in the research. Ethical approval for the study was obtained from the University of Sheffield Research Ethics Committee.

Author details

[1]Department of Psychology, Sociology & Politics, Sheffield Hallam University, Collegiate Crescent, Sheffield S10 2BQ, UK. [2]Clinical Research (Oral Care), GlaxoSmithKline Consumer Healthcare, St Georges Avenue, Weybridge, Surrey KT13 0DE, UK. [3]School of Clinical Dentistry, University of Sheffield, 19 Claremont Crescent, Sheffield S10 2TA, UK.

References

1. Cummins D. Dentin hypersensitivity: from diagnosis to a breakthrough therapy for everyday sensitivity relief. J Clin Dent. 2009;20:1–9.
2. Docimo R, Montesani L, Maturo P, DeVizio W, Zhang YP, Cummins D, Dibart S, Mateo LR. Comparing the Efficacy in Reducing Dentin Hypersensitivity of a New Toothpaste Containing 8/0% Arginine, Calcium Carbonate, and 1450ppm Fluoride to a Commercial Sensitive Toothpaste Containg 2% Potassium Ion: An Eight-Week Clinical Study in Rome, Italy. J Clin Dent. 2009;20(4):137–43.
3. Gibson B, Boiko OV, Baker SR, Robinson PG, Barlow APS, Player T, Locker D. The everyday impact of dentine sensitivity: personal and functional aspects. Soc Sci Dent. 2010;1:11–21.
4. Gillam DG, Seo HS, Bulman JS, Newman HN. Perceptions of dentine hypersensitivity in a general practice population. J Oral Rehabil. 1999;26:710–4.
5. Irwin CR, McCusker P. Prevalence of dentine hypersensitivity in a general dental population. J Ir Dent Assoc. 1997;43:7–9.
6. Porritt JM, Sufi F, Barlow A, Baker SR. The role of illness beliefs and coping in the adjustment to dentine hypersensitivity. J Clin Periodontol. 2014;41:60–9.
7. Leventhal H, Diefenbah MA, Leventhal EA. Illness Cognition: using common sense to understand treatment adherence and affect cognition interactions. Cogn Ther Res. 1992;16:143–63.
8. Leventhal H. Findings and theory in the study of fear communications. Adv Exp Soc Psychol. 1970;5:119–86.
9. Brown GK, Nicassio PM. Development of a questionnaire fot the assessment of active and passive coping strategies in chronic pain patients. Pain. 1987;31:53–64.
10. Norman SA, Thompson R, Vedhara K. A prospective examination of illness beliefs and coping in patients with type 2 diabetes. Br J Health Psychol. 2007;12:621–38.
11. Boiko OV, Baker SR, Gibson BJ, Locker D, Sufi F, Barlow APS, Robinson PG. Construction and validation of the quality of life measure for dentine hypersensitivuity (DHEQ). J Clin Periodontol. 2010;37:973–80.
12. Hagger MS, Orbell S. A Meta-analytic review of the common-sense model of illness representations. Pyschol Health. 2003;18:141–84.
13. Evans DD, Carter M, Panico R, Kimble L, Morlock JT, Spears MJ. Characteristics and predictors of short-term outcomes in individuals self-selecting yoga or physical therapy for treatment of chronic low back pain. PM R. 2010;2:1006–15.
14. Tennen H, Affleck G, Zautra A. Depression history and coping with chronic pain: a daily process analysis. Health Psychol. 2006;25:370–9.
15. Williamson GM, Schultz R. Physical illness and symptoms of depression among among elderly patients. Psychol Aging. 1992;7:343–51.
16. Zautra AJ, Marbach JJ, Raphael KG, Dohenwend BP, Lennon MC, Kenny DA. The exmaination of myofascial face pain and its relationship to psychological distress. Health Psychol. 1995;14:223–31.
17. Feldman SI, Downey G, Schaffer-Neitz R. Pain, negative mood, and perceived support in chronic pain patients: a daily diary study of people with reflex sympathetic dystrophy syndrome. J Consult Clin Psychol. 1999;67:776–85.
18. Tang NK, Salkovski PM, Hodges A, Wright KJ, Hanna M, Hester J. Effects of mood on pain responses and pain tolerance: an experimental study in chronic back pain patients. Pain. 2008;138:392–401.
19. Glover J, Dibble SL, Dodd MJ, Miaskowski C. Mood states of oncology outpatients: does pain make a difference? J Pain Symptom Manage. 1995;10:120–8.
20. Galli U, Ettlin DA, Palla S, Ehlert U, Gaab J. Do illness perceptions predict pain-related disability and mood in chronic orofacial patients? A 6-month follow-up study. Eur J Pain. 2010;14:550–8.
21. Hobro N, Weinman J, Hankins M. Using the self-regulatory model to cluster chronic pain patients: the first step towards identifying relevant treatments? Pain. 2004;108:276–83.
22. Tennen H, Affleck G. Daily processes in coping with chronic pain: methods and analytic strategies. In: Zeidner M, Endler N, editors. Handbook of coping. New York: Wiley; 1996. p. 151–80.
23. Holland GR, Narhi MN, Addy M, Gangarosa L, Orchardson R. Guidelines for the design and conduct of clinical trials on dentine hypersensitivity. J Clin Periodontol. 1997;24(11):808–13.
24. Mackinnon A, Jorm AF, Christensen H, Korten AE, Jacomb PA, Rodgers B. A short form of the Positive and Negative Affect Schedule: evaluation of factorial validity and invariance across demograohic variables in a community sample. Personal Individ Differ. 1999;27:405–16.
25. Efron B, Tibshirani R. An introduction to the bootstrap. New York: Chapman & Hall; 1993.
26. Hoyle RH, Panter AT. Writing about structural equation models. In: Hoyle RH, editor. Structural equation modelling. Thousand Oaks: Sage; 1995. p. 158–76.
27. Holtman S, Newth S, Delongis A. The role of social support in coping with daily pain among patients with rheumatoid arthritis. J Health Psychol. 2004;9:677–95.

28. Finan PH, Zautra AJ, Tennen H. Daily diaries reveal influence of pessimism and anxiety on pain prediction patterns. Psychol Health. 2008;23:551–68.
29. Charles ST, Almeida DM. Daily reports of symptoms and negative affect: Not all symptoms are the same. Psychol Health. 2006;21:1–17.
30. Watson D, Pennebaker JW. Health complaints, stress, and distress: exploring the central role of negative affectivity. Psychol Rev. 1989;96:234–54.
31. Lyons KE, Pahwa R. Electronic motor function diary for patients with Parkinson's disease: a feasibility study. Parkinsonism Relat Disord. 2007;13:304–7.
32. Quinn P, Goka J, Richardson H. Assessment of an electronic daily diary in patients with overactive bladder. BJU Int. 2003;91:647–52.
33. Affleck G, Tennen H, Armeli S, Zautra A. Multilevel daily process designs for consulting and clinical psychology: a preface for the perplexed. J Consult Clin Psychol. 1999;67:746–54.
34. Lynn P. The impact of incentives on response rates to personal interview surveys: role and perceptions of interviewers. Int J Public Opin R. 2001;13(3):326–36.
35. Goodwin L, Fairclough SH, Poole HM. A cognitive-perceptual model of symptom perception in males and females: the roles of negative affect, selective attention, health anxiety and psychological job demands. J Health Psychol. 2013;18(6):848–57.
36. Kolk AM, Hanewald GJFP, Schagen S. Gijsbers van Wijk CMT. A symptom perception approach to common physical symptoms. Soc Sci Med. 2003;57(12):2343–54.

17

Patterns of use of oral health care services and barriers to dental care among ambulatory older Chilean

Rodrigo Mariño[1*] and Rodrigo A. Giacaman[2]

Abstract

Background: This paper describes the patterns of use of oral health care services among ambulant 65-74 years or older adults, living in the Maule Region of Chile, factors associated with their use of oral health care services, and self-reported barriers to using oral health care services.

Methods: Four hundred and thirty eight older adults, aged 65–74 years, living independently in the community were orally examined and underwent an oral health interview. Recency of visits was related to the use of oral health care services within the 12 months prior to the study.

Results: 31.5% of respondents had used oral health services in the previous 12 months. In multivariate analyses, those living in rural areas (*OR* = 2.15; 95% CI:1.27–3.63), and those with secondary or higher education (*OR* = 1.65; 95% CI:1.03–2.64) visited the dentist in the last 12 months in a higher proportion. Those with more filled tooth-surfaces were more likely to have visited the dentist (*OR* = 4.02; 95% CI;3.58–4.51). Participants who self-reported dental fear, were less likely to have visited the dentist than those who did not (*OR* = 0.43; 95% CI;0.24–0.76).

Conclusion: Comparing with existing data in Chile, participants in this study appear to have a slightly lower attendance. Findings question assumptions regarding oral health services utilization by rural residents and highlight the need to identify factors that influence the use of oral health services by older Chileans.

Keywords: Oral health services utilization, Older adults, Chile

Background

Developments in medicine, improved social and economic conditions, in the Chilean population, have resulted in improvements of oral health, and, therefore, tooth retention, particularly, among Chilean older adults [1, 2], generating a growing need for them to seek regular oral health care. In addition, an increase in the life expectancy of the population, and its geographic distribution have resulted in an increased proportion of older people living in rural localities, with these regions ageing more rapidly than their counterparts in metropolitan areas [3]. This epidemiological and demographic transition has dramatically changed the nature of oral health care needs and it poses an oral health challenge. This may result in increased inequalities in access to oral health care services and in oral health outcomes, particularly among those who reside in rural areas [4, 5]. Such inequity in access to and utilization of oral health care services poses a major threat to the health and oral health of older Chileans.

Poor oral health impacts on the well-being and overall quality of life [6]. Adequate access to oral health care services becomes essential, as it provides opportunities for health promotion and disease prevention and early diagnosis, and treatment of oral diseases and conditions. Additionally, access to health care services is beneficial for the maintenance of good oral health, and health educational and awareness [7]. This is particularly the case when considering older populations. An equitable use of health care by the population is one of the most important goals of any health care system and is a human right. Consequently, achieving and maintaining the oral health of older adults is a major challenge for the Chilean health system and the society at large.

* Correspondence: r.marino@unimelb.edu.au
[1]Oral Health Cooperative Research Centre Melbourne Dental School, University of Melbourne, Melbourne, VIC 3010, Australia
Full list of author information is available at the end of the article

In 2007, the Chilean government implemented the Explicit Health Guarantee (GES) for those 60-years and older to ensure that their access to health is independent of their ability to pay [3, 8]. The GES includes 56 health conditions which are treated at no cost for the older population, including comprehensive oral health care, and some oral health conditions such as tooth loss and dental emergencies treatment for the whole population [8]. However, some health conditions are restricted to specific ages. For example, oral health care through GES is for 60 year-olds only [8].

Factors associated with the use of oral health services by older adults include: age, sex, level of education, social support and connectedness, income, general and oral health status, oral health knowledge and attitudes, perceived oral health needs, oral pain or discomfort, physical disabilities and chronic conditions [9–13]. Among older adults, underutilization of oral health services is common, with the most commonly cited barriers including the cost of dental care, shortage of professionals, and lack of familiarity with services provided and location of facilities [14, 15].

However, information on the oral health needs and oral health visit patterns of Chilean older adults is limited [8, 16, 17]. The national health survey reports that those aged 65 years and older account for 7.5% of dental visits [8]. Moreover, the data do not offer a clear picture on the use of oral health care services in rural populations, particularly those aged 65 and older. Because planning of oral health care services is dependent on the quality of current local data [18], as part of a larger study to assess the oral health profile of the Chilean Maule Region, this paper examines the patterns of use of oral health care services; factors related to the utilization of oral health care services, and barriers to using oral health services reported by in an ambulant population of older adults (65 to 74 years old) from the Maule Region. This information is necessary for adequate service planning and delivery to ensure the best possible oral health care for all Chileans. The influence of oral health on the quality of life of older adults and on the aging process, emphasizes the importance of exploring the use of oral health care services by older adults to better understand the socio-cultural context through which oral health decisions are made [19]. Providing specific information on regional populations will generate a robust advocacy instrument to argue for more oral health care resources; and place oral health within the broad concept of personal and social well-being.

Methods

A community-based cross-sectional survey was selected. In the first stage, municipalities classified as urban or rural, were randomly selected from each strata, according to population size. In the second stage, individuals participating in third age clubs and other locations where older adults gather, were selected within each municipality. Power analysis was based on the case of 15 independent variables accounting for 10% of the variance in the dependent variable, with a sample size of 437 yielding a power of 0.99, that is an 99% chance of detecting an effect of that size at the level of significance of 0.01 [20].

After approval from the University of Talca Bioethics Committee, older adults' social clubs members were invited to participate in the study. Once an individual consented to participate, he/she was asked to go through a structured interview and an oral examination at the clubs' facilities. The methods used in this study have been previously described [2]. The interview covered a range of socio-demographic characteristics and use of oral health care services. The interview also included questions about attitudes to oral health and knowledge of causes and risk factors for dental caries, periodontal disease and oral cancer adapted from previous studies [21–23]. The instrument used in this study is included as "Additional file 1". Clinical examinations were conducted by four trained and calibrated examiners (kappa statistics > 0.90) following WHO criteria and recommendations for oral health data collection [24]. Data collection extended from March to October 2011.

Measures

The behavioral model of health services framework used in this study provides an arrange of variables that predict the utilization of medical, dental, and hospital services [25–28]. The model's three domains; *predisposing variables* (demographic and attitude), *enabling variables* (e.g. income, region of residence, type of health insurance), and *need* have been found to be interrelated, and to predict personal health practices, use of professional health services, and satisfaction with one's health.

In addition to age and sex, the following socio-demographic information was collected: Marital status classified into two groups: 'Married or in a de-facto relationship'; and 'Single, widow/widower or divorced'. Participants were classified according to their educational level using three categories: 'No formal education to complete primary education'; 'Incomplete secondary education'; 'Complete secondary education or Post-secondary education'. While the questionnaire did not include a specific query on income-income was assessed though participants' status for their health insurance. Specifically, participants were asked about their health insurance, in the categories of: 'No health insurance or Government health insurance'; and 'Private health insurance'. Municipalities were classified as: 'Urban' (i.e., head of regional province); 'Non-metro centre' (i.e., municipality of more than 20,000 inhabitants); and 'Rural' (i.e., municipality or location of 20,000 or less inhabitants).

Psychosocial variables included: Oral health attitudes, measured by seven items concerned with: the inevitability of oral disease in older adults, desirability of keeping natural teeth and the efficacy of preventive behaviors, such as self-examination and dental visits. The oral health knowledge index consisted of the sum of correct responses to 38 questions about knowledge of symptoms and causes of dental caries, periodontal disease and oral cancer.

During a dental examination, examiners recorded the number of teeth present, decayed tooth surfaces, and filled tooth surfaces.

Use of oral health care services was investigated by asking participants to indicate the time interval since their last dental visit, with response option [6]: '12 months or less', '12 months to 2 years', '2 to 5 years', and 'More than 5 years'. Dental attendance was dichotomized according to whether or not a participant had visited the dentist within the last 12 months. In addition, self-perceived barriers to oral health care were assessed by asking participants to report from a list of nine commonly described categories: 'Cost'; 'Non availability of dentist'; 'Time waiting for appointments'; 'Rude behavior from staff'; 'Location of service'; 'Fear of dentist/treatment/procedures'; 'Access to health facilities'; 'Physical disability'; and 'General health problem', whether any of them prevented people from accessing dental care service. Responses were coded as 'Yes' or 'No'. A Barriers Index was created by adding positive responses.

Basic descriptive information on selected socio-demographic, psychosocial, dental status and use of oral health service variables were calculated. To establish whether differences existed between groups on dependent variables, ANOVAs and Chi-square tests were conducted. Logistic regression analysis was used to examine whether any combination of predisposing, enabling, need, and clinical variables, provided a multivariate explanation for oral health care services utilization. The final regression model was created using a stepwise selection method. Data manipulation and analyses were conducted using SPSS PC (Version 20.0).

Results

Four-hundred and thirty-eight older adults aged between 65 and 74 years participated in the study. The mean age of the sample was 69.7 years (s.d. 3.4). The majority were female (77.4%) and age ranged between 70 and 74 years (52.7%). By level of education, the majority (61.0%) had complete or incomplete primary education, with 26.9% having some secondary education, including 3.2% who had tertiary education. The remaining 12.1% had no formal education. The majority was retired or indicated not working outside home (86.4%). Only 6.6% indicated that they were still working or were looking for a job (7.1%). Almost half of the sample (49.1%) was married, another 32.9% were widow/widower and 18.0% were single or divorced. The largest proportions lived in urban areas (61.6%); 20.5% lived in non-metro centres and another 17.8% lived in rural areas. The great majority (90.6%) was under public health insurance (See Table 1).

Overall, 31.5% of participants reported having a dental visit in the previous 12 months. Seventy-five participants (17.1%) reported that their last visit had been more than 1 year, but less than 2 years ago. An additional 21.0% had not been to the dentist within the last 2 years, but not more than 5 years; and 30.4% had not been for more than 5 years ago. Amongst those who visited the dentist in the previous 12 months, the most common reasons for the visit were dental prostheses (35.5%), followed by

Table 1 Univariate associations between socio-demographic variables and use of oral health service in the previous 12 months by Chilean older adults

		Used dental service in last 12 month	
Predisposing, enabling, and need factors	n	(%) Yes	(%) No
Mean Age (years)		69.9 (3.4)[a]	69.7 (3.5)
Gender			
Male	99	35.4	64.6
Female	339	30.4	69.4
Level of education			
No formal/primary education complete	53	22.6	77.4
Some secondary education	267	33.0	67.0
Secondary education complete/some tertiary education	118	32.2	67.8
Place of residence		**	
Urban	270	29.6	70.4
Semi-urban	90	25.6	74.4
Rural	73	44.9	55.1
Health insurance			
Public	397	31.2	68.8
Other	41	34.1	65.7
Oral health knowledge		11.2 (7.1)[a]	10.6 (6.8)
Attitudes to health care*		2.8 (1.3)[a]	3.1 (1.4)
Barriers to treatment		1.4 (1.2)[a]	1.6 (1.3)
Edentulous		**	
No	333	34.8	65.2
Yes	105	21.0	79.0
Number of teeth**		12.3 (9.3)[a]	9.7 (9.9)
Missing teeth***		19.7 (9.3)[a]	22.3 (9.9)

[a]Mean and standard deviation; *$p < 0.05$; **$p < 0.01$; ***$p < 0.001$
Figures may not add due to missing values

tooth extraction (29.0%), or dental crown/filling (21.7%). A dental check-up was nominated by 5.0%. No differences were present by socio-demographic variables or reason for the last visit. However, those living in rural localities tended to be more likely ($p = 0.063$) to have visited for an extraction. Among those who had a dental visit in the previous 12 months, almost half nominated private oral health services (47.8%) a similar proportion nominated public services (46.4%). Another 5.7% indicated having attended a dental technician.

The three most frequently nominated barriers to care were cost of services (60.3%); difficulties obtaining dental appointments (32.2%); and fear of dentists (21.7%). Other commonly mentioned barriers were availability of oral health care services (18.0%), and access to oral health services (11.6%). No other category was reported by more than 5% of the sample. One-hundred and eighty-nine participants (43.2%) reported one barrier to oral health services; 21.5% and 12.1% reported two and three barriers, respectively. The remainder (7.3%), reported between four and eight barriers. Seventy participants (16.0%) reported no barriers.

Univariate associations between socio-demographic, predisposing, enabling and clinical variables and use of oral health care services are shown in Table 1. The analysis indicated that those who visited the dentist were more likely to have lower scores for oral health attitudes than those who did not (3.1 vs. 2.8, respectively; $p < 0.05$). By place of residence, those living in rural areas were more likely to have visited the dentist (44.9%) compared to those living in urban or in non-metro centres (29.5% and 25.6%, respectively; $p < 0.05$).

Concerning clinical conditions, the mean number of natural teeth was 10.5 (s.d. 9.8). On the other hand, the mean number of missing teeth was 21.5 (s.d. 9.8). One-hundred and five (24.0%) participants were fully edentulous. Edentulous participants were less likely to have been to the dentist in the previous 12 months than those with natural teeth (34.8% vs. 21.0%; $p < 0.01$; $OR = 0.82$; 95% CI: 0.73–0.94). Also those who had visited the dentist had a significantly higher mean number of filled surfaces and missing teeth than participants who had not been to the dentist recently (6.5 vs. 3.0; and 22.3 vs. 19.7; $p < 0.001$, respectively).

The probability of using oral health care services in the last 12 months, was explored with logistic regression analysis utilizing as predictors five predisposing variables (age, sex, education, marital status, and attitude to oral health), three enabling and needs variables (place of residence, oral health knowledge and type of health insurance) and three clinical variables (filled surfaces, decayed surfaces and edentulousness). In the final model four variables remained significantly associated with use of oral health care services [$\chi^2(4) = 40.82$; $p < 0.0001$]. Those who lived in rural areas were more likely to have visited the dentist ($OR = 2.15$; 95% CI: 1.27–2.63). Those who reported fear of dentists were less likely to have visited the dentist compared to those who did not report fear ($OR = 0.43$; 95% CI: 0.24–0.76). Participants with, at least, secondary education were more likely to have visited the dentist than those with lower levels of education ($OR = 1.66$; 95% CI: 1.03–2.64). Additionally, filled surfaces increased the likelihood of having had a dental visit ($OR = 1.08$; 95% CI: 1.05–1.11) Table 2 presents the results of the logistic regression. The variance in oral health care use explained by the final model was 12.5% (Nagelkerke $r^2 = 0.125$).

Discussion

Present results indicate that 31.5% of older Chilean adults participating in this study had a dental visit within the 12 months prior to the survey. This represents a somewhat lower proportion to that found in the Chilean data (33.6%) for people 65 years and older in the Valparaiso Region in 2007 and national data in 2010 (40.4%) [16, 17]. More importantly, although this was a largely dentate sample, about a third of this group (30.4%) reported not having a dental visit for 5 years or longer. This is even more significant considering that the majority of the sample had access to emergency and general oral health care through state own health services and, for those 60 years-old, access to comprehensive oral health care through the GES [3, 29]. Thus, access to public oral health care for older adults is based on whether or not they meet restrictive age criteria, or compete for access with other age groups on a "first-come first-served" basis. In Chile, approximately 23% of the 18,115 dentists work in the public system to cover 85% of the population. This represent a 40% deficit in the public

Table 2 Regression coefficient, odds ratios and 95% confidence interval for odds ratios for the factors predicting use of oral health care services among Chilean older adults

	β coefficient	Odds ratio	95% Confidence interval
Place of residence			
Rural	0.77	2.15	1.27–3.63
Urban/Semi-urban			1.00
Fear to dentist (Yes =1)	−0.85	0.43	0.24–0.76
Level of education			
Secondary complete and higher levels	0.50	1.65	1.03–2.64
Less than secondary complete			1.00
Filled tooth surfaces	0.73	1.08	1.06–1.11
Constant	−1.41		

The variance in dental visits accounted for using the full model was 12.5% ($\eta^2 = 0.125$)

versus the private system, which leaves this age group with not many choices apart from private care [30].

The results from logistic regression analysis showed that there were significant disparities in oral health services utilization by level of education, place of residence, and clinical outcomes, such as filled surfaces. These results are partly consistent with previous findings with respect to socio-demographic status (e.g., level of education). On the other hand, place of residence effects were not in the expected direction. In the present study, those living in rural areas were more likely to use oral health care services than those who lived in urban or non-metro centres. Previous studies commonly report lower use of services by rural residents [5, 31, 32]. An explanation could be that GES, may have changed oral health behaviors in this population, which may reflect public awareness campaigns. Thus, reconfirming the conclusion that the GES has improved services utilization among those who traditionally are found to have greater difficulties accessing oral health services (e.g., rural).

However, this increase in frequency does not translate into better oral health status, as demonstrated in participants' periodontal and oral health status, and use of prosthetic appliances [2]. Furthermore, there was a trend for those living in rural areas to have less conservative interventions, which suggests that interventions aimed at closing the gap in oral health services utilisation need more attention.

As demonstrated in the present study, use of oral health care services among older adults is affected by many socio-demographic, and psychosocial factors, as well as other predisposing and enabling factors. Participants identified several commonly reported barriers to accessing oral health care services (e.g., cost, availability of oral health care services, length of waiting lists, and fear of dentist) [1, 11, 21, 33], as impacting on their use of oral health services. Nonetheless, fear was the only barrier that remained significant in the multivariate model. Participants who reported fear of dentist or treatments, were less likely to have attended the dentist.

These results have important program and policy implications, as in order to increase use of oral health care services in this population, additional efforts, beyond the reduction of costs or financial barriers, would be required. The results support arguments for increasing the awareness of the need to periodically visit a dentist, and fear reduction and desensitization, at any age. This should be viewed as an appropriate and socially just intervention. Still, further is required to properly establish the relationship between rurality and oral health care services utilization. For example, no attempt was made to collect information on the participants' oral health visit experience, perspectives and influences using qualitative or mixed methods approaches. These data would have provided a better and richer appreciation of older adults' perception and ideas. In making these observations, the limitations of the study design have to be considered within. This was a sample of volunteers recruited from older persons clubs in the Maule Region who were healthy, reasonably well and autonomous, to be able to independently manage their activities and to participate in social clubs. Additionally, data were based on self-reports, and the potential for recall and social desirability biases on the frequency of visits, might also be present. Third, the data was from a regional representative sample. As such, it provides information at a regional level. The findings are not intended to be generalised to all older Chileans. Fourth, there was no differentiation between dental visits. A basic variation would be between emergency and general dental care visits. Another limitation was the socio-economic variables employed in the study may be too limited, other important predictors such as actual income, social support, or oral health literacy were not investigated.

Furthermore, although the final multivariate model provided a significant description of oral health service use, the final model accounted for 12.5% of the variance, only. Thus, predictors not considered in this study might have added further explanatory power to the model. This might include self-assessed oral health needs and status, self-efficacy and other dental and personal considerations. Alternatively, commonly described predictors might not directly apply to older Chilean populations. Also, it may be that those predictors need to be questioned since older adults keep more natural teeth and therefore, have different oral health needs and demands for services [1, 21]. Thus, this study does not claim that a definitive model has been identified; rather the study raises some potentially important predictors to be explored in future endeavors.

Nonetheless, while the present study may have limitations, due to the dearth of information regarding the oral health of older adults in Chile, it was considered important to conduct this analysis. The purpose of the study was to gain an initial understanding of, and identify factors associated with, the use of oral health services among older Chileans, and to provide relevant information for the design of future studies aimed at determining predictors of their use oral health service. Moreover, the study also has several strengths. As the proportion of edentulous people decreases, there is an increased need for oral health care services. This study contributes to a better understating of the oral health care visits of community-dwelling older adults living in the Maule Region of Chile. We explored the effect of place of residency on oral health services utilization, which may have important implications for other researchers. It is noteworthy that the direction of the rurality effect on the use of oral health care services, after adjusting for the other commonly used SES indicators, suggests the need for further understanding of the pathways that lead to the disparity in oral health. Rural communities have an impressive number of strengths and assets [33]. An improved understanding of factors related to the use of oral health care services by older adults living in urban, rural and non-metropolitan centers will also need to be met.

Future research should build on these preliminary insights and better explore the source of these discrepancies regarding predictors of the use of oral health care services described in the literature, better assess the capacity of older adults to manage their health problems, and make a distinction between types of visits. As the urban population is increasing in Chile, it is important to explore these effects with respect to other health outcomes. An equitable use of health care is an important goal within a health care system [29].

Conclusion

The study highlighted the need for additional exploration of the oral health care visit behaviors of older adults. Learning how to reach these groups and overcoming barriers to care are matters of increasing interest, given the growing size of this segment of the population and the relevance of oral health within the broad concept of oral health and wellbeing. Using information provide in this study, health planners could better develop programs and policies to address disparities in access to both preventive and restorative oral health services for all Chileans.

Abbreviations

ANOVA: Analysis of variance; CI: Confidence interval; GES: Explicit health guarantee; OR: Odds ratio; SES: Socio-economic status; WHO: World Health Organization

Acknowledgment

The authors would like to acknowledge the co-operation received from the students of the School of Dentistry, Faculty of Health Sciences, University of Talca, Chile, and the participants in the study.

Funding

This study was funded by a grant received from the International Association for Dental Research (IADR) and Internal research grant from the University of Talca, Chile.

Authors' contributions

RM contributed with the conception of the study, and the design and draft of the manuscript, and read and approved the final manuscript. RG contributed with the conception of the study, and the design and draft of the manuscript, and read and approved the final manuscript.

Authors' information

RM is an Associate professor at the Melbourne Dental School, University of Melbourne, Melbourne, Australia.
RG is Professor of Cariology, Department of Oral Rehabilitation, University of Talca, Talca, Chile.

Competing interests

The authors declare that they have no competing interest. RM is a Section Editor for BMC Oral Health.

Consent for publication

Not Applicable.

Ethics approval and consent to participate

The study has been approved by the University of Talca Bioethics Committee (Registration Number: 00038; 17-January-2011). Participation in the study was voluntary. All participants provided written informed consent to participate in this study.

Author details

[1]Oral Health Cooperative Research Centre Melbourne Dental School, University of Melbourne, Melbourne, VIC 3010, Australia. [2]Department of Oral Rehabilitation, University of Talca, Talca, Chile.

References

1. Mariño R, Cueto A, Badenier O, Acevedo R, Moya R. Oral health status and inequalities among ambulant older adults living in the central of Chile. Community Dent Health. 2011;28:143–8.
2. Mariño R, Giacaman R. Factors related to unmet oral health needs in older adults living in Chile. Arch Gerontol Geriatr. 2014;58:454–9.
3. Wallace SP, Gutiérrez VF. Equity of access to health care for older adults in four major Latin American cities. Rev Panam Salud Publica. 2005;17:394–409.
4. Kruger E, Tennant M. Oral health workforce in rural and remote Western Australia: practice perceptions. Aust J Rural Health. 2005;13:321–6.
5. Mariño R, Calache H, Whelan M. Dental status and socio-demographic profile of adults users of public oral health care services in Victoria. J Theory Pract Dent Public Health. 2013;1:6–23.
6. Australian Institute of Health and Welfare, DSRU. Geographic variation in oral health and use of dental services in the Australian population 2004–06. AIHW Department of Statistics and Research Unit Series No. 41. 2009.
7. Dolan TA, Atchison K, Huynh T. Access to dental care among older adults in the United States. J Dent Educ. 2005;69:961–74.
8. Ministerio de Salud (Chile), Programa nacional de salud del adulto mayor programa nacional de salud de las personas adultas mayores. 2014. http://web.minsal.cl/sites/default/files/files/Borrador%20documento%20Programa%20Nacional%20de%20Personas%20Adultas%20Mayores-%2004-03_14.pdf. Accessed 5 Aug 2016.
9. Luzzi L, Spencer J. Factors influencing the use of public dental services: An application of the theory of planned behaviour. BMC Health Serv Res. 2008;8:93.
10. Nitschke I, Stillhart A, Kunze J. Utilization of dental services in old age. Swiss Dent J. 2015;125:433–47.
11. Petersen PE, Holst D. Utilization of dental health services. In: Cohen L, Gift H, editors. Disease Prevention and Oral Health Promotion, Munskgaard, Copenhagen. 1995. p. 230–8.
12. Tennstedt SL, Branbilla DL, Jetter AM, McGuire HM. Understanding dental service use by older adults: sociobehavioral factors vs need. J Public Health Dent. 1994;54:211–9.
13. Kiyak HA, Reichmuth M. Barriers to and enablers of older adults' use of dental services. J Dent Educ. 2005;69:975–86.

14. Williams SA, Godson JH, Ahmed IA. Dentists' perceptions of difficulties encountered in providing dental care for British Asians. Community Dent Health. 1995;12:30–4.
15. Mariño R, Wright FAC, Minichiello V, Schofield MJ. Oral health beliefs and practices among Greek and Italian older Australians: a focus group approach. Australas J Ageing. 2002;21:93–198.
16. Badenier O, Moya R, Cueto A. Estudio de prevalencia de Enfermedades Bucodentales y necesidades de tratamiento en la V región. Informe Final. Universidad de Valparaíso, Chile. Proyecto FONIS Número: SA05I20044. Santiago, FONIS, 2007.
17. Ministerio de Salud (Chile), Encuesta Nacional de Salud. Chile 2009–2010 http://web.minsal.cl/portal/url/item/bcb03d7bc28b64dfe040010165012d23.pdf, 2011, (Accessed 1 Jan 2017).
18. Bourgeois D, Nihtila A, Mersel A. Prevalence of caries and edentulousness among 65–74 year olds in Europe. Bull WHO. 1998;76:413–7.
19. Andersen RM, Davidson PL. Ethnicity, aging and oral health outcomes: a conceptual framework. Adv Dent Res. 1997;11:203–9.
20. Cohen J. Statistical Power Analysis for the Behavioral Sciences. 2nd ed. Hillsdale: Lawrence Erlbaum Assoc publishers; 1988.
21. Mariño R, Wright FAC, Schofield MJ, Minichiello V, Calache H. Factors associated with self-reported use of dental health services among older Greek and Italian migrants. Spec Care Dentist. 2005;25:12–9.
22. Wright FAC, Gebart-Ealemont JE, Olsen CB, et al. A Longitudinal Socio-Dental Study of Adult Oral Health in Melbourne, 1985–1990. Community Dental Health Monograph Series; Number Eight. Melbourne: The University of Melbourne; 1991.
23. Mariño R, Khan A, Khew C, Stevenson C, Tham R. Pattern and factors associated with utilization of dental services among older adults in rural Victoria. Aust Dent J. 2014;59:504–10.
24. World Health Organization. Oral Health Surveys: Basic Methods. Fourthth ed. Geneva: WHO; 1997.
25. Andersen RM. Behavioral Model of Families' Use of Health Services. Research Series No. 25. Chicago: Center for Health administration Studies, University of Chicago; 1968.
26. Andersen R, Harada N, Chiu V, Makinodan T. Application of the behavioral model to health studies of Asian and Pacific Islander Americans. Asian Am Pac Isl J Health. 1995;3:128–41.
27. Andersen R, Newman J. Societal and individual determinants of medical care utilization in the United States. Milbank Mem Fund Q Health Soc. 1973;51:95–125.
28. Aday L, Awe W. Health sources utilization models. In: Gochman B, editor. Handbook of health research. Vol. Determinants of health behavior (personal and social). New York: Plenum; 1997. p. 153–72.
29. Cornejo M, Paraje G, Vásquez F, Pérez G, Carme PL, Borrell C. Changes in Socioeconomic Inequalities in the Use of Dental Care Following Major Healthcare Reform in Chile, 2004–2009. Int J Environ Res Public Health. 2015;12:2823–36.
30. Cousiño S. (2013). ¿Cuántos somos actualmente los dentistas en Chile? La burbuja odontológica. Revista Digital Contraangulo. http://www.contraangulo.com/2013/07/cuantos-somos-actualmente-los-dentistas.html. (accessed 29 Nov 2016).
31. Short L, Patterson A. Strategies to improve equity in oral health care for the rural aged. 2nd Biennial Australian Rural and Remote Health Scientific Conference. 1994.
32. Brennan D, Spencer AJ. Influence of patient, visit, and oral health factors on dental service provision. J Public Health Dent. 2002;62:48–157.
33. Averill JB. Priorities for action in a rural older adults study. Fam Community Health. 2012;35:358–72.

18

Reliability and diagnostic validity of a joint vibration analysis device

Sonia Sharma, Heidi C. Crow, Krishnan Kartha, W. D. McCall Jr.* and Yoly M. Gonzalez

Abstract

Background: This observational study was designed to evaluate the reliability and diagnostic validity of Joint Vibration Analysis (JVA) in subjects with bilateral disc displacement with reduction and in subjects with bilateral normal disc position.

Methods: The reliability of selecting the traces was assessed by reading the same traces at an interval of 30 days. The reliability of the vibrations provided by the subjects was assessed by obtaining two tracings from each individual at an interval of 30 min. The validity compared the Joint Vibration Analysis parameters against magnetic resonance imaging as the reference standard. The data were analyzed with exploratory factor analysis.

Results: The short- term reliability of the Joint Vibration Analysis outcome variables showed excellent results. Implementing factor analysis and a receiver operating characteristic as analytical methods showed that six items of the Joint Vibration Analysis outcome variables could be scaled and normalized to a composite score which presented acceptable levels of sensitivity and specificity with a receiver operating characteristic of 0.8.

Conclusion: This study demonstrated that the composite score generated from the Joint Vibration Analysis variables could discriminate between subjects with bilateral normal versus bilateral displaced discs.

Keywords: Joint vibration, Temporomandibular disorders, Reliability, Diagnostic validity, Factor analysis

Background

Temporomandibular disorders (TMD) encompass a group of musculoskeletal and neuromuscular conditions that involve the TMJ, the masticatory muscles and all associated tissues; the major symptoms are pain which is often localized in the muscles of mastication or preauricular area; joint noises, and limitation in jaw function may be present as additional complaints [1]. Based on the current Diagnostic Criteria, TMD can be classified into three major groups: pain-related; intra-articular; and degenerative joint disease and subluxation disorders [2]. Within the intra-articular group, disc displacement with reduction defines a subgroup in which diagnosis has often been based on clinical finding of joint sounds [3]. Several studies have concluded that TMJ sounds are highly variable [3–5]. Thus, the use of joint sounds as a diagnostic parameter has been questioned [6]. The reliability among calibrated examiners of such sounds has been reported to have a Kappa value of 0.63 [7]. The correct identification of intra-articular conditions using joint sounds has shown a sensitivity of 0.38 and specificity of 0.88, using the Magnetic Resonance Imaging (MRI) as the reference standard [8, 9].

Joint vibration analysis is based on principles of motion and friction by surfaces, which can be captured by accelerometers. Human joints in proper biomechanical relationship, in theory, should produce little friction and little vibration [10–14]; surface changes within the joint could cause greater friction and greater vibration. It has been postulated that different disorders can produce different vibration patterns or signatures in joint including the TMJs [15–17]. Vibration analysis of the TMJ is thus a quantitative process that measures the absolute intensity and frequency distribution of vibratory waves emanating from the joint during jaw motion.

Since there is controversy regarding the utilization of joint vibrations to characterize joint status and consequently diagnosis as presented in a recent systematic review [18], the diagnostic validity of such instrumentation

* Correspondence: wdmccall@buffalo.edu
Department of Oral Diagnostic Sciences, School of Dental Medicine, University at Buffalo, Buffalo, NY 14214, USA

used to measure and characterize this phenomenon must be tested using research designs with strong foundations including reliability evidence, blinded examiners, an acceptable reference standard such as MRI, and acceptable psychometric properties.

Furthermore the progression of joint status in participants with displaced discs has been controversial. While one report postulates a progression from disc displacement to osteoarthritis [19] there is substantial clinical evidence that most untreated patients improve and do not progress over time [20–25]. In addition there is MRI evidence that no change occurs in disc displacement over 22–80 months [26]. More recently the authors of a prospective study that assessed the stability of the temporomandibular joint in disc displacement using MRIs, found that over 8 years of follow-up, 76% of the 789 baseline joint-specific soft-tissue diagnoses did not change [27].

A systematic review [18] reported several limitations in previous reports: (1) lack of blinndness, (2) nonvalidated classification systems, (3) different imaging techniques to identify control and test groups, (4) use of joint sounds per se as evidence of pathology or as a reference standard, and (5) use of joint vibration analysis (JVA) as the reference standard even though it was the device investigated.

The premise of this research was that a more technically accurate instrument and more sophisticated analysis by using factor analysis to select variables might provide more accurate information, compared to auscultation, and more inexpensive, compared to MRI, to assess the phenomenon of joint sounds. Therefore the assessment of vibrations using instrumentation such as Joint Vibration Analysis (JVA) could have the potential to provide data that could be used to assess the phenomenon and to indicate the status of the joint. We focused on the BioJVA produced by BioResearch Associates.

The objectives of this research were, first, to determine if the data associated with joint vibrations could be selected and recorded reliably, second, to analyze the multiple correlated variables with factor analysis to determine if a smaller number of variables could represent the data, and third, to determine if the sensitivity and specificity as represented by the area under the receiver operating characteristic curve were sufficiently large for potential clinical use.

The overall goal of this research was to test the diagnostic validity of the joint vibration output variables against the reference standard of the MRI evaluation by a calibrated radiologist. The underlying analytical strategy was to examine the data with exploratory factor analysis to see (1) how many latent variables, that is, factors, were in the data, (2) whether these latent factors could be interpreted in a reasonable way, and (3) whether a composite score based on the items that survived into the interpretation could be merged into a composite score with adequate sensitivity and specificity as described by a receiver operating characteristic [28, 29].

Methods

Subjects

Thirty-six subjects who had undergone an MRI for their TMJs within the last two years agreed to participate in the study. Characterization of bilateral disc displacement or bilateral normal disc position was provided by a calibrated radiologist [8] based on MRI interpretation. The study was approved by the University at Buffalo's Health Sciences Institutional Review Board and each subject gave informed consent.

Equipment

The joint vibration analysis (JVA) in the BioPAK© system [30] was leased from Bioresearch Corporation and consisted of a headset encompassing accelerometers on each side, an amplifier, and software for a computer. The signals from the accelerometers were amplified by the small amplifier, which was placed around the subjects' neck. The amplified signals were transmitted to a PC computer where they were recorded and later analyzed with the software program. Each accelerometer consists of a metal case containing a piezoelectric crystal that has a mass resting on it. This crystal reacts to acceleration by producing a minute electric charge due to compression produced by the mass, which is directly proportional to the acceleration. This is then put into an amplifier of high input impedance prior to being recorded as a vibration signal.

JVA protocol

The subjects sat in an upright position. Their maximum unassisted opening and lateral deflections were recorded clinically and entered into the computer with the BioPAK software program. The headset device was then placed on the subject's head with the sensors positioned over the TMJs; the subjects were instructed to watch the monitor where they observed an animation illustrating opening and closing mouth movement, synchronized to a metronome. They were then instructed to open their mouth as wide as they could and close, tapping their teeth together following and matching the animation and the metronome, which they observed on the screen. As the subject performed the opening and closing with the JVA the characteristic vibrations produced by the condyles were detected by the accelerometers and recorded in the computer.

After the first set of JVA tracings were recorded the Research Diagnostic Criteria examination [31] was performed, then a second set of JVA tracings were recorded. The interval between the two sets of tracings was about 30 min.

The variables [4, 30, 32] obtained were: Total Integral I (T), representing a measure of the total amount of energy in the vibration; Integral <300 Hz which is the amount of energy in the vibration that is below 300 Hz; Integral >300 Hz which is the amount of energy in the vibration that is above 300 Hz; >300/<300 Ratio which is the ratio of the high-frequency to low-frequency energy; Peak Amplitude which indicates the highest intensity of the vibration; Peak Frequency which is the frequency at which the highest intensity of the vibration occurred and Median Frequency which is the frequency such that half of the energy is below it and half is above it. These data are provided in an Additional file 1.

Reliability

Reliability was assessed in three ways. First, the reliability of the examiners for range of motion data between the two clinical examiners was assessed by computing the intraclass correlation coefficient while lateral deviation was assessed with kappa. Second, the ability of two clinicians as a consensus to select the same traces after a three-month interval was assessed by comparing the JVA variables from those two sets of traces. Third, a test-retest protocol assessed the ability of the subjects to provide consistent data by comparing data obtained at a 30-min interval. The examiners were calibrated for Research Diagnostic Criteria for TMD [33].

Reliability of range of motion assessment

The two clinical examiners in this study were blinded to the MRI diagnosis avoiding bias to the instrumentation under evaluation; examiners were RDC/TMD calibrated [31] and provided the clinical parameters such as range of motion and deflection, which were required by the BioPAK software program to analyze the joint vibrations.

Reliability of trace selection

The selection of vibration data was done as a consensus by the two clinical examiners following the manufacturer's protocol, which included the selection of the five largest vibration amplitudes in a trace of six to eight open-close cycles. To determine if the examiners could reliably select the JVA traces with the largest time-based signals, 15 traces were randomly selected and the traces were read at two times 3 months apart.

The recorded JVA traces were then analyed for the largest vibration amplitude that consistently occurred in each joint recording from the JVA sweep. Five large vibration amplitudes were selected from each trace by both examiners and were used to calculate frequency spectrum computed by the Fast Fourier Transform algorithm. These spectra were used for this estimation of reliability.

Test-retest reliability

Data from the first recordings from the subject were compared with the recordings made 30 min later.

Factor analysis

The number of latent variables underlying the data was investigated by exploratory factor analysis. The (log) data for each item was scaled by subtracting its mean and dividing by its standard deviation to form a z-score. The mean across the six items was taken as a composite score for each subject and a receiver operating curve was generated.

Factor analysis seeks to condense a larger number of correlated variables into a smaller number of underlying, interpretable variables which explain the bulk of the relationships among the original variables. Graphical inspection of the raw data suggested that they were strongly non-Gaussian so the logarithm to the base 10 was taken of each data point. The box plot based on these logarithms suggested a better distribution for each variable (Fig. 1) and Shapiro-Wilks tests of each item within each group supported this. Due to doubts about the independence of data from the right and left joints [34], only the data from the right side were analyzed. Statistical Analysis

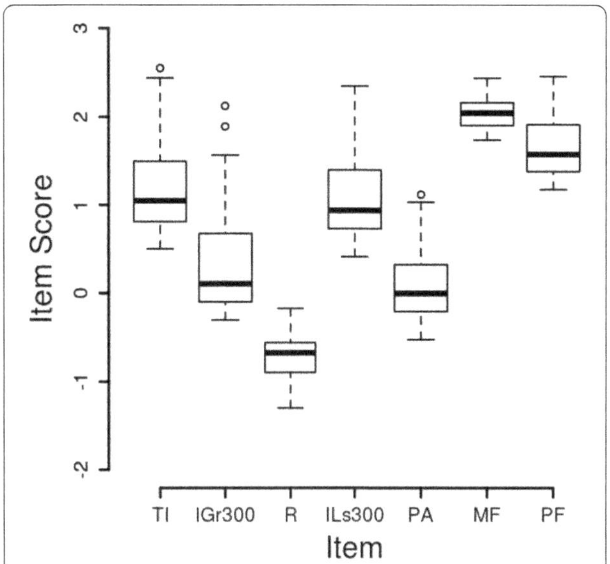

Fig. 1 Box Plot of JVA Data. The item score is the logarithm base 10 of the original data. These data, based on all 36 subjects, largely corrected the skewed distributions. The items are TI: total integral, IGr300: integral greater than 300 Hz, R: ratio of integral >300 to integral <300, ILs300: integral less than 300 Hz, PA: peak amplitude, MF: median frequency, PF: peak frequency

Reliability of dichotomous variables was assessed by percent agreement and Kappa values. Reliability of continuous variables was assessed by intraclass correlation coefficients. Validity was assessed by calculating the Receiver Operating Characteristic (ROC) using the composite score identified with the factor analysis.

The data were analysed using the R statistical and graphics package [35].

Results

Demographics

A total of 36 subjects (21 females, 15 males) participated in this study. The mean age was 39.03 ± 13.6 years. There were no statistically significant differences in age by gender. Twenty-one subjects (11 males and 10 females) had normal bilateral joints and 15 subjects (4 males and 11 females) had bilateral joints with disc displacement with reduction.

Reliability of range of motion assessment

The ability of the two clinicians to obtain reliable clinical data led to excellent intraclass correlation coefficients (ICC) as shown in Table 1.

The ICCs from traces selected at the three months interval by consensus of the two clinical examiners also showed excellent values (Table 1). These data suggest that the examiners reliably identified the joint vibrations in the traces three months apart and therefore the results obtained at the validity stage would not be biased by the ability of the examiners to identify the phenomenon using the instrumentation.

Table 1 Reliability estimates

Item	ICC or Kappa	95% CI*
Clinical Data		
Pain Free Opening	0.94	0.67 – 0.99
Maximum Unassisted Opening	0.88	0.40 – 0.98
Maximum Assisted Opening	0.98	0.89 – 1.0
Lateral Deviation	87.5% (Kappa)	
Test-Retest Reliability of Selection of JVA Traces		
Total Integral	0.99	0.98 – 1.0
Integral <300	0.99	0.97 – 0.99
Integral > 300	1.0	0.99 – 1.0
> 300/< 300 Ratio	0.91	0.82 – 0.96
Test-Retest Reliability of JVA traces provided by subject at 30 min		
Total Integral	0.90	0.84 – 0.93
Integral <300	0.89	0.83 – 0.93
Integral > 300	0.91	0.87 – 0.94
Ratio >300/< 300	0.63	0.44 – 0.76
Peak Amplitude	0.87	0.81 – 0.92
Peak Frequency	0.77	0.65 – 0.85
Median Frequency	0.70	0.54 – 0.80

*None of the confidence intervals include zero so all p's are less than 0.05

Reliability of joint vibrations by test-retest

The reliability of the joint vibrations as a phenomenon was evaluated over a period of 30 min. The ICCs for the JVA variables showed excellent values except for the Ratio >300/<300 item (Table 1). Based on the excellent reliability results, the mean between trace 1 and trace 2 was taken as the outcome variable for further analysis.

Factor analysis

Graphical inspection of the raw data suggested that they were strongly non-Gaussian so the logarithm to the base 10 was taken of each data point. The box plot based on these logarithms suggested a better distribution for each variable (Fig. 1) and Shapiro-Wilks tests of each item within each group supported this. Due to doubts about the independence of data from the right and left joints, only the data from the right side were analysed.

The Cronbach's Alpha was 0.90 with 95% confidence limits from 0.82 to 0.98. The Kaiser-Meyer-Olkin measure of sampling adequacy was 0.74 for the overall data set and the minimum item was 0.42 for the "Ratio" item. The next lowest measure of sampling adequacy (MSA) was 0.71 for the "Median Frequency" item. Notice (Table 2) that for the ratio the loading is low and the communality is low. For these reasons (supported by the low reliability in Table 1), the ratio was deleted from the subsequent analysis.

A scree plot (not shown) suggested that one or two factors might be allowed. Two factors led to several cross-loadings in the pattern matrix coefficients, some communalities greater than one, and no interpretation, so one factor was used.

The pattern loadings, communalities, means, and standard deviations for each item are shown in Table 2. A box plot of all seven items is shown in Fig. 1.

Each of the six items that were kept was scaled to a mean of zero and a standard deviation of one, a z-score (Fig. 2). The mean across the six scaled items was taken as a composite score for each subject. A plot (Fig. 3) of

Table 2 Data from exploratory factor analysis

Item	Pattern loadings	Communality	Mean	Std Dev
Total Integral	0.97	0.94	1.231	0.534
Integral > 300	0.98	0.97	0.393	0.596
Ratio	0.49	0.24	−0.752	0.260
Integral <300	0.95	0.90	1.152	0.526
Peak Amplitude	0.87	0.76	0.167	0.462
Median Freq. Frequency	0.73	0.53	2.021	0.176
Peak	0.69	0.48	1.626	0.300

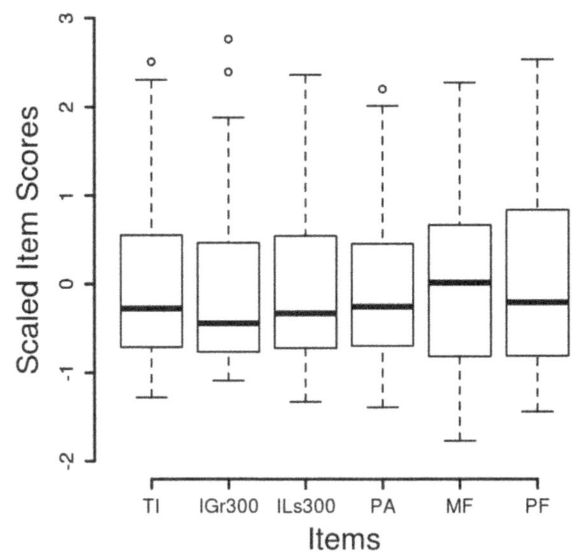

Fig. 2 Box Plot of Scaled JVA Data. In order to form a composite variable the data for each item were normalized by subtracting the mean and dividing by the standard deviation

the composite score for each subject in the disc displacement and normal groups suggested the scores differed.

The composite scores from the subjects in the two groups (Table 3) were used to generate a receiver operating curve where the scores from the subjects with bilateral disc displacement was used for the sensitivity and the scores from the subjects with bilateral normal discs were used for the specificity (Fig. 4). The area under the receiver operating characteristic curve was 0.82. A composite score of −0.04 led to a sensitivity of 0.86 and a specificity of 0.73, this score is the closest to the ideal score of 1.0 for sensitivity and 1.0 for specificity. A composite score of −0.24 led to a sensitivity of 0.67 and a specificity of 0.80, this score is the closest to the sensitivity of 0.70 and specificity of 0.95 suggested by Dworkin and LeResche ([31], pp. 318–319).

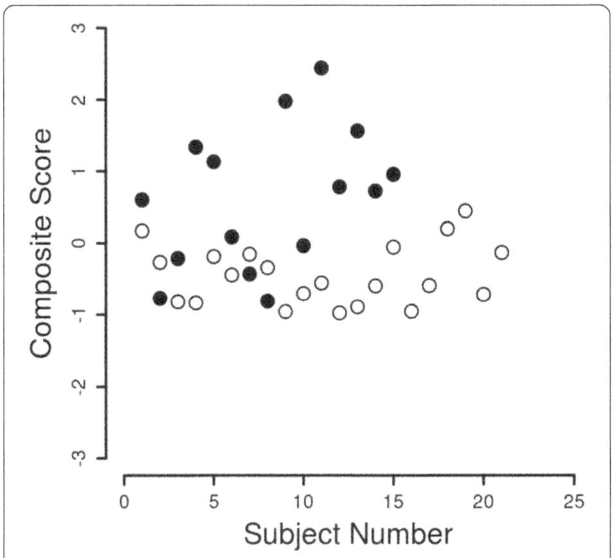

Fig. 3 Composite Scores. The filled circles are composite scores of the subjects with bilateral disc displacements and the open circles are the composite scores of the subjects with bilateral normal discs

Table 3 Composite scores of all participants by group

Normal	DDwR
0.171	0.600
−0.266	−0.769
−0.818	−0.212
−0.833	1.339
−0.185	1.133
−0.443	0.087
−0.154	−0.428
−0.341	−0.809
−0.957	1.978
−0.703	−0.033
−0.555	2.437
−0.977	0.780
−0.889	1.566
−0.595	0.723
−0.054	0.956
−0.953	
−0.591	
0.199	
0.444	
−0.716	
−0.131	
0.600	
−0.769	
−0.212	
1.339	
1.133	
0.087	
−0.428	
−0.809	
1.978	
−0.033	
2.437	
0.780	
1.566	
0.723	
0.956	

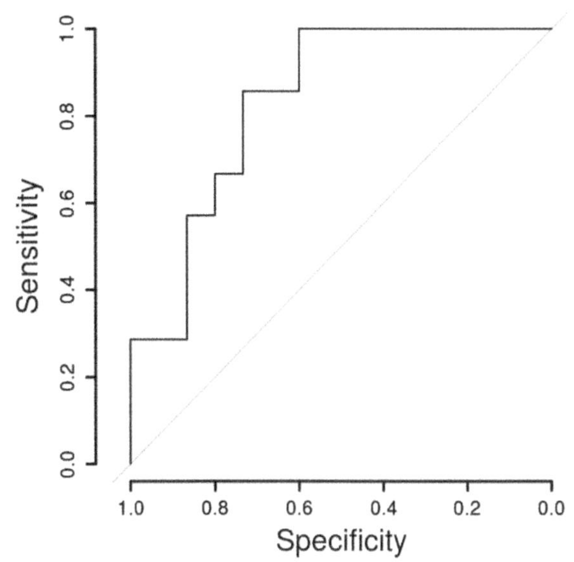

Fig. 4 Receiver Operating Characteristic. The composite scores in Fig. 3 were used to generate the Receiver Operating Characteristic curve where the subjects with bilateral normal discs were used for specificity and the subjects with bilateral displaced discs were used for sensitivity. The area under the curve is about 0.82

Discussion

The main findings of this research were that clinicians can reliably identify the tracings generated by the JVA instrumentation, that the vibration generated by the TMJs are reliable within a 30 min time period, that the data have good psychometric properties, and that exploratory factor analysis led to a composite score which had a good receiver operating characteristic.

The strengths of this research include clinical diagnostic criteria with trained and calibrated examiners, MRI TMJ soft tissue characterization by a calibrated radiologist who was blinded assessment of the data, and the use of exploratory factor analysis to assess the properties of the data and to retain relevant items from the vibration instrumentation.

We recognize that there are limitations associated with this investigation. First, this sample only included individuals with either bilateral disc displacements with reduction or bilateral normal position of the disc. This design made the results easier to interpret since there are reports that the vibration from the TMJ on one side might be detected on the other side [34, 36–38]. Clearly, unilateral disc displacement subjects need to be studied in the future, as well individuals with other intra-articular conditions in order to have a better representation of the TMD population.

Second, the imaging data and the vibration data were not concurrent. While some reports postulate a model of progression from disc displacement to osteoarthritis there are four lines of evidence that argue against the progression model. First, a large, recent, cross-sectional study failed to find evidence in favor of progression [26]. Second, several longitudinal clinical studies failed to find evidence of progression [20–25]. Third, a study with pre and post MRI imaging failed to find evidence of progression [26]. And fourth, a prospective 8 year follow-up study found that 76% of the joint diagnoses were stable [27] Therefore, although it would be preferable to have a fully parallel data set for the imaging and vibration assessment, there is no evidence that the current design jeopardized the results.

Our reliability results confirmed recent results [39], extended the short-term reliability from 3 min to 30 min, and extended the study population from healthy participants to a group of individuals with bilateral disc displacement with reduction.

While we believe that our approach is innovative, we want to clearly express that in its current format the approach is not ready for clinical diagnostic application. Future research could lead to the potential utility for characterization of disc position of the TMJs and to better understand the potential role of such vibrations in the intracapsular TMJ status and its impact in jaw function.

Conclusions

The excellent reliability obtained by the examiners reading the JVA data demonstrates that examiners can be properly trained and they can reliably identify and interpret the pertinent data produced by this technological device. In addition, the assessment of the joint vibration as phenomena can be reliably assessed within a short period of time.

Using a six-item composite score a receiver operating curve was generated (value of 0.82) suggesting that this composite score based on the vibration characterization can be used to discriminate between normal disc position and displaced disc position.

Nevertheless, the authors would like to emphasize that the results must be interpreted with caution due to the fact that the composite score is not generated by the instrumentation software, the independence of signals from each TMJ is not yet established, and because the study sample does not represent the entire spectrum of disc displacements and degenerative joint disease.

Abbreviations

ICC: Intraclass correlation coefficient; JVA: Joint vibration analysis; MRI: Vmagnetic resonance imaging; TMD: Temporomandibular disorders; TMJ: Temporomandibular joint

Acknowledgements

Not applicable.

Funding
This Research was in part supported by NIH grant# 5R01DE016417, which had no role in any part of this project.

Authors' contributions
SS contributed to data collection, statistics, and development and editing of the manuscript. HCC contributed to conception and design, supervision of data gathering, interpretation of results, and editing of the manuscript. KK interpreted the MRI data. WDM contributed to performing and interpreting statistics, and to editing the manuscript.YMG was responsible for the study design, development of the research infrastructure, and direct supervision of the data gathering by the first author. Also, she was directly involved in the data analysis, and contributed to the development and editing of the manuscript. All authors read and approved the final manuscript.

Competing interests
The authors declare that they have no competing interests.

Consent for publication
Not applicable.

Ethics approval and consent to participate
The study was approved by the University at Buffalo's Health Sciences Institutional Review Board (SIS0050203A) and each subject gave informed consent.

References
1. de Leeuw R, Klasser GD. Guidelines for assessment, diagnosis, and management. In: Temporomandibular disorders. Fifthth ed. Hanover Park: Quintessence Publishing Co; 2013. p. 129–204.
2. Schiffman E, Ohrbach R, Truelove E, Look J, Anderson G, Goulet JP, List T, Svensson P, Gonzalez Y, Lobbezoo F, et al. Diagnostic criteria for temporomandibular disorders (DC/TMD) for clinical and research applications: recommendations of the international RDC/TMD consortium network* and orofacial pain special interest groupdagger. J Oral Facial Pain Headache. 2014;28(1):6–27.
3. Brown DT, Cox 2nd LK, Hafez AA, Cox CF. True normal" TMD control subjects: a rare clinical finding. Cranio. 1998;16(2):84–9.
4. Christensen LV, Orloff J. Reproducibility of temporomandibular joint vibrations (electrovibratography). J Oral Rehabil. 1992;19(3):253–63.
5. Tallents RH, Hatala M, Katzberg RW, Westesson PL. Temporomandibular joint sounds in asymptomatic volunteers. J Prosthet Dent. 1993;69(3):298–304.
6. Greene CS. Managing the care of patients with temporomandibular disorders: a new guideline for care. JADA. 2010;141(9):1086–8.
7. Look JO, Schiffman EL, Truelove EL, Ahmad M. Reliability and validity of axis I of the research diagnostic criteria for temporomandibular disorders (RDC/TMD) with proposed revisions. J Oral Rehabil. 2010;37(10):744–59.
8. Ahmad M, Hollender L, Anderson Q, Kartha K, Ohrbach R, Truelove EL, John MT, Schiffman EL. Research diagnostic criteria for temporomandibular disorders (RDC/TMD): development of image analysis criteria and examiner reliability for image analysis. Oral Surg Oral Med Oral Pathol Oral Radiol Endod. 2009;107(6):844–60.
9. Truelove E, Pan W, Look JO, Mancl LA, Ohrbach RK, Velly AM, Huggins KH, Lenton P, Shiffman EL. The research diagnostic criteria for temporomandibular disorders. III: validity of axis I diagnoses. J Orofac Pain. 2010;24(1):35–47.
10. Ateshian GA. A theoretical formulation for boundary friction in articular cartilage. J Biomech Eng. 1997;119(1):81–6.
11. Nitzan DW. The process of lubrication impairment and its involvement in temporomandibular joint disc displacement: a theoretical concept. J Oral Maxillofac Surg. 2001;59(1):36–45.
12. Tanaka E, Dalla-Bona DA, Iwabe T, Kawai N, Yamano E, van Eijden T, Tanaka M, Miyauchi M, Takata T, Tanne K. The effect of removal of the disc on the friction in the temporomandibular joint. J Oral Maxillofac Surg. 2006;64(8):1221–4.
13. Tanaka E, Iwabe T, Dalla-Bona DA, Kawai N, van Eijden T, Tanaka M, Kitagawa S, Takata T, Tanne K. The effect of experimental cartilage damage and impairment and restoration of synovial lubrication on friction in the temporomandibular joint. J Orofac Pain. 2005;19(4):331–6.
14. Tanaka E, Kawai N, Tanaka M, Todoh M, van Eijden T, Hanaoka K, Dalla-Bona DA, Takata T, Tanne K. The frictional coefficient of the temporomandibular joint and its dependency on the magnitude and duration of joint loading. J Dent Res. 2004;83(5):404–7.
15. Chu M, Gradisar I, Mostardi R. A noninvasive electroacoustical evaluation technique of cartilage damage in pathological knee joint. Med Biol Eng Comput. 1978;16(4):437–42.
16. Chu ML, Gradisar IA, Railey MR, Bowling GF. Detection of knee joint diseases using acoustical pattern recognition technique. J Biomech. 1976;9(3):111–4.
17. Chu ML, Gradisar IA, Railey MR, Bowling GF. An electro-acoustical technique for the detection of knee joint noise. Med Res Eng. 1976;12(1):18–20.
18. Sharma S, Crow HC, McCall Jr WD, Gonzalez YM. Systematic review of reliability and diagnostic validity of joint vibration analysis for diagnosis of temporomandibular disorders. J Orofac Pain. 2013;27(1):51–60.
19. Rasmussen OC. Description of population and progress of symptoms in a longitudinal study of temporomandibular arthropathy. Scand J Dent Res. 1981;89(2):196–203.
20. Kalaykova S, Lobbezoo F, Naeije M. Two-year natural course of anterior disc displacement with reduction. J Orofac Pain. 2010;24(4):373–8.
21. Kurita K, Westesson PL, Yuasa H, Toyama M, Machida J, Ogi N. Natural course of untreated symptomatic temporomandibular joint disc displacement without reduction. J Dent Res. 1998;77(2):361–5.
22. Manfredini D, Favero L, Gregorini G, Cocilovo F, Guarda-Nardini L. Natural course of temporomandibular disorders with low pain-related impairment: a 2-to-3-year follow-up study. J Oral Rehabil. 2013;40(6):436–42.
23. Sato S, Goto S, Kawamura H, Motegi K. The natural course of nonreducing disc displacement of the TMJ: relationship of clinical findings at initial visit to outcome after 12 months without treatment. J Orofac Pain. 1997;11(4):315–20.
24. Sato S, Goto S, Nasu F, Motegi K. Natural course of disc displacement with reduction of the temporomandibular joint: changes in clinical signs and symptoms. J Oral Maxillofac Surg. 2003;61(1):32–4.
25. Yura S. Natural course of acute closed lock of the temporomandibular joint. Br J Oral Maxillofac Surg. 2012;50(7):646–9.
26. Imirzalioglu P, Biler N, Agildere AM. Clinical and radiological follow-up results of patients with untreated TMJ closed lock. J Oral Rehabil. 2005;32(5):326–31.
27. Schiffman EL, Ahmad M, Hollender L, Kartha K, Ohrbach R, Truelove EL, Zhang L, Hodges JS, Sommers E, Anderson GC, et al. Longitudinal Stability of Common TMJ Structural Disorders. J Dent Res. 2016. https://doi.org/10.1177/0022034516679396.
28. Zweig MH, Campbell G. Receiver-operating characteristic (ROC) plots: a fundamental evaluation tool in clinical medicine. Clin Chem. 1993;39(4):561–77.
29. Altman DG. Problems in dichotomizing continuous variables [letter; comment]. Am J Epidemiol. 1994;139:442–5.
30. [https://www.bioresearchinc.com/]. Accessed May 20, 2016
31. Dworkin SF, LeResche L. Research diagnostic criteria for temporomandibular disorders: review, criteria, examinations and specifications, critique. J Craniomand Disord. 1992;6:301–55.
32. Ishigaki S, Bessette RW, Maruyama T. Vibration analysis of the temporomandibular joints with degenerative joint disease. J Craniomandib Prac. 1993;11:276–83.
33. Diagnostic criteria for temporomandibular disorders (DC/TMD) clinical examination protocol: version 02June2013 [www.rdc-tmdinternational.org]. Accessed Nov 29, 2016.
34. Radke JC, Kull RS. Distribution of temporomandibular joint vibration transfer to the opposite side. Cranio. 2012;30(3):194–200.
35. R: A language and environment for statistical computing. [http://www.R-project.org/]. Accessed 14 Feb 2017.
36. Took CC, Sanei S, Rickard S, Chambers J, Dunne S. Fractional delay estimation for blind source separation and localization of temporomandibular joint sounds. IEEE Trans Biomed Eng. 2008;55(3):949–56.
37. Widmalm SE, Williams WJ, Ang BK, McKay DC. Localization of TMJ sounds to side. J Oral Rehabil. 2002;29(10):911–7.
38. Widmalm SE, Williams WJ, Yang KP. False localization of TMJ sounds to side is an important source of error in TMD diagnosis. J Oral Rehabil. 1999;26(3):213–4.
39. Zhang J, Whittle T, Wang L, Murray GM. The reproducibility of temporomandibular joint vibrations over time in the human. J Oral Rehabil. 2014;41(3):206–17.

19

Waist circumference and waist-to-height ratio are associated with periodontal pocketing—results of the Health 2000 Survey

Sanna Kangas[1], Petra Timonen[2], Matti Knuuttila[3], Antti Jula[4], Pekka Ylöstalo[3,5,6,7] and Anna-Maija Hannele Syrjälä[3,5*]

Abstract

Background: Body mass index (BMI) has been found to associate with different parameters of chronic periodontal disease in previous studies. It is reasonable to expect that central adiposity measures, such as waist circumference and waist-to-height ratio, which indirectly takes into account visceral fat, are more accurate measures of obesity-related oral health risks than BMI. The aim of this study was to examine whether central obesity is associated with periodontal pocketing, an indication of infectious chronic periodontal disease.

Methods: The study was based on a subpopulation from the national Health 2000 Survey in Finland. It included dentate, non-diabetic, never-smoking subjects aged 30–49 ($n = 1287$). The outcome variable was the number of teeth with deepened periodontal pockets (4 mm or more) and the number of teeth with deep periodontal pockets (6 mm or more). Central obesity was measured by means of waist circumference (WC) and waist-to-height ratio (WHtR). Poisson regression models were used to estimate prevalence rate ratios (PRR) and their 95% confidence intervals.

Results: Our main finding was that both WC and WHtR were associated with the number of teeth with deeper (4 mm or more) periodontal pockets; the PRR for the fifth quintile in WC was 1.5, CI: 1.2–1.9 and in WHtR 1.4, CI: 1.1–1.7, when compared to the lowest quintile. Corresponding figures for deep (6 mm or more) periodontal pockets were 2.3, CI: 0.9–6.1 for WC and 1.9, CI: 0.8–4.4 for WHtR. There were no essential differences in the strengths of the associations between WC and WHtR and the number of teeth with deepened periodontal pockets.

Conclusion: Both central adipose measures—WC and WHtR—seem to be associated with periodontal pocketing in non-diabetic, never-smoking subjects aged 30–49 years old.

Keywords: Periodontal disease, Periodontal pocketing, Waist-to-height ratio, Waist circumference, Overweight

Background

A large number of non-experimental studies have reported a weak or moderately strong association between overweight or obesity and a variety of parameters of periodontal disease [1–5]. In these studies, overweight and obesity have most often been measured by means of the body mass index (BMI), but also other measures of adiposity such as waist circumference (WC), waist-hip ratio (WHR) and waist-to-height ratio (WHtR) have been used.

A well-known shortcoming of BMI is that it does not take into account body composition nor distribution of fat. Regarding the distribution of fat tissue, it has been observed that visceral fat accumulation has harmful health effects; it increases the risk of cardiovascular disease more than does subcutaneous fat [6] and it increases the risk of cardiovascular disease regardless of BMI [7]. In some periodontal studies, adiposity measures

* Correspondence: Anna-Maija.Syrjala@oulu.fi
[3]Medical Research Center Oulu, Oulu University Hospital and University of Oulu, Oulu, Finland
[5]Periodontology and Geriatric Dentistry, Unit of Oral Health Sciences Research, P.O. Box 5281, FI-90014 Oulu, Finland
Full list of author information is available at the end of the article

such as WC and WHR that take visceral fat into account have been reported to be associated more strongly with different parameters of infectious periodontal diseases than commonly used BMI [8–11]. These findings suggest that adiposity measures that measure visceral fat accumulation accurately indicate the obesity-related health risks for periodontal health, at least more accurately than commonly used BMI.

The simplest measure of central adiposity is waist circumference, and it has been shown to be a fairly reliable indicator for periodontal disease [8, 12, 13]. However, an obvious shortcoming of waist circumference (WC) is that it relies solely on the person's waist circumference. Based on this it is expected that WHtR, which also takes into account the person's height, would be a better measure than waist circumference alone. WHtR has recently been reported to reveal several health risks including diabetes, hypertension, dyslipidaemia, metabolic syndrome and cardiovascular diseases better than BMI and WC, although in some cases the differences were small and statistically insignificant [14]. To date, only one study has analysed WHtR in relation to periodontal disease; a longitudinal study found that WHtR predicts periodontal disease progression better than BMI [15].

We have reported earlier that BMI is associated with periodontal pocketing in the Health 2000 Survey [16, 17]. Based on the known shortcomings of BMI, our aim in the present paper was to study whether central adiposity measures—WC and WHtR—are consistently associated with the number of teeth with deepened periodontal pockets, an indication of an infectious form of chronic periodontal disease among never-smoking, non-diabetic, 30–49-year-old persons.

Methods

Study design

The National Institute for Health and Welfare (formerly the National Public Health Institute of Finland) performed a Health 2000 Survey between 2000 and 2001. Data for the Health 2000 Survey were obtained from laboratory measurements, clinical health and oral examinations, self-administered questionnaires and interviews. The original survey was a nationally representative sample and consisted of 8028 subjects aged 30 or older living in continental Finland.

This cross-sectional study was restricted to subjects aged 30–49 years old. The exclusion of diabetic persons yielded a population of 2856 subjects. After further exclusion of persons who had smoked, there were 1326 persons left; of those 1297 subjects had periodontal data and 1287 subjects had both periodontal data and central obesity and height measurements available.

The clinical oral surveys were carried out by five field units (each including one dentist and one dental nurse or hygienist). They examined the condition of the periodontium and teeth using a headlamp, a mouth mirror and a WHO periodontal probe in line with WHO instructions. More information about the Health 2000 Examination Survey is reported by Heistaro [18].

Participation in this survey was voluntary and the participants gave their written consent for this study. The Ethical Committee for Epidemiology and Public Health of the Hospital District of Helsinki and Uusimaa approved the study protocol.

Outcome variables

The outcome variables were the number of teeth with deepened periodontal pockets (4 mm or more) and the number of teeth with deep periodontal pockets (6 mm or more). Periodontal pocket depth was probed on four surfaces (distobuccal, mid-buccal, mid-oral and mesio-oral) of each tooth, except third molars, and the deepest measurement on each tooth was recorded. There was 82% agreement ($\kappa = 0.32$) between a reference examiner and the field examiners [19]. For this outcome (the number of teeth with deepened periodontal pockets) no power-calculation was made.

Explanatory variables

Information on weight and height was obtained from the clinical health examination. Waist circumference (WC, in centimetres) and waist-to-height ratio (WHtR; waist circumference in centimetres divided by height in centimetres) were used as explanatory variables. Men and women were separately categorised into five categories according to the distribution of WC and WHtR, and then respective categories for men and women were combined in non-gender-specific analyses (Table 3).

Other variables

In this study, gender, age and educational level were used to describe sociodemographic background. Educational level was classified into three categories: the highest level consisted of those who had a university degree or had graduated from a polytechnic, the second level consisted of those who had graduated from high school and the lowest-level subjects had less than a high school education.

The presence of dental plaque was recorded on one side on three indicator teeth (the most posterior tooth on the upper right side, and the most posterior tooth and canine on the lower left side) [18]. The results were categorised into three categories using a modified version of the method described by Sillness and Löe [20]: no dental plaque on the indicator teeth, dental plaque in the gingival margins on the indicator teeth, and dental plaque also elsewhere on the indicator teeth. Dental visits were classified into two categories: regular *vs.* irregular check-ups. Toothbrushing was categorised into three categories: at least twice a day, daily and more seldom.

BMI (Body Mass Index; body weight in kilograms divided by the square of height in metres) was used as a categorised variable according to the WHO definition [21] of overweight and obesity: BMI < 25, 25–29.9 and ≥ 30. Lipid-lowering medication was classified into three groups: yes, no or unknown. Alcohol consumption was measured as grams of alcohol per week.

The basic characteristics of the study population as well as the basic characteristics of the study population by quintiles of waist circumference are presented in Table 1.

Table 1 Characteristics of the study population according to quintiles of waist circumference

	Waist circumference					
	Total *n* = 1287	I quintile *n* = 266 (lowest)	II quintile *n* = 255	III quintile *n* = 236	IV quintile *n* = 266	V quintile *n* = 264 (highest)
Sociodemographic variables						
Gender, proportion of males, %	42.5	42.4	42.6	41.0	43.9	42.2
Age, mean (± SD)	39.6 (±5.7)	37.5 (±5.2)	39.3 (±5.6)	39.0 (±5.9)	41.2 (±5.3)	40.9 (±5.7)
Education						
Low, %	11.9	7.8	12.4	10.0	13.3	15.7
Intermediate, %	36.9	29.7	32.2	42.3	38.7	41.9
High, %	51.2	62.5	55.4	47.7	48.0	42.3
Dental variables						
Number of teeth						
Mean (± SD)	27.1 (±3.9)	28.0 (±3.1)	27.1 (±4.2)	27.5 (±3.1)	26.9 (±3.9)	26.3 (±4.8)
Median (interquartile range)	28 (3)	28 (3)	28 (2)	28 (2)	28 (2)	28 (4)
Min, max	1, 32	4, 32	1, 32	9, 32	6, 32	3, 32
Number of teeth with periodontal pockets ≥ 4 mm						
Mean (± SD)	2.6 (±4.0)	1.8 (±2.9)	2.5 (±3.7)	2.2 (±3.5)	2.7 (±4.0)	3.6 (±5.2)
Median (interquartile range)	1 (3)	1 (3)	1 (4)	1 (3)	1 (4)	1 (5)
Min, max	0, 28	0, 14	0, 25	0, 20	0, 26	0, 28
Number of teeth with periodontal pockets ≥ 6 mm						
Mean (± SD)	0.2 (±1.2)	0.1 (±0.5)	0.1 (±0.5)	0.1 (±0.7)	0.2 (±0.9)	0.5 (±2.4)
Median (interquartile range)	0.00 (0)	0.00 (0)	0.00 (0)	0.00 (0)	0.00 (0)	0.00 (0)
Min, max	0, 26	0, 4	0, 7	0, 7	0, 9	0, 26
Dental plaque						
No dental plaque, %	40.7	46.1	43.1	46.3	38.9	29.8
Dental plaque at the gingival margins, %	50.2	46.7	48.4	45.9	52.9	56.5
Dental plaque also elsewhere, %	9.1	7.2	8.4	7.8	8.1	13.6
Dental visits						
Regular check-ups, %	69.0	75.1	71.0	70.9	67.7	60.3
Irregular, %	31.0	24.9	29.0	29.1	32.3	39.7
Toothbrushing						
At least twice a day, %	68.7	78.2	71.9	64.8	71.6	56.2
Daily, %	27.1	18.3	26.9	31.7	24.1	35.3
Less often, %	4.2	3.4	1.2	3.5	4.2	8.5
Alcohol consumption, mean (± SD)	60.3 (±97.7)	44.2 (±58.7)	66.1 (±97.7)	56.8 (±94.9)	67.0 (±101.6)	67.5 (±123.1)
BMI, mean (± SD)	25.7 (±4.4)	21.5 (±1.8)	23.4 (±1.9)	24.9 (±1.7)	26.6 (±2.0)	31.9 (±4.2)
Lipid-lowering medication, %	1.2	0.0	0.8	1.3	1.5	2.6

Statistical methods

Medians, interquartile ranges and minimum and maximum values for the number of teeth, the number of teeth with deepened periodontal pockets (4 mm or more) and the number of teeth with deep periodontal pockets (6 mm or more) were calculated.

Prevalence rate ratios (PRR) and 95% confidence intervals (95% CI) were estimated using Poisson regression models. Covariates in the regression models included potential determinants of periodontitis such as age, gender, educational level, presence of dental plaque, toothbrushing frequency, dental visits and use of lipid-lowering medication. Stratified analyses according to gender were performed.

A stratified two-stage cluster sampling design was applied in the study. The sample was weighted by post-stratification according to gender, age and region. The data analyses were performed using STATA 8.0 to take into account the two-stage cluster sampling design.

Results

The unadjusted and adjusted prevalence rate ratios (PRR) with 95% confidence intervals (CI) are shown in Tables 2 and 3.

As seen in Table 3, persons with a large WC and a high WHtR had, on average, a 40–60% higher likelihood of having teeth with periodontal pockets ≥ 4 mm than those belonging to the lowest quintile (reference category).

As seen in Table 3, persons with a large WC and a high WHtR were, on average, 30–50% more likely to have more teeth affected with pockets of more than 4 mm than those belonging to the lowest quintile (reference category). There were some deviations from linearity in the association between both WC and WHtR and the number of teeth with deepened periodontal pockets ≥ 4 mm.

The association with the number of teeth with periodontal pockets ≥ 6 mm was less consistent, showing pronounced deviations from linearity. Confidence intervals were wide and none of the risk estimates were statistically significant at a p-level of 0.05.

When comparing the associations between WC and WHtR and periodontal pockets ≥ 4 mm, there were no essential differences in the strengths of the associations (Table 3). The associations with deep periodontal pockets were difficult to compare due to the large confidence intervals, but the overall association between WHtR and deep periodontal pockets was somewhat weaker than that of WC (Table 3).

When men and women were analysed separately, the associations between both WC and WHtR and teeth with periodontal pockets of ≥ 4 mm in both men and women were close to those found in the total study population. There were inconsistent differences between genders in the association of WC and WHtR with the number of teeth with periodontal pockets ≥ 6 mm. Confidence intervals were large and the association showed pronounced deviations from linearity (data not shown).

Discussion

We expected that the measure which also takes into account the person's height would be associated more strongly with periodontal pocketing than would the simple measure of central obesity. However, to our surprise, the strength of the association between WHtR and periodontal pockets did not differ essentially from that of WC. We also expected that the WC and WHtR measures would be associated more strongly than BMI with periodontal disease. Again, to our surprise, the strength of the association was of quite the same magnitude as the association between BMI and periodontal pocketing, reported earlier by Ylöstalo and co-workers [16].

Based on the findings of the present study and the findings of the earlier one using the same data, we have to conclude that our results are somewhat different from a number of earlier studies, because the use of WHtR as a measure of obesity did not seem to provide any essential benefits compared with WC. The use of WC or WHtR did not provide any essential benefits compared with commonly used BMI, either. The reason why WC or WHtR were not superior to BMI could be that BMI may sufficiently indicate obesity-related health risks in this low-risk population. This may related to the fact that BMI appears to have a fairly high correlation with body fat among the young population, especially among women [22]. High correlations between BMI and other measures of adiposity have also been reported in these Health 2000 data [16].

There are currently a very limited number of studies where a multitude of adiposity measures including both WC and WHtR have been used. One of them is a study by Gorman and co-workers [15], who reported that WHtR was associated more strongly than WC with periodontal disease progression, measured by means of probing pocket depth, alveolar bone loss and clinical attachment loss. The fact that the results were not in line with previous studies may be related to the other properties of this study population; due to restrictions the study subjects were non-smokers and their mean age was less than 40 years. Because the data were restricted to persons who were less than 50 years old, we cannot, of course, say anything about how the central measures of obesity behave in older populations. However, habitual changes in body composition—increasing fat and decreasing muscle mass—suggest that measures which take into account these aspects are most likely better than simple measures such as absolute or relative

Table 2 Relation of study variables to the number of teeth with periodontal pockets

	Teeth with periodontal pockets ≥ 4 mm	Teeth with periodontal pockets ≥ 6 mm
	Unadjusted PRR (95% CI)	Unadjusted PRR (95% CI)
Waist circumference (*n* = 1287)		
I quintile	1	1
II quintile	1.4 (1.1–1.8)	1.1 (0.4–2.9)
III quintile	1.2 (0.9–1.6)	1.3 (0.4–3.7)
IV quintile	1.5 (1.1–2.0)	2.3 (0.8–6.2)
V quintile	2.1 (1.7–2.7)	6.0 (2.6–13.9)
Waist-to-height Ratio (*n* = 1287)		
I quintile	1	1
II quintile	1.3 (0.9–1.7)	1.1 (0.4–2.5)
III quintile	1.3 (1.0–1.7)	1.2 (0.5–3.0)
IV quintile	1.6 (1.2–2.1)	3.2 (1.3–7.5)
V quintile	2.0 (1.5–2.5)	5.9 (2.7–12.6)
Sociodemographic variables		
Gender (*n* = 1297)		
Female	1	1
Male	0.7 (0.6–0.8)	0.4 (0.2–0.7)
Age (*n* = 1297)		
30–34	1	1
35–39	1.3 (1.0–1.7)	2.4 (0.9–6.5)
40–44	1.6 (1.2–2.1)	5.6 (2.0–16.1)
45–49	2.0 (1.5–2.7)	5.2 (1.9–13.9)
Education (*n* = 1297)		
High	1	1
Intermediate	1.3 (1.1–1.5)	3.3 (1.7–6.3)
Low	1.9 (1.4–2.4)	7.2 (3.6–14.3)
Dental variables (*n* = 1297)		
Number of teeth		
≥ 25	1	1
21–24	1.5 (1.2–2.0)	2.4 (1.1–4.9)
1–20	1.9 (1.2–2.8)	3.6 (1.5–8.9)
Dental plaque (*n* = 1294)		
No dental plaque	1	1
Dental plaque at the gingival margins	2.1 (1.7–2.6)	2.7 (1.2–6.3)
Dental plaque also elsewhere	4.9 (3.7–6.6)	19.4 (7.8–48.8)
Dental visits (*n* = 1253)		
Regular check-ups	1	1
Irregular	1.5 (1.2–1.8)	3.7 (2.0–6.9)
Toothbrushing (*n* = 1253)		
At least twice a day	1	1
Daily	1.1 (0.9–1.4)	2.0 (0.9–4.5)
Less often	2.1 (1.5–2.9)	3.8 (1.8–8.0)

Table 2 Relation of study variables to the number of teeth with periodontal pockets *(Continued)*

Lipid-lowering medication (*n* = 1297)		
Yes	1	1
No	0.8 (0.5–1.3)	2.9 (0.5–17.7)
Unknown	0.9 (0.5–1.5)	4.6 (0.5–43.9)

weights, or even a simple measure of central obesity. This reasoning is supported by the study by Romero-Corral et al. [22], who reported that correlations between BMI and body fat are also somewhat lower in older age groups.

Strengths and limitations

The effect of competing risks for periodontitis such as tobacco smoking, diabetes and age was eliminated by restricting this study to those who had never smoked, had no signs of diabetes and were 30–49 years old. The confounding effect of other potential risks for periodontitis was controlled by using multivariate models. Covariates that were used to control for the effects of poor oral hygiene were dental plaque and toothbrushing frequency. These methods controlled completely for the effects of diabetes and smoking, and also to some degree for the effects of various behavioural factors associated with smoking. The methods used to control for the effect of poor oral hygiene are always more or less incomplete, and it is possible that some residual confounding related to oral hygiene exists.

The outcome variables were continuous variables—the number of teeth with pocket depth ≥ 4 mm and ≥ 6 mm—both indicative of infectious periodontal diseases, although of different severity. Regarding its registration and measurement, it should be noted that the fact that registering was done at tooth level may have caused an underestimation of the extent of periodontal disease. Also the fact that pocket measurement was done on four predetermined sites may have caused an underestimation of periodontal disease. However, the effects of the above-mentioned aspects are mostly likely small, as most of the participants had a fairly healthy periodontium, i.e., they had a very small number of teeth with deepened periodontal pockets.

Table 3 Relation of WC and WHtR to the number of teeth with periodontal pockets

	WC	WHtR
	Adjusted PRR (95% CI)	Adjusted PRR (95% CI)
	n = 1241	*n* = 1241
Teeth with periodontal pockets ≥ 4 mm		
I quintile	1.0	1
II quintile	1.3 (1.0–1.7)	1.2 (0.9–1.5)
III quintile	1.2 (0.9–1.5)	1.2 (0.9–1.5)
IV quintile	1.2 (0.9–1.6)	1.2 (0.9–1.6)
V quintile	1.5 (1.2–1.9)	1.4 (1.1–1.7)
Teeth with periodontal pockets ≥ 6 mm		
I quintile	1.0	1
II quintile	0.8 (0.3–2.3)	0.6 (0.2–1.7)
III quintile	1.1 (0.4–3.1)	0.8 (0.3–1.9)
IV quintile	1.3 (0.5–3.7)	1.6 (0.7–4.0)
V quintile	2.3 (0.9–6.1)	1.9 (0.8–4.4)

Models are adjusted for age, gender, education, dental plaque, toothbrushing, dental visiting and lipid-lowering medication
WC Waist Circumference, *WHtR* Waist-to-height Ratio

Conclusions

Based on these data, it can be estimated that the subjects who belong to the highest quintiles of WC or WHtR have a 40–60% increased likelihood of having teeth with periodontal pockets at least 4 mm deep compared with those belonging to the lowest quintiles of WC or WHtR. The typical number of teeth with deepened periodontal pockets at least 4 mm deep was two or three among lean persons, but if the person had a large waist circumference, measured either absolutely (WC) or relatively (WHtR), he/she had approximately one tooth more with a deepened periodontal pocket. This excess of periodontally affected teeth, which can be attributed to central obesity, can be compared, for example, with the excess that can be attributed to daily smoking, which in these data was about 2–3 teeth with periodontal pocketing [16].

Both WC and WHtR seemed to be associated with periodontal pocketing, an indication for infectious chronic periodontal disease among non-diabetic, never-smoking subjects aged 30–49 years old. The overall interpretation is that the findings of this study lend support to the findings of previous studies where an association between obesity and various parameters of chronic periodontitis has been found. Self-evidently this study also lends support to the current view in periodontal research that obesity may have adverse effects on the periodontium. In the present study, we could not observe any essential differences in the strengths of the associations between WC and WHtR and periodontal pocketing, indicating that additional information about other dimensions of the body does not provide any essential benefits in this age group when assessing obesity-related risks for periodontal health.

Abbreviations

BMI: Body mass index; CI: Confidence intervals; PRR: Prevalence rate ratios; WC: Waist circumference; WHR: Waist-hip ratio; WHtR: Waist-to-height ratio

Acknowledgements

The present study is part of the Health 2000 Survey, organised by the National Institute for Health and Welfare (THL), the former Public Health Institute (KTL) of Finland (http://www.terveys2000.fi/indexe.html), and partly supported by the Finnish Dental Society Apollonia and the Finnish Dental Association.

Statistician Ahti Niinimaa is acknowledged for his statistical guidance.

Funding

Health 2000 Survey is supported by National Institute for Health and Welfare (THL), the former Public Health Institute (KTL) of Finland (http://www.terveys2000.fi/indexe.html), the Finnish Dental Society Apollonia and the Finnish Dental Association. Funding covers study design of Health 2000 Survey and collection of clinical data.

Authors' contributions

SK has has compiled this article as her thesis work in dentistry. She has made partly the drafting. She has participated in the interpretation of the data, revised the article and participated in final approval of the article. PT has participated in the drafting, revised the article and participated in the final approval. MK is a dental consultant in the Health 2000 Survey and at the Medical Research Center in Oulu University. He has participated in interpretation, revision and final approval of the article. AJ is a consultant of internal medicine in the Health 2000 Survey. He has revised the article, participated in the interpretation of the data and participated in final approval. PY has supervised the writing of the manuscript. He has participated in drafting, interpretation and revision of the article and participated in final approval. A-MS has supervised the writing of the manuscript. She made partly the drafting. She has participated in the interpretation of the data and revised the article and participated in final approval of the article. All authors read and approved the final manuscript.

Competing interests

Unit of Oral Health Sciences Research, Oulu University, will cover partially or in entirely the article processing charge. The authors declare that they have no other competing of interest in this study.

Consent for publication

Not applicable.

Ethical approval and consent to participate

The Ethical Committee for Epidemiology and Public Health of the Hospital District of Helsinki and Uusimaa approved the study protocol. Participation in this survey was voluntary and the participants gave their written consent for this study.

Author details

[1]Private Dental Office Viisaudenhammas, Rovaniemi, Finland. [2]Dental Training Clinic, Social and Health Services, Oulu, Finland. [3]Medical Research Center Oulu, Oulu University Hospital and University of Oulu, Oulu, Finland. [4]National Institute for Health and Welfare (THL), Helsinki, Finland. [5]Periodontology and Geriatric Dentistry, Unit of Oral Health Sciences Research, P.O. Box 5281, FI-90014 Oulu, Finland. [6]Institute of Dentistry, University of Eastern Finland, Kuopio Campus, Kuopio, Finland. [7]Oral and Maxillofacial Department, Kuopio University Hospital, Kuopio, Finland.

References

1. Chaffee BW, Weston SJ. Association between chronic periodontal disease and obesity: a systematic review and meta-analysis. J Periodontol. 2010;81:1708–24.
2. Suvan J, D'Aiuto F, Moles DR, Petrie A, Donos N. Association between overweight/obesity and periodontitis in adults. A systematic review. Obes Rev. 2011;12:e381–404.
3. Keller A, Rohde JF, Raymond K, Heitmann BL. Association between periodontal disease and overweight and obesity: a systematic review. J Periodontol. 2015;86:766–76.
4. Muñoz-Torres FJ, Jiménez MC, Rivas-Tumanyan S, Joshipura KJ. Associations between measures of central adiposity and periodontitis among older adults. Community Dent Oral Epidemiol. 2014;42:170–7.
5. Nascimento GG, Leite FR, Do LG, Peres KG, Correa MB, Demarco FF, Peres MA. Is weight gain associated with the incidence of periodontitis? A systematic review and meta-analysis. J Clin Periodontol. 2015;42:495–505.
6. Ryo M, Funahashi T, Nakamura T, Kihara S, Kotani K, Tokunaga K, Matsuzawa Y, Shimomura I. Fat accumulation and obesity-related cardiovascular risk factors in middle-aged Japanese men and women. Intern Med. 2014;53:299–305.
7. Miyawaki T, Abe M, Yahata K, Kajiyama N, Katsuma H, Saito N. Contribution of visceral fat accumulation to the risk factors for atherosclerosis in non-obese Japanese. Intern Med. 2004;43:1138–44.
8. Saito T, Shimazaki Y, Koga T, Tsuzuki M, Ohshima A. Relationship between upper body obesity and periodontitis. J Dent Res. 2001;80:1631–6.
9. Al-Zahrani MS, Bissada NF, Borawskit EA. Obesity and periodontal disease in young, middle-aged, and older adults. J Periodontol. 2003;74:610–5.
10. Wood N, Johnson RB, Streckfus CF. Comparison of body composition and periodontal disease using nutritional assessment techniques: Third National Health and Nutrition Examination Survey (NHANES III). J Clin Periodontol. 2003;30:321–7.
11. Kim EJ, Jin BH, Bae KH. Periodontitis and obesity: a study of the Fourth Korean National Health and Nutrition Examination Survey. Periodontol. 2011;82:533–42.
12. Han DH, Lim SY, Sun BC, Paek DM, Kim HD. Visceral fat area-defined obesity and periodontitis among Koreans. J Clin Periodontol. 2010;37:172–9.
13. Palle AR, Reddy CM, Shankar BS, Gelli V, Sudhakar J, Reddy KK. Association between obesity and chronic periodontitis: a cross-sectional study. J Contemp Dent Pract. 2013;14:168–73.
14. Ashwell M, Gunn P, Gibson S. Waist-to-height ratio is a better screening tool than waist circumference and BMI for adult cardiometabolic risk factors: systematic review and meta-analysis. Obes Rev. 2012;13:275–86.
15. Gorman A, Kaye EK, Apovian C, Fung TT, Nunn M, Garcia RI. Overweight and obesity predict time to periodontal disease progression in men. J Clin Periodontol. 2012;39:107–14.
16. Ylöstalo P, Suominen-Taipale L, Reunanen A, Knuuttila M. Association between body weight and periodontal infection. J Clin Periodontol. 2008;35:297–304.
17. Saxlin T, Ylöstalo P, Suominen-Taipale L, Männistö S, Knuuttila M. Association between periodontal infection and obesity: results of the Health 2000 Survey. J Clin Periodontol. 2011;38:236–42.
18. Heistaro S, editor. Methodology report. Health 2000 Survey B26/2008. Helsinki: Publications of the National Public Health Institute; 2008.
19. Vehkalahti M, Knuuttila M, Hausen H. Kliinisten mittausten laadun varmistaminen (Quality assurance of clinical examinations). In: Suominen-Taipale L, Nordblad A, Vehkalahti M, Aromaa A, editors. Suomalaisten aikuisten suunterveys, Terveys 2000 – tutkimus (Oral Health of Finnish Adults, Health 2000 Health Examination Survey) B16/2004. Helsinki: Publications of the National Public Health Institute; 2004. p. 24–32.
20. Silness J, Löe H. Periodontal disease in pregnancy II. Correlation between oral hygiene and periodontal condition. Acta Odontol Scand. 1964;22:121–35.
21. Word Health Organization. Obesity. Preventing and managing the global epidemic. Report of a WHO consultation (WHO Technical Report Series 894). Geneva: Word Health Organization; 2000.
22. Romero-Corral A, Somers VK, Sierra-Johnson J, Thomas RJ, Collazo-Clavell ML, Korinek J, Allison TG, Batsis JA, Sert-Kuniyoshi FH, Lopez-Jimenez F. Accuracy of body mass index in diagnosing obesity in the adult general population. Int J Obes (Lond). 2008;32:959–66.

Less extrusion debris during the retreatment of curved canals using twisted files with higher rotational speeds: an *ex vivo* study

Mengdong Liu[1,2], Shijiang Xiong[1*], Fei Tan[2] and Yi Liu[2]

Abstract

Background: Debris extrusion from the apical foramen can be problematic in severely curved canals. This study aimed to assess the use of Twisted Files (TF) at different rotational speeds during retreatment, compared with manual technique using Triple-Flex Files (TFF).

Methods: Forty-eight mesiobuccal root canals were randomized to four groups ($n = 12$ per group). In groups A, B, and C, gutta-percha was removed using TF at 500, 1000, and 1500 rpm, respectively, while it was removed using TFF in group D. Apical debris was collected in a pre-weighed centrifuge tube. The weight of dry debris was assessed by comparing the pre- and post-instrumentation weight for each group.

Results: Instrumentation in group D (0.69 ± 0.04 mg) extruded significantly more debris than any of the TF groups (A: 0.54 ± 0.05 mg; B: 0.48 ± 0.04 mg; C: 0.42 ± 0.03 mg; all $P < 0.001$). In addition, increasing the rotational speed of TF decreased the amount of extruded debris (A vs. B: $P = 0.006$; B vs. C: $P < 0.001$; A vs. C: $P < 0.001$).

Conclusions: TF at 1500 rpm produced less apical extrusion debris than other TF operating speeds and TFF.

Keywords: Apical debris, Root canal therapy, Rotational speed, Tooth apex, Triple-Flex Files, Twisted Files

Background

The main goal of endodontic retreatment is to remove infected dentin and root-filling material throughout the canal length to re-establish decontamination of the root canal system and to preserve the tooth [1, 2]. Debris generated during retreatment may cause undesired consequences, such as inflammation and postoperative pain [1, 3]. Many techniques have been used to remove gutta-percha in root-filled teeth, such as hand files, heat, solvents, and rotary instruments [4]. Unfortunately there is considerable evidence that all of these techniques apically extrude some of the debris, but the amount is likely to vary according to the technique used [4–6]. Motor-driven rotary devices are associated with less dentinal debris extrusion because of their unique file design that also works as an Archimedic screw [7], but the complexity of root canal anatomy makes retreatment difficult and highlights the need for investigation of these issues. Indeed, when using rotary instruments, the high degree of root canal curvature may lead to iatrogenic damage, and this risk in increased with higher rotational speed. A proper evaluation of the different tools available would then allow appropriate and safe retreatment techniques to be selected with the lowest incidence of extrusion possible.

Twisted Files (TF; SybronEndo, Orange, CA, USA) are rotary nickel titanium endodontic files that were introduced in 2008. They can be twisted and converted back into an austenite structure by heating and cooling [8]. The manufacturer claims that TF are superior to traditional file systems due to their cyclic fatigue resistance, flexibility, and better cutting efficiency [9]. Compared with other instruments, TF can work safely at higher rotational speeds, but few studies have investigated the

* Correspondence: xiongshijiangdr@sohu.com
[1]School of Dentistry, Shandong University, 44, Wenhua West Road, Jinan 250012, Shandong Province, China
Full list of author information is available at the end of the article

behavior of TF during retreatment [10]. Previous retreatment studies have been performed on relatively straight root canals [11–13], which may not accurately represent the challenge of retreating curved canals. Furthermore, almost all rotary instruments were studied at similar speeds. Therefore, the influence of rotational speed on effective retreatment has not been assessed.

The purpose of the present study was to quantitatively evaluate the amount of debris extruded apically after endodontic retreatment with TF at different operating speeds, compared with traditional hand techniques using Triple-Flex Files in severely curved root canals.

Methods

Specimen selection

A total of 48 mandibular first molars were collected from patients with periodontal disease undergoing tooth extraction. To be included in the study, tooth had to be without a history or disease or treatment. This study was approved by the ethics committee of the Affiliated Hospital of Qingdao University.

Radiographs of each tooth were obtained, digitized, and stored electronically using the Digora Optime digital imaging system (Soredex, Tuusula, Finland). Angles and radius of curvature were measured using the proprietary software Digora for Windows (DfW version 2.7, Soredex, Tuusula, Finland). Root canal curvature was determined according to the Schneider's method [14]. The radius of each sample was measured according to Schäfer et al. [15].

The mesiobuccal root canals were used when encountering the following criteria: 1) curvature ranging between 25° and 35°; 2) a radius below 10 mm in a buccal direction; and 3) not more than 5° in a mesial to distal direction. The mesiobuccal root canals were examined under an operating microscope (Carl Zeiss, Jena, Germany) to verify the presence of a single apical foramen, with fully formed apices. The roots had no previous root canal treatment. The access cavity was prepared using high-speed diamond burs (Dentsply Maillefer, Ballaigues, Switzerland) with water cooling. After accessing the cavity, the canal patency was established with a size 10 K-file (Dentsply Maillefer, Ballaigues, Switzerland). Only canals with an initial apical size equivalent to a size 10 K-file were selected.

According to the above criteria, 48 molars with severely curved mesiobuccal root canals were collected and thoroughly cleaned by removing the calculus and the soft deposits using curettes. The teeth were stored in a saline solution before use.

Root canal preparation and obturation

Apical patencies were determined with a size 10 K-file. The K-file was introduced carefully into the canal until it was visible at the apical foramen, and the working length (WL) was established as 1 mm short of this length. The crowns were flattened, so that a final dimension of 13-mm working length was achieved for each root.

The coronal portion was initially flared with Gates Glidden drills (Dentsply Maillefer, Ballaigues, Switzerland) sizes 1–3 and was instrumented using ProTaper Universal Rotary Files (Dentsply Maillefer, Ballaigues, Switzerland) up to size F1, according to the manufacturer's instructions. Each instrument was used for the preparation of only one tooth. On withdrawal of each instrument, the canals were flushed with 5 mL of distilled water. ProTaper Universal Gutta Percha Point size F1 (Dentsply Maillefer, Ballaigues, Switzerland) was selected as the master gutta-percha cone fitted with tug-back at the WL. The root canals were dried with sterile paper points and obturated with the master cone and sealer using a continuous wave of condensation technique (System B, Elements Obturation Unit, Sybron Endo, Orange, CA, USA). The total length of the root canal filling did not exceed the level of the staging platform from the apex to the coronal aspect, and also assessed by anteroposterior and lateral view X-ray photography, in an attempt to control the amount of root filling in each tooth, so that the volume of the filling material was approximately equal in all root canals.

The teeth were radiographed (Soredex Minray, Soredex, Milwaukee, WI, USA) at different angles to confirm the quality of the filling procedure. The access cavities were temporarily filled (Cavition-GC, Tokyo, Japan). The obturated roots were stored in 100% humidity at 37°C for two weeks to allow complete setting of the sealer.

Experimental process

The instrument used to evaluate the extruded debris was a minor adaptation from a previously used design (Fig. 1) [16]. The teeth were held securely under pressure by stoppers, and the root apex was hung within the receptor tube and suspended below the upper rim of the centrifuge tube. A bent 27-gauge needle was forced alongside the stopper to use as a drainage cannula and to balance the air pressure inside and outside the tubes. The tube was held vertically by hand only by the outer vial during retreatment. In no case was the inner tube touched by the operator's fingers. All vials were covered with adhesive plaster to prevent the operator from viewing debris extrusion during retreatment. The tubes were individually preweighed three times with a 10^{-5} g precision analytic microbalance (Sartorius AG, Göttingen, Germany).

Retreatment technique

All teeth were coded and randomized to four groups (12 teeth/group). Gutta-percha in the coronal portion was removed using size 1–3 Gates Glidden drills. The rotary

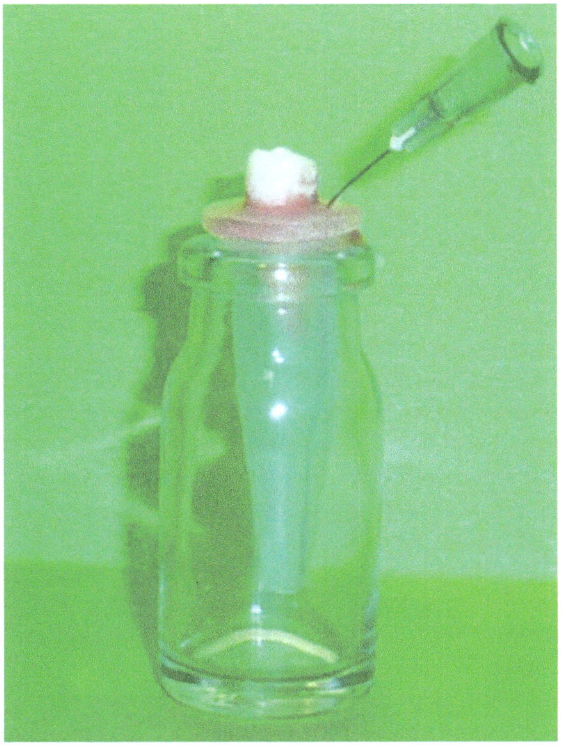

Fig. 1 Collection instrument used to evaluate the apically extruded debris

instrument was driven by an endodontic motor (NSK, Endo-Mate DT, Tokyo, Japan) with the crown-down technique at the recommended speed and torque according to the manufacturer's instructions. The final apical file was one size larger than that used in the first preparation. The four groups were then retreated according to their group allocation. No apical counter pressure was applied.

Group A: Specimens were retreated using TF at 500 rpm without torque-control, according to the manufacturer's recommendations, and using a 4:1 speed reduction and an electric motor at 2000 rpm. The instrumentation sequence was .01/#25, .06/#25, and .08/#25 at the WL. The shaping procedure began with TF size .04/#25. TF size 25/08 was inserted and used as the final apical file.

Group B: TF at 1000 rpm. The method for gutta-percha removal was the same as in group A except the motor was used with 4:1 speed reduction and was powered by an electric motor at 4000 rpm, resulting in instrument rotation speed of 1000 rpm.

Group C: TF at 1500 rpm. The method for gutta-percha removal was the same as in group A except the motor was used with 4:1 speed reduction and was powered by an electric motor at 6000 rpm, resulting in instrument rotation of 1500 rpm.

Group D: manual technique. The canals were reinstrumented sequentially using triangular Triple-Flex Files (SybronEndo, Orange, CA, USA; made of stainless steel designed for flexibility and integrity) in sizes 20 to 25, to a master apical file size of 25. The files were pre-curved according to root canal direction and gutta-percha was removed from the canal using the balance force technique and step-back in 0.625-mm increments (determined using a caliper) to a file size 55 so that the taper was determined to be 8%. Canal patency was maintained with a size 25 K-file during reinstrumentation. Consequently, the final canal diameter and taper was comparable to the samples in the other groups.

Debris collection

During all retreatment procedures, the flutes of the files were cleaned completely after each use. Canals were flushed with 20 mL of distilled water. All instruments were used for only one specimen and then discarded. Any deformed instruments were also discarded. Retreatment was deemed complete when the WL was reached and no more gutta-percha was visible on the last instrument used in every group, based on the step-back approach [17].

After retreatment, any debris (dentin and filling material) visually adherent to the external surface of the apex was scraped and collected into the tube containing the sample. The root apex was flushed with 0.5 mL of distilled water to wash any remaining debris (dentin and filling material) into its tube. No solvent was used. Each root canal was prepared, filled, and retreated by the same operator to reduce interoperator variability.

After the retreatment procedure, the centrifuge tubes were removed from the vials by handling with clean cotton forceps at all times. They were stored in an incubator at 37°C for 4 weeks to evaporate moisture before finally being weighed three times on a microbalance and the average value was used for analysis. The weight of the extruded debris was determined by subtracting the weight of the preweighed empty tube from the final weight. Evaluation was carried out by a second examiner who was blinded to group assignment.

Statistical analysis

Statistical analysis was performed using SPSS 19.0 (IBM, Armonk, NY, USA). In the preliminary analysis, the raw data followed a normal distribution (Shapiro-Wilk test); statistical analysis was thus performed using parametric one-way analysis of variance. Post-hoc pairwise comparisons were performed using the Tukey's multiple comparison test. Statistical significance was established at 0.05.

Results

Characteristics of the teeth

Table 1 presents the angle and radius of curvature, respectively, of the 48 teeth of the four groups. Results showed that the four groups were similar (all $P > 0.05$).

Table 1 Angle and radius of canal curvature of the 48 teeth

	Angle			Radius		
Group	Mean angle (degree)	SD	Range	Mean radius (mm)	SD	Range
A($n = 12$)	28.95	3.15	25.1–35.0	6.82	2.17	3.0–9.8
B($n = 12$)	34.90	29.3	25.1–34.9	6.86	1.83	3.7–9.8
C($n = 12$)	31.05	2.73	27.6–35.0	7.25	2.15	3.9–10.0
D($n = 12$)	29.43	2.99	25.0–34.0	7.21	2.21	3.2–10.0

Group A: Twisted Files at 500 rpm; Group B: Twisted Files at 1000 rpm; Group C: Twisted Files at 1500 rpm; Group D: manual technique
SD standard deviation

Amount of debris

The amount of apical debris for each group is shown in Table 2. The results indicated that all retreatment techniques used in this study caused measurable apical extrusion of debris. The manual instrumentation group (group D) extruded significantly more debris (0.69 ± 0.04 mg) than the TF groups (A: 0.54 ± 0.05 mg; B: 0.48 ± 0.04 mg; C: 0.42 ± 0.03 mg; all $P < 0.001$). In addition, increasing the rotational speed of TF decreased the amount of extruded debris (A vs. B: $P = 0.006$; B vs. C: $P < 0.001$; A vs. C: $P < 0.001$).

Discussion

The aim of this study was to evaluate the use of TF for endodontic retreatment in terms of prevention of extrusion debris and in cases of severely curved mesiobuccal root canals. To do so, three different speeds of rotation were compared when using the TF and manual treatment of curved root canals. The results showed that each of the methods used produced extrusion debris, but that TF at 1500 rpm produced the smallest amount.

Reducing extrusion debris is important for effective endodontic retreatment as it reduces the likelihood of inflammation and postoperative pain. These results are consistent with previous retreatment studies that used various nickel titanium rotary instruments compared with conventional instruments, and demonstrated that rotary instruments produced less debris [12]. This is due, at least in part, to the up-and-down motion of the manual files, which is more likely to push debris toward the apical end [12].

Previous studies on retreatments have been performed on relatively straight root canals [11–13], because their low curvatures eliminated complications likely to arise in the instrumentation of severely curved root canals. However, it can be argued that the filling materials in straight root canals are more easily removed so that canal repreparation tends to extrude less debris, and this may not accurately represent the challenge of retreating curved canals. On the contrary, teeth with high degrees of curvature may give rise to different results [18]. Therefore, studying these devices in straight root canals only does not fully reflect the differences among various technologies. It has been shown that in mandibular first molars' mesiobuccal root canals the mean curvature is 25° and the mean radius is 10.6 mm [15]. Thus, the present study investigated mesiobuccal root canals with severe curvature angles of 25–35° and a short radius of <10 mm in an attempt to simulate these challenging clinical conditions. To the best of the authors' knowledge, there have been no peer-reviewed studies in which molars with severely curved roots were used to assess the amount of dentin debris extruded during retreatment.

Table 2 Amount of Apically Extruded Debris

Group	Number	Mean Weight (mg)	SD	Range
A	12	0.54	0.05	0.45–0.61
B	12	0.48	0.04	0.42–0.56
C	12	0.42	0.03	0.38–0.49
D	12	0.69	0.04	0.62–0.76

Group A: Twisted Files at 500 rpm; Group B: Twisted Files at 1000 rpm; Group C: Twisted Files at 1500 rpm; Group D: manual technique
SD standard deviation

In previous studies, the continuous wave of condensation technique [19] has been rarely used in curved canals. We used this method before retreatment to ensure filling and to avoid filling defects, to make that the results of the investigation are more reliable. The technique has become increasingly popular because it uses heat to produce a homogenous obturation that adapts well to the canal walls and replicates the prepared root-canal space [20, 21].

Unlike previous studies, a major factor in the present study was the use of different rotational speeds. High rotational speed not only increases efficiency but also probably produces more heat [22]. This may be because rotary reinstrumentation generates frictional heat during its contact with gutta-percha and dentin. In addition, rotational speed is associated with heat generation during the formation of martensite [23]. The resulting heat could plasticize the gutta-percha, making it into a single block, thus facilitating its removal and minimizing extruded debris [24]. In addition, plasticized gutta-percha cannot pass through the apical foramen [24], which could have contributed to the differences observed at high rotational speed. Furthermore, the Archimedes screw effect due to higher rotational speed should be taken into account [25]. On the other hand, the exact same methods for coronal introduction of gutta-percha was used among all groups, and eventual differences in pressure should be counterbalanced by the standard method and randomization of the samples. Nevertheless, the plasticization of gutta-percha due to heat during retreatment could be associated with thermal damage to the teeth [26], but heat damage was not examined in the present study. Additional studies are necessary to determine if heat due to rotational speed during retreatment is associated with significant heat damage.

Although the current ground-fluted rotary instruments that are commonly used have excellent performance, there are inevitably many drawbacks due to their design. They have difficulties negotiating a severe curvature, which may increase the risk of iatrogenic damage such as bleeding and perforation of the lateral wall of the root canal. Furthermore, they must be operated in strict accordance with the speed and torque instructions, otherwise there is a risk of unexpected instrument separation, especially in curved root canals [27]. Since most devices have similar low rotational speeds, and the difference is very small, comparisons between device speeds are almost meaningless. Rotational devices that can be used effectively in curved root canals and at higher speeds could improve retreatment.

TF, which are manufactured by twisting instead of grinding the nickel titanium alloy, have been shown to have excellent performance [8]. TF with R-phase technology gives a much higher level of flexibility and can perform side-cutting with great efficiency, while still successfully negotiating a complex curvature. Above all, TF can work at speeds up to 1500 rpm, underlining that using higher rotational speed will lead to less debris. The manufacturer suggests that using a speed of 500 rpm is likely to reduce waste and increase the service life of the instrument, but our experience of using it between 900 and 1500 rpm is also positive and more efficient. We therefore tested TF at three different speeds 500, 1000, and 1500 rpm to assess whether speed would influence the amount of apical debris. The results showed that TF at the highest rotational speed produced the least debris. The results of the experiment were consistent with our inference of the benefits of increased speed and temperature. Nevertheless, other instruments use different rotational speeds and additional studies are necessary to assess these instruments.

This study has some limitations. The clinical relevance of this ex vivo study should be interpreted with caution. In vivo, the apex would be surrounded by periradicular tissues that may serve as a natural barrier preventing debris extrusion. In an early (1977) in vivo study, Salzgeber and Brilliant [28] showed that vital tissues helped control the apical and lateral penetration of an irrigating solution. In addition to the apical control of extruded debris, other factors involved in retreatment require further evaluation. For instance, the heat produced by high speed rotation may be transmitted to the outer root. It has been shown that a 10°C rise may cause irreversible thermal damage to the supporting periodontal structures [29]. Whether the heat produced in this investigation could cause damage to the surrounding tissue needs further evaluation. Finally, apart the power tool nature of TF, there was intrinsic differences between the TF and the manual instrument, such as the cross section (round for TF and triangular for manual files), alloy, and the number of files used. Nevertheless, groups A, B, and C used the same instrument. Additional research will be necessary to evaluate the cleaning efficiency of the TF at higher speeds and to determine the optimal rotational speeds (and torque values) for the removal of gutta-percha.

Conclusions

These results provide important information on preventing apical debris and should help improve retreatment outcomes. TF at high rotational speed was associated with less debris extrusion than at lower speeds, and in comparison with manual endodontic retreatment in curved root canals. Speed may be a significant factor for the retreatment results and may improve retreatment outcomes. Further research is needed to fully evaluate the effect of high rotational speed on endodontic retreatment.

Abbreviations

TF: Twisted files; TFF: Triple-flex files; WL: Working length

Acknowledgments

None.

Availability of data and materials

The de-identified data from this study can be requested from the corresponding author at: xiongshijiangdr@sohu.com. Individuals who are interested in accessing study data should submit a written request outlining their aims and analytical plans in obtaining and using the data with an address, contact and e-mail information for tracking purposes. The information provided to users should not be used for commercial purposes, and should not be distributed to third parties.

Authors' contributions

MDL participated in literature search, study design, data collection, data analysis, and wrote the manuscript. SJX conceived and coordinated the study, analyzed the data, and provided a critical revision. FT and YL carried out the data collection and statistical analysis. All authors reviewed the results and approved the final version of the manuscript.

Competing interests

The authors declare that they have no competing interests.

Consent for publication

Not applicable.

Ethics approval and consent to participate
This study was approved by the ethics committee of the Affiliated Hospital of Qingdao University. The need for informed consent was waived by the committee.

Author details
[1]School of Dentistry, Shandong University, 44, Wenhua West Road, Jinan 250012, Shandong Province, China. [2]School of Stomatology, Qingdao University, Qingdao 266021, Shandong Province, China.

References

1. Torabinejad M, Corr R, Handysides R, Shabahang S. Outcomes of nonsurgical retreatment and endodontic surgery: a systematic review. J Endod. 2009;35:930–7.
2. Kim S, Kratchman S. Modern endodontic surgery concepts and practice: a review. J Endod. 2006;32:601–23.
3. Siqueira Jr JF. Microbial causes of endodontic flare-ups. Int Endod J. 2003;36:453–63.
4. Lumley PJ, Adams N, Tomson P. Root canal retreatment. Dent Update. 2006;33:210–5.
5. Huang X, Ling J, Wei X, Gu L. Quantitative evaluation of debris extruded apically by using ProTaper Universal Tulsa rotary system in endodontic retreatment. J Endod. 2007;33:1102–5.
6. Saad AY, Al-Hadlaq SM, Al-Katheeri NH. Efficacy of two rotary NiTi instruments in the removal of Gutta-Percha during root canal retreatment. J Endod. 2007;33:38–41.
7. Ferraz CC, Gomes NV, Gomes BP, Zaia AA, Teixeira FB, Souza-Filho FJ. Apical extrusion of debris and irrigants using two hand and three engine-driven instrumentation techniques. Int Endod J. 2001;34:354–8.
8. Gambarini G, Grande NM, Plotino G, Somma F, Garala M, De Luca M, et al. Fatigue resistance of engine-driven rotary nickel-titanium instruments produced by new manufacturing methods. J Endod. 2008;34:1003–5.
9. Kim HC, Yum J, Hur B, Cheung GS. Cyclic fatigue and fracture characteristics of ground and twisted nickel-titanium rotary files. J Endod. 2010;36:147–52.
10. Marfisi K, Mercade M, Plotino G, Duran-Sindreu F, Bueno R, Roig M. Efficacy of three different rotary files to remove gutta-percha and Resilon from root canals. Int Endod J. 2010;43:1022–8.
11. Burklein S, Schafer E. Apically extruded debris with reciprocating single-file and full-sequence rotary instrumentation systems. J Endod. 2012;38:850–2.
12. Kustarci A, Akpinar KE, Er K. Apical extrusion of intracanal debris and irrigant following use of various instrumentation techniques. Oral Surg Oral Med Oral Pathol Oral Radiol Endod. 2008;105:257–62.
13. Surakanti JR, Venkata RC, Vemisetty HK, Dandolu RK, Jaya NK, Thota S. Comparative evaluation of apically extruded debris during root canal preparation using ProTaper, Hyflex and Waveone rotary systems. J Conserv Dent. 2014;17:129–32.
14. Schneider SW. A comparison of canal preparations in straight and curved root canals. Oral Surg Oral Med Oral Pathol. 1971;32:271–5.
15. Schafer E, Diez C, Hoppe W, Tepel J. Roentgenographic investigation of frequency and degree of canal curvatures in human permanent teeth. J Endod. 2002;28:211–6.
16. Myers GL, Montgomery S. A comparison of weights of debris extruded apically by conventional filing and Canal Master techniques. J Endod. 1991;17:275–9.
17. Endodontics CP. Part 7. Preparing the root canal. Br Dent J. 2004;197:603–13.
18. Tanalp J, Kaptan F, Sert S, Kayahan B, Bayirl G. Quantitative evaluation of the amount of apically extruded debris using 3 different rotary instrumentation systems. Oral Surg Oral Med Oral Pathol Oral Radiol Endod. 2006;101:250–7.
19. Buchanan LS. The continuous wave of condensation technique: a convergence of conceptual and procedural advances in obturation. Dent Today. 1994;13:80. 2, 4-5.
20. Wu MK, Kast'akova A, Wesselink PR. Quality of cold and warm gutta-percha fillings in oval canals in mandibular premolars. Int Endod J. 2001;34:485–91.
21. Lea CS, Apicella MJ, Mines P, Yancich PP, Parker MH. Comparison of the obturation density of cold lateral compaction versus warm vertical compaction using the continuous wave of condensation technique. J Endod. 2005;31:37–9.
22. Bramante CM, Fidelis NS, Assumpcao TS, Bernardineli N, Garcia RB, Bramante AS, et al. Heat release, time required, and cleaning ability of MTwo R and ProTaper universal retreatment systems in the removal of filling material. J Endod. 2010;36:1870–3.
23. Eggeler G, Hornbogen E, Yawny A, Heckmann A, Wagner M. Structural and functional fatigue of NiTi shape memory alloys. Mater Sci Eng A. 2004;378:24–33.
24. Betti LV, Bramante CM. Quantec SC rotary instruments versus hand files for gutta-percha removal in root canal retreatment. Int Endod J. 2001;34:514–9.
25. Vaudt J, Bitter K, Neumann K, Kielbassa AM. Ex vivo study on root canal instrumentation of two rotary nickel-titanium systems in comparison to stainless steel hand instruments. Int Endod J. 2009;42:22–33.
26. Chauhan A, Nilker V, Mandke LP. Effect of Temperature Rise on Periodontal Tissue During Endodontic Treatment: An In Vitro Study. Indian J Oral Health Res. 2015;1:66–71.
27. Zelada G, Varela P, Martin B, Bahillo JG, Magan F, Ahn S. The effect of rotational speed and the curvature of root canals on the breakage of rotary endodontic instruments. J Endod. 2002;28:540–2.
28. Salzgeber RM, Brilliant JD. An in vivo evaluation of the penetration of an irrigating solution in root canals. J Endod. 1977;3:394–8.
29. Eriksson AR, Albrektsson T. Temperature threshold levels for heat-induced bone tissue injury: a vital-microscopic study in the rabbit. J Prosthet Dent. 1983;50:101–7.

21

Temporal relationship between dysthymia and temporomandibular disorder: a population-based matched case-control study in Taiwan

Shang-Lun Lin[1,2], Shang-Liang Wu[3], Shun-Yao Ko[2], Ching-Yu Yen[4,5], Wei-Fan Chiang[6,7] and Jung-Wu Yang[2,8,9,10*]

Abstract

Background: Numerous studies have reported a relationship between depression and temporomandibular disorders (TMD), but the conclusions remain undefined. The aim of this article was to examine the temporal relationship between depression and TMD.

Methods: In this retrospective matched case-control study, we recruited all samples from a randomsample sub-dataset of one million insured individuals for the year 2005 (Longitudinal Health Insurance Database (LHID2005)). All beneficiaries were enrolled in the National Health Insurance (NHI) programme in Taiwan. We used propensity scoring and matched the case and control groups (1:1) by ten confounding factors to detect the effect of different types of depression on TMD.

Results: The positive correlative factors of TMD included the total number of times medical advice was sought for an unspecified anomaly of jaw size plus malocclusion (TTSMA-JS, $p = 0.045$), the total number of times medical advice was sought for an anxiety state (TTSMA-AS, $p = 0.000$), and the total number of times medical advice was sought for a panic disorder (TTSMA-P, $p = 0.009$). Dysthymia (synonymous with chronic depression) had an effect on TMD. The odds ratio (OR) of dysthymia for TMD measured by multiple logistic regression was 1.91 ($p = 0.008$) after adjusting for demographic factors, psychiatric comorbidities, and maxillofacial confounders.

Conclusions: This study demonstrated the established temporal relationship between dysthymia and TMD. The inclusion of a psychiatrist on the TMD management team is appropriate.

Background

Temporomandibular disorders (TMD) are a significant public health problem globally. A meta-analysis study reported that 30% of randomly selected subjects showed a perceived dysfunction, and 44% demonstrated a clinically assessed dysfunction of their temporomandibular joint (TMJ) pain with/without joint sound [1]. TMD has been considered a multifaceted and complex disease process [2]. Most TMD patients sought treatment because of pain involving the pre-auricular region, jaw, head, and neck [3]. The presence of pain elsewhere in the body, female gender, and pre-existing depressive symptoms are related to the onset of TMD [4]. Pain-related TMD may, therefore, have an influence on the quality of life with disability, psychosocial and behavioural consequences [5]. The clinical ICD-9 codes for TMD only focus on the physical domain of pain, joint mobility, and disc location. The diagnostic criterion for TMD (DC/TMD) includes psychosocial status evaluation (Axis II) as a necessary component [6].

Depression has been increasing over time, and it is one of the leading causes of disease-related disability worldwide [7]. A large cross-sectional epidemiological study of Portuguese college students reported that 61.4% of the students with the symptom of TMD also had signs of anxiety or depression [8]. Various studies have indicated that painful temporomandibular disorders are associated with high levels of depression [9–11].

* Correspondence: jungwuyang1979@gmail.com
[2]Graduate Institute of Medical Science, College of Health Science, Chang Jung Christian University, Tainan, Taiwan
[8]Department of Oral and Maxillofacial Surgery, Tainan Sin Lau Hospital, the Presbyterian Church in Taiwan, Tainan, Taiwan
Full list of author information is available at the end of the article

Furthermore, these conditions are often bi-directional and co-existent [9, 10]. However, these studies were unable to prove a temporal relationship between depression and TMD. Moreover, a population-based cohort study design could not determine whether depression was a source or consequence of TMD [2]; thus, this study was not supportive of evidence-based medicine. Previous TMD studies seldom mentioned the three main types of depression: (1) a major depressive disorder is a severe episodic depression for at least 2 weeks; (2)dysthymia is persistent depression for at least 2 years; and (3) a depressive disorder, not elsewhere classified, is characterized by a minor episode (different than a major depressive disorder) and a shorter course than dysthymia.

The propensity score, which is an adequate method for population allocation, can minimize the differences between groups. Propensity score analysis can reduce the bias of an observational study and adjust for the main confounders [12, 13]. No current TMD case-control studies have used the propensity score for a large population and thereby maximizing the validity.

The purpose of this study was to demonstrate the temporal relationship between depression and TMD utilizing a case-control study design. We assumed that depression is one of the crucial risk factors for TMD. Depressive patients who seek professional help for mental health care and have a willingness to seek medical resources are more likely to be diagnosed with and treated for TMD compared with the general population [14].

Methods

Data resources

The National Health Insurance system, which is a source of study data, has provided insurance coverage for more than 98% of the 23 million Taiwanese people and has contracted with more than 93% of medical institutions since 1996. The National Health Research Institute (NHRI) administered all medical claims information recorded from the contracted health care facilities. We retrieved all sampled subjects from the Longitudinal Health Insurance Database (LHID2005). The LHID2005 includes all of the original medical claims and registration files for one million enrollees in the NHI programme. The one million random-sample enrollees in the LHID2005 were taken from all insured persons registered in the 2005 registry of beneficiaries ($N = 23.72$ million) [15]. This dataset contained the registry of medical facilities, orders of inpatients and outpatients, dental services, and prescriptions linked to anonymous identifications. Thousands of published SCI papers had proven the high validity of NHI data [16, 17]. Because all patient identifications were released to the public for research purposes, the LHID was omitted from full review by the Institutional Review Board in Taiwan. We still obtained an ethical certificate (protocol number SLH919-104-007) from the Ethics Committee of Tainan Sin Lau Hospital, the Presbyterian Church in Taiwan.

Study samples

In selecting samples for analysis in this retrospective matched case-control study, we first recruited 952,728 outpatients between 2004 and 2013 from a representative onemillion sub-datasets. We selected the samples by ICD-9-CM (International Classification of Diseases, 9th revision, Clinical Modification) codes for TMD (ICD-9-CM codes 524.61, 524.60, 524.63, 524.62, and 524.69) and depression (ICD-9-CM codes 296.2X, 300.4, 296.3X, and 311). In our study design, the independent variables were three general types of depressive disorders: depressive disorders not elsewhere classified (ICD-9-CM code 311), dysthymia (ICD-9-CM code 300.4), and major depressive disorders (ICD-9-CM codes 296.3X and 296.2X). To avoid a selection bias of TMD diagnoses and depression, we only included those patients who had at least three clinical records for TMD and depression during the follow-up period after the index date. This study excluded the following cases: (1)TMD that occurred before the onset of depression (168 patients) and (2) a total of OPD visits for depression or TMD less than three (11,596 patients). A total of 13,568 TMD patients and 939,160 non-TMD patients were included in the initial pool of patients via the recruiting process. From this initial pool, 1804 TMD patients with qualified criterions and 200,000 non-TMD random-selected patients were analyzed for the study. The matching protocol (1:1) for the patients (201,804) had 10 confounding variables, including monthly income, age, sex, and the total number of times seeking medical advice (TTSMA) for the following illnesses: mandible fracture (ICD-9-CM codes 802.2 and 802.3), anxiety state (ICD-9-CM code 300.00), unspecified anomaly of jaw size plus malocclusion (ICD-9-CM codes 524.0–524.5), panic disorder (ICD-9-CM code 300.01), generalized anxiety disorder (ICD-9-CM code 300.02), obsessive compulsive disorders (ICD-9-CM code 300.03), and psychiatric diseases except the above-mentioned disorders (ICD-9-CM codes 290–319). A total of 1079 outpatients were allocated to the case group and the control group (Fig. 1). The follow-up period for the case and control groups was between January 1, 2004, and December 31, 2013. For the case group without depression, the starting point was the first ambulatory care visit (including outpatient departments of hospitals or clinics); for the case group with depression, the starting point was a time of the first diagnosis of depression. For the case unit, the end point was the time of the first diagnosis of TMD.

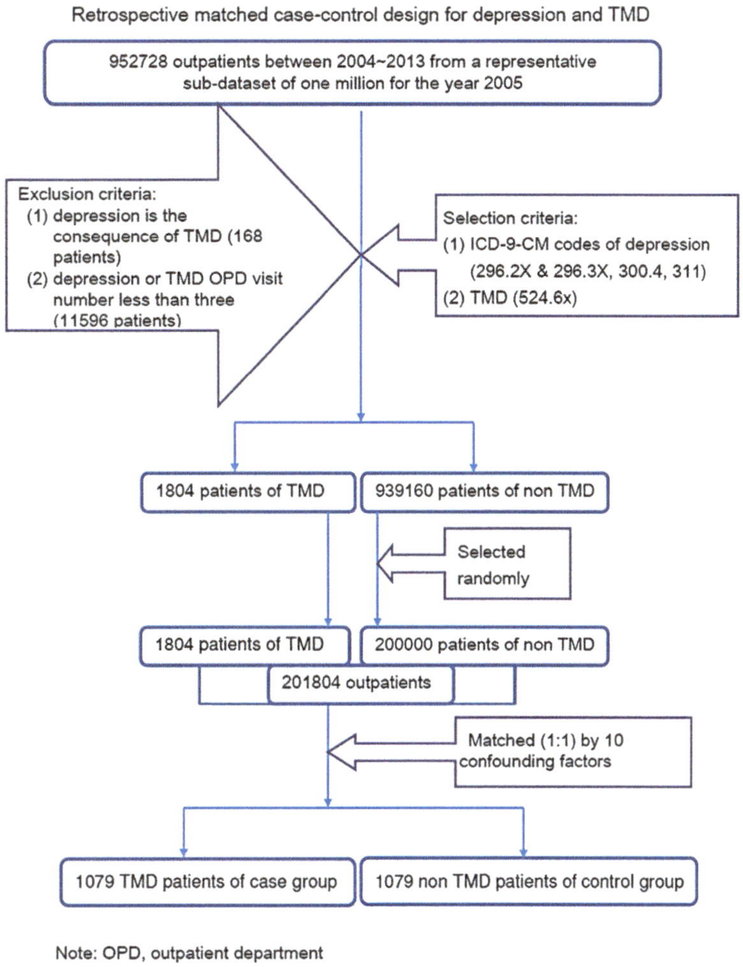

Fig. 1 Flowchart of sample selection

Statistical analysis

We used G-power 3.1.2 to determine the sample size (z-tests, logistic regression, and two tails). With an odds ratio = 1.407, X distribution = binomial, $R^2 = 0.2$, $\alpha = 0.05$, and power = 0.8, it was calculated that the total required sample size for this study was 1920 [18].

The study generated the propensity score of each case by choosing depression (yes/no) as the dependent variable and the ten confounders as independent variables in "predicted values, probabilities" of logistic regression. The matching of the propensity score ensured that the probabilities of depression were exactly equal in the TMD group and the control group.

We compared the ten confounders (no coded cases of obsessive compulsive disorders (ICD-9-CM code 300.03)) of demographic variables and comorbidities between TMD and non-TMD patients using the propensity score. Multiple logistic regression analysis with the odds ratio (OR) was used to estimate the risk of TMD associated with depression after adjusting for confounders. We executed all analyses using SPSS statistical software (version 20 for Windows; IBM; New York, USA).

Results

The gender distribution comparison of patients between the two groups was identical. There were more females than males in both the TMD and non-TMD groups (71.3% versus 28.7%, respectively).

Table 1 shows the comparisons of the continuous variables of confounders between case and control groups. There were no differences in monthly income ($p = 0.899$), age ($p = 0.431$), TTSMA-MF ($p = 0.160$), TTSMA-GA ($p = 0.299$), and TTSMA-PD ($p = 0.109$). There were differences in TTSMA-JS($p = 0.045$), TTSMA-AS ($p = 0.000$), and TTSMA-P ($p = 0.009$) between the two groups.

In Table 2, multiple logistic regression analysis shows that the risk of TMD was significantly greater in the dysthymia (ICD-9-CM code 300.4) (OR 1.91, $p = 0.008$) after adjusting for the ten confounders. Another confounder, TTSMA for anxiety state (TTSMA-AS),

Table 1 Continuous variables of confounders between two groups

variables	mean	sd	Min.	Max.	F	p
MI					0.02	0.899
control	26,422	24,287	0	182,000		
case	26,556	24,420	0	182,000		
Age					0.62	0.431
control	38.93	17.59	1.00	88.00		
case	39.53	17.81	1.00	92.00		
TTSMA-MF					1.97	0.160
control	0.00	0.00	0.00	0.00		
case	0.04	0.98	0.00	31.00		
TTSMA-JS					4.03	0.045
control	0.09	0.45	0.00	7.00		
case	0.14	0.83	0.00	15.00		
TTSMA-AS					32.43	0.000
control	1.23	6.95	0.00	132.00		
case	3.92	13.88	0.00	145.00		
TTSMA-P					6.93	0.009
control	0.05	1.04	0.00	31.00		
case	0.32	3.20	0.00	55.00		
TTSMA-GA					1.08	0.299
control	0.28	4.63	0.00	123.00		
case	0.46	3.26	0.00	45.00		
TTSMA-PD					2.57	0.109
control	1.68	12.19	0.00	218.00		
case	2.52	12.13	0.00	165.00		

Depression: 296.2, 296.3, 300.4, 311 (ICD-9 codes). MI: monthly income. TTSMA-MF: the total number of times seeking medical advice for mandible fracture. TTSMA-JS: the total number of times seeking medical advice for the unspecified anomaly of jaw size. TTSMA-AS: the total number of times seeking medical advice for anxiety state. TTSMA-P: the total number of times seeking medical advice for panic disorder. TTSMA-GA: the total number of times seeking medical advice for generalized anxiety disorder. TTSMA-PD: the total number of times seeking medical advice for psychiatric diseases (ICD-9 codes: 290.X-319) except depression

demonstrated a significant positive correlation with TMD(OR 1.03, $p = 0.000$).

The mean follow-up time was 4.71 ± 2.85 years (after matching), the minimum follow-up period was 0 years, and the maximum follow-up period was 10 years for both groups.

Discussion

Temporomandibular disorders are associated with high levels of depression [8, 9, 19]. However, studies of cross-sectional models only present a possible association and not a temporal relationship. Although Macfarlane et al. found in their case-control study that people with PDS (pain dysfunction syndrome) were characterized by high levels of psychological distress [10], they could not clarify whether depression occurred prior to the onset of TMD or as a consequence of TMD.

Table 2 Odds ratio of temporomandibular disorder in depressions adjusted for confounders in multiple logistic regression

variables	OR(95% CI)
T296(yes/no)	1.02(0.37 ~ 1.67)
T300.4(yes/no)	1.91(1.44 ~ 2.38)
T311(yes/no)	0.68(-0.06 ~ 1.42)
MI	1(-0.96 ~ 2.96)
Age	1(-0.96 ~ 2.96)
TTSMA-MF	93(-3809.01 ~ 3995.01)
TTSMA-JS	1.13(-0.34 ~ 2.6)
TTSMA-AS	1.03(1.01 ~ 1.05)
TTSMA-P	1.06(-0.51 ~ 2.63)
TTSMA-GA	1(-0.23 ~ 2.23)
TTSMA-PD	1(-0.08 ~ 2.08)
Sex(Male/Female)	1.06(0.86 ~ 1.26)

T296: Ever seeking medical advice for major depressive disorder. T300.4: Ever seeking medical advice for dysthymia. T311: Ever seeking medical advice for Depressive disorder, not elsewhere classified. MI: monthly income. TTSMA-MF: the total number of times seeking medical advice for mandible fracture. TTSMA-JS: the total number of times seeking medical advice for the unspecified anomaly of jaw size. TTSMA-AS: the total number of times seeking medical advice for anxiety state. TTSMA-P: the total number of times seeking medical advice for panic disorder. TTSMA-GA: the total number of times seeking medical advice for generalized anxiety disorder. TTSMA-PD: the total number of times seeking medical advice for psychiatric diseases (ICD-9 codes: 290.X-319) except depression

Our study was similar to previous research showing that females had a higher rate of TMD than males [2, 20], and depressive patients had an increased risk of TMD [2]. The odds ratio of dysthymia for TMD was 1.91, which was lower than that of the previous case-control study (OR = 2.5) [10]. The reason for this finding might be because other subtypes of depression and the ten confounding factors interfered with the effect of dysthymia. As confounding factors, both mandible fracture and an unspecified anomaly of jaw size with malocclusion or dentofacial deformity are not in the causal pathway of depression to TMD, but they are associated with depression [21, 22] and TMD [23–25].

The virtues of our study, which has great internal validity, are as follows: our study included a 10-year follow-up period; the definition of depression and TMD were based on diagnoses by specialists and required at least three visits; TMD occurred prior to depression was excluded; and case and control groups were strictly matched (1:1) by propensity score. Moreover, we adjusted for demographic factors, psychiatric comorbidities of depression and maxillofacial confounding factors in the multiple logistic regression analysis. All of these factors showed minimal differences between two groups and powerfully increased our internal validity. The minimal and maximal ranges of all variables represent most of the Taiwanese population and ensure external validity. Therefore, the character of TMD in our study was supportive of more validity. Additionally, we investigated dysthymia's unique effect on TMD, results of which supported that pain and mood disorders might share similar neurobiological mechanisms and neuroanatomical constructs, especially chronic mood disorder [26]. Depressed patients are inclined to have symptoms of pain and consume more health resources than non-depressed patients. Therefore, dysthymia (a synonym for chronic depression) patients with temporomandibular pain tend to acquire a diagnosis of TMD when seeking typical medical services. Our findings are consistent with the fact that dysthymia patients had the most statistically significant pain symptoms [26]. Successful depression treatment might reduce the pain of TMD [27].

There are some limitations to our study. First, orthodontic treatment and orthognathic surgery do not appear in the National Health Insurance program, and patients still have to pay without assistance from the insurance programme. Therefore, we could not provide the ICD-9-CM codes from the insurance program, with which our confounding factors of TMD would have been more complete. Second, clinically common symptoms such as bruxism, which might highly affect TMD, could not be coded using ICD-9-CM. Additionally, ICD-9-CM couldnot clearly code the following TMDs: condylysis/idiopathic condylar resorption, synovial chondromatosis, osteochondritis dissecans, osteonecrosis of the temporomandibular joint, and systematic arthritis with involvement of the temporomandibular joint. Third, our study design did not allow us to present the temporal effects of key confounders, such as the anxiety state. Further studies with different independent variables might help clarify these issues. Fourth, to reduce the differences between the case and control groups, we sacrificed 725 cases, which may have reduced our external validity. Finally, we found it difficult to categorize the subtypes of TMD found in the database using ICD-9-CM codes; therefore, evaluating the impact of depression on subtypes of TMD is an arduous undertaking.

Conclusions

This study demonstrated that dysthymia had a temporal relationship with TMD. The results suggest that a psychological evaluation should be part of the primary management of TMD, and these patients should receive a referral to a psychiatrist as needed. Further cohort studies are required to evaluate issues such as whether TMD has a causal effect on depression, how various types of depression influence different subtypes of TMD, and whether maxillofacial problems (such as mandible fracture, and the anomaly of jaw size with malocclusion) can be causative risk factors for TMD.

Acknowledgements

This study is based in part on data from the National Health Insurance Research Database provided by the Bureau of National Health Insurance, Department of Health, Taiwan and managed by the National Health Research Institutes. The interpretations and conclusions contained herein do not represent those of the Bureau of National Health Insurance, Department of Health, or the National Health Research Institutes.

Funding

No source of funding to report.

Authors' contributions

SL, Lin participated in the design of the study. SL, Wu contributed to perform the statistical analysis. SY participated in the sequence alignment. CY contributed to conceive of the study. WF contributed to draft manuscript. JW contributed to critically revise manuscript. All authors read and approved the final manuscript.

Competing interests

The authors declare that they have no competing interests.

Consent for publication

Not applicable.

Ethics approval and consent to participate

This study obtained an ethical certificate (protocol number SLH919-104-007) from the Ethics Committee of Tainan Sin Lau Hospital, the Presbyterian Church in Taiwan.

Author details

[1]Department of Psychiatry, Kaohsiung Armed Forces General Hospital, Kaohsiung, Taiwan. [2]Graduate Institute of Medical Science, College of Health Science, Chang Jung Christian University, Tainan, Taiwan. [3]School of Medicine, Griffith University, Gold Coast, Australia. [4]School of Dentistry, Taipei Medical University, Taipei, Taiwan. [5]Department of Oral and Maxillofacial Surgery, Chi-Mei Medical Center, Yongkang, Tainan, Taiwan. [6]Department of Oral and Maxillofacial Surgery, Chi-Mei Medical Center, Liouying, Tainan, Taiwan. [7]School of Dentistry, National Yang-Ming University, Taipei, Taiwan. [8]Department of Oral and Maxillofacial Surgery, Tainan Sin Lau Hospital, the Presbyterian Church in Taiwan, Tainan, Taiwan. [9]Yuan Yuan Dental Federation, Tainan, Taiwan. [10]701 No. 57, Sec. 1, East Gate Road, East Dist., Tainan City,, Taiwan, R.O.C..

References

1. De Kanter R, Truin G, Burgersdijk R, Van't Hop M, Battistuzzi P, Kalsbeek H, Kayser A. Prevalence in the Dutch adult population and a meta-analysis of signs and symptoms of temporomandibular disorder. J Dent Res. 1993; 72(11):1509–18.
2. Liao CH, Chang CS, Chang SN, Lane HY, Lyu SY, Morisky DE, Sung FC. The risk of temporomandibular disorder in patients with depression: a population-based cohort study. Community Dent Oral Epidemiol. 2011; 39(6):525–31.
3. Auvenshine RC. Temporomandibular disorders: associated features. Dent Clin N Am. 2007;51(1):105–27. vi.
4. Pereira LJ, Pereira-Cenci T, Cury AADB, Pereira SM, Pereira AC, Ambosano GMB, Gavião MBD. Risk indicators of temporomandibular disorder incidences in early adolescence. Pediatr Dent. 2010;32(4):324–8.
5. Juhl GI, Jensen TS, Norholt SE, Svensson P. Incidence of symptoms and signs of TMD following third molar surgery: a controlled, prospective study. J Oral Rehabil. 2009;36(3):199–209.
6. Schiffman E, Ohrbach R, Truelove E, Look J, Anderson G, Goulet J-P, List T, Svensson P, Gonzalez Y, Lobbezoo F. Diagnostic criteria for temporomandibular disorders (DC/TMD) for clinical and research applications: recommendations of the International RDC/TMD Consortium Network and Orofacial Pain Special Interest Group. J Orofac Pain. 2014;28:6–27.

7. Topuzoglu A, Binbay T, Ulas H, Elbi H, Aksu Tanik F, Zagli N, Alptekin K. The epidemiology of major depressive disorder and subthreshold depression in Izmir, Turkey: Prevalence, socioeconomic differences, impairment and help-seeking. J Affect Disord. 2015;181:78–86.
8. Minghelli B, Morgado M, Caro T. Association of temporomandibular disorder symptoms with anxiety and depression in Portuguese college students. J Oral Sci. 2014;56(2):127–33.
9. Fernandes G, Goncalves DAG, Siqueira JTT, Camparis CM. Painful temporomandibular disorders, self reported tinnitus, and depression are highly associated. Arq Neuropsiquiatr. 2013;71(12):943–7.
10. Macfarlane T, Gray R, Kincey J, Worthington H. Factors associated with the temporomandibular disorder, pain dysfunction syndrome (PDS): Manchester case-control study. Oral Dis. 2001;7(6):321–30.
11. Fernandes G, Selms M, Gonçalves D, Lobbezoo F, Camparis C. Factors associated with temporomandibular disorders pain in adolescents. J Oral Rehabil. 2015;42(2):113–9.
12. Tanaka S, Tanaka S, Kawakami K. Methodological issues in observational studies and non-randomized controlled trials in oncology in the era of big data. Jpn J Clin Oncol. 2015;45(4):323–7.
13. Anglemyer A, Horvath HT, Bero L. Healthcare outcomes assessed with observational study designs compared with those assessed in randomized trials. Cochrane Database Syst Rev. 2014;(4). Art. No.: MR000034. doi:10.1002/14651858.MR000034.pub2.
14. Demyttenaere K, Bonnewyn A, Bruffaerts R, Brugha T, De Graaf R, Alonso J. Comorbid painful physical symptoms and depression: prevalence, work loss, and help seeking. J Affect Disord. 2006;92(2):185–93.
15. Administration NHI. 2015. https://www.gender.ey.gov.tw/gecdb/Stat_Statistics_DetailData.aspx?sn=u4ceyDJ9iGzBYUGlJC0z7w%3D%3D&d=Rv%2B7HVE3GXFli8TeyUcZrw%3D%3D. Accessed 18 July 2015.
16. Cheng CL, Kao YHY, Lin SJ, Lee CH, Lai ML. Validation of the National Health Insurance Research Database with ischemic stroke cases in Taiwan. Pharmacoepidemiol Drug Saf. 2011;20(3):236–42.
17. Chen Y-C, Wu J-C, Chen T-J, Wetter T. A publicly available database accelerates academic production. BMJ. 2011;342:d637.
18. Faul F, Erdfelder E, Lang A-G, Buchner A. G* Power 3: A flexible statistical power analysis program for the social, behavioral, and biomedical sciences. Behav Res Methods. 2007;39(2):175–91.
19. Fernandes G, Franco A, Siqueira J, GonÇAlves D, Camparis C. Sleep bruxism increases the risk for painful temporomandibular disorder, depression and non-specific physical symptoms. J Oral Rehabil. 2012;39(7):538–44.
20. Macfarlane TV, Blinkhorn AS, Davies RM, Kincey J, Worthington HV. Oro-facial pain in the community: prevalence and associated impact. Community Dent Oral Epidemiol. 2002;30(1):52–60.
21. Islam S, Ahmed M, Walton GM, Dinan TG, Hoffman GR. The association between depression and anxiety disorders following facial trauma—A comparative study-mandible fracture-Revised cohort. Injury. 2010;41(1):92–6.
22. de Avila ED, de Molon RS, Loffredo LC, Massucato EM, Hochuli-Vieira E. Health-related quality of life and depression in patients with dentofacial deformity. Oral Maxillofac Surg. 2013;17(3):187–91.
23. Akhter R, Hassan NM, Ohkubo R, Tsukazaki T, Aida J, Morita M. The relationship between jaw injury, third molar removal, and orthodontic treatment and TMD symptoms in university students in Japan. J Orofac Pain. 2008;22(1):50–6.
24. Sonnesen L, Bakke M, Solow B. Malocclusion traits and symptoms and signs of temporomandibular disorders in children with severe malocclusion. Eur J Orthodontics. 1998;20(5):543–59.
25. Barrera-Mora JM, Espinar Escalona E, Abalos Labruzzi C, Llamas Carrera JM, Ballesteros EJ, Solano Reina E, Rocabado M. The relationship between malocclusion, benign joint hypermobility syndrome, condylar position and TMD symptoms. Cranio. 2012;30(2):121–30.
26. Agüera-Ortiz L, Failde I, Mico J, Cervilla J, Lopez-Ibor J. Pain as a symptom of depression: prevalence and clinical correlates in patients attending psychiatric clinics. J Affect Disord. 2011;130(1):106–12.
27. Kroenke K, Shen J, Oxman TE, Williams JW, Dietrich AJ. Impact of pain on the outcomes of depression treatment: results from the RESPECT trial. Pain. 2008;134(1):209–15.

The influence of adding modified zirconium oxide-titanium dioxide nano-particles on mechanical properties of orthodontic adhesive: an in vitro study

Nayef H. Felemban[1,3*] and Mohamed I. Ebrahim[2]

Abstract

Background: The purpose of this in-vitro study was to examine the effect of incorporating different concentrations of Zirconium oxide-Titanium dioxide (ZrO2-TiO2) nanoparticles, which can have antibacterial properties, on the mechanical properties of an orthodontic adhesive.

Methods: ZrO2-TiO2 (Zirconium oxide, HWNANO, Hongwu International Group Ltd, China) -Titanium dioxide, Nanoshell, USA) nanopowder were incorporated into orthodontic adhesive (Transbond XT, 3 M Unitek, Monrovia, USA) with different concentrations (0.5% weight nonofiller and 1% weight nanofiller). The size of nanoparticle was 70–80 nm for ZrO2 and less than 50 nm for TiO2. For measuring the shear bond strength of the three groups of orthodontic adhesives [Transbond (control), Transbond mixed with 0.5% weight ZrO2-TiO2, and Transbond mixed with 1% weight ZrO2-TiO2], 30 freshly extracted human first premolars were used and bonded with stainless steel metal brackets (Dentaurum®, Discovery®, Deutschland), using the 3 orthodontic adhesives and 3 M Unitek; Transbond TM Plus Self-Etching Primer (10 samples in each group). The recorded values of compressive strength and tensile strength (measured separately on 10 samples of orthodontic adhesives (add the 3 D size of sample, light cured for 40 s on both sides) of each orthodontic adhesives), as well as the shear bond strength in Mega Pascal unit (MPa) were collected and exposed to one-way analysis of variance (ANOVA) and Tukey's post-hoc tests.

Results: orthodontic adhesive with 1% weight ZrO2-TiO2 showed the highest mean compressive (73.42 ± 1. 55 MPa, p: 0.003, F: 12.74), tensile strength (8.65 ± 0.74 MPa, p: 0.001, F: 68.20), and shear bond strength (20.05 ± 0. 2 MPa, p: 0.001, F: 0.17).

Conclusions: Adding ZrO2-TiO2 nanoparticle to orthodontic adhesive increased compressive strength, tensile strength, and shear bond strength in vitro, but in vivo studies and randomized clinical trials are needed to validate the present findings.

Keywords: Orthodontic adhesives, Titanium dioxide, Zirconium oxide

* Correspondence: nfelemban@tudent.edu.sa; nfelemban@yahoo.com
[1]Orthodontic department, Faculty of Dentistry, Taif University, Taif, Saudi Arabia
[3]P.O.B. 4302, Makkah 21955, Saudi Arabia
Full list of author information is available at the end of the article

Background

Failure in the bonding system of orthodontic brackets will lead to frequent debonding of orthodontic brackets that delays treatment results. Several tooth- or material-related factors can affect the bonding systems and the failure rates of orthodontic brackets; about 5–7% of clinical bond failures occur for different reasons [1, 2].

Shear bond strength of orthodontic composite resin is greater than resin-modified glass-ionomer cement and polyacid-modified composite resin [3]. Other studies show that shear bond strength was not significantly different when tested over a period of time after orthodontic brackets bonding [4].

In order to improve the properties of resin-based composite, previous studies have focused on the pretreatment of inorganic fillers [5, 6], resin monomers [7], and the development of curing methods. Heat-curing and post-curing heat treatments both increase the degree of polymerization and improve the composite strength to some extent [8]. Nanofillers and fibers have been proposed as reinforcing fillers in dental composite, adding these fillers and fibers will result in increase in composite strength [9].

With the great development of nanotechnology and Nano-phased materials, much attention is directed toward the use of Nano-sized fillers to reinforce the denture base resins, thus producing a polymer nanocomposite with improved mechanical and physical properties as compared to those filled with micro-scale particles; furthermore, the use of multiple Nano fillers rather than a single additive develops a high performance composite that cannot be achieved by using a single filler [10]. The mechanical properties of the resultant polymer nanocomposite depend strongly on the dispersion and adhesion of the filler at the filler matrix interface, thus surface treatment of the fillers with a silane coupling agent is necessary to improve compatibility between the filler and matrix [11].

Both Zirconium oxide (ZrO_2) and Titanium dioxide (TiO_2) nanoparticles have interesting mechanical, physical, and photocatalystic properties that make them suitable additives; furthermore, many properties of these mixed nanostructured-metal oxides (ZrO_2:TiO_2) were reported to be better than single additives mainly due to the size difference between titanium and zirconium [12].

Several antibacterial components have been added to dental composite resin and adhesive system to disinfect the area around the adhesive restorations for a prolonged duration such as dodecylamine, bipyridine, tannic acid derivatives, polyhexanide, amphilic lipids, silver, Chlorhexide gluconate and fluorides, also incorporating TiO_2 to orthodontic adhesive can enhance antibacterial effect and decrease surface roughness of orthodontic adhesives [13].

The objective of this study was to evaluate the effect of incorporation of ZrO_2–TiO_2 Nano fillers which can have antibacterial effect on mechanical properties of orthodontic adhesive; compressive strength, tensile strength, and shear bond strength.

The null hypothesis was that there was a statistically significant deference between mean values of compressive, tensile and shears bond strengths in orthodontic adhesive after adding ZrO_2–TiO_2 Nano fillers in deferent concentrations.

Methods

All materials that been used in the study with manufacturer information are listed in Table 1.

Surface modification of nano fillers

Introducing the reactive groups onto the surface of Nano fillers was achieved by their action of the trimethoxysilylpropyl methacrylate (TMSPM) silane coupling agent with the Nano fillers using 5% weight (wt.) of TMSPM for surface modifications of ZrO_2 nanoparticles and 75% wt. of TMSPM for surface modifications of TiO_2 nanofillers [14]. ZrO_2 and TiO_2 (1:1) Nano fillers by weight were added into dental adhesive used in orthodontics with different concentrations (1 and 0.5% respectively).

Preparation of modified adhesives

To achieve dental adhesives containing 10% nanoparticles, 64 mg nanopowder was blended into 576 mg (Transbond™ XT Light Cure Adhesive composite, 3 M Unitek), using a mixing spatula on a glass slab in a semi-dark environment until a uniform consistency was achieved. Two hundred mg of the 10% wt. blended composite was then mixed with 200 mg of the original composite to obtain 0.5% wt. containing composite, similarly, 40 mg of 10% composite was blended with 360 mg original composite for the 1% w/w composite [15]. After mixing the particles with composite the resultant composite is passed through two roll mills for about five minutes in a mastication stage, for better distribution of nanoparticles in the matrix [16].

Grouping of the specimens

A total of 60 specimens were used in this study. The specimens of orthodontic adhesive were divided into three main groups (20 specimens each) according to the percentage of ZrO_2–TiO_2 nanopowder that was added to the dental adhesive with concentrations 0.5%, 1% and control group without any additive. Every group was further subdivided into two subgroups (10 specimens each) according to the type of test as shown in Table 2, Figs. 1 and 2.

Table 1 Materials

	Materials	Trade	Manufacturer
1	Zirconium oxide (ZrO_2) nanofiller 70–80 nm	HWNANO	China
2	Titanium oxide (TiO_2) Nanofiller < 50 nm.	Nanoshell	USA
3	Trimethoxysilylpropyl methacrylate 98%Silane	No 2530- 85-8.	Sigma- Aldrich (Germany)
4	Orthodontic Adhesive	Transbond XT, Adhesive composite 3 M Unitek, Monrovia	USA

Compressive strength

Mold construction

4 mm diameter by 6 mm height cylindrical Teflon mold was fabricated according to the International Standards Organization (ISO) No. 9917 (2000).

Specimens preparation

The orthodontic Adhesive was condensed in the Teflon mold, which was then placed on a glass plate according to each group. Specimens were covered with celluloid strips and pressed with another glass plate. All of the specimens were exposed to light cure for 40 s from both sides (BG-light-LTD, 4002 Plovdiv, 430-490 nm, Bulgaria). The specimens were stored in distilled water for 24 h prior to testing. Curing radiometer equipment (LI-189.Li-Cor Inc, Lincoln, NE68504, USA) was used to ensure steady light intensity throughout the polymerization of all specimens.

Compressive strength testing

Specimens were loaded on the Lloyd mechanical testing machine (model LRX plus II, Fareham, England) at crosshead speed of 0.5 mm/min. The specimens were placed with flat ends vertically laid between the two metal plates.

The load was applied until the specimen was crushed; the peak force required to fracture each specimen was recorded in Newton from the stress-strain curve. The compressive strength was calculated in Mega Pascal (MPa) using the following equation:

$$\text{Compressive Strength} = 4P/\pi d$$

Where (P) is the load at the fracture point in Newtons and d is the diameter of the specimen.

Diametric tensile strength

Measuring the tensile strength of orthodontic adhesive is done using an indirect tensile test, a compressive load is placed on the diameter of a cylindrical specimen. The compressive stress induces a tensile stress in the plane of the application of the force. The tensile stress is directly proportional to the compressive load.

In this test, the specimen cylinder was mounted on the Lloyd mechanical testing machine and the load was applied to the specimen using a crosshead speed of 0.5 mm/min applying a compressive force on the specimen until fracture. The diametric tensile strength was calculated in (MPa) using the following equation:

$$\text{Diametric Tensile Strength} = 2P/\pi dt$$

Where (P) is the load at the fracture point in Newtons, (d) is the diameter of the specimen, and (t) is the thickness of the specimen.

Shear bond strength

Thirty freshly extracted, human maxillary first premolars for orthodontic reasons were collected and stored in a solution of 0.1% thymol. The criteria for tooth selection included intact buccal enamel, not subjected to any pretreatment chemical agents, no cracks, and no caries [17]. The teeth were placed and mounted in metal rings using cold-cure acrylic resin and numbered randomly; then the teeth were polished for 10 s with non-fluoridated pumice using prophylactic rubber cups [18–20].

Metal brackets (Dentaurum®, Discovery®) of maxillary first premolars with an average base surface area of 10.5 mm^2 were used in this study. Then the teeth were randomly

Table 2 Orthodontic adhesive groups

Groups	Group description	Type of test	Quantity
Group A	Orthodontic adhesive without any additives (control group)	-Compressive and tensile strength	-10 specimens
		- Shear bond strength	-10 specimens
Group B	Orthodontic adhesive with 0.5% wt.	-Compressive and tensile strength	-10 specimens
	ZrO_2-TiO_2 nanofillers.	- Shear bond strength	-10 specimens
Group C	Orthodontic adhesive with 1% wt.	-Compressive and tensile strength	-10 specimens
	ZrO_2-TiO_2 nanofillers	- Shear bond strength	-10 specimens
Total			60 specimens

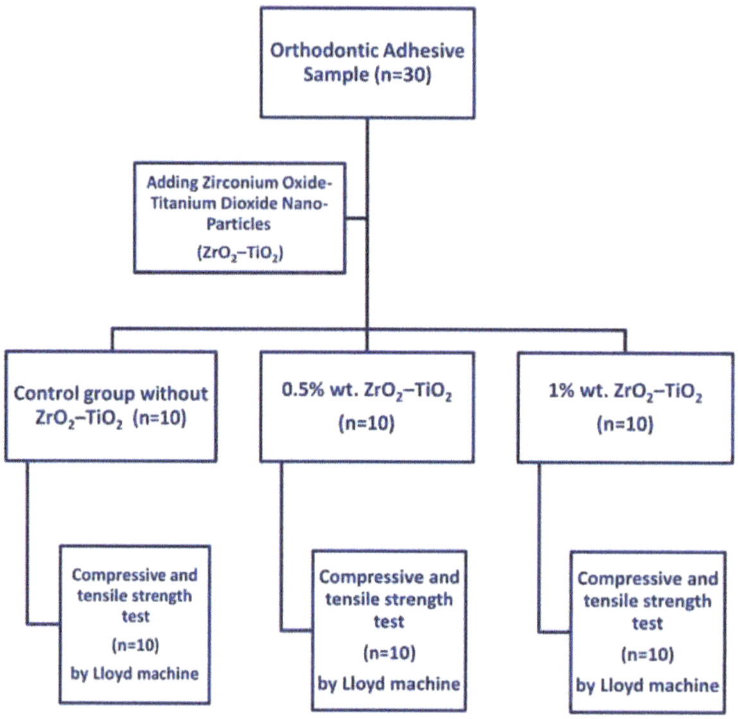

Fig. 1 Flow diagram of specimens groups for compressive and tensile strength tests

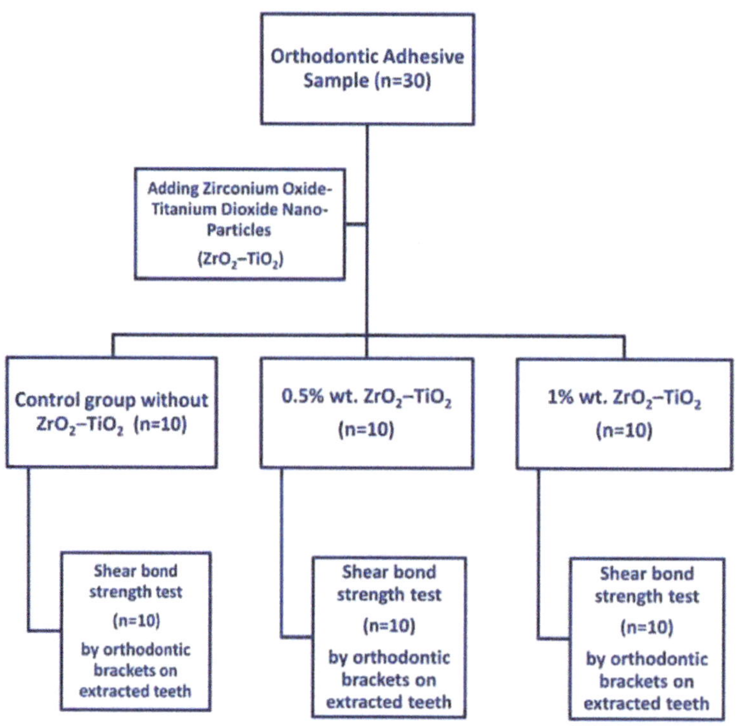

Fig. 2 Flow diagram of specimens groups for shear bond strength test

divided into three groups, each consisting of 10 teeth, and bonded as shown in Table 2 (groups A, B and C).

The groups were bonded using 3 M Unitek; Transbond™ Plus Self-Etching Primer one bottle, which was applied for 20 s then dried with mild air flow, then light cured for 10 s.

Group A (the control group), the orthodontic brackets bonded to the tooth surface using Transbond™ XT Light Cure Adhesive.

Groups B and C, the orthodontic brackets bonded to the tooth surface using the modified adhesive as described in Table 2.

The specimens were immersed in 37 °C water for 24 h, and then subjected to thermo-cycling to simulate clinical thermal stress conditions before testing. These directions are according to the American National Standards Institute/American Dental Association (ANSI/ADA) [21], and International Organization for Standardization (ISO) [22] for direct filling resins and dental adhesion.

All specimens were subjected to thermo-cycling by being stored alternatively in water reservoirs at 5 °C and 55 °C, respectively, remaining in each reservoir for 30 s [23].

Shear bond strength testing

Shear bond strength testing was done using a Lloyd universal testing machine. Upper attachment knife-edge was used; Plastic cylinders with embedded teeth and brackets were mounted on a joint (lower attachment) and aligned in the testing apparatus to ensure consistency for the point of force application and direction of the debonding force for all specimens.

The direction of the debonding force was parallel to the enamel surface in an occlusal-gingival direction. The load was applied perpendicular to the interface of the tooth and bracket at a crosshead with speed of 0.5 mm/min until debonding occurred.

The shear bond strength in kg/cm^2 was calculated based on the following equation:

$$\text{Shear Bond Strength} = P/\pi.r^2$$

Where (P) is shear load in kilograms, (r) is the radius of the specimen in millimeter.

Then the shear bond strength was converted to MPa by multiplying the results by 0.09807.

The recorded values of compressive, tensile, and shear bond strength in (MPa) were collected, and statistically analyzed. One-way analysis of variance (ANOVA) and Tukey's tests were used for testing the significance between the means of tested properties of all tested materials. This was statistically significant when the P value ≤ 0.05.

Results

The comparison between mean compressive strengths in (MPa) is shown in Table 3, comparison between mean tensile strengths in (MPa) is shown in Table 3, and comparison between mean shear bond strengths in (MPa) is shown in Table 4.

All groups of orthodontic adhesive with nanoparticles (B and C) showed compressive strength, tensile strength, and shear bond strength values higher than that of the control group (A).

The power analysis revealed that a total sample size of 30 (10 per group) was needed to detect clinically meaningful differences between the groups at a power of 85% and at 0.05 significance level.

Compressive and tensile strengths

Orthodontic adhesive specimens with ZrO_2–TiO_2 Nano fillers (groups C and B) showed significantly high compressive and tensile strengths when compared with the control group, while the increase in compressive and tensile strengths was not significant between Group C (1% wt. ZrO_2–TiO_2) and Group B (0.5% wt. ZrO_2–TiO_2).

Shear strength

Table 4 shows the comparison between the mean shear bond strength of three tested groups. Orthodontic

Table 3 Comparison between mean compressive and tensile strength in (MPa) of adhesive groups

Groups	Nanoparticle percent	N	Range	Mean (SD)	95% CI	F	*p*-value	Tukey post Hoc
Compressive strength								
Group A	without nanofillers	10	53.65 – 57.23	54.92 (4.15)	53.6–55.3	12.74	0.003	Group C < Group A, Group B < Group A
Group B	0.5 wt %	10	65.96 – 72.68	69.28 (3.76)	68.0–70.5			
Group C	1 wt %	10	69.33 – 76.58	73.42 (1.55)	71.7–74.2			
Tensile strength								
Group A	without nanofillers	10	2.21 – 6.38	4.92 (0.54)	4.1–5.7	68.20	0.001	Group C < Group A
Group B	0.5 wt %	10	6.54 – 8.35	6.14 (0.71)	5.1–6.5			
Group C	1 wt %	10	7.42 – 9.64	8.65 (0.74)	7.8–8.5			

N Number of sample, *CI* Confidence interval, *SD* Standard deviation

Table 4 Comparison between mean shear bond strength in (MPa) of adhesive groups

S hear bond strength								
Groups	Nanoparticle percent	N	Range	Mean (SD)	95% CI	F	*p*-value	Tukey Post Hoc
Group A	without nanofillers	10	13.21 - 16.79	14.75 (0.25)	13.6–15.1	0.17	0.001	Group C < Group A, Group B < Group A
Group B	0.5 wt %	10	18.34 - 22.41	20.32 (0.47)	19.4–20.9			
Group C	1 wt %	10	23.22 - 27.58	25.05 (0.2)	14.3–20.3			

N Numb er of sample, *CI* Confide nce interval, *SD* S tandard deviat ion

adhesive specimens with 1% wt. ZrO_2–TiO_2 Nano fillers (Group C) showed a significantly highest shear bond strength followed by the orthodontic adhesive specimen with 0.5% wt. ZrO_2-TiO_2 Nano fillers (Group B), while the control group was significantly lowest shear bond strength.

Therefore the null hypothesis that compares the compressive, tensile and shears bond strengths after adding ZrO_2–TiO_2 Nano fillers to orthodontic adhesive was accepted and not rejected in this study.

Discussion

Several factors, such as failure in the bonding technique, low retentiveness of certain bracket bases, masticatory forces, and reduced size of the bracket base for esthetic reasons, can result in bracket debonding [24, 25] that will prolong the treatment time and increase the treatment costs. Several solutions had been proposed, such as aluminum-oxide sand blasting and primer application [26], to minimize the unwanted debonding rates in this study by adding ZrO_2–TiO_2 to orthodontic adhesive. The results showed an increase in the shear bond strength (20.32 and 25.05 MPa), although 5.9 to 7.5 MPa is the minimum acceptable shear bond strength for routine clinic use, as considered by Reynolds [27], we don't always have an ideal situation for bonding brackets and up to 21 MPa shear bond strength is acceptable for orthodontic treatment. The failure rate of brackets with Transbond™ Plus range from 0.94% to 7.4% [28–31].

In this study, the self-etching primer had been applied for 20 s prior to the process of light curing (unlike the manufacturer's instructions) which would yield superior performance of the etching primer. This was done by prolonging the application time, as shown by dos Santos,et al [29].

In order to simulate the mastication forces that create stresses to the restoration materials a compressive strength test are used in laboratory experiments [32]. Most mastication forces are not constant and the exact values are not known [33].

Measuring the shear bond strength for bonded orthodontic brackets is very common in literatures, it is a simple test when compared to tensile bond strength tests, in which it is difficult to align the specimen in the testing machine without creating deleterious stress distributions [34, 35].

Titanium dioxide (TiO_2) nanofiller has an antibacterial effect, biocompatibility and minimum toxicity. This nanofillers beside their antibacterial effect they have been suggested as reinforcing fillers [36, 37].

Zirconium oxide (ZrO_2) was used because it has excellent biocompatibility and white color which is less likely to alter its esthetic. The nanofiller particles were used in this study as they yield a better dispersion, eliminate aggregation, and improve its compatibility with organic polymer [38].

Both ZrO_2 and TiO_2 nanoparticles were reported to be better than single additives mainly due to the size differences between titanium and zirconium [12]. In this study, compressive, tensile, and shear bond strength improvement of orthodontic adhesive containing 1% and 0.5% (w/w) ZrO_2–TiO_2 nanoparticles can be attributed to the small sizes of the ZrO_2 and TiO_2 and also to the surface modification of the nanofillers with TMSPM coupling agents which provide better dispersion of particles in matrix, avoid agglomeration, and improves interfacial adhesion of the fillers to the polymer matrix [39].

Shear bond strength can be 40% less when measured in vivo than in vitro and this makes our results in shear bond strength higher than what will be in real clinical cases, adding ZrO_2–TiO_2 nanoparticles can enhance the shear bond strength for optimum clinical use, further in vivo studies are needed [40].

Color stability, polymerization shrinkage, antibacterial effect and toxicity of adding ZrO_2–TiO_2 nanoparticles on resin-based adhesives could be studied in the future with other mechanical and physical properties in different concentrations of Nano filler.

Conclusions

On the basis of this study, we can conclude that the addition of ZrO_2–TiO_2 nanoparticles on resin-based adhesives increase the compressive, tensile, and shear bond strengths of the adhesive in vitro.

Abbreviations

MPa: Mega pascal; N: Newton; RBC: Resin-based composite; TiO_2: Titanium dioxide; Wt.: Weight; ZrO_2: Zirconium oxide; ZrO_2–TiO_2: Zirconium oxide–titanium dioxide

Acknowledgements
We would like to show our gratitude and thanks to Dr. Roshan Noor Mohamed (assistant professors, preventive dentistry department, faculty of dentistry, Taif University) and Dr. Sakeenabi Basha (assistant professors, preventive dentistry department, faculty of dentistry, Taif University) for sharing their help and assistance in statistical analysis for this research.

Authors' contributions
NF participated in the design of the study, helped in data collection and drafted the manuscript. ME collected the data, performed the statistical analysis, and helped draft the manuscript. Both authors read and approved the final manuscript.

Competing interest
The authors declare that they have no competing interests.

Consent for publication
Not applicable.

Ethics approval and consent to participate
All extracted teeth had been extracted for orthodontic treatment not for research purposes, collection of extracted teeth had been done after the approval of ethical committee in faculty of dentistry, Taif University.

Author details
[1]Orthodontic department, Faculty of Dentistry, Taif University, Taif, Saudi Arabia. [2]Restorative dentistry department, Faculty of Dentistry, Taif University, Taif, Saudi Arabia. [3]P.O.B. 4302, Makkah 21955, Saudi Arabia.

References
1. O'Brien KD, Read MJ, Sandison RJ, Roberts CT. A visible light-activated direct-bonding material: an in vivo comparative study. Am J Orthod Dentofacial Orthop. 1989;95:348–51.
2. Bakhadher W, Halawany H, Talic N, Abraham N, Jacob V. Factors affecting the shear bond strength of orthodontic brackets-a review of in vitro studies. Acta med (Hradec Králové. 2015;58(2):43.
3. Rix D, Foley TF, Mamandras A. Comparison of bond strength of three adhesives: composite resin, hybrid GIC, and glass-filled GIC. Am J Orthod Dentofacial Orthop. 2001;119:36–42.
4. Hajrassie MK, Khier SE. In-vivo and in-vitro comparison of bond strengths of orthodontic brackets bonded to enamel and debonded at various times. Am J Orthod Dentofacial Orthop. 2007;131:384–90.
5. Ruddell DE, Maloney MM, Thompson JY. Effect of novel filler particles on the mechanical and wear properties of dentalcomposites. Dent Mater. 2002;18:72–80.
6. Xu HH, Quinn JB, Smith DT, Antonucci JM, Schumacher GE, Eichmiller FC. Dental resin composites containing silica-fused whiskers - - effects of whisker-to-silica ratio on fracture toughness and indentation properties. Biomaterials. 2002;23:735–42.
7. Lu H, Stansbury JW, Nie J, Berchtold KA, Bowman CN. Development of highly reactive mono- (meth) acrylates as reactive diluents for dimethacrylate-based dental resin systems. Biomaterials. 2005;26:1329–36.
8. Loza-Herraro MA, Rueggeberg FA, Caughman WF, Schuster GS, Lefebvre CA, Gardner FM. Effect of heating delay on conversion and strength of a post-cured resin composite. J Dent Res. 1998;77:426–31.
9. Bayne SC. Mechanical property analysis of two admixed PRIMM-modified commercial dental composites. Acad Dent Mater Trans. 1996;9:238.
10. Aly AA, Zeidan EB, Alshennawy AA, El-Masry AA, Wasel WA. Friction and wear of polymer composites filled by nano-particles: a review. World J Nanosci Eng. 2012;2:32–9.
11. Asar NV, Albayrak H, Korkmaz T, Turkyilmaz I. Influence of various metal oxides on mechanical and physical properties of heat-cured polymethylmethacrylate denture base resins. J Adv Prosthodont. 2013;5:502–6.
12. Tomar LJ, Chakrabarty BS. Synthesis, structural and optical properties of TiO 2–ZrO 2 nanocomposite by hydrothermal method. Adv Mat Lett. 2013;4(1):64–7.
13. Borzabadi-Farahani A, Borzabadi E, Lynch E. Nanoparticles in orthodontics, a review of antimicrobial and anti-caries applications. Acta Odontol Scand. 2014;72(6):413–7.
14. Chaijareenont P, Takahashi H, Nishiyama N, Arksomnukit M. Effect of different amounts of 3-methacryloxypropyltrimethoxysilane on the flexural properties and wear resistance of alumina reinforced PMMA. Dent Mater J. 2012;31:623–8.
15. Mirhashemi A, Bahador A, Kassaee M, Daryakenari G, Ahmad-Akhoundi M, Sodagar A. Antimicrobial effect of nano-zinc oxide and nano-chitosan particles in dental composite used in orthodontics. J Med Bacteriol. 2015;2(3-4):1.
16. Yekrangi A, Afrasiabi M, Langari A, Hafshejani MK. Investigation of abrasion and morphology of rubber/nano titanium oxide nanocomposites. ARPN J Eng Appl Sci. 2014;9:580–5.
17. Bishara SE, Oonsombat C, Soliman MM, Warren JJ, Laffoon JF, Ajlouni R. Comparison of bonding time and shear bond strength between a conventional and a new integrated bonding system. Angle Orthod. 2005;75(2):237.
18. Saito K, Sirirungrojying S, Meguro D, Hayakawa T, Kasai K. Bonding durability of using self-etching primer with 4-META/MMA-TBB resin cement to bond orthodontic brackets. Angle Orthod. 2005;75(2):260.
19. Cehreli Z, Kecik D, Kocadereli I. Effect of self–etching primer and adhesive formulations on the shear bond strength of orthodontic brackets. Am J Orthod Dentofacial Orthop. 2005;127:573–9.
20. Bishara SE, Ostby AW, Laffoon JF, Waren J. Shear bond strength comparison of two adhesive systems following thermocycling. A new self-etch primer and a resin-modified glass ionomer. Angle Orthod. 2007;77:337–41.
21. American National Standards Institute and American Dental Association. Specification no. 27: resin-based filling materials. Chicago: American Dental Association; 1993.
22. International Organization of Standardization. Dental materials: testing of adhesion to tooth structure. 2003. ISO/TS 11405.
23. Janda R, Roulet JF, Latta M, Rüttermann S. The effects of thermocycling on the flexural strength and flexural modulus of modern resin-based filling materials. Dent Mater. 2006;22:812–7.
24. Labella R, Lambrechts P, Van Meerbeek B, Vanherle G. Polymerization shrinkage and elasticity of flowable composites and filled adhesives. Dent Mater. 1999;15:128–37.
25. Katona TR, Long RW. Effect of loading mode on bond strength of orthodontic brackets bonded with 2 systems. Am J Orthod Dentofacial Orthop. 2006;129:60–4.
26. Özcan M, Vallittu PK, Peltomäki T, Huysmans M, Kalk W. Bonding polycarbonate brackets to ceramic: effects of substrate treatment on bond strength. Am J Orthod Dentofacial Orthop. 2004;126:220–7.
27. Reynolds IR. A review of direct orthodontic bonding. Br J Orthodont. 1975;2:171–8.
28. Pandis N, Eliades T. A comparative in vivo assessment of the long-term failure rate of 2 self-etching primers. Am J Orthod Dentofacial Orthop. 2005; 128:96–8.
29. dos Santos JE, Quioca J, Loguercio AD, Reis A. Six-month bracket survival with a self-etch adhesive. Angle Orthod. 2006;76(5):863.
30. Aljubouri YD, Millett DT, Gilmour WH. Six and 12 months' evaluation of a self-etching primer versus two-stage etch and prime for orthodontic bonding: a randomized clinical trial. Eur J Orthod. 2004;26:565–71.
31. Ireland AJ, Knight H, Sherriff M. An in vivo investigation into bond failure rates with a new self-etching primer system. Am J Orthod Dentofacial Orthop. 2003;124:323–6.
32. Peutzfeldt A, Roulet JF. Restorative materials for the direct technique in: adhesion the silent revolution in dentistry. 1st ed. Chicago: Quintessence Publishing Co. Inc; 2000. Chap5:61-80.
33. Wang L, D'Alpino PH, Lopes LG, Pereira JC. Mechanical properties of dental restorative materials: relative contribution of laboratory tests. J Appl Oral Sci. 2003;11:162–7.

34. Sudsangiam S, van Noort R. Do dentin bond strength tests serve a useful purpose? J Adhes Dent. 1999;1(1):57.
35. Kemp-Scholte CM, Davidson CL. Marginal sealing of curing contraction gaps in class V composite resin restorations. J Dent Res. 1988;67:841–5.
36. Xia Y, Zhang F, Xie H, Gu N. Nanoparticle-reinforced resin-based dental composites. J Dent. 2008;36:450–5.
37. Garcia-Contreras R, Scougall-Vilchis RJ, Contreras-Bulnes R, Sakagami H, Morales-Luckie RA, Nakajima H. Mechanical, antibacterial and bond strength properties of nano-titanium-enriched glass ionomer cement. J Appl Oral Sci. 2015;23:321–8.
38. Sun L, Gibson R, Gordaninejad F, Suhr J. Energy absorption capability of nanocomposites: a review. CompSci Tech. 2009;69:2392–409.
39. Liu X, Han Y, Gao G, Li Z, Liu F. Effect of silane coupling agent on the mechanical, thermal properties and morphology of tremolite/PA1010 composites. Chinese J Polymer Sci. 2008;26:255–62.
40. Eslamian L, Borzabadi-Farahani A, Mousavi N, Ghasemi A. A comparative study of shear bond strength between metal and ceramic brackets and artificially aged composite restorations using different surface treatments. Eur J Orthod. 2012;34(5):610.

23

Response of human dental pulp cells to a silver-containing PLGA/TCP-nanofabric as a potential antibacterial regenerative pulp-capping material

Barbara Cvikl[1,3], Samuel C. Hess[2], Richard J. Miron[1,6], Hermann Agis[3], Dieter Bosshardt[4], Thomas Attin[5], Patrick R. Schmidlin[1,5*] and Adrian Lussi[1]

Abstract

Background: Damage or exposure of the dental pulp requires immediate therapeutic intervention.

Methods: This study assessed the biocompatibility of a silver-containing PLGA/TCP-nanofabric scaffold (PLGA/Ag-TCP) in two in vitro models, i.e. the material adapted on pre-cultured cells and cells directly cultured on the material, respectively. Collagen saffolds with and without hyaluronan acid (Coll-HA; Coll) using both cell culturing methods and cells growing on culture plates served as reference. Cell viability and proliferation were assessed after 24, 48, and 72 h based on formazan formation and BrdU incorporation. Scaffolds were harvested. Gene expression of interleukin(IL)-6, tumor necrosis factor (TNF)-alpha, and alkaline phosphatase (AP) was assessed 24 h after stimulation.

Results: In both models formazan formation and BrdU incorporation was reduced by PLGA/Ag-TCP on dental pulp cells, while no significant reduction was found in cells with Coll and Coll-HA. Cells with PLGA/Ag-TCP for 72 h showed similar relative BrdU incorporation than cells stimulated with Coll and Coll-HA. A prominent increase in the pro-inflammatory genes IL-6 and TNF-α was observed when cells were cultured with PLGA/Ag-TCP compared to the other groups. This increase was parallel with a slight increase in AP expression. Overall, no differences between the two culture methods were observed.

Conclusions: PLGA/Ag-TCP decreased viability and proliferation rate of human dental pulp cells and increased the pro-inflammatory capacity and alkaline phosphatase expression. Whether these cellular responses observed in vitro translate into pulp regeneration in vivo will be assessed in further studies.

Keywords: Dental pulp, Regeneration, Capping, In vitro techniques

Background

The dental pulp represents the vital core of teeth and lays largely hidden under a protective shell, which forms the teeth, i.e. dentin, cementum and enamel [1]. The cells physiologically constitute together with the lining layer of odontoblasts to the cellular aspect of the pulp-dentin complex, which allows for several complex adaptive and reactive processes during all stages of tooth development and life [2, 3]. Several factors may lead to gene up- or down-regulation or even to cause cell death–in the worst-case. In the latter scenario, odontoblastoid cells have to differentiate first from the subodontoblast layer or have to be recruited from specific progenitor cells from the pulp core. The formation of reactionary or reparative dentin is the result of these self protecting reactions during injury [4, 5]. Reparative dentin forms at a highly variable degree [6] depending on the specific physical or chemical influences. Irrespective of the pathological agent, dentinogenesis would be a desirable therapeutic endpoint of healing or even

* Correspondence: patrick.schmidlin@zzm.uzh.ch
[1]Department of Preventive, Restorative and Pediatric Dentistry, School of Dentistry, University of Bern, Bern, Switzerland
[5]Clinic of Preventive Dentistry, Periodontology and Cariology, Center of Dental Medicine, University of Zurich, Plattenstrasse 11, Zurich CH-8032, Switzerland
Full list of author information is available at the end of the article

regeneration. But in many cases, exposure of the pulp requires immediate therapeutic intervention as it mostly relates to maceration of this highly vulnerable and susceptible organ. In addition, any pathological changes including microbial contamination have probably preceded and the pulp-dentin complex has been infected. Therefore, agents applied in such cases should exhibit both, antibacterial and mineralizing activity. The mineralizing activity may be – classically – achieved by some irritating action of the selected material or induction of release of biologically active molecule or a combination thereof [7].

As the development of mineralized tissues in the human body, i.e. bone, cementum or dentin is based on calcification processes within a fiber arrangement, the use of modern scaffolds in the form of fibers may potentially offer some advantages, especially if these materials are doped with particles that show distinct antibacterial and mineralizing characteristics. In this context, biodegradable polymers, such as poly(lactic acid) (PLA) and the co-polymerpoly(lactic-co-glycolic acid) (PLGA) have been widely investigated and applied to fabricate porous scaffolds in order to restore damaged tissues [8]. A flexible, moldable, electrospun cotton wool-like nanocomposite has been developed [9–11], which contains amorphous calcium phosphate nanoparticles embedded in a biodegradable synthetic PLGA. It is prepared through an electrospinning process, which gives it the typical cotton wool-like appearance. The incorporation of inorganic substances and organic substances within composite scaffolds has been shown to enhance biomineralization. In addition, L-poly(lactic acid) and PLGA composite scaffolds, especially when combined with basic substances like hydroxyapatite, tricalcium phosphate or demineralized bone powder, have also shown not to induce inflammatory tissue reactions in vivo, thus seem to be highly biocompatible [12]. These materials can be optionally doped with silver, which has shown to result in enhanced antimicrobial properties against *Escherichia coli* when compared to tetracycline controls [13]. Furthermore, a preclinical study in sheep showed indirect evidence that–besides its extraordinary in vitro bioactivity – a silver containing nanocomposite material (0.4 wt.% total silver concentration) could provide additional antimicrobial properties for treating bone defects exposed to microorganisms and the absence of clusters of lymphocytes, plasma cells and spindle type fibroblasts further confirmed its biocompatibility [14].

Type I collagen from dentinal tissue on the other hand has also the ability to self-assemble and to form repetitive structures and extended networks of aligned fibers [15]. Its interactions with non-collagenous proteins [16] and its positional relationship with mineral crystals within mature tissues [17] provide convincing evidence that the preassembled collagen matrix could serve as a template for organize d mineralization in dentin.

It was the aim of this in vitro study to assess the response of human dental pulp cells to a novel silver-containing nanofabric (PLGA/Ag-TCP) and compare it to collagen (Coll) scaffolds with or without the addition of hyaluronan acid (HA). The cell viability, proliferation, and expression of the pro-inflammatory genes interleukin(IL)-6, tumor necrosis factor (TNF)-alpha as well as alkaline phosphatase (AP) expression were assessed in two in vitro models: Cells were cultured in presence of the scaffold (Model I), which might more closely represent the in vivo situation of a pulp capping and the cells were cultured directly on the scaffold (Model II).

We hypothesized that PLGA/Ag-TCP induces minor cellular responses with regards to viability, proliferation, and pro-inflammatory capacity when compared to Coll scaffolds with and without hyaluronan acid, which is known in the research field of wound healing [18] and that the differences are more pronounced in the model I than in model II.

Methods

Scaffolds and materials

For the fabrication of the silver-containing nanofabric, clinically approved poly(lactide-co-glycolide) (PLGA) with a copolymer ratio of 85:15 (Resomer Sample MD Type RG) was purchased from Boehringer Ingelheim with a weight and number average molecular weight of 380,300 and 181,900 g mol^{-1}, respectively. Fibers with PLGA/Ag-TCP containing 2% silver in a 70:30 ratio were fabricated by an electrospinning process [13]. Each electrospinning solution was prepared with a concentration of 5.9% (w/w) PLGA in chloroform (Riedel de Haen, Ph. Eur.) containing 6.4% (w/w) of the surfactant Tween20 (Polysorbate20, Fluka, Ph. Eur.) referred to the polymer. For the preparation of the electrospinning solution, corresponding amounts of the nanoparticles were first dispersed in a chloroform/Tween20 stock solution using an ultrasonic processor at 70 W for 5 min. PLGA was subsequently added and dissolved for 15 h by magnetic stirring. Electrospinning was performed by feeding the solutions through four capillaries (inner diameter 1.0 mm) using a syringe pump. The feeding rate was set to 8 mL h^{-1}. A voltage of 24 kV was applied to the needle tips, which was kept in a chloroform–air stream (160 $mlmin^{-1}$) by a concentrically mounted polyetheretherketone (PEEK) adapter. A positively charged jet was formed from the Taylor cone and was sprayed onto a rotating (100 rpm) collection tube covered by an aluminium foil. The distance between the needle tip and the collection tube (diameter 8 cm) was kept constant at 17 cm. The as-spun scaffolds were dried and stored in vacuum at room temperature.

As reference, a collagen scaffold with and without hyaluronan acid (Coll-HA, Coll) was used in the present study (Bio-Gide®, Geistlich, Wolhusen, Switzerland; LOT 81500056; molecular weight of collagen 1 300 KDa). The hyaluronan acid (Regedent, Zurich, Switzerland; LOT MK2-1714/1) applied on the membrane contained 2 mg sodium hyaluronate (molecular weight 2.5 MDa), 16 mg cross-linked sodium hyaluronate (molecular weight 1 MDa), 6.9 mg sodium chloride and water for injection ad 1 ml (Vol. 1.2 ml).

Cell culture

Human dental pulps of two anonymous donors below 30 years were isolated from caries-free third molars after informed consent was obtained (Ethics Committee of the Medical University Vienna; EK 631/2007). Dental pulp tissues were left in Dulbecco's Modified Eagle Medium (DMEM, Invitrogen Corporation, Carlsbad, CA, USA) supplemented with 10% fetal bovine serum (FCS; PAA Laboratories, Linz, Austria) and antibiotics (Invitrogen) at 37 °C, 5% CO_2, and 95% humidity. Dental pulp cells grown out from the pulp were cultured. Cells that had not undergone more than five passages were used and cell seeding for indicated experiments was performed in growth medium at 30,000 cells/cm^2. The cell density was based on previous in vitro studies on the impact of biomaterials on cell activity [19]. Experiments on viability and proliferation were performed with two different cell donors, each in duplicates. Gene expression analyses were performed twice, each time in duplicates, using pooled dental pulp cells of the two donors.

Preparation and pretreatment of the scaffolds

For MTT tests and BrdU incorporation assays silver-containing nanofabric (PLGA/Ag-TCP) scaffolds and collagen (Coll) scaffolds of Ø 6 mm were gained from corresponding scaffolds using a biopsy punch. For gene expression, analysis scaffolds of Ø 2.2 cm were cut. One half of the collagen scaffolds was soaked in cross-linked hyaluronan acid for 1 min and thoroughly washed with PBS for 2 min (Coll-HA) immediately before stimulation of the cells.

In vitro models (Model I, Model II)

Two different in vitro models were used. Cells were pre-cultured and the scaffold was placed thereon (Model I – scaffold on cells) and cells were cultured directly on the scaffold (Model II cells on scaffold). In both models cell viability and proliferation was assessed based on formazan formation (MTT test) and BrdU incorporation, respectively, after 24, 48, and 72 h. Gene expression of IL-6, TNF-α and AP was analyzed after 24 h.

MTT assay

For model I, where cells were cultured in the presence of the scaffolds, the latter were removed from the plates just before 3-[4,5-dimethythiazol-2-yl]-2,5-diphenyltetrazolium bromide (MTT, 0.5 mg/ml, Sigma-Aldrich, St. Louis, MO, USA) was added. In model II, where the cells were cultured directly on the scaffold, MTT was added in each well and incubated for 2 h at 37 °C. Afterwards, formazan crystals, formed by the NAD(P)H-dependent oxidoreductases, were dissolved in dimethyl sulfoxide. Optical density was measured with a microplate reader (EL 808, Biotek Instruments, Winooski, VT, USA) and normalized to untreated cells.

BrdU incorporation assay

For model I similarly to the MTT assay, scaffolds were removed from the culture plates before the BrdU incorporation assay was performed. For model II growth medium was removed, dental pulp fibroblasts were washed with PBS and serum-free media containing 5-bromo-2′-deoxyuridine (BrdU) was added to the cells for 2 h. BrdU incorporation was determined following the manufacturer's instructions (Cell Proliferation ELISA, BrdU colorimetric kit from Roche; Basel, Switzerland) and normalized to untreated cells.

Scanning electron microscopy

Surface structure topography of the scaffolds was examined by a scanning electron microscope at magnifications of × 500 at the Center of Microscopy and Image Analysis, University of Zurich (scanning electron microscopy (SEM); Carl Zeiss Supra 50 VP FESEM, Carl Zeiss). For this purpose, the samples were fixed for 24 h in 2.5% glutaraldehyde solution. Afterward, the scaffolds were rinsed with PBS and dehydrated in ascending concentrations of alcohol (50, 70, 80, and 90%) twice for 15 min. Finally, the scaffolds were immersed three times for 15 min in 94% and 60 min in 100% ethanol. Samples were then subjected to critical point drying (Bal-Tec CPD030), mounted on SEM mounts (Bal-Tec AG, Blazers, Liechtenstein), and were gold sputtered (Balzers SCD 030, Balzers Union, Balzers, Liechtenstein) for 60 s in an argon gas atmosphere at a target distance of 50 mm, at pressure of 5 Pascal (Pa) at 45 mA. SEM images were taken at a working distance of an acceleration voltage of 10 kV.

Gene expression analysis

Twenty-four hours after stimulation, the scaffolds were either removed (Model I) or retained (Model II) for gene expression analysis. Total cellular RNA was isolated with the High Pure RNA Isolation Kit (Roche F. Hoffmann-La Roche, Basel, Switzerland). Reverse transcription (RT) was performed with Transcriptor Universal cDNA

Master (Roche) and PCR was performed with the FastStart Universal SYBR Green Master (Roche) on a 7500 Real-Time PCR System (Applied Biosystems, Life Technologies Corporation, Carlsbad, CA, USA). Primers against the pro-inflammatory cytokines human IL-6 and TNF-α representing first reaction to an inflammation, as well as against AP as an early differentiation marker [20], and GAPDH, the house-keeping gene were designed in the online Universal ProbeLibrary Assay Design Center (Roche). The mRNA levels were calculated by normalizing to GAPDH using the ΔΔCt method.

Statistical analysis

Data obtained by MTT and BrdU incorporation assays were reported as median, 25% percentile, 75% percentile, minimum and maximum of two independent experiments, each performed in duplicates. Differences between cells stimulated with the three scaffolds were tested using a non-parametric Kruskal-Wallis test followed by a post-hoc Mann-Whitney *U*-test. Furthermore differences between the two cell seeding methods and the three different stimulation periods were statistically analyzed (SPSS version 19.0, SPSS Inc., Chicago, IL, USA). Statistical significance was considered at $p < 0.05$. Data obtained by RT PCR, showing the differences in mRNA expression of target genes between cells stimulated with the different scaffolds and unstimulated cells were described by the mean and standard deviation.

Results

Dental pulp cells in all groups except for the Ag containing scaffold groups had a fibroblast like morphology without any signs of malaise and were attached over the whole period of 72 h (Fig. 1). In the Ag containing scaffold groups, cells were rounded up and most of them did not attach.

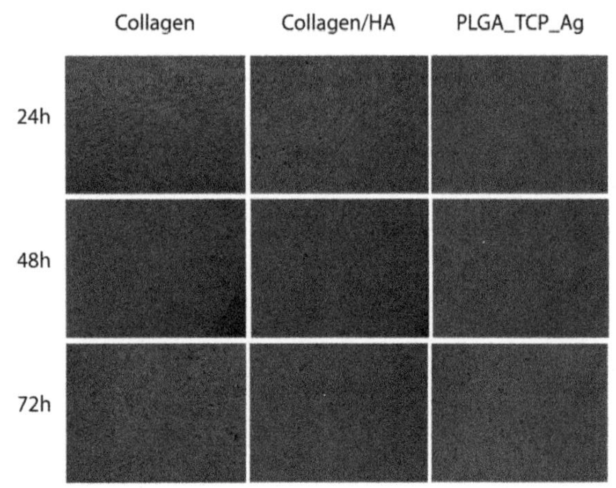

Fig. 1 Morphology of dental pulp cells after stimulation with PLGA/Ag-TCP, Coll, and Coll-HA scaffolds for 24, 48, and 72 h, respectively

PLGA/Ag-TCP scaffolds decrease formazan formation in human dental pulp-derived cells

Formazan formation as indicator for viability of dental pulp fibroblasts incubated with the scaffolds after 24, 48, and 72 h are shown in Fig. 2a and b.

When cells were cultured in the presence of the scaffolds (Model I) (Fig. 2a) the absolute viability values were higher than when the cells were cultured directly on the scaffolds (Model II) (Fig. 2b) while the overall trend with regard to the impact of the scaffold was the same. Formazan formation of cells incubated with PLGA/Ag-TCP was decreased after 24 h compared to the unstimulated control (w/o) ($p < 0.05$). In contrast, cells stimulated with Coll or Coll/HA using Model I did not show any differences compared to the unstimulated control (w/o) ($p > 0.05$) (Fig. 2a). After 48 and 72 h, all cells stimulated with scaffolds showed reduced levels of formazan formation, most prominently, when stimulation was performed with PLGA/Ag-TCP. When directly comparing the formazan formation of the cells that were stimulated with the three different scaffolds, substantial differences between the Ag containing scaffold and both collagen scaffolds were found. After 24, 48, and 72 h viability was significantly reduced when cells were stimulated with PLGA/Ag-TCP as compared to cells stimulated with Coll or Coll/HA (all $p < 0.05$). Comparing Coll and Coll/HA, no differences could be revealed at all times (all $p > 0.05$).

PLGA/Ag-TCP scaffolds decrease BrdU incorporation in human dental pulp-derived cells

BrdU incorporation as indicator for proliferation of cells incubated with the scaffolds after 24, 48, and 72 h are shown in Fig. 3a and b.

In model II the PLGA/Ag-TCP scaffolds showed false positive reactions with the substrate solution TMB (3,3′,5,5′-Tetramethylbenzidine) of the BrdU assay. Nevertheless, the results of the BrdU assay from Coll and Coll-HA support the results in model I.

In model I, where cells were cultured in the presence of the scaffolds, incorporation of BrdU in dental pulp fibroblasts was decreased when cells were stimulated with PLGA/Ag-TCP or Coll compared to the unstimulated control (w/o) ($p < 0.05$). After 48 h, proliferation only decreased in the group with PLGA/Ag-TCP, whereas after 72 h, a decrease was again detectable in both groups (PLGA/Ag-TCP and Coll). A comparison of the proliferation rate of cells stimulated with the three different scaffolds showed that cells of the PLGA/Ag-TCP group achieved significantly lower values than both collagen groups (Coll and Coll/HA) after 24 and 48 h (all $p < 0.05$). Interestingly, after 72 h of stimulation, no significant differences between all three groups were detectable. Comparing Coll and Coll-HA, no differences could be revealed at all time points of stimulation (all $p > 0.05$; Fig. 3).

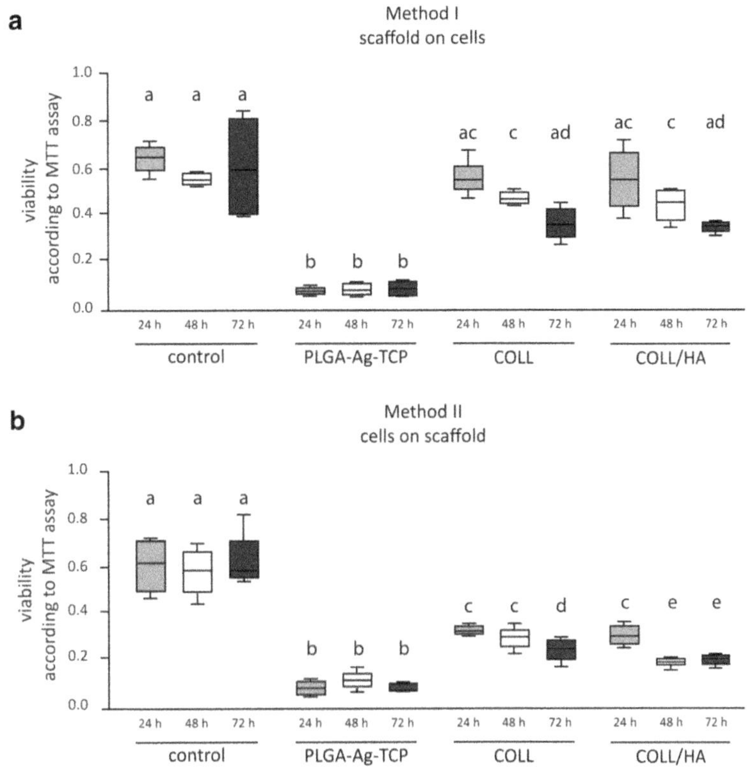

Fig. 2 Viability of dental pulp fibroblasts measured by MTT assay after stimulation for 24h, 48h or 72h with PLGA/Ag-TCP, Coll, and Coll-HA scaffolds using two different seeding methods (**a**) the scaffolds were placed on the cells; (**b**) the cells were seeded on the scaffolds. Unstimulated cells acted as control. Different letter indicate statistically significant differences

Scanning electron microscopy

Representative SEM demonstrated the typical woven appearance of the PLGA/Ag-TCP scaffold and the collagen structure of the resorbable scaffold. On a surface level, there was no difference between the untreated and hyaluronan treated scaffold surface, as the hyaluronan represents a material, which is very hydrophilic and thus spreads very well on the surface. Therefore, the surface of the scaffold was not affected. Furthermore, there is no chemical interaction between hyaluronan and scaffold, which might lead to a surface modification. Hyaluronan spreads on the scaffold and will act on cellular level due to its biochemical properties. The cross-linked hyaluronan will be absorbed on a very low level to its long molecular chain and due to the cross-linking (Fig. 4).

PLGA/Ag-TCP scaffolds increase IL-6, TNF-α, and AP expression in human dental pulp-derived cells

Data for IL-6, TNF-α and AP gene expression are shown in Fig. 5a and b.

After stimulation of the dental pulp fibroblasts using cell seeding method I, i.e. scaffold on cells, expression of IL-6 and TNF-α substantially increased when PLGA/Ag-TCP was used, whereas the expression of IL-6 and TNF-α was compareable with no stimulation when Coll or Coll/HA were used. Regarding AP, cells stimulated with PLGA/Ag-TCP showed a slight increase in mRNA expression, while cells stimulated with Coll or Coll/HA showed a slightly decreased expression (Fig. 5a).

Gene expression values of the cell seeding method II, i.e. cells on scaffold, confirmed the results of cell seeding method I (Fig. 5b).

Discussion

This proof of principle study assessed the cell viabilty and proliferation as well as the pro-inflammatory and metabolic capacity of human dental pulp cells in response to a novel silver-containing PLGA/TCP-nanofabric and compared it to collagen scaffold with and without hyaluronan acid (Coll and Coll-HA). It was hypothesized that PLGA/Ag-TCP induce minor reduction of cell viability and cell proliferation, which are comparable to the Coll and Coll-HA. Based on our results this hypothesis was rejected.

Considering also that the exposed dental pulp is a wound, the structure of the wound is important for the determination, differentiation, proliferation, survival, polarity and migration of cells [21]. Progresses in biomaterial science have significantly advanced, and scaffold materials have been tailored to mimic extracellular

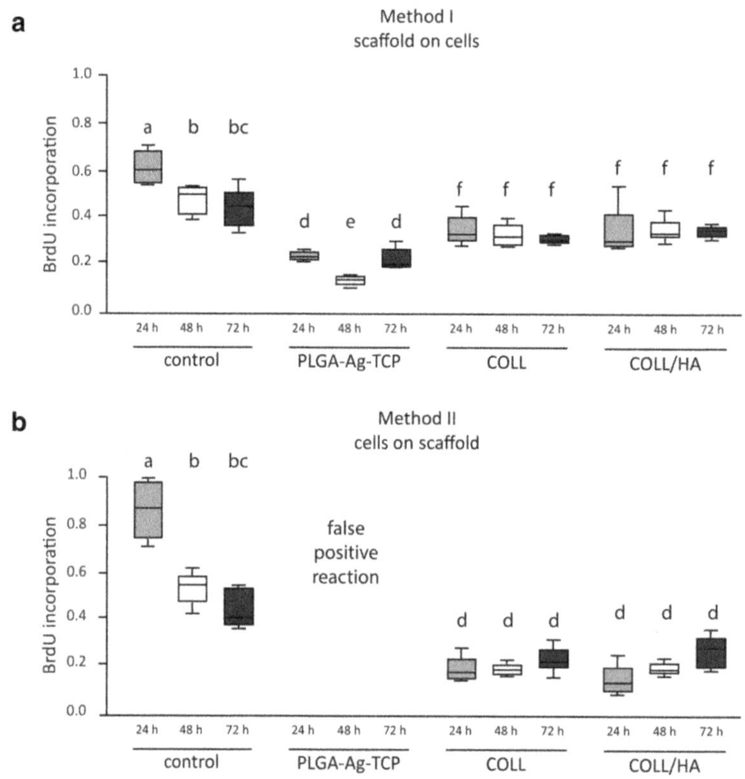

Fig. 3 Proliferation of dental pulp fibroblasts measured by BrdU incorporation assay after stimulation for 24h, 48h or 72h with PLGA/Ag-TCP, Coll, and Coll-HA scaffolds using two different seeding methods (**a**) the scaffolds were placed on the cells; (**b**) the cells were seeded on the scaffolds). Unstimulated cells acted as control. Different letters indicate statistically significant differences

microenvironments of tissues or even organs to promote tissue regeneration under specific requirements in vivo [22]. In a recent study, Chen and co-workers tested the hypothesis that dental pulp/dentin complexes would contribute to the regeneration of tooth root and fabricated aligned PLGA/gelatin electrospun sheets (APES), treated dentin matrix (TDM) and native dental pulp extracellular matrix (DPEM), which were combined for periodontal or pulp regeneration, respectively [23]. Seeded with stem cells, the sandwich composites (APES/TDM/DPEM) generated tooth root-like tissues after being transplanted in porcine jaws for 12 weeks. In dental pulp/dentin complex-like tissues, columnar odontoblasts-like layer even arranged along the interface between newly formed predentin matrix and dental pulp-like tissues in which blood vessels could be found. This conceptual study showed that fibrous scaffolds are able to act as a potent control structure leading to a well-organized tissue formation of even original quality. However, under clinical conditions, such healing may be hampered by simple infections. Thus antimicrobial strategies have to be envisaged, which allow for appropriate cell homing.

Therefore, when thinking about the management of deep carious lesions and pulp affections in terms of capping procedures, bridging mechanisms are still warranted that encounter the effective disinfection and mineralization of the wound area. This study was based on this concept as well. A smart scaffold was designed, which combined antibacterial and bioactive properties, which seemed ideal for this indication. The nanofabric doped with silver has been shown to result in enhanced antimicrobial properties [13] when compared to tetracycline controls whilst being biocompatible in preclinical studies [14]. However, the immediate cell response within the limitations of the present in vitro investigation were shown to reduce cell viability and proliferation, while inducing a tremendous pro-inflammatory response and an increase in AP. This is in accordance with other findings with antimicrobial agents, which show evident cytotoxic effects in fibroblasts or osteoblasts [24, 25]. Long-term effects of the differentiation status of surviving cells, however, have not been investigated yet. These cells, despite being under stress and struggling for survival, can recover and form even mature osteoblasts even without external addition of growth factors and continue to deposit osteogenic cues into the newly formed extracellular matrix [26].

Summarizing the data of the present study, PLGA/Ag-TCP showed a toxic potential for dental pulp cells, while the collagen scaffolds with and without hyaluronan acid were well tolerated by the cells. This is particularly true for the 24 h data. However, after 72 h of stimulation a significant decrease in viability occurred in all groups. Whether this is of clinical significance could not be answered with the present in vitro testing method yet. Further investigations including a simulation of the physiological circulation might elucidate whether the cytotoxicity of PLGA/Ag-TCP is reversible or less dramatic, for instance by simple changing of the media.

The results of the BrdU assay may support the MTT findings. Over the entire study period of 72 h, the proliferation in the unstimulated control group substantially decreased. In the experimental groups, however, the proliferation remained at the same level during the entire investigative period, irrespective of the scaffold used. After 72 h, cells stimulated with PLGA/Ag-TCP even showed proliferation rates comparable to cells stimulated with Coll and Coll/HA. Two possible explanations could be drawn from these findings: either Ag is released from the scaffold and thereby affecting the assay, which might result in false positive results, or the cells enter a kind of "rescue state" and strongly attempt to proliferate. The latter assumption is strengthened by the results of the viability assay, and by the fact that the non-stimulated cells rather showed a decrease in the proliferation after 72 h, while all stimulated cells kept the proliferation rate at the same level over the entire period. Furthermore, the supernatant was removed directly before the assay. Together, it has to be stated that PLGA/Ag-TCP is toxic in this experimental set-up. Therefore, important questions still remain to be answered after this first proof of principle study. One critical question that needs to be further elucidated is whether the experimental outcome would have been the same when initial cell seeding would have been performed with fewer cells. In our results regarding viability and proliferation cells that were incubated with collagen or collagen with hyaluronan acid showed no dramatic changes over a period of 72 h. In contrast, with regard to cells incubated with PLGA/Ag-

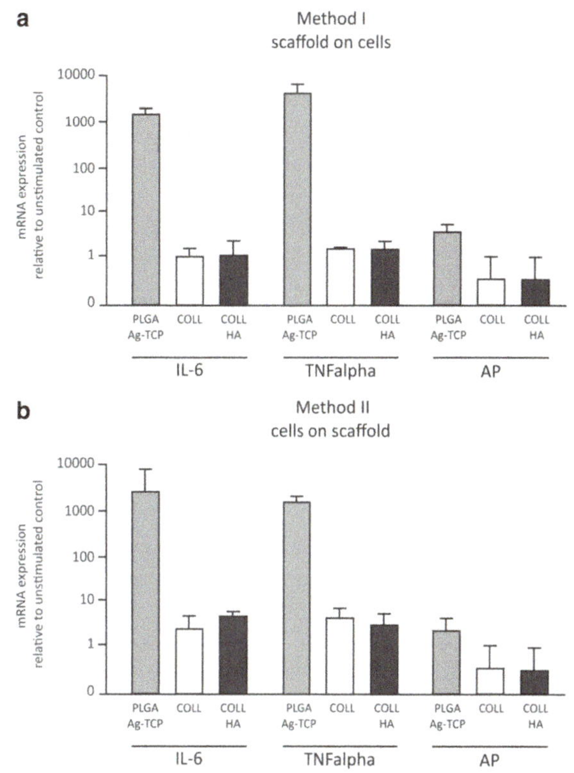

Fig. 5 mRNA expression of dental pulp fibroblasts after stimulation with PLGA/Ag-TCP, Coll, and Coll-HA scaffolds using two different seeding methods (**a**) the scaffolds were placed on the cells; (**b**) the cells were seeded on the scaffolds. Unstimulated cells acted as control

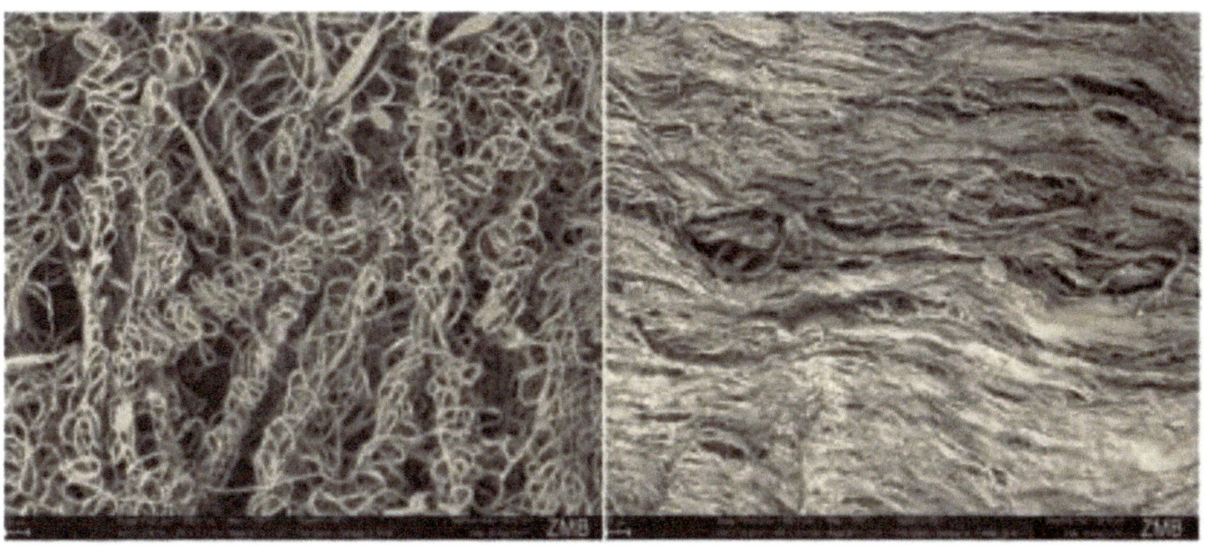

Fig. 4 Scanning electron microscopy images of representative PLGA/Ag-TCP (*left*) and Coll scaffolds (*right*), respectively

TCP we detected a decrease in the proliferation assay after 48 h, combined with an increase after 72 h. Our explanation of entering a "rescue state" might be indirectly checked by reducing the numbers of cells in the initial seeding in the other groups, where also an increase in proliferation might be seen. Our seeding density was 30,000 cells/cm^2, which was based on previous in vitro studies [19]. Future studies will need to address the impact of the seeding density, especially since the literature on initial seeding density is divergent [27].

In this study, the MTT assay was used to assess cell cytotoxicity, which is a widely used approach [28]. In the MTT assay, the cellular activity with regard to the activity of NAD(P)H-dependent cellular oxidoreductase enzymes is certainly decreased under toxic conditions. However, the assay does not directly distinguish between the increase in cell numbers in the control vs. inhibition of cell division or reduction of cell numbers in the control group. Hence, enzyme release assays like the lactate dehydrogenase release assay or the Glyceraldehyde-3-Phosphate Dehydrogenase release assay where the enzymatic activity of soluble, cytosolic enzymes correlates with cell death would be a feasible approach [29]. However, the stable formazan formation and the reduction of BrdU incorporation over the 72 h observation period in the control group due to the chosen in vitro setup does not suggest that proliferation confounds our interpretation regarding the toxic effect. This is further supported by the morphological evaluation in the microscope. In addition, we have tried to determine the amount of silver in the medium, but there was either no silver ions released from the scaffolds or the concentration was below the detection limit of the applied method, i.e. in this case atomic absorption spectrometry.

Not surprisingly though, based on the toxic effects, the data of the RT-PCR showed an enhanced increase in inflammatory genes when cells were stimulated with PLGA/Ag-TCP for 24 h, thus the idea of entering a "rescue state" is supported. However, a slight increase in ALP was detected. In further studies it would be interesting to additionally evaluate the inflammatory response as well as a possible mineralization activity by using longer stimulation periods, maybe with osteogenic medium and to investigate these results also on a protein level. Furthermore, to reduce the toxicity of PLGA/Ag-TCP, while maintaining the known bactericidal effect and cause positive counter reaction of the cells. In a best-case scenario this might result in an increased migration of cells to the area of the exposed pulp, as well as an increased proliferation of the cells and tertiary dentin formation under a clinical situation. Besides, it would be interesting to know, if sorted stem cells from the dental pulp would show other reactions than the fibroblast like cells that were used in the experiments containing only 2–6% of cells that are positive for STRO-1 [30, 31].

A conceptual combination of hyaluronan acid and a silver scaffold, however, could also bear some benefits but also bear some problems as a recent article suggested [32]: Peritendinous adhesions, one of the common complications after tendon injury and subsequent surgery has led to the interesting development and investigation on a physical barrier between the injured site and the surrounding tissue using silver (Ag) nanoparticles embedded in electrospun hyaluronan acid (HA)/polycaprolactone (PCL) nanofibrous scaffolds (NFMs) (HA/PCL + Ag NFMs) to prevent peritendinous adhesions and bacterial infection after tendon surgery. This in vitro cell culture experiments revealed that HA/PCL + Ag NFMs exhibited the highest inhibition of fibroblast attachment and proliferation. Interestingly, in contrast to our findings, no significant cytotoxicity was observed, which was explained by the synergistic effect of Ag and HA and a lubrification effect. In the present study, this protective finding was not observed. Since a regeneration of tissues wants to be achieved, which includes the formation of the original tissues in dense contact to each other, the above mentioned contact inhibition seems not a desirable goal in this indication. Therefore, a combination of HA and Ag has to be carefully studied. Hyaluronan acid was chosen as potential candidate for improved wound healing in this screening study [18]. But the overall adjunctive beneficial effects of HA when on the collagen scaffolds in the present investigation were not that impressive within the limitations of this study. This might be due to the fact that the scaffolds were soaked in HA for a relatively short time of 1 min to stimulate the direct use in the clinical application for pulp capping procedures [33]. Maybe an incorporation of hyaluronan directly in the scaffolds or a pre-treating over a longer time period would change the cellular response, however, a longer pre-treatment is clinically not always possible, e.g. in the case of a direct pulp capping.

Regarding the two seeding methods investigated in this study, it became apparent that both methods are feasible since the outcomes are equal in all tested methods, which means that our second hypothesis was also rejected. Method I (scaffold on cells) appeared, however, better for this type of material testing. Firstly, this method better represents the clinical situation, since, for example at a direct pulp capping, the capping material has to be put on to the pulp tissue and not vice versa. Secondly, the direct comparison to the control group is more accurate in model I "scaffold on cells", because always the same conditions are present. The other method (cells on scaffold) often misses a direct comparison group. Another advantage of the method I "scaffold on cells" is the easier implementation in the experimental procedure. The experiments are more accurate, faster and easier, thus less error-prone. In addition, considering the results of the proliferation assay, influence of the testing methodology by the scaffold can be excluded since the scaffold is removed directly before the investigations.

Conclusion

Within the limitations of this in vitro study the following conclusions can be drawn:

PLGA/Ag-TCP initially decreased the viability and proliferation rate of human dental pulp cells while increasing the pro-inflammatory capacity and alkaline phosphatase expression. Whether surviving cells can enter a rescue state and therefore support the long-term survivability has to be determined in future studies. Furthermore a possible bactericidal effect has to be demonstrated.

Regarding the two different models it was obvious that Method I (scaffold on cells) was preferably using the presented study design.

Acknowledgment
The authors thank Catherine Solioz for her careful technical assistance in helping with the experiments. The support from the Functional Materials Laboratory of the Federal Institute of Technology in Zurich for the preparation of the Ag/TCP based materials was also greatly appreciated (Prof. Dr. Wendelin Stark).

Funding
This study was supported–in part–by the Swiss Dental Association SSO Grant [project number 286–15].

Authors' contributions
BC and PRS conceived the study, participated in its design and drafted the manuscript. SCH prepared the material for this study. RJM, HA and DB helped to supervise the methodological correctness of the performed study and the coordination. TA and AL supported the study design. All authors carefully read and approved the final text.

Competing interests
PRS declares a financial interest in the form of a patent application (WO2008/049242) on electrospun, biodegradable implant material licensed to Zurich Biomaterials llc., of which PRS is a shareholder. All other authors declare that they have no competing interests.

Consent for publication
Not applicable.

Ethics approval and consent to participate
Isolation of human dental pulps was approved by the Ethics Committee of the Medical University Vienna with the number EK 631/2007. All participants signed the consent form.

Author details
[1]Department of Preventive, Restorative and Pediatric Dentistry, School of Dentistry, University of Bern, Bern, Switzerland. [2]Institute for Chemical and Bioengineering, Department of Chemistry and Applied Biosciences, ETH Zurich, Zurich, Switzerland. [3]Department of Conservative Dentistry & Periodontology, Medical University of Vienna, Vienna, Austria. [4]Robert K. Schenk Laboratory of Oral Histology, Department of Periodontology, Department of Oral Surgery and Stomatology, University of Bern, Bern, Switzerland. [5]Clinic of Preventive Dentistry, Periodontology and Cariology, Center of Dental Medicine, University of Zurich, Plattenstrasse 11, Zurich CH-8032, Switzerland. [6]Department of Periodontology, College of Dental Medicine, Nova Southeastern University, Fort Lauderdale, Florida, USA.

References
1. Arana-Chavez VE, Massa LF. Odontoblasts: the cells forming and maintaining dentine. Int J Biochem Cell Biol. 2004;36:1367–73.
2. Cooper PR, Holder MJ, Smith AJ. Inflammation and regeneration in the dentin-pulp complex: a double-edged sword. J Endod. 2014;40:S46–51.
3. Bleicher F. Odontoblast physiology. Exp Cell Res. 2014;325:65–71.
4. Yamamura T. Differentiation of pulpal cells and inductive influences of various matrices with reference to pulpal wound healing. J Dent Res. 1985; 64 Spec No:530–40.
5. Murray PE, Hafez AA, Windsor LJ, Smith AJ, Cox CF. Comparison of pulp responses following restoration of exposed and non-exposed cavities. J Dent. 2002;30:213–22.
6. Smith AJ, Cassidy N, Perry H, Begue-Kirn C, Ruch JV, Lesot H. Reactionary dentinogenesis. Int J Dev Biol. 1995;39:273–80.
7. Sangwan P, Sangwan A, Duhan J. Tertiary dentinogenesis with calcium hydroxide: A review of proposed mechanisms. Int Endod J. 2013;46:3–19.
8. Rezwan K, Chen QZ, Blaker JJ, Boccaccini AR. Biodegradable and bioactive porous polymer/inorganic composite scaffolds for bone tissue engineering. Biomaterials. 2006;27:3413–31.
9. Schneider OD, Loher S, Brunner TJ. Cotton wool-like nanocomposite biomaterials prepared by electrospinning: In vitro bioactivity and osteogenic differentiation of human mesenchymal stem cells. J Biomed Mater Res B Appl Biomater. 2008;84:350–62.
10. Schneider OD, Weber F, Brunner TJ, Loher S. In vivo and in vitro evaluation of flexible, cottonwool-like nanocomposites as bone substitute material for complex defects. Acta Biomater. 2009;5:1775–84.
11. Buschmann J, Härter L, Gao S, Hemmi S, Welti M, Hild N, Schneider OD, Stark WJ, Lindenblatt N, Werner CM, Wanner GA, Calcagni M. Tissue engineered bone grafts based on biomimetic nanocomposite PLGA/ amorphous calcium phosphate scaffold and human adipose-derived stem cells. Injury. 2012;43:1689.
12. Holderegger C, Schmidlin PR, Weber FE, Mohn D. Preclinical in vivo Performance of Novel Biodegradable, Electrospun Poly(lactic acid) and Poly(lactic-co-glycolic acid) Nanocomposites: A Review. Materials. 2015;8:4912–31.
13. Schneider OD, Loher S, Brunner TJ. Flexible, silver containing nanocomposites for the repair of bone defects: antimicrobial effect against E. coli infection and comparison to tetracycline containing. J Mater Chem. 2008;18:2679–84.
14. Schneider OD, Mohn D, Fuhrer R, Klein K. Biocompatibility and bone formation of flexible, cotton wool-like PLGA/calcium phosphate nanocomposites in sheep. Open Orthop J. 2011;5:63–71.
15. Kadler K. Extracellular matrix. 1: fibril-forming collagens. Protein Profile. 1994; 1:519–638.
16. Beniash E, Traub W, Veis A, Weiner S. A transmission electron microscope study using vitrified ice sections of predentin: structural changes in the dentin collagenous matrix prior to mineralization. J Struct Biol. 2000;132:212–25.
17. Landis WJ, Hodgens KJ, Song MJ, Arena J, Kiyonaga S, Marko M, Owen C, McEwen BF. Mineralization of collagen may occur on fibril surfaces: evidence from conventional and high-voltage electron microscopy and three-dimensional imaging. J Struct Biol. 1996;117:24–35.
18. Price RD, Myers S, Leigh IM, Navsaria HA. The role of hyaluronic acid in wound healing: assessment of clinical evidence. Am J Clin Dermatol. 2005;6:393–402.
19. Al Mustafa M, Agis H, Müller HD, Watzek G, Gruber R. In vitro adhesion of fibroblastic cells to titanium alloy discs treated with sodium hydroxide. Clin Oral Implants Res. 2015;26:15–9.
20. Klein MO, Bijelic A, Ziebart T, Koch F, Kämmerer PW, Wieland M, Konerding MA, Al-Nawas B. Submicron scale-structured hydrophilic titanium surfaces promote early osteogenic gene response for cell adhesion and cell differentiation. Clin Implant Dent Relat Res. 2013;15:166–75.
21. Hynes RO. The extracellular matrix: not just pretty fibrils. Science. 2009;326: 1216–9.
22. Atala A, Kasper FK, Mikos AG. Engineering complex tissues. Sci Transl Med. 2012;4:160rv12.
23. Chen G, Chen J, Yang B, Li L, Luo X, Zhang X, Feng L. Combination of aligned PLGA/Gelatin electrospun sheets, native dental pulp extracellular matrix and treated dentin matrix as substrates for tooth root regeneration. Biomaterials. 2015;52:56–70.

24. Wilken R, Botha SJ, Grobler A, Germishuys PJ. In vitro cytotoxicity of chlorhexidine gluconate, benzydamine-HCl and povidone iodine mouthrinses on human gingival fibroblasts. SADJ. 2001;56:455–60.
25. Cabral CT, Fernandes MH. In vitro comparison of chlorhexidine and povidone-iodine on the long-term proliferation and functional activity of human alveolar bone cells. Clin Oral Investig. 2007;11:155–64.
26. Schmidlin PR, Imfeld T, Sahrmann P, Tchouboukov A, Weber FE. Effect of short-time povidone-iodine application on osteoblast proliferation and differentiation. Open Dent J. 2009;3:208–12.
27. Issa RI, Engebretson B, Rustom L, McFetridge PS, Sikavitsas VI. The effect of cell seeding density on the cellular and mechanical properties of a mechanostimulated tissue-engineered tendon. Tissue Eng Part A. 2011; 17:1479–87.
28. Sumantran VN. Cellular chemosensitivity assays: an overview. Methods Mol Biol. 2011;731:219–36.
29. Decker T, Lohmann-Matthes ML. A quick and simple method for the quantitation of lactate dehydrogenase release in measurements of cellular cytotoxicity and tumor necrosis factor (TNF) activity. J Immunol Methods. 1988;115:61–9.
30. Huang GT, Shagramanova K, Chan SW. Formation of odontoblast-like cells from cultured human dental pulp cells on dentin in vitro. J Endod. 2006;32: 1066–73.
31. Pisciotta A, Carnevale G, Meloni S, Riccio M, De Biasi S, Gibellini L, Ferrari A, Bruzzesi G, De Pol A. Human dental pulp stem cells (hDPSCs): isolation, enrichment and comparative differentiation of two sub-populations. BMC Dev Biol. 2015;15:14.
32. Chen CH, Chen SH, Shalumon KT, Chen JP. Prevention of peritendinous adhesions with electrospun polyethylene glycol/polycaprolactone nanofibrous membranes. Colloids Surf B: Biointerfaces. 2015;133:221–30.
33. Mueller A, Fujioka-Kobayashi M, Mueller HD, Lussi A, Sculean A, Schmidlin PR, Miron RJ. Effect of hyaluronic acid on morphological changes to dentin surfaces and subsequent effect on periodontal ligament cell survival, attachment, and spreading. Clin Oral Investig. 2016 May 19. [Epub ahead of print]

24

Prevalence of *Candida albicans* and non-*albicans* on the tongue dorsa of elderly people living in a post-disaster area

Toshiro Sato[1], Mitsuo Kishi[1*], Miki Suda[1], Kiyomi Sakata[2], Haruki Shimoda[2], Hiroyuki Miura[3], Akira Ogawa[4] and Seiichiro Kobayashi[4]

Abstract

Background: *Candida* species are normal commensal organisms of the mouth. However, they can cause oral mucosal and severe systemic infections in persons with reduced immune function, which is common in the very elderly. In post-disaster areas, the number of elderly residents rapidly increases due to the outflow of younger generations. Hence, we examined the prevalence of *Candida albicans* and non-*albicans* in association with oral and systemic conditions, life style, medications, and living conditions.

Methods: This study was performed in 2014. Participants of this study were 266 community dwellers aged 60 years or older in Otsuchi town, which was severely damaged by the Great East Japan Earthquake and Tsunami in 2011. Oral specimens were collected from tongue dorsa by swabbing. After 48 h incubation on CHROMagar™ medium, *C. albicans* and non-*albicans* were identified by the morphology and pigmentation of the colonies. Oral and systemic health check-ups were performed to assess the following: number of remaining teeth and periodontal status, oral hygiene, use of dentures, obesity, hypertension, hyperlipidemia, and hyperglycemia. A questionnaire addressed lifestyle, medications, and living conditions. Using the variables above, the relative factors involved in the colonization and the amounts of each type of *Candida* were determined.

Results: *C. albicans* and non-*albicans* were detected in 142 (53.4%) and 63 (23.7%) participants, respectively. Multinomial logistic regression analyses revealed that the significant factors of colonization by *C. albicans* were "having decayed teeth" and "relocation from home". Factors related to non-*albicans* colonization were "age over 80 years", "number of remaining teeth", "use of dentures", and "obesity". On the contrary, none of the parameters were related to the amount of non-*albicans* in the carrier, and the amount of *C. albicans* was significantly associated with "number of teeth" and "hypertension".

Conclusions: Prevalence-related factors differed between *C. albicans* and non-*albicans* colonization. In addition, other than oral status, systemic and living conditions affected the prevalence of both *C. albicans* and non-*albicans* in elderly people living in a post-disaster area.

Keywords: *Candida albicans*, Non-*albicans*, Elderly, Post-disaster area

* Correspondence: mkishi@iwate-med.ac.jp
[1]Division of Preventive Dentistry, Department of Oral Medicine, School of Dentistry Iwate Medical University, 1-3-27 Chuo-dori, Morioka, Iwate 020-8505, Japan
Full list of author information is available at the end of the article

Background

Over 40 species of *Candida* yeasts, the most common of which is *Candida albicans,* can cause infections in humans. In addition, *C. tropicalis, C. parapsilosis,* and *C. glabrata* are major pathogenic *Candida* species collectively referred to as non-*albicans* [1–4]. Several *Candida* species colonize mucosal surfaces in the oral cavity, digestive tract, and vagina. *Candida* are normal commensal organisms of the mouth and generally cause no problems in healthy people. In the general population, carriage rates are reported to be in the range 3 to 75% without any symptoms [5]. However, the overgrowth of *Candida* in oropharyngeal or esophageal mucosa causes a burning sensation, taste disorders, severe mucositis, or dysphagia and results in poor nutrition. From these symptoms, oral candidiasis is the most common human fungal infection, especially in the elderly or hospitalized patients [5–7]. Once the oral cavity is colonized, it becomes easier for the yeasts to reach the respiratory system, and since it is a commensal species of the gut lumen and the cutaneous surfaces, the colonization index is increasing [7, 8]. Thus, oral *Candida* poses a risk of systemic disorders as well as local mucosal infections in the elderly. Previous studies indicate that the risk factors involved in oral *Candida* colonization in the elderly include wearing dentures, poor oral/denture hygiene, and low local saliva flow [9–15]. Furthermore, elderly individuals are at risk of overgrowth of *Candida* due to several predisposing factors, such as systemic disease, decreased immune function, and the use of various medicines [7, 10, 16–19]. Therefore, the risks of *Candida* colonization should be clarified in terms of both systemic and oral conditions, especially in elderly people who are likely to harbor *Candida* and are more likely to receive hospital care.

In 2011, Japan experienced the Great East Japan Earthquake, a catastrophic disaster. Most of the severely damaged areas were rural and consisted of already aging communities compared with other areas of Japan, which has one of the largest aging populations in the world [20]. Moreover, the rate of growth of the elderly population has rapidly increased due to the outflow of the younger generation in post-disaster areas, and a considerable number of elderly people are still displaced from their homes 5 years after the disaster [21]. The extraordinary lifestyle after the disaster has had negative effects on systemic, mental, and oral health [22–24], and could affect the prevalence of oral *Candida* colonization in elderly community dwellers in the disaster areas.

The primary aim of this study was to assess the prevalence of oral *Candida* colonization and distinguish non-*albicans* from *C. albicans* in elderly community dwellers of a post-disaster area because non-*albicans* has recently been detected more frequently [25].

A second aim was to identify the factors associated with oral *Candida* colonization among demographic, oral, and systemic conditions, lifestyle, medication status, and living conditions.

Methods

Study design and population

This was a cross-sectional study involving clinical surveys, a questionnaire, and microbiological examinations using culture methods. The participants were community dwellers aged 60 years or over in Otsuchi, located on the Pacific Coast of Iwate Prefecture, which experienced some of the most severe damage from the Great East Japan Earthquake and Tsunami. However, the area suffered no effects of radiation from the Fukushima Daiichi Nuclear Disaster because the distance from the power station was over 200 km. In 2014, from individuals who attended an annual oral health checkup that we had carried out since 2011, 266 candidates aged 60 years or older who lived in the tsunami inundated area at the disaster site, were randomly recruited to an additional examination to detect *Candida* species (Fig. 1). Detailed methods of initial subject recruitment were reported in our previous paper [24]. All the candidates gave informed consent to participate in this study after receiving sufficient information. The mean age and standard deviation of our participants were 72.3 and 7.0. None of the participants used antibiotics, or antifungal medications during the survey.

The study protocol was approved by the Medical Ethics Committee of Iwate Medical University School of Medicine (H23-69) and School of Dentistry (01214).

Sample collection and identification of *Candida* species

Oral samples were collected by swabbing 10 times vertically from the circumvallate papillae to the tip of the tongue with a sterile cotton swab. Each swab was immediately immersed into 2 mL of sterile phosphate buffered

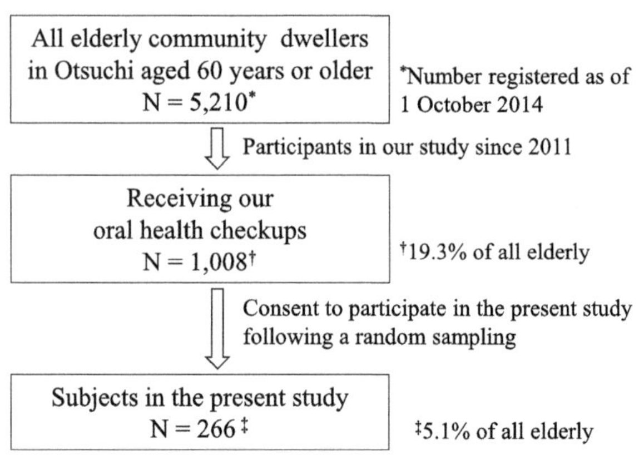

Fig. 1 Sample selection and description of the study population

saline (PBS, pH 7.4) in a stock tube and stored on ice until inoculation. After stirring with a Vortex® Mixer, the cotton swab was removed from the PBS and the suspension was inoculated onto a CHROMagar Candida™ plate (CHROMagar Microbiology, Paris, France) within 8 h of collection, because we confirmed in our preliminary study that the time elapsed would not affect the culture results. After 48 h of incubation, all colonies observed on CHROMagar™ were identified by their morphology and pigmentation according to the manufacturer's instructions and a previous study [26]. In addition, the colony forming unit/mL (CFU) was calculated for both *C. albicans* and non-*albicans*.

Oral examinations

Oral examinations were performed by a skilled dentist. Dental caries status was assessed according to the World Health Organization (WHO) method [27] with some modifications as follows: (1) a tooth with treated or untreated root caries was recorded as a filled or decayed, and (2) a remaining root without a crown was counted as a present tooth. Periodontal conditions were assessed using the Community Periodontal Index (CPI) procedures and diagnostic criteria, which are also recommended by the WHO. In addition, oral hygiene status was assessed as one of three grades: poor, fair, or good. Information on denture use was obtained from both oral examination and interview. In later analyses, participants with a CPI code of 3 or 4 (having periodontal pockets) were summarized, and oral hygiene status was categorized as poor or other status.

Systemic data

Body mass index (BMI, kg/m^2), blood pressure (BP, mmHg) and biochemical data, including high-density lipoprotein cholesterol (HDLC; mg/dL), low-density lipoprotein cholesterol (LDLC; mg/dL), and glycated hemoglobin (HbA1c, %) were obtained from the results of health check-ups that the municipality supplied as a public health service. The health check-up was performed according to a Japanese national guideline (the Specific Health Checkups) [28]. Participants were placed in one of two groups depending on the measurements, using the following cutoff values: BMI $\geq$25 (obesity), systolic BP $\geq$ 140 or diastolic BP $\geq$90 (hypertension), HDLC $\leq$ 34 or LDLC $\geq$140 (dyslipidemia), and HbA1c $\geq$5.6% (hyperglycemia).

Self-reported data

Self-report questionnaires were administrated to assess lifestyle (smoking and drinking status), daily medications (antihypertension drugs, diabetes drugs, hypnotics), and whether the participants' current accommodation was the same as that before the disaster (relocation from home). The choices of answers for smoking status were current smoker, past smoker, and non-smoker. We categorized those choices into current smoker or other in our statistical analyses. Similarly, choices for drinking status (daily drinker, occasional drinker, and no drinker) were summarized into daily drinker or other.

Statistical analyses

The prevalence of *Candida* was examined in all 266 participants. In subsequent factor analyses, two participants were excluded because certain data was missing. To determine the factors related with colonization of *C. albicans* or non-*albicans*, we assessed risk measurements by multinomial logistic regression models followed by crude analyses using Chi-squared tests. To compare the amounts of *Candida* species between the parameters, the Mann-Whitney *U* test or Kruskal-Wallis test was used, since the distribution of *Candida* amounts were non-normal after logarithmic transformation. Post hoc multiple comparisons after the Kruskal-Wallis test were performed using the Mann-Whitney *U* test with Bonferroni correction. To reveal the relationship between number of remaining teeth and log CFUs of *C. albicans* and non-*albicans*, Spearman's rank correlation analysis and logistic regression analysis using a cutoff value (log CFU = 1.5) were performed. A two-sided *p*-value of less than 0.05 was considered statistically significant. All statistical analyses were conducted using the software program SPSS version 24.0 for Windows (IBM).

Results

Prevalence of *C. albicans* and non-*albicans*

Candida species in tongue dorsa were detected in 162 participants (60.9%). *C. albicans* was the most frequently detected in (n = 142; 53.4%) participants, followed by *C. glabrata* (n = 60; 22.6%), *C. tropicalis* (n = 5; 1.8%), and *C. parapsilosis* (n = 2; 0.7%). *C. krusei* were not detected in any of our participants. At least one non-*albicans* species were detected in 63 (23.7%) of the participants (Table 1). In addition, 61.1% and 11.7% of *Candida* carriers exclusively harbored either *C. albicans* or *C. glabrata*, respectively. A combination of *C. albicans* and *C. glabrata* was found in 23.5% of *Candida* carriers, and other combinations were found in only 3.7%.

Factors associated with colonization by *C. albicans* and non-*albicans*

Tables 2 and 3 show the significant factors related to colonization by *C. albicans* and non-*albicans* in the demographic data and the parameters measured in this study (see Additional file: 1 for complete data). A crude odds ratio (COR) with a 95% confidence interval (CI) was calculated from a bi-variable Chi-squared test, and the adjusted odds ratio (AOR) with 95% CI was

Table 1 Detection rates of *Candida* in elderly community dwellers ($n = 266$) in a post-disaster area

Candida spp.	Number of carriers	% of entire subjects	% of carriers of any *Candida*
C. albicans	142	53.4	87.7
C. glabrata	60	22.6	37.0
C. tropicalis	5	1.8	3.1
C. parapsilosis	2	0.7	1.2
C. krusei	0	0	0
Any non-*albicans*	63	23.7	38.9
Any *Candida* spp.	162	60.9	-

calculated from multinomial logistic regression analysis in which the variables were all adjusted for each other. In the bi-variable models, participants "having one or more decayed teeth", "poor oral hygiene" and "relocation from home" harbored *C. albicans* at a significantly higher frequency (COR = 3.35; 95% CI = 1.70–6.63, COR = 2.42; 95% CI = 1.18–4.99 and COR = 1.45; 95% CI = 1.06–1.99, respectively). For colonization of non-*albicans*, "over 80 years old", "less than 20 remaining teeth/edentulous", "use of dentures" and "obesity" were significant factors associated with colonization (COR = 2.21; 95% CI = 1.36–5.34, COR = 1.84/2.39; 95% CI = 1.51–2.42/1.83–3.12, COR = 1.56; 95% CI = 1.37–1.77 and COR = 1.45; 95% CI = 1.06–2.00, respectively). In the multivariable models, "having one or more decayed teeth" and "relocation from home" were significant factors for colonization by *C. albicans* similarly to bi-variable analyses, although "poor oral hygiene" was not significant (AOR = 3.51; 95% CI = 1.60–7.67, AOR = 2.17; 95% CI = 1.25–3.78 and AOR = 2.01; 95% CI = 0.77–5.24, respectively). The same factors were significant to colonization by non-albicans in bi-variable analyses, excluding "less than 20 teeth" (AOR = 3.37; 95% CI = 0.88–12.9). In addition, the odds ratios of "over 80 years old", "edentulous", "use of dentures" and "obesity" were raised after adjustment for each other (AOR = 2.58; 95% CI = 1.12–5.71, AOR = 5.99; 95% CI = 1.37–26.3, AOR = 4.02; 95% CI = 1.05–15.4 and AOR = 2.25; 95% CI = 1.15–4.40, respectively).

Factors related to the amounts of *C. albicans* and non-*albicans* among the carriers

We compared the amounts (log CFU) of *Candida* between same parameters as the examination for colonization-related factors of each *Candida* carrier. Larger amounts of *C. albicans* were detected in edentulous subjects than in dentate subjects among *C. albicans* carriers. In addition, participants with hypertension and a daily drinking habit harbored greater amounts of *C. albicans*. However, the amounts of non-*albicans* among the carriers were no different between any of the categories (Table 4).

Correlation between amounts of *C. albicans* and non-*albicans* with number of remaining teeth in denture wearers

Spearman's correlation coefficient between amounts (log CFU) of *Candida*, number of remaining teeth and age were examined in each *Candida* carrier wearing a denture (Table 5). There were significant correlations between log CFU and number of remaining teeth in both groups of carriers ($\rho = -0.40$, p-value < 0.01 for *C. albicans*; $\rho = -0.38$, p-value < 0.01 for non-*albicans*), although we also found significant relationships between age and number of remaining teeth ($\rho = -0.34$, p-value < 0.01 for *C. albicans*; $\rho = -0.40$, p-value < 0.01 for non-*albicans*). To adjust for possible confounders, we applied logistic regression models using a cutoff value. In these models, the dependent variable was a high amount of each type of *Candida* (CFU ≥ 1.5) and the independent variables were number of remaining teeth and age in years. As Table 6 shows, after a stepwise procedure, the number of remaining teeth was selected as a significant factor of high amounts of both *C. albicans* and non-*albicans* (adjusted

Table 2 Significant factors related to colonization of *C. albicans* in surveyed parameters in this study ($N = 264$)

Parameter	*n*	COR (95% CI) *p*-value	AOR (95% CI) *p*-value	Number of positive (%)
Having one or more decayed teeth				
Yes	53	3.35 (1.70–6.63) <0.01	3.51 (1.60–7.67) <0.01	40 (75.5)
No[a]	211	1.00	1.00	101 (47.9)
Oral hygiene				
Poor	34	2.42 (1.18–4.99) <0.01	2.01 (0.77–5.24) 0.15	25 (73.5)
Fair/Good	230		1.00	116 (50.4)
Relocation from home				
Yes	104	1.45 (1.06–1.99) 0.02	2.17 (1.25–3.78) <0.01	65 (62.5)
No	160	1.00	1.00	76 (47.5)

Parameters include significant factors in either bivariate or multivariate analysis, *COR* crude odds ratio from bivariate analysis, *AOR* adjusted odds ratio from multinomial logistic regression analysis; *CI* confidence interval

[a]The reference categories are in the last row for all explanatory variables

Table 3 Significant factors related to colonization of Non-*albicans* in surveyed parameters in this study ($N = 264$)

	n	COR (95% CI) *p*-value	AOR (95% CI) *p*-value	Number of positive (%)
Age (in years)				
≥ 80	44	2.21 (1.36–5.34) <0.01	2.58 (1.12–5.71) 0.02	18 (40.9)
< 80[a]	220	1.00	1.00	45 (20.5)
Number of remaining teeth				
Edentulous	73	2.39 (1.83–3.12) <0.01	5.99 (1.37–26.3) 0.02	27 (37.0)
1-19	107	1.84 (1.51–2.42) <0.01	3.37 (0.88–12.9) 0.08	32 (29.9)
20 or more	84	1.00	1.00	4 (4.8)
Use of dentures				
Yes	180	1.56 (1.37–1.77) <0.01	4.02 (1.05–15.4) 0.04	59 (32.8)
No	84	1.00	1.00	4 (4.8)
Obesity (BMI ≥ 25)				
Yes	99	1.45 (1.06–2.00) 0.04	2.25 (1.15–4.40) 0.02	31 (31.3)
No	165	1.00	1.00	32 (19.4)

Parameters include significant factors in either bivariate or multivariate analysis, *COR* crude odds ratio from bivariate analysis, *AOR* adjusted odds ratio from multinomial logistic regression analysis; *CI* confidence interval
[a]The reference categories are in the last row for all explanatory variables

partial regression coefficient = 0.94; 95% CI = 0.88–0.99 and adjusted partial regression coefficient = 0.91; 95% CI = 0.83–0.98).

Discussion

In this study, the subjects were community dwellers in a post-disaster area. There have been several reports on prevalence of *Candida* species, mainly in institutionalized elderly, or in patients with HIV, carcinoma, or diabetes [9, 29–34]. However, information on the carriage rates of oral *Candida* in community dwellers is limited. Wang et al. [18] reported that 68.6% of community-dwelling elderly Japanese people aged 75 years were positive for total *Candida*. In addition, Goto et al. [35] reported prevalence rates of 63.6% for total *Candida*, and 53.4% for *C. albicans* in an elderly population aged 65–74. These rates are very close to those of our subjects (60.9% for total *Candida* and 53.4% for *C. albicans*); however, *Candida* prevalence varies widely in the oral cavities of healthy individuals according to several previous studies [5, 25, 36]. The factors associated with *Candida* colonization in the oral cavities of elderly people include age, use of dentures, poor oral/denture hygiene, and low saliva flow, in addition to systemic diseases [9–15]. The similar overall carriage rates of *Candida* found in these studies and ours in similarly aged Japanese elderly people may indicate that differences among oral or systemic conditions do not affect the colonization status of *Candida* even in post-disaster areas.

We found differences among the factors associated with oral colonization between *C. albicans* and non-*albicans* (Tables 2 and 3). The oral factors affecting colonization presented in previous studies, such as use of dentures or number of remaining teeth, were associated exclusively with non-*albicans* in our subjects. On the contrary, quantitative analysis revealed that none of the parameters were associated with the colony counts of non-*albicans,* although edentulous subjects harbored significantly greater amounts of *C. albicans*. In addition, denture users tended to have a greater amount of *C. albicans* although this was not statistically significant (Table 4). The dissimilarities between *Candida* species both in our qualitative and quantitative analyses suggested differences in the time of colonization by *C. albicans* and non-*albicans*. Elderly subjects might harbor stable non-progressive colonization by *C albicans*, while non- *albicans* colonization could be progressive. Therefore, despite the number of remaining teeth, or use of dentures being common factors in the prevalence of both *Candida* species, they might have largely affected colonization by non-*albicans* and growth of *C. albicans,* at least in our subjects. On the other hand, colonization by *C. albicans* related significantly to "having one or more decayed teeth". The relationship between *Candida* carriage and dental caries status has mainly been reported in children [37–39]. In these studies, *C. albicans* or total *Candida* carriage was generally associated with the prevalence of dental caries. However, race, age, country, and the oral status of the subjects in these previous studies were very different from our study, which makes it difficult for us to compare our results. In addition, the previous studies aimed to clarify the etiology of *Candida* in dental caries. Rather, we presumed that "having decayed teeth" was a consequence of poor living conditions after the disaster. Affected individuals were exempt from medical insurance premiums and

Table 4 Comparisons of colony amounts of *Candida* species by demographic characteristics, oral conditions, systemic conditions, lifestyle, medications, and relocation from home in carriers

	C. albicans			Non-*albicans*		
	No. of carriers	Mean log CFU (SD)	*p*-value[a]	No. of carriers	Mean log CFU (SD)	*p*-value
Sex						
Female	78	1.44 (0.65)	0.72	42	1.91 (0.92)	0.63
Male[a]	63	1.44 (0.66)		21	1.73 (0.74)	
Age (in years)						
≥ 80	29	1.59 (0.74)	0.24	18	1.87 (0.88)	0.84
< 80	112	1.40 (0.63)		45	1.85 (0.86)	
Having one or more decayed teeth						
Yes	40	1.45 (0.60)	0.77	13	1.56 (0.62)	0.31
No	101	1.43 (0.68)		50	1.93 (0.90)	
Number of remaining teeth						
Edentulous	33	1.88 (0.67)	<0.01[b]	27	2.17 (0.93)	0.09
1-19	60	1.35 (0.61)		32	1.62 (0.78)	
20 or more	48	1.25 (0.56)		4	1.55 (0.24)	
Having periodontal pockets						
Yes	41	1.32 (0.66)	0.16	14	1.69 (0.71)	0.55
No	100	1.49 (0.65)		49	1.90 (0.60)	
Oral hygiene						
Poor	25	1.39 (0.65)	0.70	8	1.69 (0.73)	0.75
Fair/Good	116	1.45 (0.66)		55	1.88 (0.88)	
Use of denture						
Yes	93	1.52 (0.68)	0.07	59	1.88 (0.88)	0.49
No	48	1.29 (0.58)		4	1.45 (0.40)	
Obesity (BMI ≥ 25)						
Yes	11	1.42 (0.72)	0.86	31	1.93 (0.89)	0.50
No	130	1.44 (0.65)		32	1.78 (0.84)	
Hypertension (systolic BP ≥ 140 or diastolic BP ≥90)						
Yes	38	1.61 (0.63)	0.04	24	1.84 (0.77)	0.96
No	103	1.37 (0.65)		39	1.86 (0.92)	
Dyslipidemia (HDLC ≤ 34 or LDLC ≥140)						
Yes	37	1.31 (0.57)	0.20	14	1.90 (0.92)	0.99
No	104	1.48 (0.68)		49	1.84 (0.85)	
Hyperglycemia (HbA1c ≥5.6)						
Yes	31	1.58 (0.67)	0.14	17	2.07 (0.71)	0.50
No	110	1.40 (0.65)		46	1.77 (0.90)	
Current smoker						
Yes	11	1.42 (0.72)	0.86	5	1.63 (0.88)	0.58
No	130	1.44 (0.65)		58	1.87 (0.86)	
Daily drinker						
Yes	19	1.72 (0.67)	0.40	7	1.81 (1.26)	0.54
No	122	1.39 (0.64)		56	1.86 (0.81)	

Table 4 Comparisons of colony amounts of *Candida* species by demographic characteristics, oral conditions, systemic conditions, lifestyle, medications, and relocation from home in carriers *(Continued)*

Taking antihypertensive drugs						
Yes	83	1.48 (0.65)	0.30	38	1.98 (0.83)	0.09
No	58	1.37 (0.66)		25	1.65 (0.88)	
Taking diabetes drugs						
Yes	8	1.45 (0.60)	0.80	5	2.11 (0.82)	0.41
No	133	1.43 (0.66)		58	1.83 (0.87)	
Taking hypnotics						
Yes	25	1.49 (0.76)	0.81	12	2.15 (0.79)	0.14
No	116	1.42 (0.63)		51	1.78 (0.87)	
Relocation from home						
Yes	65	1.40 (0.65)	0.50	25	1.82 (0.84)	0.72
No	76	1.47 (0.66)		38	1.88 (0.89)	

[a]Statistical differences were examined by Mann-Whitney *U* test for bivariate combinations, and Kruskal-Wallis test for comparison of 3 groups
[b]Post-hoc multiple comparisons using Bonferroni adjustment indicated that there was statistical significance between edentulous and others

payments at medical institution counters, including dental facilities, by the Japanese government and the local municipalities [40]. However, despite the existence of these services, subjects with decayed teeth did not appear to have received dental care for some reason, perhaps due to lack of transportation, social networks, and so on. *C. albicans* was also found more frequently in subjects living in a different house from their own home (many of them were in temporary housing). Moreover, significant trends in the prevalence of *Candida* species were also found in general health conditions such as obesity and colonization by non-*albicans*, and hypertension and colony counts of *C. albicans* in *C. albicans* carriers. The reasons are unclear, however, such symptoms tend to originate from an unhealthy lifestyle. Therefore, our findings suggested that living conditions and systemic disorders derived from lifestyle other than oral factors could affect the prevalence of *Candida* elderly people living in post-disaster areas.

Analyses of denture wearers harboring *C. albicans* or non-*albicans* revealed negative correlations between number of remaining teeth and the colony counts of both *C. albicans* and non-*albicans* after adjusting for the confounders number of remaining teeth and age (Table 5 and 6). Thus, positive correlations were found between the number of missing teeth and the quantities of *Candida*. Accordingly, dentures covering large areas of oral mucosa could be a risk factor for high amounts of both *C. albicans* and non-*albicans*. Although studies on the relationship between dentures and the amount of *Candida*, or denture size and frequency of *Candida* colonization have occasionally been reported [41, 42], our research might be the first study on denture size and the amount of *Candida*, especially in subjects without symptoms. However, it is unclear whether the colony counts of *Candida* is a risk factor for the incidence of candidiasis. Further investigation into the significance of amounts of the colonization of *Candida* is needed.

This study had several limitations. First, the number of subjects represented a small proportion of the entire community (population of 60 years or older was 5,210 on 1 October 2014, according to a government report). However, our subjects were probability samples recruited from all participants who took part in our dental health check-ups. We believe they represented all residents to a reliable degree because the total number of participants ($n = 1{,}008$, Fig. 1) were sufficient to represent the entire elderly population. Second, we did

Table 5 Relationships between colony amounts of *Candida* species, age, and number of remaining teeth in carriers wearing dentures

	C. albicans (*n*=93)			Non-*albicans* (*n*=59)		
	Log CFU	Number of remaining teeth	Age	Log CFU	Number of remaining teeth	Age
Log CFU		−0.40 (<0.01)	−0.18 (0.09)		−0.38 (<0.01)	0.10 (0.45)
Number of remaining teeth	−0.40 (<0.01)		−0.34 (<0.01)	−0.38 (<0.01)		−0.40 (<0.01)
Age	−0.18 (0.09)	−0.34 (<0.01)		0.10 (0.45)	−0.40 (<0.01)	

Value shows Spearman's correlation coefficient (*p*-value)

Table 6 Relationship between age, number of remaining teeth, and colony amounts of *Candida* by logistic regression models[a]

C. albicans (*n* = 93)					
	Variable	Crude partial regression coefficient	Adjusted partial regression coefficient	95% CI	*p*-value
First step	Number of remaining teeth	-0.06	0.94	0.53–0.94	0.053
	Age	0.01	1.02	0.95–1.08	0.65
Second (final) step	Number of remaining teeth	-0.07	0.94	0.88–0.99	0.03
Non- albicans (*n* = 59)					
	Variable	Partial regression coefficient	Adjusted partial regression coefficient	95% CI	*p*-value
First step	Number of remaining teeth	-0.11	0.90	0.82–0.98	0.02
	Age	-0.02	0.62	0.90–1.06	0.62
Second (final) step	Number of remaining teeth	-0.10	0.91	0.83–0.98	0.02

[a]Dependent variable: log CFU ≥ 1.5; 1, log CFU < 1.5; 0

not assess dryness of the mouth since this could not be conducted in our field survey. Based on the previous studies, this factor is frequently associated with *Candida* prevalence. Our models accounting for the prevalence of *Candida* would have been more accurate if this factor had been included. Third, being a cross-sectional study, it essentially lacked data from the affected region before the disaster, although we expect to provide supplemental data in a follow-up study. Finally, whether our findings are specific to post-disaster areas remains unclear given the lack of comparative data from non-disaster situation. This study was conducted as part of a large-scale cohort study aimed at supporting victims of the Great East Japan Earthquake. Since the research design did not include control areas at the beginning of the study in 2011 [22–24], it was not possible to establish control areas during the present survey because of time and budget constraints. However, compared to some previous studies for similarly aged elderly people living in ordinary conditions, our results partially identified relative post-disaster risks for the prevalence of *Candida* and can be generalized to some degree.

Conclusions

In our participants, the factors related to colonization or amounts differed between *C. albicans* and non-*albicans*. It is suggested that there is a difference in the time of colonization between *Candida* species. In addition, the amounts of both *Candida* types were related to greater numbers of missing teeth. Perhaps the amount of *Candida* on the tongue dorsa increased with increases in size of the area covered by the denture. Further, systemic and living conditions, other than oral status, could affect the prevalence of both *C. albicans* and non-*albicans* among elderly people living in a post-disaster area.

Additional file

Additional file 1: Relationships of demographic character, oral conditions, systemic conditions, lifestyle, medications and relocation from home with colonization of *C. albicans* and non-*albicans* (*N* = 264). Results of multinomial logistic regression analysis for colonization of *C. albicans* and non-*albicans*. Relationships of *C. albicans* and non-*albicans* colonization with all independent variables examined in this study are presented in this table. (DOCX 22 kb)

Abbreviations

AOR: Adjusted odds ratio; BMI: Body mass index; BP: Blood pressure; CFU: Colony forming unit/mL; CI: Confidential interval; COR: Crude odds ratio; CPI: Community Periodontal Index; HbA1c: Glycosylated hemoglobin; HDLC: High-density lipoprotein cholesterol; LDLC: Low-density lipoprotein cholesterol; SD: Standard deviation; WHO: World Health Organization

Acknowledgements

We sincerely thank all of the staff in the town of Otsuchi for their support. We also thank Dr. Yuki Yonekura for useful advice while writing the manuscript.

Funding

The current study was supported by Grant-in-Aid from the Ministry of Health, Labor and Welfare, Health and Labor Sciences Research Grants, Japan [H23-Tokubetsu-Shitei-002; H24-Kenki-Shitei-001, H25-Kenki-Shitei-001(Fukkou)], and JSPS KAKENHI Grant number 15 K11425. The funding body had no role in the study design, the collection, analysis, and interpretation of data, writing the manuscript, or in the decision to submit the manuscript for publication.

Authors' contributions

TS conceived this study, executed almost all parts of the survey, and drafted the manuscript. MK administered the study, and contributed to data analysis. MS contributed to data acquisition. HS administered data other than oral data. HM organized dental health survey team. KS, SK and AO planned and supervised this study. All authors read and approved the final manuscript.

Competing interests

The authors declare that they have no coompeting interest.

Consent for publication

Not applicable.

Ethics approval and consent to participate

We obtained informed consent from all participants who took part in our study. This study protocol was approved by the Medical Ethics Committee of Iwate Medical University School of Medicine (H23-69) and School of Dentistry (01214).

Author details

[1]Division of Preventive Dentistry, Department of Oral Medicine, School of Dentistry Iwate Medical University, 1-3-27 Chuo-dori, Morioka, Iwate 020-8505, Japan. [2]Department of Hygiene and Preventive Medicine, Iwate Medical University, School of Medicine, 2-1-1 Nishitokuta, Yahaba, Iwate 028-3694, Japan. [3]Division of Dental Education, Department of Oral Medicine, School of Dentistry Iwate Medical University, 1-3-27 Chuo-dori, Morioka, Iwate 020-8505, Japan. [4]Iwate Medical University, 19-1 Uchimaru, Morioka, Iwate 020-8505, Japan.

References

1. Johnson EM. Rare and emerging Candida species. Curr Fungal Infect Rep. 2009;3:152–9.
2. Lucas VS. Association of psychotropic drugs, prevalence of denture-related stomatitis and oral conditions. Community Dent Oral Epidemiol. 1993;21: 313–6.
3. Arendorg TM, Walker DM. The prevalence and intra-oral distribution of *Candida albicans* in man. Arch Oral Biol. 1980;254:1–10.
4. Pfaller MA, Diekema DJ. Epidemiology of invasive candidiesis : a persistent public health problem. Clin Microbiol Rev. 2007;20:133–63.
5. Scully C, El-Kabir M, Samaranayake LP. Candida and oral candidosis : A review. Crit Rev Oral Biol Med. 1994;5:125–57.
6. Abu-Elteen KH, Rm A-A. The prevalence of candida albicans populations in the mouths of complete denture wearers. New Microbiol. 1998;21:41–8.
7. Fanello S, Bouchara JP, Sauteron M, et al. Predictive value of oral colonization by Candida yeasts for the onset of a nosocomial infection in elderly hospitalized patients. J Med Microbiol. 2006;55:223–8.
8. Wisplinghoff H, Bischoff T, Tallent SM, Seifert H, Wenzel RP, Edmond MB. Nosocomial bloodstream infections in US hospitals: analysis of 24,179 cases from a prospective nationwide surveillance study. Clin Infect Dis. 2004;39: 309–17.
9. Grimoud AM, Marty N, Bocquet H, Andrieu S, Lodter JP, Chabanon G. Colonization of the oral cavity by candida species: risk factors in long-term geriatric care. J Oral Sci. 2003;45:51–5.
10. Dongari-Bagtzoglou A, Dwivedi P, Ioannidou E, Shaqman M, Hull D. Burleson J Oral *Candida* infection and colonization in solid organ transplant recipients. Oral Microbiol Immunol. 2009;24:249–54.
11. Budtz-Jörgensen E, Stenderup A, Grabowski M. An epidemiologic study of yeasts in elderly denture wearers. Community Dent Oral Epidemiol. 1975;3: 115–9.
12. Epstein JB, et al. Quantitative relationships between Candida albicans in saliva and the clinical status of human subjects. J Clin Microbiol. 1980;12: 475–6.
13. Navazesh M, et al. Relationship between salivary flow rates and *Candida albicans* counts. Oral Surg Oral Med Oral Pathol Oral Radiol Endod. 1995;80: 284–8.
14. Torres SR, et al. Relationship between salivary flow rates and Candida counts in subjects with xerostomia. Oral Surg Oral Med Oral Pathol Oral Radiol Endod. 2002;93:149–54.
15. Shimizu C, Kuriyama T, Williams DW, Karasawa T, Inoue K, Nakagawa K, Yamamoto E. Association of oral yeast carriage with specific host factors and altered mouth sensation. Oral Surg Oral Med Oral Pathol Oral Radiol Endod. 2008;105:445–51.
16. Aizen E, Feldman PA, Madeb R, Steinberg J, Merlin S, Sabo E, Perlov V, Srugo I. *Candida albicans* colonization of dental plaque in elderly dysphagic patients. Isr Med Assoc J. 2004;6:342–5.
17. Vargas KG, Joly S. Carriage frequency, intensity of carriage, and strains of oral yeast species vary in the progression to oral candidiasis in human immunodeficiency virus-positive individuals. J Clin Microbiol. 2002;40:341–50.
18. Wang J, Ohshima T, Yasunari U, Namikoshi S, Yoshihara A, Miyazaki H, Maeda N. The carriage of Candida species on the dorsal surface of the tongue: the correlation with the dental, periodontal and prosthetic status in elderly subjects. Gerodontology. 2006;23:157–63.
19. Yano A, Abe A, Aizawa F, Yamada H, Minami K, Matsui M, Kishi M. The effect of eating sea cucumber jelly on Candida load in the oral cavity of elderly individuals in a nursing home. Mar Drugs. 2013;11:4993–5007.
20. Annual Report on the Aging Society: 2016; Cabinet Office: Tokyo, Japan, 2016.
21. Annual Report of Reconstruction Agency, Japanese government. 2016. http://www.reconstruction.go.jp/english/. Accessed 30 Jan 2017.
22. Takahashi S, Nakamura M, Yonekura Y, Tanno K, Sakata K, Ogawa A, Kobayashi S. Association between relocation and changes in cardiometabolic risk factors: a longitudinal study in tsunami survivors of the 2011 Great East Japan Earthquake. BMJ Open. 2016;12:6.
23. Yokoyama Y, Otsuka K, Kawakami N, Kobayashi S, Ogawa A, Tannno K, Onoda T, Yaegashi Y, Sakata K. Mental health and related factors after the Great East Japan earthquake and tsunami. PLoS ONE. 2014;24:9.
24. Kishi M, Aizawa F, Matsui M, Yokoyama Y, Abe A, Minami K, Suzuki R, Miura H, Sakata K, Ogawa A. Oral health-related quality of life and related factors among residents in a disaster area of the Great East Japan Earthquake and giant tsunami. Health Qual Life Outcomes. 2015;13:143.
25. Pfaller MA, Diekema DJ, Gibbs DL, et al. Results from the ARTEMIS DISK Global Antifungal Surveillance Study, 1997 to 2007; a 10.5 year analysis of susceptibilities of Candida species to fluconazole and voriconazole as determined by CLSI standardized disk diffusion. J Clin Microbiol. 2010;48: 1366–77.
26. Odds FC, Bernarets R. CHROMagar Candida, a new differential isolation medium for presumptive identification of clinically important *Candida* species. J Clin Microbiol. 1994;32:1923–9.
27. World Health Organization. Oral health surveys: basic methods. 4th ed. Geneva: World Health Organization; 1997.
28. Specific Health Checkups and Specific Health Guidance. http://www.mhlw.go.jp/english/wp/wp-hw3/dl/2-007.pdf. Accessed 30 Jan 2017.
29. Samaranayake LP, Wilkieson CA, Lamey PJ, MacFarlane TW. Oral disease in the elderly in long-term hospital care. Oral Dis. 1995;1:147–51.
30. Tortorano AM, Peman J, Bernhardt H, Klingspor L, Kibbler CC, Faure O, Biraghi E, Canton E, Zimmermann K, Seaton S, Grillot R. ECMM Working Group on Candidaemia. Epidemiology of candidaemia in Europe: results of 28-month European Confederation of Medical Mycology (ECMM) hospital-based surveillance study. Eur J Clin Microbiol Infect Dis. 2004;23:317–22.
31. Sanitá PV, Pavarina AC, Giampaolo ET, Silva MM, Mima EG, Ribeiro DG, Vergani CE. *Candida* spp. prevalence in well controlled type 2 diabetic patients with denture stomatitis. Oral Surg Oral Med Oral Pathol Oral Radiol Endod. 2011;111:726–33.
32. Sangeorzan JA, Bradley SF, He X, Zarins LT, Ridenour GL, Tiballi RN, Kauffman CA. Epidemiology of oral candidiasis in HIV-infected patients: colonization, infection, treatment, and emergence of fluconazole resistance. Am J Med. 1994;97:339–46.
33. Wadhwa A, Kaur R, Agarwal SK, Jain S, Bhalla P. AIDS-related opportunistic mycoses seen in a tertiary care hospital in North India. J Med Microbiol. 2007;56:1101–6.
34. Belazi M, Velegraki A, Koussidou-Eremondi T, Andreadis D, Hini S, Arsenis G, Eliopoulou C, Destouni E, Antoniades D. Oral *Candida* isolates in patients undergoing radiotherapy for head and neck cancer: prevalence, azole susceptibility profiles and response to antifungal treatment. Oral Microbiol Immunol. 2004;19:347–51.
35. Goto J, Yamazaki Y, Sato J, Hata H,Oouchi M, Moriya S, Kitagawa Y. Research on carriage of *Candida* species in oral cavities of the home-independent elderly. Hokkaido J Dent Sci. 2012;32:210–21 (*in Japanese*).
36. Oliver DE, Shillitoe EJ. Effects of smoking on the prevalence and intraoral distribution of *Candida albicans*. J Oral Pathol. 1984;13:265–70.
37. Srivastava B, Bhatia HP, Chaudhary V, Aggarwal A, Kumar Singh A, Gupta N. Comparative Evaluation of Oral *Candida albicans* Carriage in Children with and without Dental Caries: A Microbiological in vivo Study. Int J Clin Pediatr Dent. 2012;5:108–12.
38. Al-Hebshi NN, Al-Maswary EA, Al-Hammadi ZO, Ghoname N. Salivary *Candida* species carriage patterns and their relation to caries experience among yemeni children. Oral Health Prev Dent. 2015;13:41–9.
39. De-la-Torre J, Marichalar-Mendia X, Varona-Barquin A, Marcos-Arias C, Eraso E, Aguirre-Urizar JM, Quindós G. Caries and *Candida* colonisation in adult patients in Basque Country (Spain). Mycoses. 2016. doi:10.1111/myc.12453 [Epub ahead of print].

40. Response to the Great East Japan Earthquake By the Ministry of Health, Labour and Welfare, the Government of Japan. 23 October 2012 Ministry of Health, Labour, and Welfare (MHLW) Government of Japan. http://www.mhlw.go.jp/bunya/kokusaigyomu/asean/2012/dl/Introduction_Dr.Yamauchi.pdf. Accessed 30 Jan 2017.
41. Kato T, Yamazaki Y, Sato J, Hata H, Oouchi M, Moriya S, Kitagawa Y. Reinvestigation of the carriage of *Candida* species in oral cavities of home-independent elderly. Hokkaido J Dent Sci. 2013;33:121–39 (*in Japanese*).
42. Lockhart SR, Joly S, Vargas K, Swails-Wenger J, Enger L, Soll DR. Natural defenses against Candida colonization breakdown in the oral cavities of the elderly. J Dent Res. 1999;78:857–68.

Effects of various debonding and adhesive clearance methods on enamel surface: an in vitro study

Xiao-Chuan Fan[1], Li Chen[2] and Xiao-Feng Huang[1*]

Abstract

Background: The purpose of this study was to evaluate orthodontic debonding methods by comparing the surface roughness and enamel morphology of teeth after applying two different debonding methods and three different polishing techniques.

Methods: Forty eight human maxillary premolars, extracted for orthodontic reasons, were randomly divided into three groups. Brackets were bonded to teeth with RMGIC (Fuji Ortho LC, GC, Tokyo, Japan) (two groups, $n = 18$ each) after acid etching (30s), light cured for 40 s, exposed to thermocycling, then underwent 2 different bracket debonding methods: debonding pliers (Shinye, Hangzhou, China) or enamel chisel (Jinzhong, Shanghai, China); the third group ($n = 12$) comprised of untreated controls, with normal enamel surface roughness. In each debonded group, three cleanup techniques ($n = 6$ each) were tested, including (I) diamond bur (TC11EF, MANI, Tochigi, Japan) and One-Gloss (Midi, Shofu, Kyoto, Japan), (II) a Super-Snap disk (Shofu, Kyoto, Japan), and (III) One-Gloss polisher. The debonding methods were compared using the modified adhesive remnant index (ARI, 1–5). Cleanup efficiencies were assessed by recording operating times. Enamel surfaces were qualitatively and quantitatively evaluated with scanning electron microscopy (SEM) and surface roughness tester, respectively. Two surface roughness variables were evaluated: Ra (average roughness) and Rz (10-point height of irregularities).

Results: The ARI scores of debonded teeth were similar with debonding pliers and enamel chisel (Chi-square = 2.19, $P > 0.05$). There were significant differences between mean operating time in each group ($F = 52.615$, $P < 0.01$). The diamond bur + One-Gloss took the shortest operating time (37.92 ± 3.82 s), followed by the Super-Snap disk (56.67 ± 7.52 s), and the One-Gloss polisher (63.50 ± 6.99 s). SEM appearance provided by the One-Gloss polisher was the closest to the intact enamel surface, and surface roughness (Ra: 0.082 ± 0.046 μm; Rz: 0.499 ± 0.200 μm) was closest to the original enamel (Ra: 0.073 ± 0.048 μm; Rz: 0.438 ± 0.213 μm); the next best was the Super-Snap disk (Ra: 0.141 ± 0.073 μm; Rz: 1.156 ± 0.755 μm); then, the diamond bur + One-Gloss (Ra: 0.443 ± 0.172 μm; Rz: 2.202 ± 0.791 μm).

Conclusions: Debonding pliers were safer than enamel chisels for removing brackets. Cleanup with One-Gloss polisher provided enamel surfaces closest to the intact enamel, but took more time, and Super-Snap disks provided acceptable enamel surfaces and efficiencies. The diamond bur was not suitable for removing adhesive remnant.

Keywords: Orthodontic debonding, Adhesive clearance, Enamel damage, Resin modified glass ionomer cement (RMGIC), Surface roughness, Scanning electron microscope (SEM)

* Correspondence: hxf1998@hotmail.com; huangxf1998@163.com
[1]Department of Stomatology, Beijing Friendship Hospital, Capital Medical University, No.95 Yong'an Road, Xicheng District, Beijing 100050, China
Full list of author information is available at the end of the article

Background

The acid etch technique and direct bonding technique, first described by Buonocore [1] in 1955 and Newman [2] in 1965, were major improvements in daily orthodontic practice. Once orthodontic therapies with fixed appliances are completed, the bonded brackets and residual adhesive must be removed. Ideally, the debonding procedure would lead to restitution of the tooth enamel, or at least, the enamel surface could be restored, as closely as possible, to its original state [3, 4]. However, when the bracket debonding process is inadequate, the enamel is injured, which results cracks and fractures in the enamel surface. This condition leads tooth sensitivity, and it increases the risk of caries and pulp inflammation [5, 6]. Therefore, it is important to evaluate an appropriate debonding process for removing brackets used in orthodontic practice. Restoration of the enamel after orthodontic treatment includes two major steps: debonding and enamel surface polishing.

Previous studies reported different methods for removing brackets, such as mechanical methods; chemical solvents; ultrasonic scalars; and lasers [7–12]. Among these methods, the mechanical removal methods are most widely used in clinical practice. Successful debonding process relies on maintaining an intact enamel structure without producing iatrogenic damage. Bishara suggested that excessive debonding strength (>11.3 MPa) may cause enamel cracks, and that cracks are less likely to appear with lower forces (7.3 MPa) [13]. Moreover, Su and colleagues established three standardized bracket removal techniques, which are commonly applied in the clinic [8]. Those results suggested that lifting forces are more acceptable for clinical use than shearing forces. Brosh and colleagues compared in vivo the bracket debonding forces of two different debonding techniques [7]. In one technique, the blades of pliers were placed between the wings and base of the bracket (wings model); in the other technique, the pliers' blades were placed between the base of the bracket and the enamel surface (base model). The results indicated that lower loads were required with the wings model and tensile forces developed at the interface with this technique. Zarrinnia et al. also demonstrated that bracket-removing pliers can apply a pulling force on the bracket wing, which avoids unnecessary torque on the tooth, when the beak rested on the labial enamel surface [14]. However, those studies lacked an evaluation of the micro-structure of the enamel surface after removing the adhesive.

In previous studies, numerous finishing and polishing procedures were tested, including a diamond bur, a tungsten carbide bur, polishing cups with pumice, and ultrasonic scalars [14–18]. Most recently, new enamel cleanup methods, such as sand blasting, polishing disks, silicone dioxide particle polishers, and a Nd: YAG laser, have been introduced into the orthodontics clinic [4, 14, 18–23]. The diamond finishing bur or tungsten carbide bur was a highly efficient (least time-consuming) surface cleaning method. However, burs can produce grooves and superimposed abrasion marks on the enamel [4, 14, 24, 25]. Therefore, these kinds of instruments require following secondary polishing treatment [26, 27]. One-Gloss polishers, could provide good tooth polishing after bracket debonding [21, 22]. However, Ye et al. reported that more color change occurred when One-Gloss polishers were used for polishing after carbide bur debonding [28]. Bonetti et al. [20] and Zarrinia et al. [14] suggested that removing resin with a 12-bladed tungsten carbide bur, followed by polishing with Sof-Lex disks, could produce the smoothest enamel surface. With scanning electron microscope (SEM) images, the smoothest surface was obtained when Sof-Lex disks were used alone [4]. Tufekci reported that the enamel loss was not significantly different between the Sof-Lex disk and tungsten carbide bur methods [29].

To our knowledge, most previous studies only focused on one stage of removing fixed appliances after orthodontic treatment (debonding or enamel surface polishing), and mostly performed subjective evaluations of SEM images without a quantitative evaluation that is necessary for accurate comparisons. Few studies described the removal of resin modified glass ionomer cement (RMGIC), although is commonly used in clinic. Due to the bonding properties of RMGIC, two curing systems may be applied. One is the polymerization of composite resin, which is similar to the method used for resin adhesives. The second is an acid–base reaction [30, 31], which is different from that used for resin adhesives.

Therefore, our objective is to compare the surface roughness and enamel morphology of teeth after applying two different debonding methods and three different polishing techniques, and to identify the most appropriate, efficient method of debonding after orthodontic treatments with fixed appliances.

Methods

Specimen preparation

A total of 48 human maxillary premolars were extracted from 12- to 18-year-old patients for orthodontic reasons. The study has been approved by the ethics committee of Beijing Stomatological Hospital. Guardians of all patients provided written authorizations for use of the extracted teeth in this study. To determine eligibility for the study, teeth were examined under 10× magnification with a stereomicroscope (SMZ-1500, NIKON, Tokyo, Japan). This study included only teeth that had intact buccal enamel, no surface cracks from extraction forces, no caries, and no exposure to chemical agents (e.g., H_2O_2). All selected teeth were cleaned with flowing water and tissue debris were removed with scalpel. Then, teeth were stored in a 0.5% (weight/volume) chloramine-T solution at room temperature to inhibit bacterial growth for 24 h. After that, all specimens were stored in distilled water at 4 °C, which was refreshed weekly, for a maximum of 6 months after extraction.

Bonding and thermocycling

The buccal surfaces of each crown were cleaned with fluoride-free pumice, then sprayed with water, and dried for 10s. Out of 48 specimens, 12 served as untreated controls, and 36 were treated with an etching procedure with 35% phosphoric acid gel (Gluma, Heraeukulzer, Hanau, Germany) for 30s. After etching, teeth were rinsed with water for 30s and dried with an oil-free stream until the etched surfaces appeared chalky white. Before bonding, the enamel surfaces of etched teeth were moistened with distilled water. RMGIC bonding materials (Fuji Ortho LC, GC, Tokyo, Japan) were handled according to the manufacturers' instructions. Stainless steel maxillary premolar brackets (0.024-in. twin, TOMY, Tokyo, Japan) were placed at the Facial Axis point (FA) on the midbuccal surface of the tooth along the Facial Axis of the clinical crown (FACC). The RMGIC adhesive were light-cured for a total of 40 s, which included 10s each at the mesial, distal, gingival, and occlusal margins. The light source came from a curing light CL-628 (Beyond, Houston, USA). The original bulb was used with wavelength of 400–480 nm and a minimum output light intensity of 900 mW/cm^2. All bonding procedures were carried out by a single operator, with a standard technique.

After storing the specimens in water at 37 ± 2 °C for 24 h, thermocycling was performed for 500 cycles from 5 to 55 °C, with a dwell time of 20s; the transfer time between the two baths was 5–10s. This procedure followed the recommendations of the International Organization for Standardization [32].

Debonding process and evaluation of ARI

The specimens bonded with brackets ($n = 36$) were randomly divided into two groups of 18 specimens. One group was debonded with orthodontic debonding pliers (Shinye, Hangzhou, China). The blades of the pliers were placed between the wings and the base of the bracket, according to the 'wings model' introduced by Brosh [7]. The other group was debonded with an enamel chisel (Jinzhong, Shanghai, China). The blade of the chisel was also placed between the wings and the base of the bracket. During the debonding process, an impact force transferred to the bracket through the chisel, and the instantaneous shear force causes the bracket to fall off.

After debonding, the enamel surfaces were examined at 10× magnification with a stereomicroscope. A modified adhesive remnant index (ARI), described by Bishara, was used to quantify the amount of adhesive on the tooth surface [33]. The ARI scale was: 1 = no adhesive remaining; 2 = less than 10% of adhesive remaining; 3 = 10 to 90% of adhesive remaining; 4 = over 90% of adhesive remaining; and 5 = all adhesive remaining on the tooth.

Cleanup process

Each debonding test group was further randomly divided into three subgroups, each with 6 specimens, which received one of three cleanup methods: The first cleanup process implemented a high-speed diamond finishing bur (TC-11EF, MANI, Tochigi, Japan) cooled with water, for removing gross remnants of adhesive (only a few adhesive left on enamel surface); then, a One-Gloss polisher (Midi, Shofu, Kyoto, Japan) was used for further removal of the remaining adhesive and to polish the enamel until no visible residue left (the diamond bur + One-Gloss method). The second cleanup process implemented Super-Snap disks (Shofu, Kyoto, Japan) with three grades: the medium grade (purple disk), which was used for removing gross remnants of adhesive, and the fine (green disk) and superfine (red disk) grades, which were used to remove the remaining adhesive and to polish the enamel until no visible residue left (Super-Snap method). The third cleanup process implemented the One-Gloss polisher for removing adhesive and polishing the enamel till no visible residue left alone (One-Gloss method). The operating times required for the cleanup processes were recorded.

Surface roughness measurements

The enamel surfaces of the three cleanup process groups and one control group ($n = 12$ in each group) were evaluated with a surface roughness taster (JB-4C, Temin Optical Instrument Corp., Shanghai, China). The roughness taster sensor was placed on the enamel surface to measure the surface roughness. Five recordings were performed over a distance of 0.25 mm that the probe travels across the enamel surface (surface distance) for each specimen. The mean values of two surface roughness variables were evaluated. The first variable was the average roughness (Ra), defined as the arithmetic mean of the absolute surface roughness, measured from the centre line, over the surface distance, after removing the shape error and any large waviness content. The Ra reflected the overall roughness of the enamel surface. The second variable was the 10-point height of irregularities (Rz), defined as the average distance between the 5 highest peaks and the 5 deepest valleys, measured from a line parallel to the mean line, over the surface distance. The Rz is a useful value, when only a short surface distance is available for assessment, such as the surface distance evaluated in this study [34].

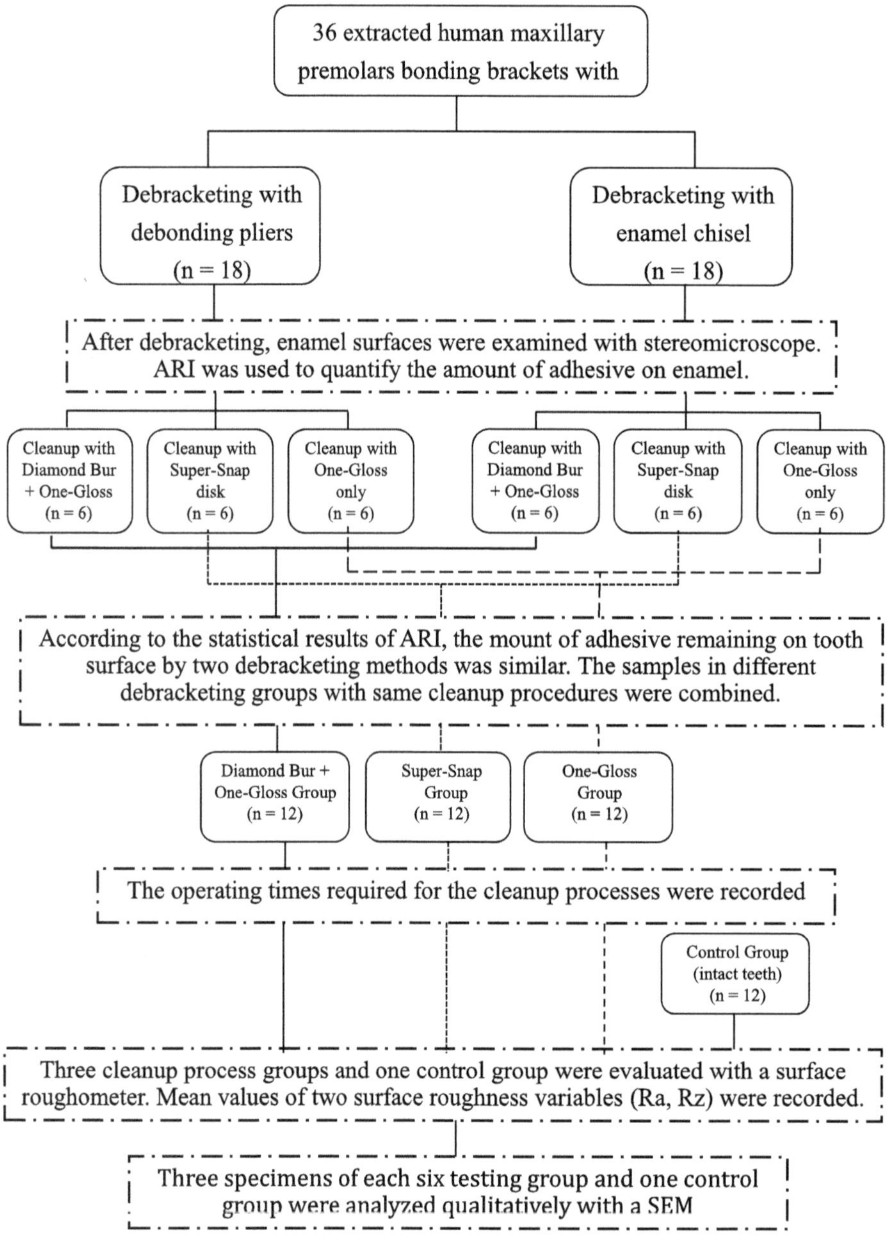

Fig. 1 The consort type diagram of the study process and variables measured

Scanning electron microscopy observations

Three specimens of each group were vacuum-dried in a vacuum dryer (JFD-310, JEOL, Tokyo, Japan) for 48 h at room temperature. Then, each specimen was coated with approximately 460 Å of a gold palladium mixture. The specimens were analyzed qualitatively with a SEM (S-4800, HITACHI, Tokyo, Japan), operated at 2.0KV, to evaluate the damaged area on the enamel surface.

Statistical analysis

Statistical analysis was performed with the IBM SPSS Statistics software (Version 20.0, IBM, New York, USA).

Table 1 Distribution of ARI scores for different debonding methods

Group	Sample Size	ARI					Chi-square value	*P*-value
		1	2	3	4	5		
Enamel chisel	18	0	0	4	3	11	2.190	0.534
Debonding pliers	18	0	2	3	3	10		

ARI score: 1 = no adhesive remaining; 2 = less than 10% of adhesive remaining; 3 = 10 to 90% of adhesive remaining; 4 = over 90% of adhesive remaining; and 5 = all adhesive remaining on the tooth

Table 2 Operating times for cleanup (s)

Group	Sample Size	Mean (SD)	*F*-value	*P*-value
Diamond bur + One-Gloss	12	37.92 (3.82)	52.615	<0.001
Super-Snap	12	56.67 (7.52)		
One-Gloss	12	63.50 (6.99)		

The modified ARIs of the two debonding groups were evaluated with the chi-square test to determine statistical differences. The one-way analysis of variance (ANOVA) and the Bonferroni multiple comparisons test were used to analyze statistical differences in operating times among the three cleanup groups and in surface roughness parameters (Ra, Rz) among the three cleanup groups and the control group. The significance threshold for all statistical tests was predetermined at $P < 0.05$.

The consort type diagram of the study process and variables measured was shown in Fig. 1.

Results

Adhesive remnant index

The modified ARIs remnant of the two groups treated with different debonding processes are presented in Table 1. The chi-square test showed no statistical difference between the ARIs of the two groups ($P > 0.05$).

Operating time

Table 2 shows the time required for the cleanup process with each of the three methods tested. A one-way ANOVA of the time required for cleanup showed an F value of 52.615, indicating a significant difference ($P < 0.01$) between groups. A Bonferroni multiple comparisons test (Table 3) showed that the time for cleanup with the diamond bur + One-Gloss method was significantly ($P < 0.01$) shorter than that of the other two methods. Similarly, the cleanup time with the Super-Snap method was significantly ($P < 0.05$) shorter than that with the One-Gloss method.

Surface roughness measurement

The data of Ra and Rz for each cleanup process are presented in Table 4. A one-way ANOVA of the surface roughness, measured after the different cleanup processes, showed F values of 37.245 for the Ra and 25.158 for the Rz, indicating a significant difference among methods ($P < 0.01$). A Bonferroni multiple comparisons test (Table 5) showed that the Ra and Rz values for the diamond bur + One-Gloss method were significantly higher ($P < 0.01$) than those found with the other methods. Similarly, the Rz value for the Super-Snap method was significantly higher ($P < 0.05$) than that found for untreated controls and for teeth treated with the One-Gloss method. There were no significant differences in surface roughness among the other methods tested.

Scanning electron microscopy observations

Figure 2 shows SEM images of the original, intact enamel. The enamel had cross-striations (Fig. 2a) and craters (Fig. 2b). Figures 3 and 4 show the enamel condition after debonding with an enamel chisel and debonding pliers, respectively, then applying the three different cleanup methods. After cleanup with the diamond bur + One-Gloss (Figs. 3a and 4a), the enamel surfaces showed the worst scratches, with thick, deep grooves and scars. After cleanup with the Super-Snap method (Figs. 3b and 4b), the enamel surfaces were smoother, with shallow scratches, and deep scars were rare. After cleanup with the One-Gloss method (Figs. 3c and 4c) the enamel surface was smoothest, with only a few, shallow scratches.

Discussion

Debonding process

The principle of mechanical removal method is to make a stress fracture at the enamel-adhesive-bracket interface. In the present study, we chose debonding pliers and enamel chisel for removing brackets by using pulling and shear forces respectively, and explored the effects of these two types of forces on the enamel surfaces. The modified ARI with five gradesis an internationally recognized scale for evaluating resin fracture by Bishara [33]. The higher scores indicate fractures that are closer to the adhesive-bracket interface. The ARI scores were broadly similar for the two debonding methods tested; both methods showed high frequencies of scores in the 3 to 5 range, which suggested that debonding with either the debonding pliers or the enamel chisel caused the bond to fail at the bracket-adhesive interface or within the adhesive. This location can be advantageous for the clinician. When the bond is broken at the adhesive-enamel interface, the enamel may fracture during debonding [35].

Table 3 Bonferroni test results for comparing operating times

Group	Group Compared	Mean difference	*P*-value	95% Confidence Interval
Diamond bur + One-Gloss	Super-Snap	−18.750	<0.001	−25.264/−12.236
	One-Gloss	−25.583	<0.001	−32.097/−19.070
Super-Snap	One-Gloss	−6.833	0.037	−13.347/−0.320

Table 4 Surface roughness for each cleanup process (μm)

Group	Sample Size	Mean (SD)		*F*-value (Ra/Rz)	*P*-value (Ra/Rz)
		Ra	Rz		
Control	12	0.073 (0.048)	0.438 (0.213)	37.245/25.158	<0.001/<0.001
Diamond bur + One-Gloss	12	0.443 (0.172)	2.202 (0.791)		
Super-Snap	12	0.141 (0.073)	1.156 (0.755)		
One-Gloss	12	0.082 (0.046)	0.499 (0.200)		

Ra average roughness, *Rz* 10-point height of irregularities

ARI can be used to reflect the fracture position but not to record any damage on the enamel surface. In order to test damage to the enamels, more studies are needed [36, 37]. Based on SEM observations at 50× magnification, 5 out of 9 teeth in the enamel chisel group exhibited cracks on the enamel surface after removing the remnant adhesive (Fig. 5). Moreover, 1 out of 5 cracked teeth also exhibited enamel fracture (Fig. 6). These types of enamel damage were not observed in any of the teeth in the debonding pliers group. Bishara suggested that excessive debonding force (>11.3 MPa) may cause enamel cracks [13]. In this study, for the debonding pliers group, we place the blades of the pliers the area between the wings and the base of the bracket (wings model), but not between the base of the brackets and the enamel surface (base model). According to the investigation by Brosh and colleagues [7], the moment that develops by drawing the point of application away from the bracket-adhesive-enamel interface decreases the force required to detach the bracket. Consequently, lower stress is applied in the wings model, and no cracks on the enamel surface were observed in pliers group. While, the enamel chisel mainly requires impact forces to detach the brackets, and large, instantaneous impact forces may case enamel damage.

Cleanup process

A roughened enamel surface may facilitate bacterial plaque retention, which produces superficial staining and gingival inflammation. Moreover, the acidic byproduct initiated by a bacterial plaque results in a lower pH, which leads to the chemical dissolution of mineralized hard tissue, and promotes dental caries [38]. Therefore, a smooth tooth surface is important, both for aesthetic reasons, and for resisting demineralization. The purpose of the secondary cleanup process is to restore the natural smooth enamel surface after removing directly bonded brackets in orthodontic treatments.

The diamond-finishing bur and tungsten carbide bur were previously reported to be used for removing adhesive. But burs should not be used alone in orthodontic debonding processes. Abrasion marks by burs increase the roughness on the enamel surface. Therefore, a secondary polishing instrument should be used later [26, 27]. Tungsten carbide bur is a more common instrument for debonding. Based on the review of previous literature, it might produce parallel grooves during the debonding of orthodontic attachments [4, 24, 25]. This clinic characteristic of the diamond bur was similar to tungsten carbide bur [14, 24, 26], and the diamond bur has higher efficiency. In this study, we selected diamond bur as a representative to study the effects of high-speed rotating instrument to enamel surface. Consistent with other studies [4, 25], we found that the least time was spent with the diamond bur + One-Gloss method. However, the enamel appearance was the worst in the diamond bur + One-Gloss method by evaluation of the SEM and surface roughness, compared to the other polishing processes. Indiamond bur + One-Gloss group, the deep grooves and scars caused by diamond-finishing bur could not be reduced or cleared with the One-Gloss polisher. Ye reported that the colour change produced when RMGIC was polished with a carbide bur + One-Gloss was less pronounced than that produced with a

Table 5 Bonferroni test results for comparing Ra & Rz values

Group	Group Compared	Ra			Rz		
		Mean difference	*P*-value	95% Confidence Interval	Mean difference	*P*-value	95% Confidence Interval
Control	Diamond bur + One-Gloss	−0.370	<0.001	−0.482/−0.258	−1.765	<0.001	−2.403/−1.126
	Super-Snap	−0.068	0.609	−0.180/0.044	−0.719	0.020	−1.357/−0.080
	One-Gloss	−0.009	1.000	−0.121/0.103	−0.062	1.000	−0.700/0.577
Diamond bur + One-Gloss	Super-Snap	0.302	<0.001	0.190/0.414	1.046	<0.001	0.408/1.684
	One-Gloss	0.361	<0.001	0.249/0.473	1.703	<0.001	1.064/2.341
Super-Snap	One-Gloss	0.059	0.914	−0.053/0.171	0.657	0.041	0.018/1.295

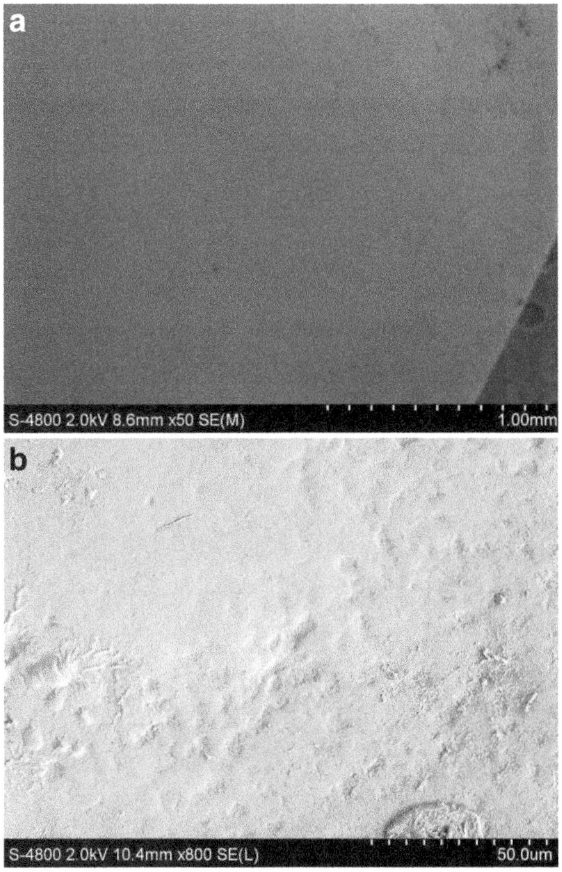

Fig. 2 Representative scanning electron microscope (SEM) images of intact enamel surfaces. **a** SEM 50×; **b** SEM 800×

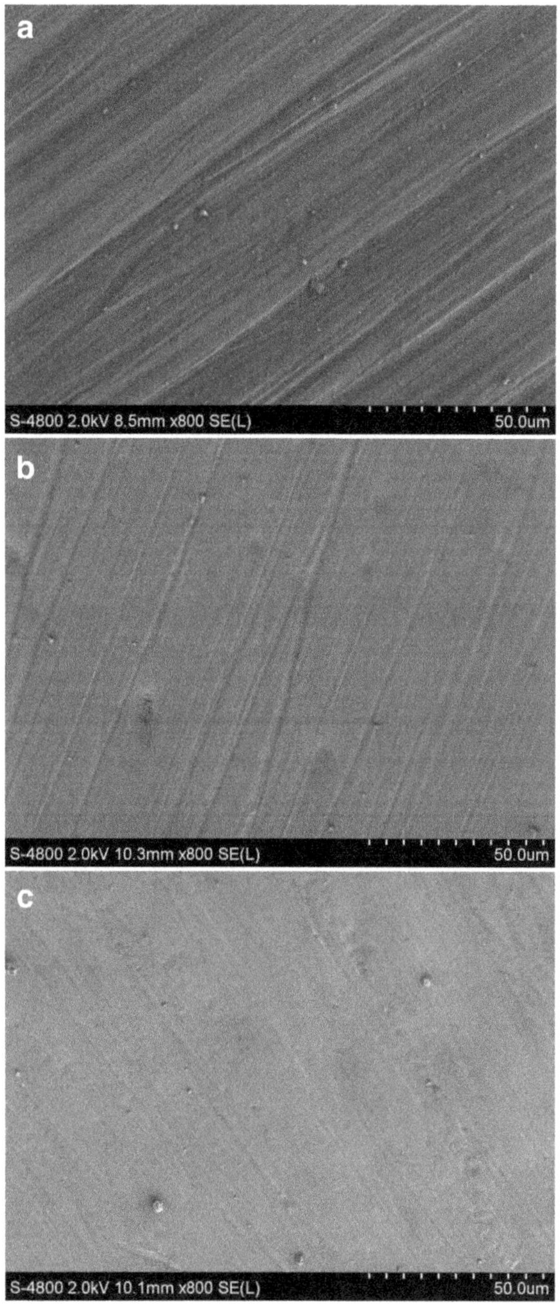

Fig. 3 Representative scanning electron microscope (SEM) images of enamel surfaces after debonding with an enamel chisel. SEM magnification: 800×. **a** Diamond bur + One-Gloss; **b** Super-Snap; **c** One-Gloss method

carbide bur alone, but significantly more pronounced than that produced with a carbide bur + Sof-Lex or with the PoGo polisher under the same conditions [28]. Those findings suggested that One-Gloss polishers only provided limited improvement over a finishing bur, and that the various combinations of finishing bur and silicone particle polishers were inadequate for removing adhesive. The finding was also consistent with observation from Odaira [22].

In the One-Gloss polisher group, it produced the smoothest surface, with very few shallow scratches. Enamel surfaces after polishing were closest to the original enamel surface by SEM. But it also required the longest operating time, and thus, it exhibited the least efficiency in three cleanup processes tested. Previous studies reported that Sof-Lex, an aluminium-oxide-coated abrasive disk, which is similar to Super-Snap, produced surfaces with the closest appearance to the original enamel surface [4, 39]. In the present investigation, the micromorphological images of surfaces by Super-Snap exhibited some deep scars, apart from the shallow scratches, but the result was far superior to that produced with the diamond bur + One-Gloss. The process by Super-Snap only required moderate operating times. The operating times observed in our study were much longer than those reported in other previous investigations [4, 25]. This difference might result from the fact that we only applied light pressure when polishing.

We used SEM images to gain a better understanding of how the enamel surfaces changed with different

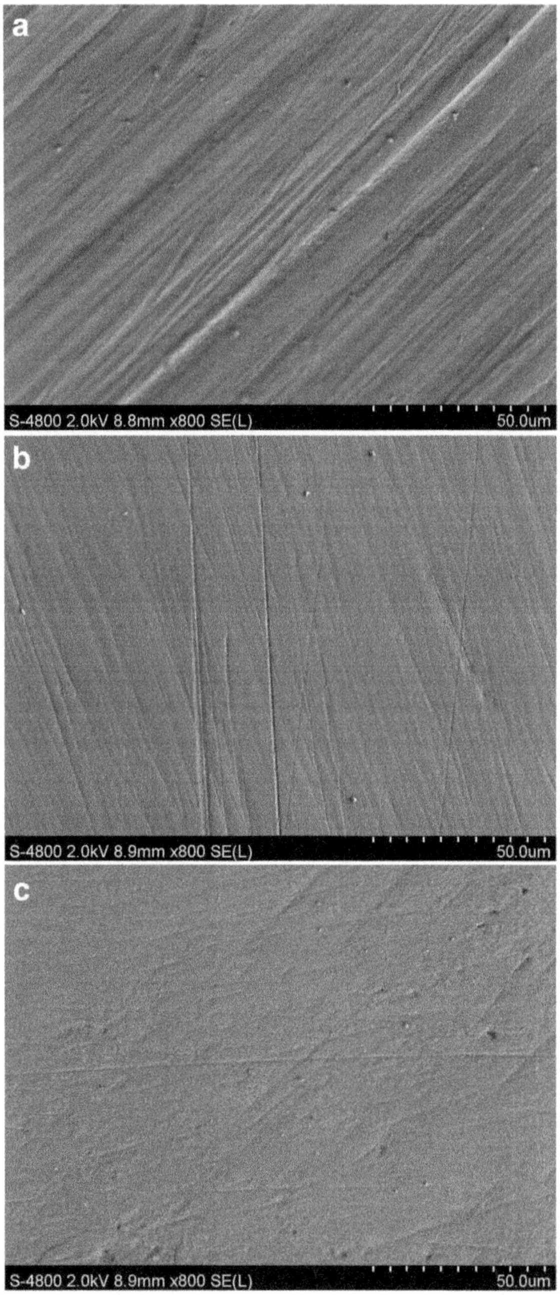

Fig. 4 Representative scanning electron microscope (SEM) images of enamel surfaces after debonding with debonding pliers. SEM magnification: 800×. **a** Diamond bur + One-Gloss, **b** Super-Snap, **c** One-Gloss method

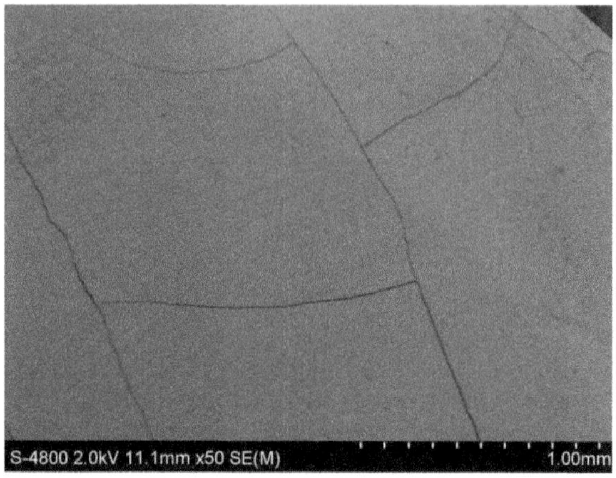

Fig. 5 Representative scanning electron microscope (SEM) image of cracks on the enamel surface after debonding with an enamel chisel. SEM magnification: 50×

adhesive removal methods. However, SEM requires subjective inspection, and cannot be used for comparative assessments alone [40]. Alternatively, quantitative techniques, such as surface roughness tester, can provide more reliable comparisons of different cleanup processes. The Ra value reflects the overall roughness of the enamel surface, as shown in previous studies [4, 19, 39]. However, the Ra value does not fully describe surface roughness [41, 42], because it cannot indicate the depth of irregularities or differentiate between shallow and deep grooves [4]. Therefore, we introduced an additional variable, Rz, to evaluate the degree of scratching caused by polishing. Rz was defined as the average distance from the mean line to the five highest peaks and the five deepest valleys. The Rz value is more stable than the distance between the highest and lowest points (Rt or Rmax).

According to the statistical results of ARI, both debonding methods showed high frequencies of ARI scores in the 3 to 5 range and the chi-square test showed no difference between two groups. These results suggested that the amount of adhesive remaining on tooth surface by two debonding methods was similar before cleanup process. So we combined the samples in different debonding groups with same cleanup procedures for statistical

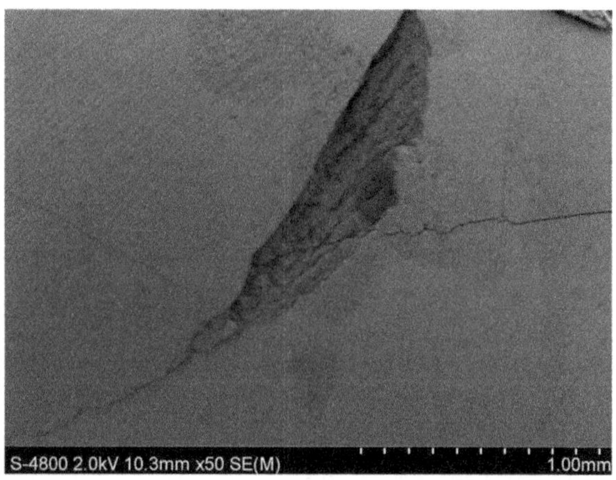

Fig. 6 Scanning electron microscope (SEM) image of a fracture on the enamel surface after debonding with an enamel chisel. SEM magnification: 50×

analysis of surface roughness measurement. The results showed that the diamond bur + One-Gloss produced the roughest surfaces. The Ra and Rz values were 0.443 ± 0.172 μm and 2.202 ± 0.791 μm, respectively. These values were significantly higher than those in the other two polishing methods. The SEM observations showed similar results. Previous studies reported Ra values of 0.125–0.260 μm for nanofilled composites polished with Al_2O_3 abrasive grain discs [43, 44]. In the present study, the Ra value after polishing with Super-Snap was 0.141 ± 0.073 μm, which was close to the value achieved with the Al_2O_3 discs, but lower than that reported in other studies that tested on enamel surfaces [4]. The One-Gloss polisher exhibited the least roughness, which showed no significant difference from the intact enamel surface, both in Ra and Rz values. The Super-Snap method also produced an Ra value similar to that of the intact enamel surface, but the Rz value was significantly higher than those observed with the One-Gloss method and the control. This implied that cleanup with Super-Snap produced an acceptable enamel surface, but it left a number of deep scratches. These findings were confirmed in the SEM images. The results of our study were based on the removal of RMGIC. Due to the different bonding properties of RMGIC and resin adhesive [30, 31], our data may not accurately reflect the actual situation of the removal of the resin adhesive from enamel. The comparison study of debonding different materials such as RMGIC and resin might be done in the future.

Conclusions

On the basis of our investigation, the following conclusions could be drawn:

1. Debonding with debonding pliers can reduce the risk of enamel cracks; therefore, this method is safer than the enamel chisel method for removing brackets.
2. Diamond finishing burs produced the worst enamel appearances, and the deep grooves and scars caused by the finishing bur could not be reduced or smoothed with a One-Gloss polisher.
3. Cleanup with Super-Snap produced acceptable results, but a number of deep scratches were left on the enamel surfaces.
4. One-Gloss silicone particle polishing alone produced enamel surfaces that were closest to the intact enamel surface, but the polishing efficiency was the lowest of all the methods tested.

Abbreviations

ANOVA: Analysis of variance; ARI: Adhesive remnant index; Ra: Average roughness; RMGIC: Resin modified glass ionomer cement; Rz: 10-point height of irregularities; SEM: Scanning electron microscope

Acknowledgement

Not Applicable.

Funding

This study was supported by the Beijing Science and Technology Committee (z131107002213047) to Li Chen and the Capital Health Research and Development of Special Funding (2011-2002-01) and the achievement promotion project from Beijing Health and Family Planning Commission (TG-2015-018) to Xiaofeng Huang.

Authors' contributions

XH participated in the research design, data analysis and interpretation, critical revision of the paper. LC collected the extracted teeth and performed the debonding and clean-up process of specimens. XF performed most of the experiments, and was a major contributor in writing the manuscript. All authors read and approved the final manuscript.

Competing interests

The authors declare that they have no competing interests.

Consent for publication

Not applicable.

Ethics approval and consent to participate

The study has been approved by the ethics committee of Beijing Stomatological Hospital. Guardians of all patients provided written authorizations for use of the extracted teeth in this study.

Author details

[1]Department of Stomatology, Beijing Friendship Hospital, Capital Medical University, No.95 Yong'an Road, Xicheng District, Beijing 100050, China. [2]Department of Orthodontics, Capital Medical University School of Stomatology, No.4 Tiantan Xili, Dongcheng District, Beijing 100050, China.

References

1. Buonocore MG. A simple method of increasing the adhesion of acrylic filling materials to enamel surfaces. J Dent Res. 1955;34:849–53.
2. Newman GV. Epoxy adhesives for orthodontic attachments: progress report. Am J Orthod. 1965;51:901–12.
3. Shuler FS, van Waes H. SEM-evaluation of enamel surface after removal of fixed orthodontic appliances. Am J Dent. 2003;16:390–4.
4. Ozer T, Basaran G, Kama JD. Surface roughness of the restored enamel after orthodontic treatment. Am J Orthod Dentofac Orthop. 2010;137:368–74.
5. Dovgan JS, Walton RE, Bishara SE. Electrothermal debracketing: patient acceptance and effects on the dental pulp. Am J Orthod Dentofac Orthop. 1995;108:249–55.
6. Ireland AJ, Hosein I, Sherriff M. Enamel loss at bond-up, debond and clean-up following the use of a conventional light-cured composite and a resin-modified glass polyalkenoate cement. Eur J Orthod. 2005;27:413–9.
7. Brosh T, Kaufman A, Balabanovsky A, Vardimon AD. In vivo debonding strength and enamel damage in two orthodontic debonding methods. J Biomech. 2005;38:1107–13.
8. Su MZ, Lai EH, Chang JZ, Chen HJ, Chang FH, Chiang YC, et al. Effect of simulated debracketing on enamel damage. J Formos Med Assoc. 2012;111:560–6.
9. Larmour CJ, McCabe JF, Gordon PH. An ex vitro investigation into the effects of chemical solvence on the debond behaviour of ceramic orthodontic brackets. Br J Orthod. 1998;25(1):35–9.
10. Boyer DB, Engelhardt G, Bishara SE. Debonding orthodontic ceramic brackets by ultrasonic instrumentation. Am J Orthod Dentofac Orthop. 1995;108(3):262–6.
11. Ma T, Marangoni RD, Flint W. In vitro comparison of debonding force and intrapulpal temperature changes during ceramic orthodontic bracket removal using a carbon dioxide laser. Am J Orthod Dentofac Orthop. 1997;111(2):203–10.
12. Olszowska JJ, Tandecka K, Szatkiewicz T, Sporniak-Tutak K, Grocholewicz K. Three-dimensional quantitative analysis of adhesive remnants and enamel loss resulting from debonding orthodontic molar tubes. Head Face Med. 2014;10:37.

13. Bishara SE, Fonseca JM, Boyer DB. The use of debonding pliers in the removal of ceramic brackets: force levels and enamel cracks. Am J Orthod Dentofac Orthop. 1995;108(3):242–8.
14. Zarrinnia K, Eid NM, Kehoe MJ. The effect of different debonding techniques on the enamel surface: An in vitro qualitative study. Am J Orthod Dentofac Orthop. 1995;108(3):284–93.
15. Oliver RG, Griffiths J. Different techniques of residual composite removal following debonding time taken and surface enamel appearance. Br J Orthod. 1992;19(2):131–7.
16. Hosein I, Sherriff M, Ireland AJ. Enamel loss during bonding, debonding, and cleanup with use of a self-etching primer. Am J Orthod Dentofac Orthop. 2004;126:717–24.
17. Burapavong V, Marshall GW, Apfel DA, Perry HT. Enamel surface characteristics on removal of bonded orthodontic brackets. Am J Orthod. 1978;74:176–87.
18. Olszowska JJ, Tandecka K, Szatkiewicz T, Stepien P, Sporniak-Tutak K, Grocholewicz K. Three-dimensional analysis of enamel surface alteration resulting from orthodontic clean-up comparison of three different tools. BMC Oral Health. 2015;15:146.
19. Kim SS, Park WK, Son WS, Ahn HS, Ro JH, Kim YD. Enamel surface evaluation after removal of orthodontic composite remnants by intraoral sandblasting: A 3-dimensional surface profilometry study. Am J Orthod Dentofac Orthop. 2007;132:71–6.
20. Bonetti GA, Zanarini M, Parenti S, Lattuca M, Marchionni S, Gatto MR. Evaluation of enamel surfaces after bracket debonding: An in-vivo study with scanning electron microscopy. Am J Orthod Dentofac Orthop. 2011;140:696–702.
21. Chen L, Zhang JJ, Zhao BJ. Research of three adhesive removal methods influences on tooth surface after metal brackets debonding. Chinese J Aesthet Med. 2011;20(1):126–9.
22. Odaira C, Itoh S, Ishibashi K. Clinical evaluation of a dental color analysis system: the crystaleye Spectrophotometer. J Prosthodont Res. 2011;55:199–205.
23. Alexander R, Xie J, Fried D. Selective removal of residual composite from dental enamel surfaces using the third harmonic of a Q-switched ND:YAG laser. Lasers Surg Med. 2002;30:240–5.
24. Campbell PM. Enamel surfaces after orthodontic bracket debonding. Angle Orthod. 1995;65(2):103–10.
25. Eminkahyagil N, Arman A, Cetinsahin A, Karabulut E. Effect of resin-removal methods on enamel and shear bond strength of rebonded brackets. Angle Orthod. 2006;76:314–21.
26. Bishara SE, Trulove TS. Comparisons of different debonding techniques for ceramic brackets: an in vitro study. Part II. Findings and clinical implications. Am J Orthod Dentofac Orthop. 1990;98:263–73.
27. Eliades T, Kakaboura A, Eliades G, Brantley TG. Comparison of enamel colour changes associated with orthodontic bonding using two different adhesive. Eur J Orthod. 2001;23:85–90.
28. Ye C, Zhao Z, Zhao Q, Du X, Ye J, Wei X. Comparison of enamel discoloration associated with bonding with three different orthodontic adhesives and cleaning-up with four different procedures. J Dent. 2013;4:e35–40.
29. Tufekci E, Merrill TE, Pintado MR, Beyer JP, Brantley WA. Enamel loss associated with orthodontic adhesive removal on teeth with white spot lesions: An in vitro study. Am J Orthod Dentofac Orthop. 2004;125:733–40.
30. Silverman E, Cohen MS, Demke RS, Silverman M. A new light-cured glass ionomer cement that bonds brackets to teeth without etching in the presence of saliva. Am J Orthod Dentofac Orthop. 1995;108:231–6.
31. Sfondrini MF, Cacciafesta V, Pistorio A, Sfondrini G. Effects of conventional and high-intensity light-curing on enamel shear bond strength of composite resin and resin-modified glass-ionomer. Am J Orthod Dentofac Orthop. 2001;119(1):30–5.
32. International Organization for Standardization. Dental Materials Guidance on Testing on Adhesion to Tooth Structure. Geneva, Switzerland ISO TR 11405. 2004.
33. Bishara SE, Gordan VV, VonWald L, Jakobsen JR. Shear bond strength of composite, glass ionomer, and acidic primer adhesive systems. Am J Orthod Dentofac Orthop. 1999;115(1):24–8.
34. Stout KJ. Surface roughness: measurement, interpretation and significance of data. Mater Eng. 1981;2:260–5.
35. Bishara SE, Gordan VV, VonWald L, Olson ME. Effect of an acidic primer on the shear bond strength of orthodontic brackets. Am J Orthod Dentofac Orthop. 1998;114:243–7.
36. Eslamian L, Borzabadi-Farahani A, Mousavi N, Ghasemi A. A comparative study of shear bond strength between metal and ceramic brackets and artificially aged composite restorations using different surface treatments. Eur J Orthod. 2012;34:610–7.
37. Eslamian L, Borzabadi-Farahani A, Tavakol P, Tavakol A, Amini N, Lynch E. Effect of multiple debonding sequences on shear bond strength of new stainless steel brackets. J Orthod Sci. 2015;4(2):37.
38. Reis AF, Giannini M, Lovadino JR, dos Santos Dias CT. The effect of six polishing systems on the surface roughness of two packable resin-based composites. Am J Dent. 2002;15:193–7.
39. Janus J, Fauxpoint G, Arntz Y, Pelletier H, Etienne O. Surface roughness and morphology of three nanocomposites after two different polishing treatments by a multitechnique approach. Dent Mater. 2010;26:416–25.
40. Eliades T, Gioka C, Eliades G, Makou M. Enamel surface roughness following debonding using two resin grinding methods. Eur J Orthod. 2004;26:333–8.
41. Grossman ES, Rosen M, Cleaton-Jones PE, Volchansky A. Scientific surface roughness values for resin based materials. SADJ. 2004;59(7):274.
42. Marigo L, Rizzi M, La Torre G, Rumi G. 3-D surface profile analysis: different finishing methods for resin composites. Oper Dent. 2001;26(6):562–8.
43. Senawongse P, Pongprueksa P. Surface roughness of nanofill and nanohybrid resin composites after polishing and brushing. J Esthet Restor Dent. 2007;19(5):265–75.
44. Attar N. The effect of finishing and polishing procedures on the surface roughness of composite resin materials. J Contemp Dent Pract. 2007;8(1):27–35.

26

Assessing the progression of chronic periodontitis using subgingival pathogen levels: a 24-month prospective multicenter cohort study

E. Kakuta[1], Y. Nomura[2*], T. Morozumi[3], T. Nakagawa[4], T. Nakamura[5], K. Noguchi[5], A. Yoshimura[6], Y. Hara[6], O. Fujise[7], F. Nishimura[7], T. Kono[8], M. Umeda[8], M. Fukuda[9], T. Noguchi[9], N. Yoshinari[10], C. Fukaya[4], S. Sekino[11], Y. Numabe[11], N. Sugano[12], K. Ito[12], H. Kobayashi[13], Y. Izumi[13], H. Takai[14], Y. Ogata[14], S. Takano[15], M. Minabe[15,16], A. Makino-Oi[17], A. Saito[17], Y. Abe[18], S. Sato[19], F. Suzuki[20], K. Takahashi[21], T. Sugaya[22], M. Kawanami[22], N. Hanada[2], S. Takashiba[23] and H. Yoshie[3]

Abstract

Background: The diagnosis of the progression of periodontitis presently depends on the use of clinical symptoms (such as attachment loss) and radiographic imaging. The aim of the multicenter study described here was to evaluate the diagnostic use of the bacterial content of subgingival plaque recovered from the deepest pockets in assessing disease progression in chronic periodontitis patients.

Methods: This study consisted of a 24-month investigation of a total of 163 patients with chronic periodontitis who received trimonthly follow-up care. Subgingival plaque from the deepest pockets was recovered and assessed for bacterial content of *Porphyromonas gingivalis*, *Prevotella intermedia*, and *Aggregatibacter actinomycetemcomitans* using the modified Invader PLUS assay. The corresponding serum IgG titers were measured using ELISA. Changes in clinical parameters were evaluated over the course of 24 months. The sensitivity, specificity, and prediction values were calculated and used to determine cutoff points for prediction of the progression of chronic periodontitis.

Results: Of the 124 individuals who completed the 24-month monitoring phase, 62 exhibited progression of periodontitis, whereas 62 demonstrated stable disease. The *P. gingivalis* counts of subgingival plaque from the deepest pockets was significantly associated with the progression of periodontitis ($p < 0.001$, positive predictive value = 0.708).

Conclusions: The *P. gingivalis* counts of subgingival plaque from the deepest pockets may be associated with the progression of periodontitis.

Keywords: Progression of periodontitis, Periodontal stability, *Porphyromonas gingivalis*, Subgingival plaque

Background

Periodontitis is a chronic inflammation, which is leaded by periodontal bacteria and host immune response [1]. Periodontitis results in loss of connective tissue and bone support and is a major cause of tooth loss in adults [2]. The maintenance care following the initial active therapy phase plays an essential part in periodontal treatment to prevent disease progression based on the patient's individual needs [3].

The clinical diagnosis of chronic periodontal disease is based on visual and radiographic assessment of the periodontal tissues and on measurements of the space between the tooth and gum [2]. However, traditional clinical criteria are often insufficient for determining sites of active disease, for monitoring quantitatively the response to therapy or for measuring the degree of susceptibility to future disease progression [4]. Therefore, it is

* Correspondence: nomura-y@tsurumi-u.ac.jp
[2]Department of Translational Research, Tsurumi University School of Dental Medicine, 2-1-3 Tsurumi, Tsurumi-ku, Yokohama 230-8501, Japan
Full list of author information is available at the end of the article

necessary to establish effective markers indicating periodontitis progression.

The role of salivary biomarkers and periodontal pathogens were determined during periodontal disease progression [5]. Salivary *Porphyromonas gingivalis* ratio (ratio: *P. gingivalis* counts/Total bacteria counts) may be potential indicators for the progression of periodontitis. Such a salivary test could be a useful diagnostic tool for predicting periodontal disease progression [6]. And also, our previous report suggested the *P. gingivalis* ratio would be an indicator for the progression of periodontitis [7]. Therefore, salivary periodontal pathogens were suggested as useful marker of periodontitis progression.

While, several previous studies determined the subgingival plaque pathogens were useful indicators of periodontal progression. Monitoring the proportions of *P. gingivalis* and *Treponema denticola* in subgingival plaque had the potential to help identify sites at significant risk for progression of periodontitis [8]. The levels of red complex bacteria (*P. gingivalis*, *Tannerella forsythia*, and *T. denticola*) in subgingival plaque had a strong relationship with the clinical parameters [9]. Higher levels of *P. gingivalis*, *Prevotella intermedia* and *Aggregatibacter actinomycetemcomitans* in subgingival plaque appear to be related to an increased risk of periodontitis progression [10–12]. Similarly, *A. actinomycetemcomitans*, *P. gingivalis*, and *P. intermedia* may be useful as indicators of periodontitis activity [13]. In addition, presence of *A. actinomycetemcomitans* in subgingival plaque was a risk marker for periodontitis progression at the full mouth level [14, 15]. The increase in the number of *P. gingivalis*, *P. intermedia* in subgingival plaque of adolescents depends on the severity of gingivitis and appears to be a contributing factor for the shift from gingivitis to periodontitis [16, 17]. Thus, periodontal pathogens of subgingival plaque were valuable risk markers for periodontitis progression.

The bacterial tests or serum IgG tests were used to monitor periodontitis progress [5, 6, 18]. However, it remains unclear what periodontal bacteria from subgingival plaque are the most useful for estimation of periodontitis progression during regular follow-ups after initial therapy. In addition, previous reports did not test for possible correlations between the levels of periodontal bacteria in saliva and those in subgingival plaque from the deepest pockets.

The aims of this multicenter study were two-fold. The first goal was to evaluate subgingival bacteriological markers among patients treated for chronic periodontitis who exhibited or lacked subsequent disease progression during 24 months of regular follow-ups. The second goal was to define diagnostic values for indicating periodontitis progression and stability, including comparison between the levels of periodontal pathogens in subgingival plaque from the deepest pockets compared to those in saliva.

Methods

Study design

This study was performed as a clinical research project for diagnosis of periodontitis, as sponsored by the Japanese Society of Periodontology. Subjects were recruited in cooperation with 17 facilities (16 university hospitals and one clinic) in Japan, and were registered between February 2009 and February 2012. An additional file shows this in more detail [see Additional file 1]. The study enrolled a total of 163 follow-up patients, that is, individuals with chronic periodontitis who had completed active treatments such as initial therapy or periodontal surgery. Each diagnosis was based on the Guidelines of the American Academy of Periodontology [19]. All individuals were of age ≥ 30 years, systemically healthy, possessed at least 20 teeth, and had not taken systemic antibiotics, anti-inflammatory drugs, or immunosuppressive drugs within 3 months prior to enrollment.

Clinical assessment

The follow-up patients were seen trimonthly over a 24-month period. At each visit, the patients received treatment only to remove supragingival plaque and calculus, if detected. To identify disease progression, a full-mouth periodontal examination, except for the third molars, was performed every 6 months. The following clinical parameters were recorded: plaque index (PlI), bleeding on probing (BOP), probing pocket depth (PPD), and clinical attachment level (CAL). PlI was recorded at 4 sites per tooth (mesial, buccal, distal, and lingual). PPD, CAL, and BOP were recorded at 6 sites per tooth (mesiobuccal, buccal, distobuccal, mesiolingual, lingual, and distolingual). Patients with at least one site of CAL loss of ≥ 3 mm at a given site over the 24-month study period were considered to be exhibiting periodontitis progression [6, 7, 20, 21]. Intra and inter-examiner calibration sessions were conducted at the beginning and middle of the study period.

Sample collection

At baseline, samples of subgingival plaque from the deepest pockets, saliva, and blood were collected from each patient. Samplings were carried out according to the following order; blood samples, saliva samples, and subgingival plaque samples. Whole saliva was collected from each subject by having the individual chew on a gum base, containing neither fragrance nor flavored ingredients, for 5 min. The subgingival plaque was collected as follows: after removal of the supragingival plaque, samples of subgingival plaque from the deepest pockets (except for those at the third molars) were obtained by consecutive insertion (at a given site) of two sterile number-40 paper points (Zipperer Absorbent Paper Points, VDW GmbH, Munich, Germany) into the periodontal pocket for 10 s per point [22]. The plaque and saliva samples were sent immediately to a medical laboratory (BML Corporation, Tokyo, Japan) for bacterial analysis [6, 17, 23]. Blood sampling was performed using a commercial kit (DEMECAL Blood Test Set; Sunstar Inc, Osaka, Japan). In brief, device-treated serum was obtained from a 50-μL sample of whole capillary blood collected from the middle fingertip. The samples of sera were sent immediately to a commercial laboratory (Leisure Inc., Tokyo, Japan) for immune analysis [7, 24–27].

Quantification of periodontal bacteria in subgingival plaque from the deepest pockets and in saliva

Quantitative analysis of the total bacterial count and periodontopathic bacterial counts, including *P. gingivalis*, *P. intermedia*, and *A. actinomycetemcomitans*, was performed using a modification of the Invader PLUS assay [7, 22, 28, 29]. Briefly, bacterial DNA was extracted from samples of the subgingival plaque from the deepest pockets by suspending each plaque sample in 1 mL of phosphate-buffered saline, pH 7.4 and processing using the MagNA Pure LC Total Nucleic Acid Isolation Kit (Roche, Basel, Switzerland) according to the manufacturer's instructions. Similarly, bacterial DNA was extracted from the 100-μl whole saliva samples using the MagNA Pure LC Total Nucleic Acid Isolation Kit. The individual sequences of each bacterial species were obtained from a public database (National Center for Biotechnology Information, Bethesda, MD). Primers for each species were designed based on a region of the 16S rRNA gene. A pair of universal primers and a universal probe were used to determine the total number of bacteria. Primary probes and Invader oligos were designed using the Invader technology creator (HOLOGIC, Madison, WI) and were based on sequences in the amplified regions [7, 28–30].

Template DNA was added to a 15-μL reaction mixture containing primers for each species, 50 μM dNTPs, 700 nM primary probe, 70 nM Invader oligo, 2.5 U polymerase chain reaction (PCR) enzyme (EagleTaq DNA polymerase, Roche, Basel, Switzerland), and the Invader core reagent kit (Cleavase XI Invader core reagent kit, HOLOGIC, Madison, WI) containing a fluorescence resonance energy transfer (FRET) mix and an enzyme/$MgCl_2$ solution. The reaction mixture was preheated at 95 °C for 20 min, and a 2-step PCR reaction (95 °C for 1 s and 63 °C for 1 min) was performed for 35 cycles using an ABI PRISM 7900 thermocycler (Applied Biosystems, Foster City, CA). Fluorescence values of carboxyfluorescein (FAM; wavelength/bandwidth: excitation, 485/20 nm; emission, 530/25 nm) were measured at the end of the incubation/extension step at 63 °C for each cycle.

The limit of detection for this method was determined for each species with dilutions of bacterial DNA. Standard curves were constructed based on a crossing point determined by the fit point method.

Next, the proportions of the 3 pathogens within the total bacterial counts were determined [10, 31]. Bacterial ratios (%) and bacterial counts ($\log_{10}$) for each species also were used in various comparison and diagnostic analyses.

Measurement of IgG titers against periodontal bacteria

Serum IgG antibody titers against periodontal pathogens were determined by Leisure Inc. using enzyme-linked immunosorbent assay (ELISA) [32]. The method and selection of bacterial antigens were based on previous reports [7, 24–27]. Briefly, sonicated preparations of *P. gingivalis* FDC381, *P. intermedia* ATCC25611, and *A. actinomycetemcomitans* ATCC29523 were used as representative bacterial antigens. Each antigen was diluted to 10 μg/mL with 0.1 M carbonate buffer (pH 9.6). An aliquot of this diluted solution (100 μL) then was added to each well in a flat-bottomed microtiter plate (Greiner Co. Ltd., Frickenhausen, Germany) and the plate was stored overnight at 4 °C. Each well with immobilized antigen was washed three times with PBS containing 0.05% Tween-20 (PBST). Subsequently, a diluted serum sample (3100-fold dilution with PBST) was added to each well. After incubation at 37 °C for 2 h, each well was washed three times with PBST and bound/free (B/F) separation was carried out. Next, a 100-μl aliquot of 1:5000 diluted alkaline phosphatase-conjugated goat antihuman IgG antibody (Jackson Immuno Research Laboratories, Inc., Baltimore, MD) was added to each well. After incubation at 37 °C for 2 h, each well was washed three times with PBST and B/F separation was carried out. Thereafter, 50 μl of *p*-nitrophenyl phosphate (Wako Pure Chemical Industries, Ltd., Osaka, Japan) adjusted to 1 mg/ml with 10% diethanolamine buffer (pH 9.8) was added to each well as substrate. The plate then was incubated at room temperature for 10–20 min. The enzymatic reaction was terminated by adding 50 μl of 3 M NaOH, and optical density (measurement at 405 nm; reference at 490 nm) was measured in a Micro ELISA Auto Reader (Bio-Rad Laboratories, Hercules, CA).

The standard titration curves were formulated using serial dilutions of pooled control serum collected from participants without periodontitis. The absorbance of each sample after reaction was defined as an ELISA unit (EU), such that 100 EU corresponded to 1:3200 dilution of the control sample. The antibody titers were expressed as standardized values calculated as follows: (EU for study serum samples—EU for control samples)/2 standard deviations (SD), using SDs as determined based on ELISA of the control samples [25].

Statistical analysis

Descriptive analysis of the collected data was performed; the results are presented as medians. The Mann Whitney U test was used to compare clinical parameters, periodontal bacterial amounts, and IgG titers with or without progression of chronic periodontitis (CP). Only correlation with sex was performed using the Fisher's exact test. To determine an optimal test for distinguishing follow-up patients with periodontal progression or stability, we constructed receiver operating characteristic (ROC) curves and set the cutoff point based on the minimum difference between sensitivity and specificity [6, 25]. On the basis of the calculated cutoff point, we then made appropriate cross-tabulations. Diagnostic values were calculated by the Fisher's exact test to identify statistically significant differences. To check the correlation of periodontal bacteria with disease progression, logistic regression analysis was carried out to eliminate possible confounding variables. This study was originally designed to evaluate the diagnostic salivary levels of *P. gingivalis* in patients with or without the progression of CP. Calculation of the sample size was described in our previous report [7]. For the present study, post-hoc power analysis calculation using the cross table for patients with or without progression of CP against positive or negative for *P. gingivalis* suggested that groups would have to consist of at least 41 subjects each. A similar analysis revealed that groups of at least 26 subjects each would be required to detect differences in *P. gingivalis* counts ($\log_{10}$) in subgingival plaque from the deepest pockets. All analyses were performed by independent statisticians (Y.N., E.K., and N.H.) using IBM SPSS Statistics ver. 19.0 software (IBM Japan, Tokyo, Japan) and S-plus (ver. 6.0, NTT DATA, Tokyo, Japan).

Results

Of the 163 follow-up patients enrolled in the study, 32 dropped out during the study period due to a variety of causes (including occurrence of the Great East Japan Earthquake), and 7 others withdrew because of the use during the study of antimicrobial agents for the treatment of acute periodontal abscesses. In the end, 124 subjects successfully completed the study protocol. Of the 124 patients who completed the study protocol, 62 follow-up patients (50%) presented with disease progression, whereas the same number of patients (50%) demonstrated stable disease.

Demographic characteristics and biological variables of the study participants at baseline are shown in Table 1.

Table 1 Clinical parameters and bacterial levels at baseline in the patients with stable CP and progressive CP

	Stable CP patients ($n = 62$)	Progressive CP patients ($n = 62$)	p-value
Gender (male/female)	23/39	26/36	0.199
Age (year)	60.0 (56.0–66.0)	61 (52.5–68.0)	0.193
Smoking (non-smoker/smoker)	59/3	61/1	0.619
PII	0.12 (0.06–0.30)	0.17 (0.07–0.45)	0.291
BOP (% positive)	3.62 (1.53–11.28)	6.54 (2.48–10.45)	0.022*
PPD (mm)	2.15 (1.80–2.53)	2.26 (1.76–2.57)	0.885
The deepest PPD (mm)	4.0 (4.00–6.00)	5.0 (4.25–7.75)	<0.001*
CAL (mm)	2.8 (2.34–3.33)	2.87 (2.78–3.62)	0.710
The deepest CAL (mm)	7.00 (5.25–8.00)	7.5 (6.25–9.00)	0.042*
P. gingivalis counts ($\log_{10}$) Subgingival plaque	1.00 (1.00–3.17)	1.64 (1.00–4.29)	<0.001*
P. gingivalis counts ($\log_{10}$) Saliva	2.59 (1.00–3.66)	3.34 (2.67–4.08)	0.002*
P. gingivalis IgG titers (EU)	1.28 (0.32–4.26)	1.63 (0.95–6.34)	0.503
P. intermedia counts ($\log_{10}$) Subgingival plaque	1.00 (1.00–1.63)	1.00 (1.00–2.72)	0.049*
P. intermedia counts ($\log_{10}$) Saliva	1.87 (1.00–3.65)	3.02 (1.41–4.05)	0.038*
P. intermedia IgG titers (EU)	−0.39 (0.47–0.13)	−0.27 (0.45–0.21)	0.173
A. actinomycetemcomitans counts ($\log_{10}$) Subgingival plaque	1.00 (1.00–1.00)	1.00 (1.00–1.00)	0.164
A. actinomycetemcomitans counts ($\log_{10}$) Saliva	1.00 (1.00–1.00)	1.00 (1.00–1.50)	0.065
A. actinomycetemcomitans IgG titers (EU)	−0.26 (0.41–0.03)	−0.30 (0.40–0.10)	0.278

Value represent median value (25–75 percentile). *CP* chronic periodontitis, *PII* plaque index, *BOP* bleeding on probing, *PPD* probing pocket depth, *CAL* clinical attachment level, *EU* enzyme-linked immunosorbent assay unit

The deepest PPD and the deepest CAL indicate the value of the sites which is the deepest PPD and the deepest CAL in each subject, respectively. p values for gender were calculated using the Fisher's exact test, and all others were Mann Whitneys' U tests. The *mark represent statistical significance between stable CP patients and progressive CP patients ($p < 0.05$)

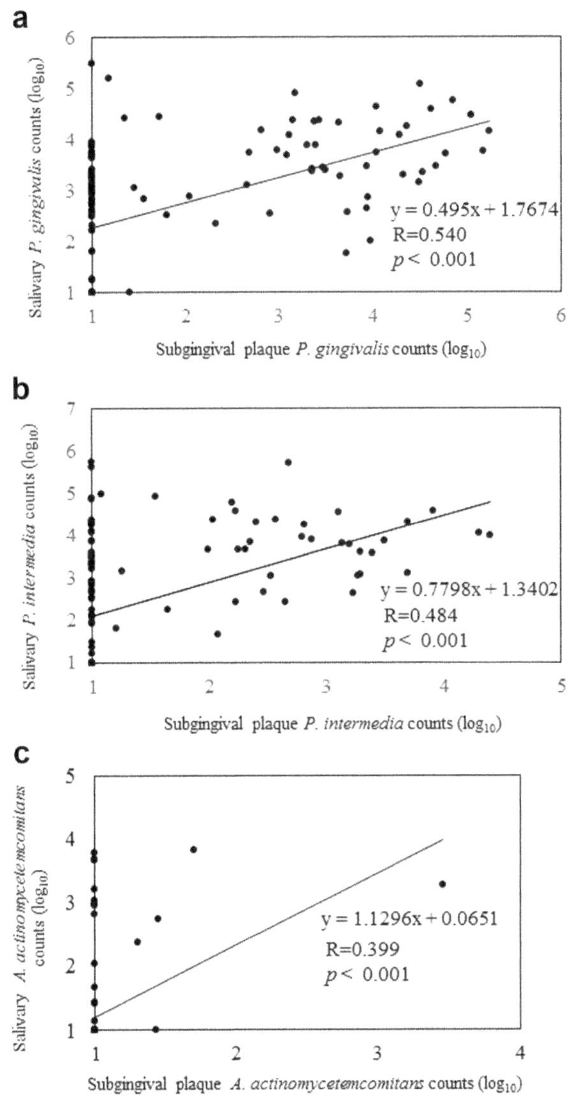

Fig. 1 Scatter plots of periodontal pathogen counts from salivary and subgingival plaque from the deepest pockets for individual subjects. Correlations of periodontal pathogen counts in saliva and subgingival plaque from the deepest pockets were statistically significant. The correlation coefficient of bacterial counts in saliva and subgingival plaque from the deepest pockets was the highest for *P. gingivalis* (panel **a**) when compared with other pathogens (panel **b**, **c**). Note, for each of the three bacterial species, that bacterial counts were below the limit of detection in some subgingival plaque samples; this observation was most notable for *A. actinomycetemcomitans*, which could not be detected in >95% of samples (panel **c**).

BOP, the deepest PPD, and the deepest CAL were significantly higher in subjects who exhibited progressive CP compared to patients with stable CP. For the pathogens, *P. gingivalis* counts in subgingival plaque from the deepest pockets, *P. intermedia* counts in subgingival plaque from the deepest pockets, *P. gingivalis* counts in saliva, and *P. intermedia* counts in saliva were significantly higher in subjects who exhibited progressive CP compared to patients with stable CP.

Figure 1 shows the scatter plots of periodontal pathogen counts in saliva compared to those in subgingival plaque from the deepest pockets. Correlation coefficients of bacterial counts from saliva and subgingival plaque from the deepest pockets were 0.540 ($p < 0.001$) for *P. gingivalis*, 0.484 ($p < 0.001$) for *P. intermedia*, and 0.399 ($p < 0.001$) for *A. actinomycetemcomitans*. However, in some samples of subgingival plaque from the deepest pockets, bacterial counts were below the limit of detection. Notably, *A. actinomycetemcomitans* was not detected in 95.7% of samples of subgingival plaque from the deepest pockets.

To determine an optimal test for distinguishing follow-up patients with periodontal progression from those with stable CP, we constructed receiver operating characteristic curves and set the cutoff points on the basis of the minimum differences between sensitivity and specificity [6, 25]. Furthermore, on the basis of the cutoff point, we made appropriate cross-tabulations.

Table 2 shows the cutoff points, sensitivity, specificity, positive predictive value, negative predictive value, likelihood, and area under the curve for the periodontal bacterial counts and IgG titers. Among the 3 periodontal pathogens, only *P. gingivalis* yielded counts that demonstrated significant correlation with CP status (cutoff point = 1.370 ($p < 0.001$), sensitivity = 0.548, specificity = 0.774, positive predictive value = 0.708, negative predictive value = 0.632, likelihood ratio = 2.429, AUC = 0.666).

The area under the curve of the *P. gingivalis* counts was the largest amongst all markers evaluated. The specificity of *P. gingivalis* counts in subgingival plaque from the deepest pockets was higher than that for salivary *P. gingivalis* counts (0.323) [7].

To check the importance of periodontal bacteria in the progression of periodontal disease, logistic regression analysis was carried out to eliminate possible confounding variables. As shown in Table 3, the crude odds ratio of the deepest CAL in each subject, and *P. gingivalis* count were statistically significant. According to the multivariate adjusted odds ratio, only *P. gingivalis* counts exhibited a significant ($p = 0.034$) correlation with CP status.

Discussion

In this study, we evaluated potential markers for periodontitis progression during a 24-month study interval. The results suggested associations between periodontitis progression and bacterial levels in subgingival plaque recovered from the deepest pockets. We previously used PCR to examine the presence of each of six species of periodontopathic bacteria in whole saliva and subgingival plaque [33]. A statistical relationship was found between the presence of *P. gingivalis*, *P. intermedia*, *Prevotella nigrescens*, and *T. denticola* in saliva and in periodontal pocket samples; in

Table 2 Diagnostic values of subgingival plaque bacterial levels and serum IgG titers for periodontal bacteria

	Cutoff	*p*-value	Sensitivity	Specificity	Positive predictive value	Negative predictive value	Likelihood ratio	AUC
P. gingivalis counts (log_{10})	1.370	<0.001	0.548	0.774	0.708	0.632	2.429	0.666
P. intermedia counts (log_{10})	1.040	0.077	0.371	0.774	0.622	0.552	1.643	0.568
A. actinomycetemcomitans counts (log_{10})	1.151	0.171	0.065	0.984	0.800	0.513	4.000	0.478
P. gingivalis IgG titer[a]	1.355	>0.999	0.516	0.500	0.508	0.508	1.032	0.444
P. intermedia IgG titer[a]	−0.345	0.281	0.565	0.548	0.556	0.557	1.250	0.535
A. actinomycetemcomitans IgG titer[a]	−0.275	0.590	0.452	0.484	0.467	0.469	0.875	0.571

Fisher's exact test was used for statistical analysis ($p < 0.05$). The *P. gingivalis* counts was statistically significant
The area under the curve of the *P. gingivalis* counts was the largest amongst all markers. Subgingival plaque *P. gingivalis* counts specificity was higher than salivary *P. gingivalis* counts (0.323) [7]
EU enzyme-linked immunosorbent assay unit, *AUC* area under the curve
[a]: J Periodontal Res. 2016 Dec;51(6):768–778

the event of disagreement, the organisms were more frequently present in saliva than in periodontal pockets (p <0.001). Meanwhile, *A. actinomycetemcomitans* and *T. forsythia* were not reliably detected by sampling of either saliva or periodontal pockets [31].

Our results indicated that The *P. gingivalis* counts of subgingival plaque from the deepest pockets might be used as indicators of the progression of periodontitis. The results of the present study, along with those of our previous study [7], suggest the value of *P. gingivalis* in assessing the progression of CP. Specificity of *P. gingivalis* counts in subgingival plaque from the deepest pockets was higher than that in saliva. The absolute pathogen burden is clearly more informative than merely a dichotomization between carriers and noncarriers [34]. *P. gingivalis*, alone or in combination with *T. forsythia* and *T. denticola*, has been reported to exhibit the deepest mean pocket depths [9]. The thresholds predictive of progressive periodontitis correspond to 0.01% for *A. actinomycetemcomitans*, 0.1% for *P. gingivalis*, and 2.5% for *P. intermedia* [13]. In an 18-month-long study, the presence of *P. gingivalis* and *P. intermedia* in subgingival plaque at proportions exceeding 2% was a significant predictor of periodontitis progression in older adults [35]. These results support the appropriateness using *P. gingivalis* as a marker for the progression of CP, and are consistent with the results obtained in the present study. In the work described here, we evaluated the diagnostic value for periodontal disease of the levels of bacteria in subgingival plaque from the deepest pockets (Table 2), in extension of our previous report [7] showing the diagnostic value for periodontal disease of salivary bacterial levels. Specificity, positive predictive value, likelihood ratio, and AUC of *P. gingivalis* counts for the progression of periodontal disease

Table 3 Multiple logistic regression analysis for progression of chronic periodontitis

	Crude OR (95% CI)	*p*-value	Multivariate adjusted OR (95% CI)	*p*-value
Gender (male/female)	0.62 (0.30–1.29)	0.200	1.06 (0.43–2.65)	0.893
Age (years)	1.02 (0.98–1.07)	0.271	1.03 (0.97–1.08)	0.324
PII	2.15 (0.37–12.48)	0.393	0.88 (0.10–8.10)	0.909
BOP (% positive)	1.04 (1.00–1.08)	0.077	1.03 (0.98–1.08)	0.285
CAL (mm)	1.14 (0.69–1.87)	0.603	0.72 (0.33–1.58)	0.415
The deepest CAL (mm)	1.25 (1.01–1.54)	0.039*	1.35 (0.99–1.85)	0.059
P. gingivalis counts (log_{10})	4.163 (1.913–9.06)	<0.001*	1.56 (1.03–2.34)	0.034*
*P. gingivalis*IgG titers (EU)	1.01 (0.98–1.05)	0.422	1.01 (0.99–1.03)	0.276
P. intermedia counts (log_{10})	2.022 (0.92–4.443)	0.080	0.99 (0.52–1.76)	0.973
P. intermedia IgG titers (EU)	1.45 (0.46–4.60)	0.531	2.04 (0.50–8.22)	0.318
A. actinomycetemcomitans counts (log_{10})	4.207 (0.457–38.757)	0.205	44.70 (0.05–36,574)	0.267
A. actinomycetemcomitans IgG titers (EU)	0.78 (0.33–1.85)	0.581	0.52 (0.15–1.76)	0.291

The crude odds ratio of the deepest CAL in each subject, P. gingivalis count, and the combination of P. gingivalis counts and P. gingivalis IgG titers were statistically significant. According to the multivariate adjusted odds ratio, only P. gingivalis counts was statistically significant ($p = 0.034$)
OR odds ratio, *95% CI* confidence interval with 95% significance level, *PII* plaque index, *BOP* bleeding on probing, *CAL* clinical attachment level;Counts, each bacteria counts in subgingival plaque, *EU* enzyme-linked immunosorbent assay unit
*$p < 0.05$

in subgingival plaque were higher than the respective parameters for bacterial counts in saliva. However, we note that bacterial counts could not be determined in numerous samples of subgingival plaque from the deepest pockets, with detection failing for *P. gingivalis*, *P. intermedia*, and *A. actinomycetemcomitans* in 59.7, 70.2, and 95.7% of samples, respectively.

Subgingival plaque samples from the deepest pockets did not yield detectable levels of periodontal bacteria in several individuals enrolled in this study; however, the salivary samples were able to detect periodontal bacteria in these cases. An inherent limitation of sampling subgingival plaque from the deepest pockets is that these specimens only reflect the condition of sampling site. Notably, however, *P. gingivalis* counts in subgingival plaque from the deepest pockets yielded greater sensitivity and specificity for periodontal progression than did *P. gingivalis* counts in saliva. In this context, it is worth noting that sampling of subgingival plaque from the deepest pockets is more difficult than sampling of saliva. Clinicians using these tests should consider these merits and demerits when considering the use of sampling for periodontal bacteria in subgingival plaque from the deepest pockets. Further investigations will be needed to assess the utility of salivary bacteria levels as markers of periodontal condition.

Conclusions

The *P. gingivalis* counts of subgingival plaque from the deepest pockets may be associated with the progression of periodontitis.

Acknowledgements
Not applicable.

Funding
This study was supported by a grant of the clinical research project for the diagnosis of periodontitis from the Japanese Society of Periodontology.

Authors' contributions
We confirmed that all authors have read and approved the final version of the manuscript, and agreed with this submission to your journal. Also, we are confident that all authors meet conditions the ICMJE authorship criteria. EK performed statistical analysis and prepared the manuscript. TM performed follow-up care of patients, data collection and prepared the manuscript. TNakag planed study design and managed recruitment of subjects. TNakam, KN, AY, YH, OF, TK, MF, TNog, NY, CF, SSek, YNuma, NS, KI, HK, YI, HT, YO, STakan, MM, AM-O, YA, SSa, FS, and TS, MK, NH performed follow-up care of patients and data collection. FN, MU, AS and KT advised regarding bacterial and serum aspects, and divided the preparation of the manuscript. YNomu and NH performed statistical analysis. STakash managed database administration. HY planed study design and gave scientific advices on the study.

Competing interests
The authors declare that they have no competing interests.

Consent for publication
Not applicable.

Ethics approval and consent to participate
Subjects were recruited in cooperation with 17 facilities (16 university hospitals and one clinic) in Japan, and were registered between February 2009 and February 2012. Informed written consent was obtained from each subject, and the protocol was approved by the Institutional Review Board of each participating institution. An additional file shows this in more detail [see Additional file 1].

Author details
[1]Department of Oral Microbiology, Tsurumi University School of Dental Medicine, 2-1-3 Tsurumi, Tsurumi-ku, Yokohama, Japan. [2]Department of Translational Research, Tsurumi University School of Dental Medicine, 2-1-3 Tsurumi, Tsurumi-ku, Yokohama 230-8501, Japan. [3]Division of Periodontology, Department of Oral Biological Science, Niigata University Graduate School of Medical and Dental Sciences, 2-5274 Gakkocho-dori, Chuo-ku, Niigata, Japan. [4]Department of Dentistry and Oral Surgery, School of Medicine, Keio University, 35 Shinano-machi, Shinjuku-ku, Tokyo, Japan. [5]Department of Periodontology, Kagoshima University Graduate School of Medical and Dental Sciences, 8-35-1 Sakuragaoka, Kagoshima, Japan. [6]Department of Periodontology, Unit of Translational Medicine, Nagasaki University Graduate School of Biomedical Sciences, 1-12-4 Sakamoto, Nagasaki, Japan. [7]Section of Periodontology, Division of Oral Rehabilitation, Faculty of Dental Science, Kyushu University, 3-1-1 Maidashi, Higashi-ku, Fukuoka, Japan. [8]Department of Periodontology, Osaka Dental University, 8-1 Kuzuhahanazonocho, Hirakata, Japan. [9]Department of Periodontology, School of Dentistry, Aichi Gakuin University, 2-11 Suemori-doori,Chikusa-ku, Nagoya, Japan. [10]Department of Periodontology, School of Dentistry, Matsumoto Dental University, 1780 Hirokagobara, Shiojiri, Nagano, Japan. [11]Department of Periodontology, School of Life Dentistry at Tokyo, The Nippon Dental University, 1-9-20 Fujimi, Chiyoda-ku, Tokyo, Japan. [12]Department of Periodontology, Nihon University School of Dentistry, 1-8-13 Kanda-Surugadai, Chiyoda-ku, Tokyo, Japan. [13]Department of Periodontology, Graduate School of Medical and Dental Sciences, Tokyo Medical and Dental University, 1-5-45 Yushima, Bunkyo-ku, Tokyo, Japan. [14]Department of Periodontology, Nihon University School of Dentistry at Matsudo, 2-870-1 Sakae-cho-nishi, Matsudo-shi, Chiba, Japan. [15]Bunkyo-Dori Dental Clinic, 2-4-1 Anagawa, Inage-ku, Chiba, JAPAN. [16]Division of Periodontology, Department of Oral function and Restoration, School of Dentistry, Kanagawa Dental University, 82 Inaokacho, Yokosuka, Kanagawa, Japan. [17]Department of Periodontology, Tokyo Dental College, 2-9-18 Misakicho, Chiyoda-ku, Tokyo, Japan. [18]Comprehensive Dental Care, The Nippon Dental University Niigata Hospital, 1-8 Hamaura-cho, Chuo-ku, Niigata, Japan. [19]Department of Periodontology, School of life Dentistry at Niigata, The Nippon Dental University, 1-8 Hamaura-cho, Chuo-ku, Niigata, Japan. [20]Division of Dental Anesthesiology, Department of Oral Surgery, School of Dentistry, Ohu University, 31-1 Misumido, Tomita, Koriyama, Fukushima, Japan. [21]Division of Periodontics, Department of Conservative Dentistry, School of Dentistry, Ohu University, 31-1 Misumido, Tomita, Koriyama, Fukushima, Japan. [22]Division of Periodontology and Endodontology, Department of Oral Health Science, Hokkaido University Graduate School of Dental Medicine, Kita 13, Nishi 7, Kita-ku, Sapporo, Japan. [23]Department of Pathophysiology-Periodontal Science, Okayama University Graduate School of Medicine, Dentistry and Pharmaceutical Sciences, 2-5-1 Shikata-cho, Okayama, Japan.

References

1. Salvi GE, Lang NP. Host response modulation in the management of periodontal diseases. J Clin Periodontol. 2005;32:108–29.
2. Pihlstrom BL, Michalowicz BS, Johnson NW. Periodontal diseases. Lancet. 2005;366:1809–20.
3. Jansson L, Lagervall M. Periodontitis progession in patients subjected to supportive maintenance care. Swed Dent J. 2008;32:105–14.

4. Giannobile WV, Beikler T, Kinney JS, Ramseier CA, Morelli T, Wong DT. Saliva as a diagnostic tool for periodontal disease: current state and future directions. Periodontol 2000. 2009;50:52–64.
5. Kinney JS, Morelli T, Braun T, et al. Saliva/pathogen biomarker signatures and periodontal disease progression. J Dent Res. 2011;90:752–8.
6. Nomura Y, Shimada Y, Hanada N, et al. Salivary biomarkers for predicting the progression of chronic periodontitis. Arch Oral Biol. 2012;57:413–20.
7. Morozumi T, Nakagawa T, Nomura Y, et al. Salivary pathogen and serum antibody to assess the progression of chronic periodontitis: a 24-mo prospective multicenter cohort study. J Periodontal Res. 2016 Jan 20. doi: 10.1111/jre.12353. [Epub ahead of print]
8. Byrne SJ, Dashper SG, Darby IB, Adams GG, Hoffmann B, Reynolds EC. Progression of chronic periodontitis can be predicted by the levels of *Porphyromonas gingivalis* and Treponema denticola in subgingival plaque. Oral Microbiol Immunol. 2009;24:469–77.
9. Socransky SS, Haffajee AD, Cugini MA, et al. Microbial complexes in subgingival plaque. J Clin Periodontol. 1998;25:134–44.
10. Haffajee AD, Socransky SS, Smith C, Dibart S. Relation of baseline microbial parameters to future periodontal attachment loss. J Clin Periodontol. 1991; 18:744–50.
11. Haffajee AD, Socransky SS. Microbial etiological agents of destructive periodontal diseases. Periodontol. 1994;5:78–111. Review.
12. Wang X, Li L, Yang M, Geng Y, Chen H, Xu Y, Sun Y. Prevalence and distribution of Aggregatibacter actinomycetemcomitans and its cdtB gene in subgingival plaque of Chinese periodontitis patients. BMC Oral Health. 2014;14:37. doi:10.1186/1472-6831-14-37.
13. Bragd L, Dahlén G, Wikström M, Slots J. The capability of *Actinobacillus actinomycetemcomitans, Bacteroides gingivalis* and *Bacteroides intermedius* to indicate progressive periodontitis; a retrospective study. J Clin Periodontol. 1987;14:95–9.
14. Van der Velden U, Abbas F, Armand S, Loos BG, Timmerman MF, et al. Java project on periodontal diseases. The natural development of periodontitis: risk factors, risk predictors and risk determinants. J Clin Periodontol. 2006;33:540–8.
15. Timmerman MF, Van der Weijden GA, Abbas F, et al. Untreated periodontal disease in Indonesian adolescents. Longitudinal clinical data and prospective clinical and microbiological risk assessment. J Clin Periodontol. 2000;27:932–42.
16. Papapanou PN, Baelum V, Luan WM, et al. Subgingival microbiota in adult Chinese: prevalence and relation to periodontal disease progression. J Periodontol. 1997;68:651–66.
17. Yang NY, Zhang Q, Li JL, Yang SH, Shi Q. Progression of periodontal inflammation in adolescents is associated with increased number of *Porphyromonas gingivalis, Prevotella intermedia, Tannerella forsythensis*, and *Fusobacterium nucleatum*. Int J Paediatr Dent. 2014;24:226–33.
18. Sugi N, Naruishi K, Kudo C, et al. Prognosis of periodontitis recurrence after intensive periodontal treatment using examination of serum IgG antibody titer against periodontal bacteria. J Clin Lab Anal. 2011;25:25–32.
19. Krebs KA, Clem 3rd DS. American Academy of Periodontology, Guidelines for the management of patients with periodontal diseases. J Periodontol. 2006;77:1607–11.
20. Beck JD. Methods of assessing risk for periodontitis and developing multifactorial models. J Periodontol. 1994;65:468–78.
21. Ogawa H, Yoshihara A, Hirotomi T, Ando Y, Miyazaki H. Risk factors for periodontal disease progression among elderly people. J Clin Periodontol. 2002;29:592–7.
22. Morozumi T, Kubota T, Abe D, Shimizu T, Komatsu Y, Yoshie H. Effects of irrigation with an antiseptic and oral administration of azithromycin on bacteremia caused by scaling and root planning. J Periodontol. 2010;81: 1555–63.
23. Morozumi T, Kubota T, Abe D, Shimizu T, Nohno K, Yoshie H. Microbiological effect of essential oils in combination with subgingival ultrasonic instrumentation and mouth rinsing in chronic periodontitis patients. Int J Dent. 2013;2013:146479.
24. Takeuchi K, Furuta M, Takeshita T, et al. Serum antibody to *Porphyromonas gingivalis* and periodontitis progression: the Hisayama Study. J Clin Periodontol. 2015;42:719–25.
25. Kudo C, Naruishi K, Maeda H, et al. Assessment of the plasma/serum IgG test to screen for periodontitis. J Dent Res. 2012;91:1190–5.
26. Kudo C, Shin WS, Minabe M, et al. Analysis of the relationship between periodontal disease and atherosclerosis within a local clinical system: a cross-sectional observational pilot study. Odontology. 2015;103:314–21.
27. Furuta M, Shimazaki Y, Tanaka S, et al. Gender-specific associations of serum antibody to *Porphyromonas gingivalis* and inflammatory markers. Biomed Res Int. 2015;2015:897971.
28. Tadokoro K, Yamaguchi T, Kawamura K, et al. Rapid quantification of periodontitis-related bacteria using a novelmodification of Invader PLUS technologies. Microbiol Res. 2010;165:43–9.
29. Tada A, Takeuchi H, Shimizu H, et al. Quantification of periodontopathic bacteria in saliva using the invader assay. Jpn J Infect Dis. 2012;65:415–23.
30. Lyons SR, Griffen AL, Leys EJ. Quantitative real-time PCR for *Porphyromonas gingivalis* and total bacteria. J Clin Microbiol. 2000;38:2362–5.
31. Tomita S, Komiya-Ito A, Imamura K, et al. Prevalence of Aggregatibacter actinomycetemcomitans, Porphyromonas gingivalis and Tannerella forsythia in Japanese patients with generalized chronic and aggressive periodontitis. Microb Pathog. 2013;61–62:11–5.
32. Murayama Y, Nagai A, Okamura K, et al. Serum immunoglobulin G antibody to periodontal bacteria. Adv Dent Res. 1988;2:339–45.
33. Umeda M, Contreras A, Chen C, Bakker I, Slots J. The utility of whole saliva to detect the oral presence of periodontopathic bacteria. J Periodontol. 1998;69:828–33.
34. Papapanou PN, Neiderud AM, Papadimitriou A, Sandros J, Dahlén G. "Checkerboard" assessments of periodontal microbiota and serum antibody responses: a case-control study. J Periodontol. 2000;71:885–97.
35. Brown LF, Beck JD, Rozier RG. Incidence of attachment loss in community-dwelling older adults. J Periodontol. 1994;65:316–23.

27

Prevalence of oral manifestations in children and adolescents with cancer submitted to chemotherapy

Deise Berger Velten*, Eliana Zandonade and Maria Helena Monteiro de Barros Miotto

Abstract

Background: Oral complications may be observed during chemotherapy and are important side effects that may directly affect the anticancer treatment, even causing septicaemia in some cases. This research was done in order to evaluate changes in oral lesions during follow-up of children and adolescents in chemotherapy at Hospital Estadual Infantil Nossa Senhora da Glória (HEINSG).

Methods: The study design was longitudinal, 45 patients were evaluated and monitored for 1 month after the initiation of chemotherapy. Twenty-eight patients were male and 17 female, ranging from 3 months to 18 years old.

Results: The results show an increase in the number of mucositis cases and a decrease in xerostomia cases after the initiation of treatment, and other oral lesions were also found in low numbers.

Conclusions: It is possible to avoid oral complications by maintaining a good oral health, and reducing infectious outbreaks. It is also feasible to obtain an early diagnosis of, and treat these oral complications, preventing them from following a more severe clinical course that may negatively affect the individual's treatment. This outcome requires the presence of a dental surgeon on the multidisciplinary cancer treatment team.

Keywords: Chemotherapy, Oral manifestations, Oncology

Background

Cancer is a term used to describe a group of diseases that involve the uncontrolled growth of cells [1]. In recent decades, cancer has become a serious global public health problem. The World Health Organisation (WHO) has estimated that in the year 2030, there will be 27 million incident cases of cancer, 17 million deaths from cancer, and 75 million people each year living with cancer. The regions most affected by these increases are developing countries [2].

Infant-juvenile cancers differ from adult cancers in many respects, such as types, sites, aetiologies, characteristics and treatments [1].

Neoplasms were the leading cause (7%) of deaths due to morbidity in children and adolescents (1–19 years) in 2011 and were surpassed by only deaths due to external causes. This fact is particularly troubling when one considers that younger individuals comprise a large proportion of the Brazilian population. According to information from the last population census in 2010, approximately 30% of the population is below the age of 19 [3].

According to population-based cancer records (Registros de Câncer de Base Populacional), the percentage of paediatric tumours observed in Brazil is 3%. Approximately 11,840 new cases of cancer in children and adolescents up to 19 years of age have been estimated in Brazil for 2014 [3].

There has been an improvement in the survival rates of children with cancer due to dosage intensification and the combination of chemotherapy drugs, which has also led to success in the cancer treatment healing response [4, 5]. Chemotherapy acts by destroying or inhibiting the growth of rapidly multiplying cells, without differentiating cancer cells, which proliferate rapidly, from normal cells, such as the oral mucosa [6].

Chemotherapy is used to treat approximately 70% of cancer patients [5, 7]. Of these patients, 40% develop oral manifestations, and this number increases to over 90% in children under 12 years of age [6, 8].

* Correspondence: deisebergervelten@yahoo.com.br
Federal University of Espírito Santo, Av. Mal. Campos, 1468 - Maruípe, Vitória, ES 29043-900, Brazil

The following oral manifestations related to anticancer treatment are commonly found: mucositis, xerostomia [9, 10], infections, salivary gland dysfunction, dysgeusia and pain [11].

Given that most infant-juvenile patients with malignancies receive chemotherapy, which is often associated with side effects consisting of oral complications, this study aimed to evaluate changes over the course of two monitoring sessions in the oral manifestations of children and adolescents receiving chemotherapy at the Hospital Estadual Infantil Nossa Senhora da Glória (HEINSG).

Methods

This study had a longitudinal design and was performed by monitoring children and adolescents aged up to 18 years and 364 days who had received their first cancer diagnosis and had started chemotherapy at HEINSG between April 2013 and April 2014. The individuals were evaluated on two occasions approximately 1 month after the initiation of chemotherapy.

When individuals were admitted to HEINSG and diagnosed with a malignant neoplasm, at the first study stage, an interview and clinical examination were performed before or within 3 days of starting chemotherapy. At this stage, data regarding oral health and sociodemographic characteristics, such as gender, age, place of birth, education, maternal education and socioeconomic status, were collected.

The HEINSG serves its patients only by the Unified Health System (SUS) and it is located the only reference center of public state network for cancer treatment in children and adolescents. Being a public referral hospital usually the patients treated are less favored socioeconomic status.

The Economic Classification of individuals followed the New Economic Classification Standard Criteria of Brazil, which aims to discriminate large groups of people according to their consumption capacity of accessible products and services to a significant portion of the population and classify households, assuming, as an assumption that the class is a familiar feature among others. According to this criterion individuals can be classified into five classes A, B, C, D and E and class A is the best economic status and class E the worst economic condition [12].

Some information, such as the indicated treatment and diagnosis, was collected from the patient's medical records.

For information about xerostomia, mucositis, oral candidiasis, herpes simplex and cold sore, a clinical examination was conducted after completing the interview. All patients were examined in HEINSG dependencies by the same operator, which was a dentist (DBV), thus, diminishing the interobserver variation. A preparation was made through pictures of the most common oral alterations that would be expected to be found in the study group.

Through sialometry it is possible to evaluate the production of unstimulated saliva, or by chemical, mechanical or gustatory stimulation [13]. Individuals commonly produce 0.3 ml/min of saliva without stimulation; when secretion is less than or equal to 0.1 ml/min, it is characterised as hyposalivation [14].

An adaptation was made to the criteria proposed by the World Health Organization [15], a scale test that consists in measuring the production of saliva produced for 1 min in a graph vessel (0 to 3 ml), to diagnose hyposalivation [13]. The test was performed after 1.5–2 h in which the patient should not have smoked, drunk, washed his mouth or swallowed food.

When the sialometry test performed in patients obtained a measure less than 0.3 ml/min. saliva, and moreover were present the symptoms described in any of degrees of severity scale used to quantify the xerostomia as a side effect (Table 1) proposed by the World Health Organization (WHO) xerostomia was considered present and was considered absent when the test there was a greater extent 0.3 ml/min and was also not observed any symptoms.

Xerostomia was only evaluated in children aged 6 years or more and in adolescents.

Mucositis was diagnosed via clinical examination by evaluating the appearance of the oral mucosa. Mucositis was not graded according to severity but was considered absent or present according to whether a change in the mucosa was noted on any of the severity scales (discoloration, erythema, pseudomembrane or deep ulceration) proposed by the WHO [15].

Complications including oral candidiasis, labial herpes simplex and mouth ulcers were evaluated by visual clinical examination [16].

Statistical analysis

A descriptive analysis was performed on the sociodemographic characteristics and oral manifestations of the participants at the three study stages, according to their

Table 1 Quantification of xerostomia as a side effect according to WHO

	Degrees of severity of xerostomia
Grade 1	Symptomatic (thick or sparse saliva) without significant dietary changes, saliva production unstimulated > 0.2 ml/min.;
Grade 2	Symptomatic with significant changes in the oral intake (copious intake of water or use of other lubricants, limited to purees diet and/or soft and wet food); unstimulated saliva production from 0.1 to 0.2 ml/min.;
Grade 3	Symptoms leading to inability to feed orally; need for administration of intravenous fluids, enteral or parenteral nutrition; unstimulated saliva flow <0,1 ml/min.

Fonte. World Health Organization. Nacional Cancer Institute. Common Terminology Criteria for Adverse Events [15]

respective frequencies and percentages. The Kappa statistic was used to measure concordance in cases in which a particular individual presented an oral manifestation at the next stage.

McNemar's test was used to verify changes in the number of cases of oral manifestations (direction of disagreement) between stages. A significance level of 5% was adopted, and the software used in all analyses was IBM (SPSS) version 21.

All parents or guardians of the participants signed the consent form and previously clarified data collection. The study was approved on 20 February 2013 by the Research Ethics Committee of the Health Sciences Center (Health Sciences Center) of the Federal University of Espirito Santo (Federal University of Espirito Santo - UFES) by the number opinion 201,117.

Results

Between the months April 2013 and April 2014, a total of 66 children and adolescents were admitted to HEINSG diagnosed with cancer to make chemotherapy. In 15 of these patients it was not possible to approach (Fig. 1). The initial study population was composed of 51 individuals so.

The final sample size was 45 children and adolescents at the second evaluation (1 month after the initial examination). It was not possible to follow six patients between the 1st and 2nd moments described in Fig. 1.

Table 2 shows the sociodemographic characteristics and diagnosis of the 45 individuals monitored during the study who were evaluated approximately 30 days after the initial examination, showing that most of the individuals were in the one- to 4-year-old age group (31.1%), were male (62.2%), resided in greater Vitória (46.7%), belonged to

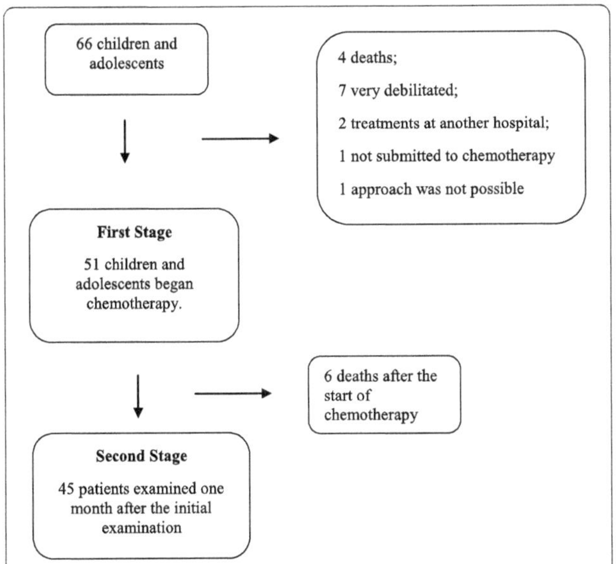

Fig. 1 Deaths during the monitoring of patients at HEINSG

Table 2 Sociodemographic characteristics and diagnosis of 45 children and adolescents who were monitored in the study (2013 and 2014, HEINSG)

Category		*n*	%
Age group	Less than 1 year	4	8.9
	1–4 years	14	31.1
	5–9 years	11	24.4
	10–14 years	6	13.3
	15–18 years	10	22.2
Gender	Male	28	62.2
	Female	17	37.8
City of residence/ Home location	Greater Vitória – ES state	21	46.7
	City in ES state (other than the capital city)	18	40.0
	Bahia state	4	8.9
	Minas Gerais state	2	4.4
Socioeconomic class	B	7	15.6
	C	28	62.2
	D	9	20.0
	E	1	2.2
Head of household	Father	28	62.2
	Mother	3	6.7
	Grandfather/ Grandmother	3	6.7
	Other	11	24.4
Education of household head (years of study)	0–4 years of study	4	8.9
	4–8 years of study	18	40.0
	8–12 years of study	12	26.7
	More than 12 years of study	11	24.5
Mother's education (years of study)	0–4 years of study	3	6.6
	4–8 years of study	15	33.3
	8–12 years of study	10	22.2
	More than 12 years of study	16	35.5
	Not known	1	2.0
Diagnosis	Leukaemia	17	37.7
	Lymphomas	10	22.2
	Renal tumours	4	8.8
	CNS tumours	4	8.8
	Sympathetic NS tumours	3	6.6
	Bone tumours	2	4.4
	Other	5	11.1

socioeconomic class C (62.2%), attended school (73.3%), and had up to 4 years of education (24.4%). Regarding the children's and adolescents' families, the heads of most households were fathers (62.2%). The education data clearly show that most household heads had up to 8 years of education (40%), and most of the mothers had more than 12 years of education (35.5%).

Table 2 also shows that leukaemia was the most common diagnosis, occurring in 37.7% of cases.

Table 3 shows the prevalence of oral complications found during the clinical examinations conducted during the three research stages. The prevalence of mucositis considerably increased between the first and second study stages, rising from 3.9 to 17.8%. The prevalence of Xerostomia considerably decreased between the first and second stages, falling from 31 to 7.4% of cases.

Table 4 shows the changes in oral manifestations between the first and second study stages. A reduction in the number of cases of xerostomia was observed between the first and second stages, and the result of McNemar's test was very close to the significance level, with a *p*-value of 0.06.

Discussion

Approximately 40% of adult cancer patients and more than 90% of children under 12 years of age undergoing cancer treatment have oral manifestations that directly or indirectly arise from stomatotoxicities, such as mucositis; xerostomia; fungal infections, such as candidiasis; and viral infections, such as labial herpes simplex [6, 8].

Many national and international studies in the literature show a correlation between anticancer treatments, particularly chemotherapy and the occurrence of oral complications in infant-juvenile patients and adults [7, 10, 17–26], and the magnitude of these side effects depends on a number of factors related to the treatment, tumour and patient [22].

A less favored socioeconomic status is usually related to a greater number of oral diseases such as caries, i.e., a more unfavorable oral condition, which increases the risk of oral manifestations during chemotherapy [27]. In this study, however this association was not proven statistically, probably because patients studied belonged mostly to classes B, C and D, with a greater concentration in class C, which made it difficult to compare the classes. Our results therefore showed that oral manifestations were not related to the socioeconomic status of patients.

Table 3 Prevalence of oral manifestations at the two research stages

	Stages			
	1°		2°	
	n	%	n	%
Mucositis	2	3.9	8	17.8
Xerostomia	9	31	2	7.4
Cold sores	1	2	1	2.2
Candidiasis	2	3.9	4	8.9
Herpes simplex	0	0	1	2.2

Table 4 Changes in oral manifestations between the first and second study stages

	Stage 1	Stage 2		*Kappa*	*P* value	McNemar
		Yes	No			*P* value
Mucositis	Yes	0	2	−0.077	0.999	0.109
	No	8	35			
Xerostomia	Yes	2	5	0.369	0.065	0.063
	No	0	19			
Cold sores	Yes	0	1	−0.023	0.999	0.999
	No	1	43			
Candidiasis	Yes	2	0	0.646	0.006	0.500
	No	2	41			

Oral mucositis is defined as an inflammation and ulceration of the oral mucosa [28–32] and is one of the most common and frequent lesions in cancer patients undergoing chemotherapy. It is a major cause of pain and also represents a distressing experience for cancer patients [27, 33].

In this study, an increase in oral mucositis cases was observed between the first and second stages. In addition, mucositis was the most common oral manifestation found in the clinical examination conducted 1 month after the beginning of chemotherapy. This result is similar to those found in other studies [22, 23, 26, 34] conducted in Brazil (Recife, Juiz de Fora, São José dos Campos and João Pessoa) and abroad (China). Other authors [25] have observed mucositis percentages higher than those found in this study. The results of research conducted in São Luis (Brazil) [17] were different than those of this study, as few cases of mucositis occurred during anticancer treatment for leukaemia. This finding was likely due to the small sample, which included only 12 individuals. The literature varies regarding the prevalence of oral mucositis induced by chemotherapy, which has been reported to be 40 [21], 65 [32] and between 52 and 81% [32]. However, in general, the results reported in the literature have been higher than those found in this study, which is likely due to favourable oral health conditions before the initiation of treatment, with a low percentage of oral diseases, which reduces the risk of developing oral manifestations during treatment [6]. In this study, children and adolescents with various types of cancer were examined, which may, to some extent, be responsible for the low prevalence of mucositis, whereas in studies concentrating solely on leukaemia patients, generally speaking, a higher prevalence of oral manifestations was encountered because leukaemia is characterised by a high incidence of oral lesions during treatment [34].

Tests used in this study for measuring salivary flow were an adaptation of the standards proposed by the World Health Organization for quantification of xerostomia as a side effect of chemotherapy. Usually, authors recommend saliva collection for 5 min to measure the flow, but in adults [13]. In the present study, patients evaluated were children and adolescents who showed a severe general condition, sometimes incapacitating, so we chose to perform this adaptation in sialometry test, reducing saliva collection time.

In this study, the number of xerostomia cases declined between the first and second stages. Different results were found by other estudos [10, 23] of leukaemic patients [26] in which there was an increase in the number of cases of xerostomia between stages. It is likely that in this study, the reduction in xerostomia cases after the start of chemotherapy (which was close to the significance level, reaching 6%) was due to the care given during treatment, as an increased number of cases of leukaemia can be observed among patients, and the majority of individuals with leukaemia remained hospitalised, received continuous intravenous hydration and also followed guidelines regarding the need for extensive water and liquid intake in the first month of treatment.

A low prevalence of oral candidiasis was found in this study, which is consistent with other studies [23] and differs from the results obtained in one study [26] of leukaemia patients. The low prevalence of oral candidiasis (a result of the myelosuppression caused by chemotherapy agents) was likely due to the use of antifungal drugs that act topically and also systemic during the treatment [34] of most patients. Antifungal medicaments used were fluconazole 100 mg, once a day and nystatin, three times daily. These medicaments were prescribed by the hospital crew at the first signs of oral candidiasis, perhaps this influenced the low prevalence of this disease. These antifungals are not known to cause salivary flow reduction.

Patients with better oral health conditions and satisfactory oral hygiene develop fewer oral manifestations, and those conditions that do occur have a more rapid clinical course [34]. Studies have reinforced the importance of oral health for the prevention and reduction of oral complications of cancer treatment [9, 31], so prior to chemotherapy it is important to perform a Stomatological evaluation and dental care to reduce infectious outbreaks, such as removal of carious lesions and extensive restorations, treatment of periodontal disease and even tooth extractions in cases of teeth that require prolonged treatment, as all infectious processes originated in the oral cavity present a high risk of systemic infection, which can lead to septic episodes in immunocompetent patients compromised by oncologic therapy.

The presence of a dental surgeon working directly on the medical team is essential for the prevention and treatment of oral manifestations resulting from antineoplastic treatment. This dental surgeon can assist with preventing the development of a more severe clinical course, which can even result in the suspension of antineoplastic treatment [23, 34, 35].

The sample size was a limitation of this study. However, in Brazil, the observed percentage of paediatric tumours is 3%, demonstrating the low prevalence of this disease, which makes allocating a large number of individuals difficult in a primary data study.

Conclusions

Based on the results observed in this study, it can be concluded that oral manifestations were present, including mucositis, which increased and xerostomia, which showed a reduction in the number of cases after the start of chemotherapy. Oral complications, despite their relatively low prevalence, were nonetheless present and are among the most devastating complications in both the short and long term, affecting basic human activities such as eating and communicating. Furthermore, these lesions may interfere with cancer treatment, causing more serious infections or even sepsis.

The presence of an active dental surgeon on the multidisciplinary oncology team is therefore indispensable, as they can assist in the prevention, early diagnosis and treatment of oral manifestations. A dental surgeon can prevent lesions from escalating, thereby improving the patient's quality of life during treatment.

Acknowledgements
We declare that there was no significant contribution in addition to the authors themselves in the making of the article.

Funding
All spending on research were paid for by the authors.

Authors' contributions
D B V: a) the design and design, analysis and interpretation of data, b) drafting the article or revising it critically e c) approval of the version to be published. E Z: a) the design and design, analysis and interpretation of data, b) revising it critically. M H M B M: a) the design and design, analysis and interpretation of data, b) revising it critically e c) approval of the version to be published. All authors read and approved the final manuscript.

Authors' information
Ms. Deise Berger Velten – Dental Surgeon - Master in Public Health and teacher at the Federal University of Espírito Santo. Dr. Eliana Zandonade – PhD in statistics and teacher at the Federal University of Espírito Santo. Dr. Maria Helena Monteiro de Barros Miotto – Dental Surgeon - Doctor of Public Health and teacher at the Federal University of Espírito Santo.

Competing interests
The authors declare that they have no competing interests.

Consent for publication
Consent for publication is included in the consent to participate in research.

Ethics approval and consent to participate

All parents or guardians of the participants signed the consent form and previously clarified data collection. The study was approved on 20 February 2013 by the Research Ethics Committee of the Health Sciences Center (Health Sciences Center) of the Federal University of Espirito Santo (Federal University of Espirito Santo - UFES) by the number opinion 201,117.

References

1. Brasil Ministério da Saúde, Secretaria Nacional de Assistência à Saúde, Instituto Nacional do Câncer. Estimativa 2010: incidência do câncer no Brasil. Rio de Janeiro: INCA; 2009.
2. Brasil Instituto Nacional do Câncer. Estimativa/2012: incidência do câncer no Brasil. Rio de Janeiro: INCA; 2011. [acessado 2012 set 23]. Disponível em: http://portal.saude.sp.gov.br/resources/ses/perfil/gestor/homepage/estimativas-de-incidencia-decancer-2012/estimativas_incidencia_cancer_2012.pdf.
3. Câncer BINd. Estimativa/2014: incidência do câncer no Brasil. Rio de Janeiro: INCA; 2014. [acessado 2014 abr 20] Disponível em: http://www.saude.sp.gov.br/resources/ses/perfil/gestor/homepage/outros-destaques/estimativa-deincidencia-de-cancer-2014/estimativa_cancer_24042014.pdf.
4. Cheng KKF, Molassiotis A, Chang AM, Wai WC, Cheung SS. Evaluation of an oral care protocol intervention in the prevention of chemotherapy-induced oral mucositis in paediatric cancer patients. Eur J Cancer. 2001;37:2056–63.
5. Barbosa AM, Ribeiro DM, Caldo-Teixeira AS. Conhecimentos e práticas em saúde bucal com crianças hospitalizadas com câncer. Ciênc saúde coletiva. 2010;15(Supl.1):1113–22.
6. Sonis ST, Fazio RC, Fang L. Complicações bucais da terapia do câncer. In: Sonis ST, Fazio RC, Fang L, editors. Princípios e prática de medicina oral. 2nd ed. Rio de Janeiro: Guanabara Koogan; 1996. p. 358–83.
7. Osterne RLV, Brito RGM, Nogueira RLM, Soares ECS, Alves APNN, Moura JFB, et al. Saúde bucal em pacientes portadores de neoplasias malignas: estudo clínico-epidemiológico e análise de necessidades odontológicas de 421 pacientes. Rev bras cancerol. 2008;54(3):221–26.
8. Martins ACM, Caçador NP, Gaeti WP. Complicações bucais da quimioterapia antineoplásica. Acta Scientiarum. 2002;4(3):663–70.
9. Sasada INV, Cancino CMH, Petersen RC, Hellwing I, Dillenburg CS. Prevenção de intercorrências estomatológicas em oncologia pediátrica. RFO. 2015;20(1):105–09.
10. Lula ECO, Lula CEO, Alves CMCA, Lopes FF, Pereira AAP. Chemotherapy-induced oral complications in leukemic patients. Int J Pediatr Otorhinolaryngol. 2007;71:1681–85.
11. National Cancer Institute. Oral complications of chemotherapy and head/neck radiation (PDQ) – Health Professional Version. 2014. [Acessado 2014 abr 25]. Disponível em: http://www.ncbi.nlm.nih.gov/pubmedhealth/PMH0032604/.
12. Brasil. Critério de Classificação Econômica Brasil/2012. ABEP: Associação Brasileira de Empresas de Pesquisa. Disponível em: http://www.abep.org/criterio-brasil. Acesso em: 30 Jan. 2013.
13. Feio M, Sapeta P. Xerostomia em cuidados paliativos. Acta Med Port. 2005; 18:459–66.
14. Jensen SB, Pedersen AM, Reibel J, et al. Xerostomia and hypofunction of the salivary glands in câncer therapy. Support Care Cancer. 2003;11:207–25.
15. Organização Mundial de Saúde, Nacional Cancer Institute. Common Terminology Criteria for Adverse Events v3.0. 2006. [Acessado 2014 set 2]. Disponível em: http://ctep.cancer.gov/protocolDevelopment/electronic_applications/docs/ctcaev3.pdf.
16. Neville BW, Damm DD, Allen CM, Bouquot JE. Patologia oral & maxilofacial. 3rd ed. Rio de Janeiro: Ed. Elsevier; 2009.
17. Ye Y, Carlsson G, Agholme MB, Sjoberg JK, Lindberg KP, Putsep K, et al. Pretherapeutic plasma pro- and anti-inflammatory mediators are related to high risk of oral mucositis in pediatric patients with acute leukemia: A prospective cohort study. Plos One. 2013;8(5):1–7.
18. Paiva MDEB, Biase RCCG, Moraes JJC, Ângelo AR, Honorato MCTM. Estudo retrospectivo das complicações orais decorrentes da terapia antineoplásica em pacientes do Hospital Napoleão Laureano, PB. Odontologia clín científ. 2007;6(1):51–5.
19. Thomaz EBAF, Mouchrek Jr JCE, Silva AQ, Guerra RNM, Libério SA, Cruz MCFN. Longitudinal assessment of immunological and oral clinical conditions in patients undergoing anticancer treatment for leukemia. Int J Pediatr Otorhinolaryngol. 2013;77:1088–93.
20. Kreuger MRO, Savoldi LW, Hoffmann S, Diegoli NM. Complicações orais em pacientes em tratamento quimioterápico na UNACON, no município de Itajaí/SC. Revista da Faculdade de Odontologia de Lins. 2009; 21(1).
21. Arisawa EAL, Silva CMOM, Cardoso CAC, Lemos NRPL, Pinto MC. Efeitos colaterais da terapia antitumoral em pacientes submetidos à quimio e à radioterapia. Rev biociên. 2005;11(1–2):55–61.
22. Albuquerque RA, Morais VLL, Sobral APV. Avaliação clínica da frequência de complicações orais e sua relação com a qualidade de higiene bucal em pacientes pediátricos submetidos a tratamento antineoplásico. Arq Odontol. 2007;43(2):9–16.
23. Hespanhol FL, Tinoco EMB, Teixeira HGC, Falabella MEV, Assis NMSP. Manifestações bucais em pacientes submetidos à quimioterapia. Ciência & Saúde Coletiva. 2010;15(Supl. 1):1085–94.
24. Alberth M, Majoros L, Kovalecz G, Borbás E, Szegedi I, Márton IJ, et al. Significance of oral cândida infections in children with cancer. Pathology Oncology Research. 2006;12(4):237–41.
25. Otmani N, Alami R, Hessissen L, Mokhtari A, Soulaymani A, Khattab. Determinants of severe oral mucositis in paediatric cancer patients: a prospective study. Int J Pediatr Otorhinolaryngol. 2011;21:210–16.
26. Santos VI, Anbinder AL, Cavalcante ASR. Leucemia no paciente pediátrico: atuação odontológica. Cienc Odontol Bras. 2003;6(2):49–57.
27. Cheng KKF, Goggins WB, Lee VWS, Thompson DR. Risk Factors for oral mucositis in children undergoing chemotherapy: A matched case–control study. Oral Oncol. 2008;44:1019–25.
28. Volpato LER, Silva TC, Oliveira TM, Sakai VT, Machado MAAM. Radiation therapy and chemotherapy-induced oral mucositis. Rev Bras Otorrinolaringol. 2007;73(4):562–68.
29. Qutob AF, GUE S, Revesz T, Logan RM, Keefe D. Prevention of oral mucositis in children receiving cancer therapy: A systematic review and evidence-based analysis. Oral Oncol. 2013;49:102–07.
30. Belfield PM, Dwyer AA. Oral complications of childhood cancer and its treatment: current best practice. Eur J Cancer. 2004;40:1035–41.
31. Plevová P. Prevention and treatment of chemotherapy and radiotherapy induced oral mucositis: a review. Oral Oncol. 1999;35:453–70.
32. Ribeiro Júnior O, Borba AM, Guimarães JJ. Prevenção e tratamento da mucosite bucal: o papel fundamental do cirurgião dentista: Revisão. Rev clín pesq odontol. 2010;6(1):57–62.
33. Cruz LB, Ribeiro AS, Rech A, Rosa LGN, Castro Júnior CG, Brunetto AL. Influence of Low-Energy Laser in the Prevention of Oral Mucositis in Children with Cancer receiving Chemotherapy. Pediatr Blood Cancer. 2007;48:435–40.
34. Trindade AKF, De Biase RCCG, Filho GG, Pereira BC, Sousa EMD, Queiroga AS. Manifestações orais em pacientes pediátricos leucêmicos. Arq odontol. 2009;41(1):22–9.
35. Ramirez-Amador V, Esquivel-Pedraza L, Mohar A, Reynoso-Gómez E, Volkow-Fernández P, Guarner J, et al. Chemotherapy-associated oral mucosal lesions in patients with leukaemia or lymphoma. Oral Oncol. 1996;32B(5):322–27.

Permissions

All chapters in this book were first published in OH, by BioMed Central; hereby published with permission under the Creative Commons Attribution License or equivalent. Every chapter published in this book has been scrutinized by our experts. Their significance has been extensively debated. The topics covered herein carry significant findings which will fuel the growth of the discipline. They may even be implemented as practical applications or may be referred to as a beginning point for another development.

The contributors of this book come from diverse backgrounds, making this book a truly international effort. This book will bring forth new frontiers with its revolutionizing research information and detailed analysis of the nascent developments around the world.

We would like to thank all the contributing authors for lending their expertise to make the book truly unique. They have played a crucial role in the development of this book. Without their invaluable contributions this book wouldn't have been possible. They have made vital efforts to compile up to date information on the varied aspects of this subject to make this book a valuable addition to the collection of many professionals and students.

This book was conceptualized with the vision of imparting up-to-date information and advanced data in this field. To ensure the same, a matchless editorial board was set up. Every individual on the board went through rigorous rounds of assessment to prove their worth. After which they invested a large part of their time researching and compiling the most relevant data for our readers.

The editorial board has been involved in producing this book since its inception. They have spent rigorous hours researching and exploring the diverse topics which have resulted in the successful publishing of this book. They have passed on their knowledge of decades through this book. To expedite this challenging task, the publisher supported the team at every step. A small team of assistant editors was also appointed to further simplify the editing procedure and attain best results for the readers.

Apart from the editorial board, the designing team has also invested a significant amount of their time in understanding the subject and creating the most relevant covers. They scrutinized every image to scout for the most suitable representation of the subject and create an appropriate cover for the book.

The publishing team has been an ardent support to the editorial, designing and production team. Their endless efforts to recruit the best for this project, has resulted in the accomplishment of this book. They are a veteran in the field of academics and their pool of knowledge is as vast as their experience in printing. Their expertise and guidance has proved useful at every step. Their uncompromising quality standards have made this book an exceptional effort. Their encouragement from time to time has been an inspiration for everyone.

The publisher and the editorial board hope that this book will prove to be a valuable piece of knowledge for researchers, students, practitioners and scholars across the globe.

List of Contributors

Fabienne A. Gerber, Philipp Sahrmann, and Patrick R. Schmidlin
Clinic of Preventive Dentistry, Periodontology and Cariology, Center of Dental Medicine, University of Zurich, Plattenstrasse 11, CH-8032 Zurich, Switzerland

Oliver A. Schmidlin and Jürg Hans Beer
Department of Internal Medicine, Cantonal Hospital Baden, Baden, Switzerland. 3Department of

Christian Heumann
Statistics, Ludwig-Maximilians-University of Munich, Munich, Germany

Marc J. Mathews, Edward H. Mathews and George E. Mathews
CRCED, North-West University, P.O. Box 11207, Silver Lakes 0054, South Africa

Wael Sabbah
Population and Patient Health, King's College London Dental Institute, Denmark Hill Campus, Bessemer Road, London SE5 9RS, UK

Easter Joury
Population and Patient Health, King's College London Dental Institute, Denmark Hill Campus, Bessemer Road, London SE5 9RS, UK
Oral Medicine Department, Faculty of Dentistry, Damascus University, Damascus, Syria

May Khairallah
Oral Medicine Department, Faculty of Dentistry, Damascus University, Damascus, Syria

Kanaan Elias
Eastman Dental Institute, University College London, London WC1X 8LD, UK

Raman Bedi
Centre for International Child Oral Health, King's College London, 26-29 Drury Lane, Rooms 329-331, London WC2B 5RL, UK

Josef J. M. Bruers
Department of Social Dentistry and Behavioural Sciences, Academic Centre for Dentistry Amsterdam (ACTA), University of Amsterdam and VU University, Gustav Mahlerlaan 3004, 1081 LA Amsterdam, The Netherlands
Department of Research and Information, Royal Dutch Dental Association (KNMT), Nieuwegein, The Netherlands

Ronald C. Gorter and Michiel A. J. Eijkman
Department of Social Dentistry and Behavioural Sciences, Academic Centre for Dentistry Amsterdam (ACTA), University of Amsterdam and VU University, Gustav Mahlerlaan 3004, 1081 LA Amsterdam, The Netherlands

Brigitte A. F. M. van Dam
Department of Research and Information, Royal Dutch Dental Association (KNMT), Nieuwegein, The Netherlands

Shiwei Cai and Wei Chen
Department of Endodontics, University of Texas School of Dentistry at Houston, 7500 Cambridge Street, Suite 5366, Houston, TX 77054, USA

Wenjian Zhang
Department of Diagnostic and Biomedical Sciences, University of Texas School of Dentistry at Houston, 7500 Cambridge Street, Suite 5366, Houston, TX 77054, USA

Toshimitsu Iinuma, Tomoka Ito, Yugaku Kondo and Nobuhito Gionhaku
Department of Complete Denture Prosthodontics, Nihon University School of Dentistry, Tokyo, Japan

Yasumichi Arai, Yukiko Abe and Nobuyoshi Hirose
Center for Supercentenarian Medical Research, Keio University School of Medicine, Tokyo, Japan

Michiyo Takayama
Center for Preventive Medicine, Keio University School of Medicine, Tokyo, Japan

H. M. Ali, S. A. Lie and M. S. Skeie
Department of Clinical Dentistry, Faculty of Medicine and Dentistry, University of Bergen, Bergen, Norway

M. Mustafa
Oral Health Centre of Expertise in Western Norway, Hordaland, Bergen, Norway

E. F. Nasir
Oral Health Centre of Expertise in Western Norway, Hordaland, Bergen, Norway
Department of Community Dentistry, University of Science and Technology, Khartoum, Sudan

S. Hasabalrasol
Ahmed Gasim hospital, Khartoum Teaching Hospital, Khartoum, Sudan

O. H. Elshazali
Ahmed Gasim hospital, Faculty of Medicine University of Khartoum, Khartoum, Sudan

R. W. Ali
Department of Periodontics, University of Science and Technology, Khartoum, Sudan

Muzaffer Emir Dinçol, Hakan Ozbas, Bulent Yılmaz, Handan Ersev and Selcuk Gokyay
Faculty of Dentistry, Department of Endodontics, Istanbul University, 34093, Fatih, Istanbul, Turkey

Vakur Olgac
Institute of Oncology, Department of Tumor Pathology and Cytology, Istanbul University, 34093, Fatih, Istanbul, Turkey

Zhao Wei1, Zhi Cui and Ping Yan
Department of Endodontics, School and Hospital of Stomatology, Wuhan University, 237 Luoyu Road, Wuhan 430079, China

Han Jiang
The State Key Laboratory Breeding Base of Basic Science of Stomatology (Hubei-MOST) and Key Laboratory of Oral Biomedicine Ministry of Education, School and Hospital of Stomatology, Wuhan University, Luoyu Road 237, Wuhan 430079, China

P. Bottenberg
Department of Oral Health Sciences, Vrije Universiteit Brussel, Laarbeeklaan 103, 1090 Brussels, Belgium

W. Jacquet
Department of Oral Health Sciences, Vrije Universiteit Brussel, Laarbeeklaan 103, 1090 Brussels, Belgium
Depatment of Educational Sciences EDWE-LOCI, Vrije Universiteit Brussel, Pleinlaan 2, 1050 Ixelles, Brussels, Belgium

C. Behrens and A. Jablonski-Momeni
Dental School, Department of Pediatric and Community Dentistry, Philipps University of Marburg, Marburg, Germany

V. Stachniss
Dental School, Department of Restorative Dentistry, Philipps University of Marburg, Georg-Voigt-Straße 3, D-35039 Marburg, Germany

Po-Ren Teng and Miao-Jean Lin
Department of Psychiatry, Chang Bing Show Chwan Memorial Hospital, No. 6, Lu-Gong Road, Lu-Gang Township, Changhwa County, Taiwan

Ling-Ling Yeh
Department of Healthcare Administration, Asia University, No. 500, Lioufong RdWufeng, Taichung 41354, Taiwan

Gunnel Hänsel Petersson
Department of Cariology, Faculty of Odontology, Malmö University, SE-205 06 Malmö, Sweden

Svante Twetman
Department of Odontology, Faculty of Health and Medical Sciences, University of Copenhagen, Copenhagen, Denmark

Bo Zhang
Department of Pathogenic Microbiology and Immunology, School of Basic Medical Sciences, Xi'an Jiaotong University, Yanta West Road No.76, Xi'an 710061, ShaanXi, China
Clinical Laboratory, AnKang City Central Hospital, Jinzhou South Road No.85, AnKang 725000, ShaanXi, China

Yi-jie Guo, Xue-song Feng, Hui-xun Ren and Ji-ru Xu
Department of Pathogenic Microbiology and Immunology, School of Basic Medical Sciences, Xi'an Jiaotong University, Yanta West Road No.76, Xi'an 710061, ShaanXi, China
Key Laboratory of Environment and Genes Related to Diseases, Ministry of Education of China, Xi'an Jiaotong University, Yanta West Road No.76, Xi'an 710061, ShaanXi, China

A. Vasiliou
Faculty of Dentistry, University of Toronto, Toronto, ON, Canada

K. Shankardass
Department of Health Sciences, Wilfrid Laurier University, 75 University Ave West, Waterloo, ON N2L 3C5, Canada
Centre for Urban Health Solutions, LiKa Shing Knowledge Institute, St Michael's Hospital, Toronto, ON, Canada
Dalla Lana School of Public Health, University of Toronto, Toronto, ON, Canada

R. Nisenbaum
Centre for Urban Health Solutions, LiKa Shing Knowledge Institute, St Michael's Hospital, Toronto, ON, Canada
Dalla Lana School of Public Health, University of Toronto, Toronto, ON, Canada

C. Quiñonez
Faculty of Dentistry, University of Toronto, Toronto, ON, Canada
Dalla Lana School of Public Health, University of Toronto, Toronto, ON, Canada

Antonio Fallea
Unit of Dentistry, IRCCS Associazione Oasi Maria SS, Troina (EN), Italy

Rosa Zuccarello
Unit of Pedagogy, IRCCS Associazione Oasi Maria SS, Troina (EN), Italy

Francesco Calì
Laboratory of Molecular Genetics, Unit of Medical Genetics, IRCCS AssociazioneOasi Maria SS, Troina (EN), Italy

Jenny M. Porritt
Department of Psychology, Sociology & Politics, Sheffield Hallam University, Collegiate Crescent, Sheffield S10 2BQ, UK

Farzana Sufi
Clinical Research (Oral Care), GlaxoSmithKline Consumer Healthcare, St Georges Avenue, Weybridge, Surrey KT13 0DE, UK

Sarah R. Baker
School of Clinical Dentistry, University of Sheffield, 19 Claremont Crescent, Sheffield S10 2TA, UK.

Rodrigo Mariño
Oral Health Cooperative Research Centre Melbourne Dental School, University of Melbourne, Melbourne, VIC 3010, Australia

Rodrigo A. Giacaman
Department of Oral Rehabilitation, University of Talca, Talca, Chile

Sonia Sharma, Heidi C. Crow, Krishnan Kartha, W. D. McCall Jr and Yoly M. Gonzalez
Department of Oral Diagnostic Sciences, School of Dental Medicine, University at Buffalo, Buffalo, NY 14214, USA

Sanna Kangas
Private Dental Office Viisaudenhammas, Rovaniemi, Finland

Petra Timonen
Dental Training Clinic, Social and Health Services, Oulu, Finland

Matti Knuuttila
Medical Research Center Oulu, Oulu University Hospital and University of Oulu, Oulu, Finland

Antti Jula
National Institute for Health and Welfare (THL), Helsinki, Finland

Pekka Ylöstalo
Medical Research Center Oulu, Oulu University Hospital and University of Oulu, Oulu, Finland
Periodontology and Geriatric Dentistry, Unit of Oral Health Sciences Research, P.O. Box 5281, FI-90014 Oulu, Finland
Institute of Dentistry, University of Eastern Finland, Kuopio Campus, Kuopio, Finland
Oral and Maxillofacial Department, Kuopio University Hospital, Kuopio, Finland

Anna-Maija Hannele Syrjälä
Periodontology and Geriatric Dentistry, Unit of Oral Health Sciences Research, P.O. Box 5281, FI-90014 Oulu, Finland
Medical Research Center Oulu, Oulu University Hospital and University of Oulu, Oulu, Finland

Mengdong Liu
School of Dentistry, Shandong University, 44, Wenhua West Road, Jinan 250012, Shandong Province, China
School of Stomatology, Qingdao University, Qingdao 266021, Shandong Province, China

Shijiang Xiong
School of Dentistry, Shandong University, 44, Wenhua West Road, Jinan 250012, Shandong Province, China

Fei Tan and Yi Liu
School of Stomatology, Qingdao University, Qingdao 266021, Shandong Province, China

Shang-Lun Lin
Department of Psychiatry, Kaohsiung Armed Forces General Hospital, Kaohsiung, Taiwan
Graduate Institute of Medical Science, College of Health Science, Chang Jung Christian University, Tainan, Taiwan

Shang-Liang Wu
School of Medicine, Griffith University, Gold Coast, Australia

Shun-Yao Ko
Graduate Institute of Medical Science, College of Health Science, Chang Jung Christian University, Tainan, Taiwan

Ching-Yu Yen
School of Dentistry, Taipei Medical University, Taipei, Taiwan
Department of Oral and Maxillofacial Surgery, Chi-Mei Medical Center, Yongkang, Tainan, Taiwan

Wei-Fan Chiang
Department of Oral and Maxillofacial Surgery, Chi-Mei Medical Center, Liouying, Tainan, Taiwan
School of Dentistry, National Yang-Ming University, Taipei, Taiwan

Jung-Wu Yang
Graduate Institute of Medical Science, College of Health Science, Chang Jung Christian University, Tainan, Taiwan
Department of Oral and Maxillofacial Surgery, Tainan Sin Lau Hospital, the Presbyterian Church in Taiwan, Tainan, Taiwan
Yuan Yuan Dental Federation, Tainan, Taiwan
701 No. 57, Sec. 1, East Gate Road, East Dist., Tainan City,, Taiwan, R.O.C

Nayef H. Felemban
Orthodontic department, Faculty of Dentistry, Taif University, Taif, Saudi Arabia
P.O.B. 4302, Makkah 21955, Saudi Arabia

Mohamed I. Ebrahim
Restorative dentistry department, Faculty of Dentistry, Taif University, Taif, Saudi Arabia.

Barbara Cvikl
Department of Preventive, Restorative and Pediatric Dentistry, School of Dentistry, University of Bern, Bern, Switzerland
Department of Conservative Dentistry & Periodontology, Medical University of Vienna, Vienna, Austria

Adrian Lussi
Department of Preventive, Restorative and Pediatric Dentistry, School of Dentistry, University of Bern, Bern, Switzerland

Samuel C. Hess
Institute for Chemical and Bioengineering, Department of Chemistry and Applied Biosciences, ETH
Zurich, Zurich, Switzerland

Richard J. Miron
Department of Preventive, Restorative and Pediatric Dentistry, School of Dentistry, University of Bern, Bern, Switzerland
Department of Periodontology, College of Dental Medicine, Nova Southeastern University, Fort Lauderdale, Florida, USA

Hermann Agis
Department of Conservative Dentistry & Periodontology, Medical University of Vienna, Vienna, Austria

Dieter Bosshardt
Robert K. Schenk Laboratory of Oral Histology, Department of Periodontology, Department of Oral Surgery and Stomatology, University of Bern, Bern, Switzerland

Toshiro Sato, Mitsuo Kishi and Miki Suda
Division of Preventive Dentistry, Department of Oral Medicine, School of Dentistry Iwate Medical University, 1-3-27 Chuo-dori, Morioka, Iwate 020-8505, Japan

Kiyomi Sakata and Haruki Shimoda
Department of Hygiene and Preventive Medicine, Iwate Medical University, School of Medicine, 2-1-1 Nishitokuta, Yahaba, Iwate 028-3694, Japan

Hiroyuki Miura
Division of Dental Education, Department of Oral Medicine, School of Dentistry Iwate Medical University, 1-3-27 Chuo-dori, Morioka, Iwate 020-8505, Japan

Akira Ogawa and Seiichiro Kobayashi
Iwate Medical University, 19-1 Uchimaru, Morioka, Iwate 020-8505, Japan

Xiao-Chuan Fan and Xiao-Feng Huang
Department of Stomatology, Beijing Friendship Hospital, Capital Medical University, No.95 Yong'an Road, Xicheng District, Beijing 100050, China

Li Chen
Department of Orthodontics, Capital Medical University School of Stomatology, No.4 Tiantan Xili, Dongcheng District, Beijing 100050, China

E. Kakuta
Department of Oral Microbiology, Tsurumi University School of Dental Medicine, 2-1-3 Tsurumi, Tsurumi-ku, Yokohama, Japan

Y. Nomura and N. Hanada
Department of Translational Research, Tsurumi University School of Dental Medicine, 2-1-3 Tsurumi, Tsurumi-ku, Yokohama 230-8501, Japan

T. Morozumi and H. Yoshie
Division of Periodontology, Department of Oral Biological Science, Niigata University Graduate School of Medical and Dental Sciences, 2-5274 Gakkocho-dori, Chuo-ku, Niigata, Japan

T. Nakagawa and C. Fukaya
Department of Dentistry and Oral Surgery, School of Medicine, Keio University, 35 Shinano-machi, Shinjuku-ku, Tokyo, Japan

T. Nakamura and K. Noguchi
Department of Periodontology, Kagoshima University Graduate School of Medical and Dental Sciences, 8-35-1 Sakuragaoka, Kagoshima, Japan

A .Yoshimura and Y. Hara
Department of Periodontology, Unit of Translational Medicine, Nagasaki University Graduate School of Biomedical Sciences, 1-12-4 Sakamoto, Nagasaki, Japan

O. Fujise and F. Nishimura
Section of Periodontology, Division of Oral Rehabilitation, Faculty of Dental Science, Kyushu University, 3-1-1 Maidashi, Higashi-ku, Fukuoka, Japan

T. Kono and M. Umeda
Department of Periodontology, Osaka Dental University, 8-1 Kuzuhahanazonocho, Hirakata, Japan

M. Fukuda and T. Noguchi
Department of Periodontology, School of Dentistry, Aichi Gakuin University, 2-11 Suemori-doori,Chikusa-ku, Nagoya, Japan

N. Yoshinari
Department of Periodontology, School of Dentistry, Matsumoto Dental University, 1780 Hirokagobara, Shiojiri, Nagano, Japan

S. Sekino and Y. Numabe
Department of Periodontology, School of Life Dentistry at Tokyo, The Nippon Dental University, 1-9-20 Fujimi, Chiyoda-ku, Tokyo, Japan

N. Sugano and K. Ito
Department of Periodontology, Nihon University School of Dentistry, 1-8-13 Kanda-Surugadai, Chiyoda-ku, Tokyo, Japan

H. Kobayashi and Y. Izumi
Department of Periodontology, Graduate School of Medical and Dental Sciences, Tokyo Medical and Dental University, 1-5-45 Yushima, Bunkyo-ku, Tokyo, Japan.

H. Takai and Y. Ogata
Department of Periodontology, Nihon University School of Dentistry at Matsudo, 2-870-1 Sakae-cho-nishi, Matsudo-shi, Chiba, Japan

S. Takano
Bunkyo-Dori Dental Clinic, 2-4-1 Anagawa, Inage-ku, Chiba, JAPAN

M. Minabe
Bunkyo-Dori Dental Clinic, 2-4-1 Anagawa, Inage-ku, Chiba, JAPAN

Division of Periodontology, Department of Oral function and Restoration, School of Dentistry, Kanagawa Dental University, 82 Inaokacho, Yokosuka, Kanagawa, Japan

A. Makino-Oi1 and A. Saito
Department of Periodontology, Tokyo Dental College, 2-9-18 Misakicho, Chiyoda-ku, Tokyo, Japan

Y. Abe
Comprehensive Dental Care, The Nippon Dental University Niigata Hospital, 1-8 Hamaura-cho, Chuo-ku, Niigata, Japan

S. Sato
Department of Periodontology, School of life Dentistry at Niigata, The Nippon Dental
University, 1-8 Hamaura-cho, Chuo-ku, Niigata, Japan

F. Suzuki
Division of Dental Anesthesiology, Department of Oral Surgery, School of Dentistry, Ohu
University, 31-1 Misumido, Tomita, Koriyama, Fukushima, Japan

K. Takahashi
Division of Periodontics, Department of Conservative Dentistry, School of Dentistry, Ohu
University, 31-1 Misumido, Tomita, Koriyama, Fukushima, Japan

T. Sugaya and M. Kawanami
Division of Periodontology and Endodontology, Department of Oral Health Science Hokkaido University Graduate School of Dental Medicine, Kita 13, Nishi 7, Kita-ku, Sapporo, Japan

S. Takashiba
Department of Pathophysiology-Periodontal Science, Okayama University Graduate School of Medicine, Dentistry and Pharmaceutical Sciences, 2-5-1 Shikata-cho, Okayama, Japan

Deise Berger Velten, Eliana Zandonade and Maria Helena Monteiro de Barros Miotto
Federal University of Espírito Santo, Av. Mal. Campos, 1468 - Maruípe, Vitória, ES 29043-900, Brazil

Thomas Attin
Clinic of Preventive Dentistry, Periodontology and Cariology, Center of Dental Medicine, University of Zurich, Plattenstrasse 11, Zurich CH-8032, Switzerland

Patrick R. Schmidlin
Department of Preventive, Restorative and Pediatric Dentistry, School of Dentistry, University of Bern, Bern, Switzerland
Clinic of Preventive Dentistry, Periodontology and Cariology, Center of Dental Medicine, University of Zurich, Plattenstrasse 11, Zurich CH-8032, Switzerland

Deise Berger Velten, Eliana Zandonade and Maria Helena Monteiro de Barros Miotto
Federal University of Espírito Santo, Av. Mal. Campos, 1468 - Maruípe, Vitória, ES 29043-900, Brazil

Index

A

Adipokines, 2, 15-16, 19
Adipose Tissue, 2
Alveolar Bone, 2, 10, 26, 165, 198
Antimicrobial Activity, 86, 115, 118, 121-122

B

Bariatric Surgery, 11, 16, 18
Bleeding Gums, 69
Body Mass Index, 1, 3, 11, 16, 58, 60, 162, 164, 168, 201, 206
Borderline Intellectual Functioning, 131-133, 135

C

Cancer Treatment, 227-228, 230-231
Cardiovascular Disease, 17, 19, 22, 28-30, 60, 77, 124, 162
Cell Membrane, 121
Chewing Ability, 59-60, 64-65
Chronic Periodontitis, 1-3, 6, 10-11, 15-19, 26, 29, 168, 219-226
Computed Tomography, 87-88, 93
Coronary Heart Disease, 2, 19, 21-25, 27-30, 60, 62-63, 107, 129

D

Dental Anxiety, 131-136
Dental Care, 46, 67, 69, 75-77, 102-110, 112-114, 123, 125-132, 135, 148-154, 205, 225, 231
Dental Caries, 33, 37, 68, 75, 77, 100, 114-115, 149-150, 203, 207, 214
Dental Check-ups, 67, 105-106
Dental Composite, 182, 187
Dental Health, 16, 36, 62, 64, 66, 75, 77, 107-109, 113, 123, 128, 151, 153-154, 205-206
Dental Plaque, 163-167, 207
Dental Pulp Cells, 47-49, 51, 54-57, 189-195, 197-198
Dental Pulp Tissue, 47, 57
Dental Pulpal Stem Cells, 47, 55
Dental Treatment, 45, 75, 106, 108, 115, 131-132
Dentine Hypersensitivity, 137-141, 143-147
Dentition, 47-48, 55, 65, 76
Denture, 58-59, 61, 64, 182, 187, 200-207
Depression, 22, 39, 146, 175-180
Diabetes, 2-6, 16-19, 22, 29-30, 36, 58, 60, 62, 64, 107, 124, 146, 163, 167, 201, 205
Dietary Patterns, 32, 35, 37
Discoloration, 95, 98-99, 218
Dyslipidemia, 2, 201, 204

E

Edentulous, 59-61, 64, 150-152, 202-205
Enamel Surfaces, 209, 211, 213, 215-218

F

Fluorescence Activated Cell Sorting, 48, 51, 55
Fluoride Toothpaste, 33, 72

H

Hypertension, 2, 16, 29, 163, 199, 201-202, 204-205

I

Incisors, 47, 52, 55, 68
Intellectual Disabilities, 131-133, 135-136

L

Lipoteichoic Acids, 115, 121

M

Magnetic Resonance Imaging, 155
Malocclusion, 175, 178-180
Maximum Occlusal Force, 58-59, 61, 63-65
Metabolic Syndrome, 2-3, 17, 64
Myeloperoxidase, 22, 24, 26, 28-29

O

Obesity, 1-20, 29, 36, 124, 162-165, 167-168, 199, 201-205
Odontoblasts, 47, 54, 56-57, 189, 194, 197
Oral Cavity, 18, 115, 124, 200, 207, 231
Oral Diseases, 29, 67, 73, 106, 108, 110, 115, 148, 230
Oral Health, 2, 16-19, 21-23, 25, 27-29, 31-37, 44, 48, 58-59, 62, 64, 66-71, 73-77, 94, 100, 102, 105-114, 123-130, 135, 137-154, 162, 168, 174, 200, 207, 218, 225-228, 230-231
Oral Hygiene, 6, 12-13, 20, 36-37, 59, 65-67, 69, 71, 76, 102, 111, 167-168, 199, 201-202, 204, 231
Oral Manifestations, 227-231
Oral Pain, 123, 125-128, 130, 145, 149
Orthodontic Brackets, 182, 185, 187, 217-218
Orthodontic Treatment, 180, 186-187, 210, 217
Osteoprotegerin, 22, 24, 26, 28-29

P

Pain Intensity, 139, 143-144
Periodontal Disease, 2, 16-30, 107, 124, 129, 150, 162-163, 165, 167-168, 170, 219-220, 223-224, 226, 231
Periodontal Therapy, 1-2, 5-7, 9-20

Planktonic Cells, 118, 120-121
Primary Teeth, 68, 76
Probing Depth, 9-12
Progenitor Cells, 48, 55, 189

R
Retreatment Technique, 170
Root Canal Transplantation, 47, 50

S
Scanning Electron Microscopy, 115, 117, 121, 191, 193, 195, 209, 212-213, 218
Sensitive Teeth, 137-138, 140
Sensitivity Toothpaste, 139, 143-144
Soft Tissues, 2
Surface Roughness, 182, 209, 211, 213-214, 216-218

T
Temporomandibular Disorders, 155, 160-161, 175, 178-180
Tissue Regeneration, 47-48, 194
Tooth Brushing, 69, 111, 127
Tooth Decay, 69
Tooth Loss, 64-65, 114, 129, 149, 219
Tooth Retention, 148
Tooth Surfaces, 95, 99, 115, 150-151

V
Vaccination, 31-33, 36
Visceral Fat, 162-163, 168